Video 13-9 Septal subendocardial fibrosis in a cat with hypertrophic cardiomyopathy (HCM) (apical 4 chambers view).
Video 13-10 Left ventricular remodeling in a cat with hypertrophic cardiomyopathy (HCM) (right parasternal long axis 4 chambers view).
Video 13-11 Spontaneous echocardiographic contrast of the left atrium in a cat with restrictive cardiomyopathy (RCM) (right parasternal long axis view, optimized for the atria).
Video 13-12 Color Doppler in a cat with obstructive hypertrophic cardiomyopathy (HCM) showing a dynamic obstruction of the left ventricular outflow tract (apical 5 chambers view).
Video 13-13 Dynamic obstruction of the right ventricular outflow tract in a cat with hypertrophic cardiomyopathy (HCM) (right parasternal short axis view, heart base level).
Video 13-14 Dynamic obstruction of the left ventricular outflow tract and mitral regurgitation in a cat with hypertrophic cardiomyopathy (HCM) and systolic anterior movement (SAM) (apical 4 chambers view).
Video 13-15 Restrictive cardiomyopathy (RCM) in a cat (right parasternal long axis 4 chambers view).
Video 13-16 Restrictive cardiomyopathy (RCM) in a cat (right parasternal long axis 4 chambers view).
Video 13-17 Focal dyskinesia of the left ventricular free wall in a cat with restrictive cardiomyopathy (RCM) (right parasternal short axis view at the chordae tendineae level).
Video 13-18 Biatrial dilation in a cat with restrictive cardiomyopathy (RCM) (apical 4 chambers view).
Video 13-19 Dilated cardiomyopathy (DCM) in a cat (right parasternal long axis 4 chambers view).
Video 13-20 End-stage cardiomyopathy in a cat (right parasternal long axis 4 chambers view).
Video 13-21 Hypocontractile dilated left atrium with spontaneous echo contrast (SEC) in a cat (right parasternal short axis view at the level of the heart base).

Chapter 14 Pulmonary Arterial Hypertension

Video 14-1 Severe pulmonary hypertension in a dog with right ventricular dilation and hypertrophy and septal flattening (right parasternal long axis 4 chambers view).
Video 14-2 Severe pulmonary hypertension in a dog with right ventricular dilation and hypertrophy and septal flattening (right parasternal transventricular short axis view).
Video 14-3 Tricuspid regurgitation associated with major systolic pulmonary arterial hypertension (PAH) (122 mm Hg) in a young Belgian Shepherd Malinois (left parasternal long axis 4 chambers view).
Video 14-4 Marked pulmonic regurgitation with aliasing in a dog with pulmonary hypertension (right parasternal short axis view, at the level of the heart base).

Chapter 16 Cardiac Manifestations of Systemic Diseases

Video 16-1 Aortic regurgitation associated with systemic arterial hypertension (SHT) in a dog (color Doppler mode, right parasternal long axis 5 chambers view).

Chapter 17 Pericardial Diseases

Video 17-1 Pericardial effusion in a dog (right parasternal long axis 4 chambers view).
Video 17-2 Pericardial effusion in a dog (right parasternal short axis view at the level of the base of the heart).
Video 17-3 Small pericardial effusion in a cat with hypertrophic cardiomyopathy (right parasternal long axis 4 chambers view).
Video 17-4 Mild pericardial effusion in a dog with severe mitral regurgitation (right parasternal long axis 4 chambers view).
Video 17-5 Examination of the right atrial appendage in a dog with pericardial effusion (right parasternal long axis view of the aortic arch).
Video 17-6 Examination of the right atrial appendage in a dog with pericardial effusion (oblique apical 4 chambers view).

Chapter 18 Cardiac Tumors

Video 18-1 Pericardial effusion (PE) secondary to a cardiac hemangiosarcoma (HSA) in a dog (oblique right parasternal transventricular short axis view).
Video 18-2 Pericardial effusion (PE) secondary to a cardiac hemangiosarcoma (HSA) in a dog (left parasternal cranial view).
Video 18-3 Pericardial effusion (PE) secondary to a cardiac hemangiosarcoma (HSA) invading the right ventricular free wall in a dog (apical 4 chambers view).
Video 18-4 Pericardial effusion (PE) secondary to a cardiac hemangiosarcoma (HSA) invading the right ventricular free wall in a dog (right parasternal short axis transventricular view).
Video 18-5 Heart base tumor (HBT) with pericardial effusion (PE) in a dog (oblique right parasternal long axis view).
Video 18-6 Heart base tumor (HBT) invading the main pulmonary artery in a dog (right parasternal short axis view at the level of the heart base).
Video 18-7 Large heart base tumor (HBT) invading the atria in a dog (apical 4 chambers view).

Chapter 19 Congenital Cardiopathies

Video 19-1 Type 2 subaortic stenosis (SAS) in a dog (right parasternal long axis 5 chambers view).
Video 19-2 Turbulent aortic flow in a dog with subaortic stenosis (SAS) (right parasternal long axis 5 chambers view).
Video 19-3 Pulmonic valve stenosis in a dog (right parasternal short axis view at the level of the base of the heart).
Video 19-4 Left ventricular dilation in a dog with patent ductus arteriosus (PDA) (right parasternal long axis 4 chambers view).
Video 19-5 Patent ductus arteriosus (PDA) in a dog (right parasternal short axis view at the level of the base of the heart).
Video 19-6 Perimembranous ventricular septal defect (VSD) in a dog (right parasternal long axis 5 chambers view).
Video 19-7 Mitral valve dysplasia (MVD) in a dog (apical 4 chambers view).
Video 19-8 Mitral valve dysplasia (MVD) with mitral stenosis (MS) in a cat (apical 4 chambers view).
Video 19-9 Tricuspid valve dysplasia (TVD) in a dog (apical 4 chambers view).
Video 19-10 Tetralogy of Fallot (ToF) in a dog (right parasternal long axis view).
Video 19-11 Cor triatriatum sinister (CTS) in a cat (apical 4 chambers view).
Video 19-12 Turbulent intraatrial flow in a cat with cor triatriatum sinister (CTS) (right parasternal long axis 4 chambers view).
Video 19-13 Complete atrioventricular (AV) canal (type A) with common atria in a cat (right parasternal long axis 4 chambers view).
Video 19-14 Mitral regurgitation (MR) in a cat with a complete atrioventricular (AV) canal (apical 4 chambers view).

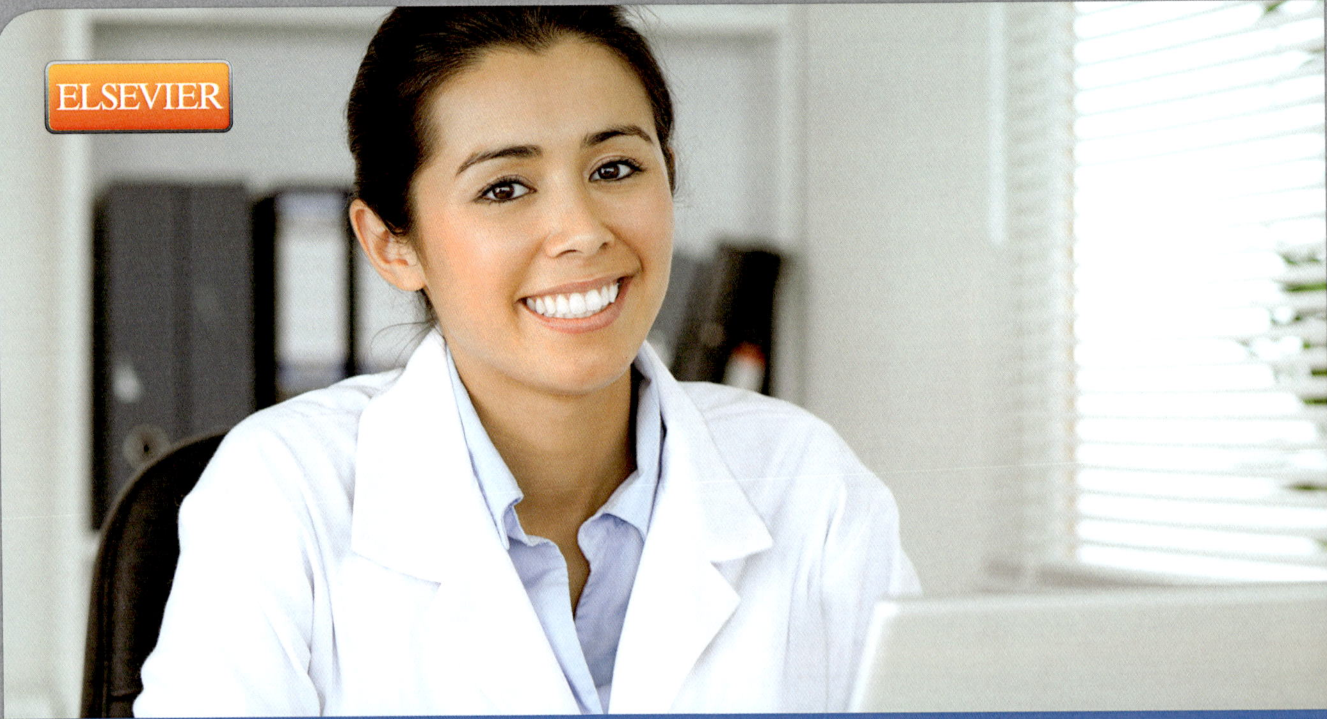

Clinical Echocardiography of the Dog and Cat

Related Elsevier Titles

Visit http://www.us.elsevierhealth.com/ for a complete listing of Veterinary titles.

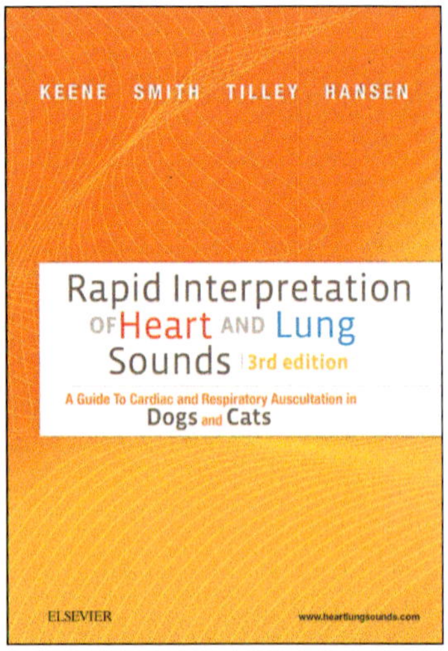

Rapid Interpretation of Heart and Lung Sounds: A Guide to Cardiac and Respiratory Auscultation in Dogs and Cats, 3rd Edition

By Bruce W. Keene, Francis W. K. Smith, Jr., Larry P. Tilley, and Bernie Hansen

ISBN: 978-0-323-32707-7

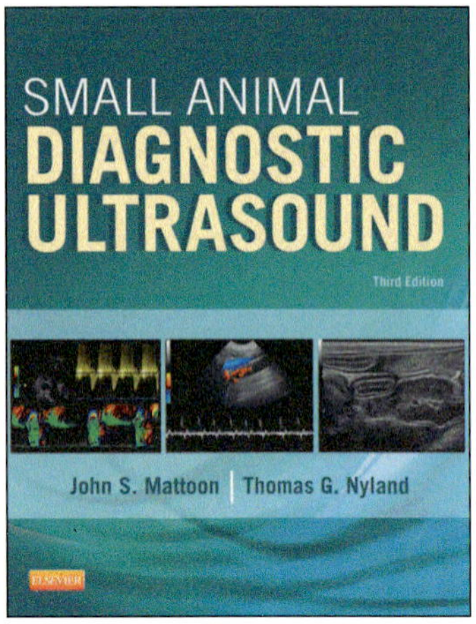

Small Animal Diagnostic Ultrasound, 3rd Edition

By John S. Mattoon and Thomas G. Nyland

ISBN: 978-1-4160-4867-1

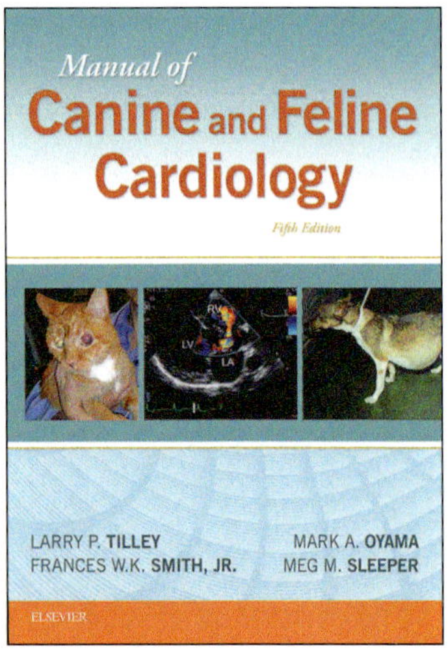

Manual of Canine and Feline Cardiology, 5th Edition

By Larry P. Tilley, Francis W. K. Smith, Jr., Mark Oyama, and Meg M. Sleeper

ISBN: 978-0-323-18802-9

Clinical Echocardiography of the Dog and Cat

Edited by Éric de Madron

Valérie Chetboul
Claudio Bussadori
Éric de Madron

In collaboration with:
Oriol Domenech
Chiara Locatelli
Antonia Mavropoulou
Danitza Pradelli
Joel Silva

ELSEVIER

ELSEVIER

3251 Riverport Lane
St. Louis, Missouri 63043

CLINICAL ECHOCARDIOGRAPHY OF THE DOG AND CAT ISBN: 978-0-323-31650-7

Library of Congress Cataloging-in-Publication Data

Echocardiographie clinique du chien et du chat. English
Clinical echocardiography of the dog and cat / edited by Eric de Madron (English edition).
p. ; cm.
Originally published as: Echocardiographie clinique du chien et du chat : techniques et applications pratiques, copyright (c) 2012, Elsevier Masson SAS.
Includes bibliographical references and index.
ISBN 978-0-323-31650-7 (hardcover : alk. paper)
I. Madron, Eric de, editor. II. Title.
[DNLM: 1. Echocardiography--veterinary. 2. Cats. 3. Dogs. SF 811]
SF811
636.089'61207543--dc23

2015001657

Content Strategy Director: Penny Rudolph
Professional Content Development Manager: Jolynn Gower
Senior Content Development Specialist: Courtney Sprehe
Publishing Services Manager: Jeff Patterson
Senior Project Manager: Tracey Schriefer
Design Direction: Julia Dummitt

Printed in the United States of America

Last digit is the print number: 9 8 7 6

The Authors

Valérie Chetboul is a doctor of veterinary medicine, a fellow of pathologic veterinary medicine, who graduated from the European College of Veterinary Internal Medicine (ECVIM-CA, degree in cardiology). She has a Doctorate in Science and is an accredited research director. She is a professor of cardiology and director of the Alfort cardiology division in charge of cardiovascular ultrasound imaging at Inserm (French Institute of Health and Medical Research) U955. She is the former editor of the *Journal of Veterinary Cardiology* and the author of several works and nearly 300 scientific articles, 100 of which were published in international, indexed journals.

Claudio Bussadori is a doctor of veterinary medicine, PhD in cardiovascular pathophysiology. He is a graduate of the European College of Veterinary Internal Medicine (ECVIM-CA) with a degree in cardiology. Dr. Bussadori is director of the Gran Sasso Veterinary Clinic (Milan, Italy) and a researcher in the department of pediatric cardiology at the San Donato Hospital in Milan, Italy.

Éric de Madron is a doctor of veterinary medicine (DVM), graduate of the American College of Veterinary Internal Medicine (ACVIM) in cardiology and of the European College of Veterinary Internal Medicine (ECVIM-CA) in internal medicine. He is a cardiologist and internist at the Alta Vista Veterinary Hospital in Ottawa, Canada.

Collaborators

Oriol Domenech is a doctor of veterinary medicine with a degree in veterinary medicine from the Autonomous University of Barcelona (Spain), and he graduated from the European College of Veterinary Internal Medicine (ECVIM-CA) in cardiology. Dr. Domenech currently works at the Veterinary Institute of Novara (Italy) and at the Survet Diagonal Carvet. He specializes in veterinary emergency and intensive care in Barcelona, Spain.

Chiara Locatelli is a doctor of veterinary medicine and a PhD in internal medicine and cardiology. She currently works at the Veterinary University in Milan (postdoctorate, cardiology department).

Antonia Mavropoulou is a doctor of veterinary medicine with a diploma from the University of Parma. She was a cardiology intern in diagnostic imaging and internal medicine at the same university. She earned a Master's degree in the clinical aspects of cardiovascular diseases. Dr. Mavropoulou is a resident at the Gran Sasso Veterinary Clinic in Milan, Italy, working in the ECVIM-CA residency program (cardiology).

Danitza Pradelli is a doctor of veterinary medicine with a PhD in animal health (Department of Medicine at the University of Parma, Italy) and has a European Master's degree in pharmaceuticals. She is the author of several articles on cardiology and veterinary echocardiography. Dr. Pradelli currently works at the Gran Sasso Veterinary Clinic in Milan, Italy.

Joel Silva graduated from the Veterinarian Faculty of Medicine in Lisbon, Portugal, and has worked for several years in Lisbon in small animal surgery and medicine. He is a resident at the Gran Sasso Veterinary Clinic in Milan, Italy, working in the ECVIM-CA residency program (cardiology).

Abbreviations

2D bidimensional
3D tridimensional
ACDO Amplatz® Canine Duct Occluder device *(Amplatz® canine duct occluder)*
AFI automated function imaging
AOSV aortic stroke volume
APW aortopulmonary window
AR aortic regurgitation
ASD atrial septal defect
ASO Amplatzer® septal occluder
AT acceleration time
ATP adenosine triphosphate
AVC aortic valve closing
AVO aortic valve opening
BCV balloon catheter valvuloplasty
BNP brain natriuretic peptide
bpm beats per minute
CHD congenital heart disease
CHF congestive heart failure
CKCS Cavalier King Charles Spaniel
CS coronary sinus
CT cardiac tumor
CTD cor triatriatum dexter
CTS cor triatriatum sinister
CV coefficient of variation
DCM dilated cardiomyopathy
DMVD degenerative mitral valve disease
DTE deceleration time of the E wave
ECWS end-systolic circumferential wall stress
EDVI end-diastolic volume index
EF ejection fraction
ESVI end-systolic volume index
ESVC European Society of Veterinary Cardiology
ET ejection time
GRMD Golden Retriever muscular dystrophy
HBT heart base tumor
HCM hypertrophic cardiomyopathy
HSA hemangiosarcoma
IMP index of myocardial performance
ISACHC International Small Animal Cardiac Health Council
IVCT isovolumic contraction time
IVRT isovolumic relaxation time
IVS interventricular septum
LA left atrium
LAP left atrial pressure
LV left ventricle
LVFP left ventricular filling pressure
LVFW left ventricular free wall
LVOT left ventricular outflow tract
MAM mitral annulus movement
MD minimal diameter
MDD minimal ductal diameter
MPA main pulmonary artery
MR mitral regurgitation
MS mitral stenosis
MVD mitral valve dysplasia
NV nuclear ventriculography
PAH pulmonary arterial hypertension
PAP pulmonary artery pressure
PAPd diastolic pulmonary artery pressure
PAPs systolic pulmonary artery pressure
PCWP pulmonary capillary wedge pressure
PDA patent ductus arteriosus
PDCM primary dilated cardiomyopathy
PET pre-ejection time
PFO patent foramen ovale
PISA proximal isovelocity surface area
PR pulmonic regurgitation
PS pulmonic stenosis
PSS portosystemic shunt
PV pulmonic valve
RA right atrium
RCM restrictive cardiomyopathy
RF regurgitant fraction
RFR regurgitant flow rate
ROA regurgitant orifice area
ROI region of interest
RV regurgitant volume
RV right ventricle
RVOT right ventricular outflow tract
SAM systolic anterior motion of the mitral valve
SAS subaortic stenosis
SEC spontaneous echo contrast

SF shortening fraction
SFe endocardial shortening fraction
SFmw mid-wall shortening fraction
SHT systemic arterial hypertension
SI sphericity index
SPAP systolic pulmonary artery pressure
SV stroke volume
TAPSE tricuspid annular plane systolic excursion
TDI tissue Doppler imaging
TEE transesophageal echocardiography
TM time-motion
ToF tetralogy of Fallot
TR tricuspid regurgitation
TS tricuspid stenosis
TTE transthoracic echocardiography
TVD tricuspid valve dysplasia
UCM undetermined cardiomyopathy
VSD ventricular septal defect
VTI velocity-time integral
WHWT West Highland White Terrier

Preface

This publication offers a complete update on the modern applications of echocardiography in cats and dogs.

The echocardiographic exam of cats and dogs has made remarkable progress in the past few years. Tissue Doppler and speckle tracking imaging have opened up new horizons. High-resolution imaging of the cardiac structures has become more sophisticated with the emergence of transesophageal echocardiography. The three-dimensional architecture of these structures can now be studied using three-dimensional echocardiography. Even traditional time-motion (TM) mode measurements have been recently updated. All of these technical improvements have transformed the echocardiographic examination, making it more quantitative.

This publication is thoroughly illustrated and complemented with videos, as well as tables and diagrams, that offer abundant numerical data of normal and abnormal values for a given pathology. The fundamental purpose of this publication is to integrate all this new knowledge to the daily clinical practice of echocardiography. Therefore, a multi-modal approach is discussed in-depth.

A synthesis of new TM methods, as well as the latest normal values updates are presented. One chapter is dedicated to interoperator and intraoperator variability of these values, as this topic is gaining attention from teams that use echocardiographic parameters as disease markers.

Novel modalities allowing regional myocardial function evaluation, such as Tissue Doppler and speckle tracking are presented. They allow a much more in-depth evaluation of global and regional systolic and diastolic ventricular myocardial function. Their contribution to the functional evaluation of different cardiopathies is discussed in their respective chapters.

The current echocardiographic exam cannot be limited to the diagnosis of the type of cardiopathy but also must stage the level of disease severity by quantifying all its parameters. A great deal of attention is therefore devoted to the quantitative evaluation of the various facets of cardiopathies: regurgitant fraction measurement, atrial pressure evaluation, pulmonary artery pressure, and global and regional systolic and diastolic function of the ventricle.

This book also discusses principles of hemodynamic evaluation in order to better understand the growing number of indices used in echocardiography to evaluate ventricle performance. New global indices, such as the Tei index, are analyzed and an entire chapter is devoted to the evaluation of the right ventricle function.

A chapter is dedicated to the cardiac evaluation of left atrial pressure and prediction of risk of congestive heart failure. Thromboembolic risk is also covered in the chapter on feline cardiopathies.

The diagnosis and evaluation of complex congenital cardiopathies is presented in detail. Recent advances in interventional veterinary cardiology, now allowing transcatheter occlusion of patent ductus arteriosus and interatrial or interventricular septal defects with occluding devices, require very precise measurements and diameters of the orifices as well as interoperative monitoring. For this purpose, a full chapter is dedicated to preintervention and postintervention evaluation of congenital cardiopathies.

This publication presents the most recent advances in echocardiography in cats and dogs and integrates them into the echocardiographic exam, always keeping in mind staging of the disease and evaluation of risk of a clinical event.

Éric de Madron

Video Credits

Videos credited to Éric de Madron

1-8, 1-9, 1-10, 1-11, 1-12, 1-13, 1-14, 1-15, 1-16, 1-17, 1-18, 1-19, 11-1, 11-2, 11-3, 11-4, 11-5, 11-6, 11-7, 11-8, 11-9, 11-10, 12-1, 13-1, 13-2, 13-3, 13-4, 13-5, 13-6, 13-7, 13-8, 13-9, 13-10, 13-11, 13-12, 13-13, 13-14, 13-15, 13-16, 13-17, 13-18, 13-19, 13-20, 13-21, 14-1, 14-2, 17-1, 17-2, 17-3, 17-4, 17-5, 17-6, 18-1, 18-2, 18-3, 18-4, 18-5, 18-6, 18-7, 19-1, 19-4, 19-8, 19-11, 19-12, 19-13, 19-14

Videos credited to Valérie Chetboul

1-1, 1-2, 1-3, 1-4, 1-5, 1-6, 1-7, 4-1, 4-2, 4-3, 12-2, 12-3, 12-4, 14-3, 14-4, 16-1

Videos credited to Claudio Bussadori

6-1, 6-2, 19-2, 19-3, 19-5, 19-6, 19-7, 19-9, 19-10

Contents

Part I: Normal Echocardiographic Examination

1 Normal Views: 2D, TM, Spectral, and Color Doppler 3
Éric de Madron
The Different Modes 4
General Considerations 5
Normal Bidimensional Views 6
Normal TM Views 16
Normal Spectral Doppler Examination 17
Color Doppler 18

2 Normal Echocardiographic Values: TM, 2D, and Doppler Spectral Modes 21
Éric de Madron
Normal TM and 2D Mode Values 22
Spectral Wave Doppler Normal Values 32

3 Intra- and Interoperator Variability 39
Valérie Chetboul
Repeatability, Reproducibility, and Operators 40
Operator's Effect on the Variability of Echocardiographic Measurements 40
Practical Consequences 41
Conclusion 43

Part II: New Cardiac Ultrasound Imaging Techniques

4 Myocardial Tissue Doppler, Derived Techniques, and Speckle Tracking Imaging 47
Valérie Chetboul
Normal Myocardial Kinetics 48
Myocardial Tissue Doppler or Tissue Doppler Imaging 50
TDI-Derived Techniques (Tissue Tracking Imaging, Strain Imaging, and Strain Rate Imaging) 62
Speckle Tracking Imaging 74
Conclusion 82

5 Transesophageal Echocardiography 85
Claudio Bussadori in collaboration with Oriol Domenech
Introduction and Technical Considerations 86
Considerations Regarding the Echocardiographer 86
Complications 87
TEE Examination Protocol 87
TEE Indications and Applications 90
Conclusion 93

6 Veterinary Applications of the Tridimensional Echocardiography 95
Claudio Bussadori in collaboration with Antonia Mavropoulou and Joel Silva
3D Echocardiography Technology 96
The Different 3D Echocardiography Methods 96
3D Echocardiography in Veterinary Medicine 98
3D Transesophageal Echocardiography 102

Part III: Hemodynamic Evaluation

7 Global Left Ventricular Systolic Function Assessment 111
Éric de Madron
Left Ventricular Anatomy 112
Radial Systolic Function: Shortening Fraction 112
Systolic Indices Derived from Ventricular Volumes 115
Assessment of the Longitudinal Systolic Function 118
Systolic Indices Obtained by Spectral Wave Doppler: Systolic Time Intervals and Index of Myocardial Performance (Tei Index) 120
Speckle Tracking–Derived Indices 121
Conclusion 122

8 Assessment of Diastolic Function 127
Éric de Madron
Diastole Phases and Determinants 128
Types of Diastolic Dysfunction 129
Echocardiographic Indices of Diastolic Function 130

9 Echocardiographic Evaluation of the Left Ventricle Filling Pressure 139
Éric de Madron
Left Atrial Pressure Curve 140
Left Atrial Pressure Echocardiographic Indices 141
Other Echocardiographic Criteria 147

10 Evaluation of the Right Ventricular Global Systolic Function 151
Éric de Madron
Evaluation of the Radial Systolic Function of the Right Ventricle: Shortening Fraction of the Right Ventricle 152
Evaluation of the Longitudinal Systolic Function 152
Indices Derived from Right Ventricular Tissue Doppler 154
Conclusion 155

Part IV: Echocardiography of Acquired Cardiopathies

11 Assessment and Quantification of Acquired Valvular Regurgitation in Dogs 159
Éric de Madron
Mitral Regurgitation 160
Tricuspid Regurgitation 175
Aortic Regurgitation 176
Pulmonic Regurgitation 177

12 Dilated Cardiomyopathy and Other Cardiomyopathies in Dogs 181
Valérie Chetboul
Primary Dilated Cardiomyopathy 182
Other Cardiomyopathies 194

13 Evaluation of Feline Cardiomyopathies 207
Éric de Madron
Hypertrophic Cardiomyopathies 208
Restrictive Cardiomyopathies 218
Dilated Cardiomyopathies 222
Atypical Cardiomyopathies 224
Thrombotic Risk Assessment 225

14 Pulmonary Arterial Hypertension 229
Valérie Chetboul
Etiology and Pathogenesis of PAH 230
Conventional Echocardiography and PAH 231
Conventional Doppler and PAH 234
New Imaging Techniques and PAH 237

15 Dirofilariasis: Specific Bidimensional Aspects 241
Éric de Madron
Echocardiographic Aspects of *Dirofilaria* 242
Other Echocardiographic Anomalies Associated with Dirofilariasis 242

16 Cardiac Manifestations of Systemic Diseases 245
Valérie Chetboul and Éric de Madron
Systemic Arterial Hypertension 246
Hyperthyroid Cardiopathy 252
Anemia 254

17 Pericardial Diseases 259
Éric de Madron
Pericardium Anatomy and Function 260
Pericardial Effusions 260
Constrictive Pericarditis 268
Congenital Anomalies of the Pericardium 269

18 Cardiac Tumors 271
Claudio Bussadori
Types of Tumors and Prevalence 272
Goals of Echocardiography in Assessing Cardiac Tumors 272
Specific Echocardiographic Presentation 273

Part V: Congenital Cardiopathies

19 Congenital Cardiopathies 285
Claudio Bussadori in collaboration with Danitza Pradelli
Left Ventricular Outflow Tract Obstructions/ Subaortic Stenosis 286
Pulmonic Stenosis 291
Patent Ductus Arteriosus 298
Ventricular Septal Defect 303
Atrial Septal Defect 305
Mitral Valve Dysplasia 308
Tricuspid Valve Dysplasia 310
Tetralogy of Fallot 312
Cor Triatriatum 313
Endocardial Cushion Defect 316

20 Echocardiographic Evaluation of Congenital Cardiopathies Before and After Intervention 323
Claudio Bussadori in collaboration with Danitza Pradelli
Pulmonic Valve Stenosis 324
Patent Ductus Arteriosus 331
Ventricular Septal Defect 336
Atrial Septal Defect 339

PART I

Normal Echocardiographic Examination

1 Normal Views: 2D, TM, Spectral, and Color Doppler, 3

2 Normal Echocardiographic Values: TM, 2D, and Doppler Spectral Modes, 21

3 Intra- and Interoperator Variability, 39

1
Normal Views: 2D, TM, Spectral, and Color Doppler

ÉRIC DE MADRON

The Different Modes, 4
General Considerations, 5
Normal Bidimensional Views, 6
Normal TM Views, 16
Normal Spectral Doppler Examination, 17
Color Doppler, 18

The Different Modes

Bidimensional Mode

Bidimensional (2D) echocardiography provides anatomic cross-sections of the heart via the emission of a wide ultrasound beam through the thorax and the reception of the echoes reflected by its different structures. This wide beam allows viewing of a large part of the organ. It is shaped in such a manner as to travel between the ribs and the pulmonary lobes. Several views or projections are used in order to observe all of the cardiac structures. 2D echocardiography allows real-time visualization of the movement and deformation of these structures in two dimensions. Bidimensional harmonic echocardiography integrates secondary harmonics of reflected echoes. This improves the visualization of structures with low levels of reflectivity, such as the myocardium.

Time-Motion Mode

Historically, time-motion (TM) mode (or M-mode) was the first mode developed. A line is selected on the 2D ultrasound cone and a series of points moving in time can then be obtained. These points correspond to the echoes reflected by the different acoustic interfaces of each cardiac structure being penetrated. The point of origin and orientation of this line can be modified if the device is equipped with "anatomic" or "free-angle" M-mode capabilities. Because of the contraction and dilation of the heart, the position of these points will vary according to the cardiac cycle phases. This appears on the screen as undulating lines corresponding to the movement of the points over time. Due to high sampling frequency, TM mode enables the recording of very rapid cardiac movements such as valve motion [1,2]. It also allows measurement of the dimensions of the heart (wall thickness and endocavitary diameters in systole and diastole) and analysis of the motion of different structures of the organ during the cardiac cycle.

Spectral Doppler Mode

When an ultrasound beam of a particular frequency encounters a flow of erythrocytes moving at speed S, part of these ultrasounds is reflected toward the transducer at a modified frequency. This is defined as the Doppler effect [3,4]. This change in frequency, or shift, is proportional to the speed of the erythrocytes (i.e., the blood flow speed) and to the angle cosine (referred to as θ) formed by the ultrasound beam and the blood flow axis of displacement according to the equation:

$$V = (\Delta F \times C)/(2F_0 \times \cos\theta)$$

where ΔF is the measured frequency shift, C is the initial ultrasound speed in the soft tissue, and F_0 is the initial beam frequency [3]. The Doppler examination, by measuring this ΔF frequency shift, allows the determination of the blood flow velocity and its direction. To best measure real flow velocity without underestimating it, the θ angle must be as close to 0 degrees as possible. The ultrasound beam must then be aligned as much as possible to the axis of the flow movement.

The Doppler examination allows the study of the characteristics of the intracardiac flows, the detection of abnormal flows, and the measurement of transvalvular or transorifice stroke volumes.

The spectral Doppler exam includes pulsed and continuous wave Doppler modes, which complement each other perfectly. In both cases, the frequency shift is analyzed and filtered by the cardiac ultrasound machine, which transforms it into acoustic and graphic signals. The graphic signal represents the spectral analysis through fast Fourier transform of all reported frequency shifts in the flow under study. A velocity "envelope" changing in time can thus be obtained. As a rule, when erythrocytes move toward the transducer, their velocities are coded as positive. Inversely, they are coded as negative when moving away from the transducer. Not all red cells within a blood flow move at the same velocity. The Doppler signal will indicate through its intensity the relative prevalence of these velocities. In a normal transvalvular flow, the erythrocytes move in the same direction and at the same speed. The flow is then considered to be "laminar."

Pulsed Wave Spectral Doppler

The unique transducer crystal emits at a certain frequency (known as recurrence frequency), then listens between each ultrasound blast. Knowing the ultrasound propagation speed through soft tissue (1540 m/s), it becomes possible to set the emission and reception so as to record only frequencies reflected from a certain depth of the beam [3]. The pulsed wave Doppler examination requires selecting a small zone, called sample volume, on the Doppler cursor line positioned on the 2D echocardiographic image. This sample volume contains erythrocytes whose velocities are to be analyzed. Thus this examination enables the analysis of the blood flow characteristics in a specific area of the heart or great arteries [3]. The time allocated to reception of the reflected waves limits the measurable maximum velocities. The maximum recordable frequency shift (known as the Nyquist limit) is equal to half of the recurrent frequency of the wave train emitted by the transducer. Frequency shifts that go beyond this limit lead to an artifact known as "aliasing" or "ambiguous velocity." When this artifact is produced, the part of the Doppler envelope exceeding this limit is truncated and appears at the opposite edge of the screen. When this phenomenon becomes very pronounced, it can interfere with the measurement of maximum velocities and even prevent the determination of flow direction. To increase the Nyquist limit, one can modify the baseline, use a lower frequency transducer, increase the recurrence frequency by purposefully selecting a sample volume very close to the transducer, or even use a high pulse repetition frequency (PRF) technique known as a high PRF. The latter involves setting the transducer in a nearly continuous emission and reception mode, allowing the capture of the entirety of the Doppler signals encountered along the beam without the interference of a now very high Nyquist limit. However, high PRF mode does not allow one to know the exact depth at which the measured velocities were recorded (ambiguous range). This becomes extremely close to continuous Doppler (see below) [3-5].

Continuous Wave Spectral Doppler

Continuous wave spectral Doppler is characterized by the use of two crystals working in a simultaneous and continuous manner, one emitting and one receiving. This continuous work by both crystals abolishes the Nyquist limit and allows the recording of any velocity value. However, with all velocities along the beam being recorded, it becomes impossible to pinpoint the exact location of the origin of the flow. Pairing the pulsed wave and continuous wave modes allows one to locate the flows and to record the highest velocities without any artifacts, respectively.

Color Doppler Mode

In color Doppler mode, the cardiac flow is directly visible in color on the 2D image. As a rule, flows moving toward the transducer appear in red whereas those moving away from it appear in blue. This color representation is obtained through the velocity spectrum obtained by fast Fourier transform. The different velocities recorded by the device are represented by a series of small colored squares (vertical axis) moving in time (horizontal axis). The greater the quantity of erythrocytes moving at the same speed at the same time, the more the Doppler signals will coincide (i.e., in the same square), leading to greater square color intensity. This type of representation is known as "amplitude analysis" because the different intensity amplitudes are displayed. If the Nyquist limit is reached, as in the case of pulsed wave spectral Doppler, an aliasing phenomenon will appear. It is characterized by a change in color: red becoming blue and vice versa. Another important concept is variance. Variance expresses the degree of difference between the varying velocities within a sample volume and the average velocity. In a normal laminar flow, variance is very low and maximum velocities are generally lower than the Nyquist frequency limit. The flow then is coded in a homogeneous red or blue color. On the other hand, turbulent flows are characterized by a widened velocity spectrum—in other words, by a wide variance. This leads to multiple colors that cover the spectrum between red and blue (known as a mosaic aspect) [6,7]. Color Doppler mode is very useful for locating flows and is able to accurately determine their extent within the cardiac cavities (colorimetric extent). The measurement of flow velocities is performed using spectral modes (pulsed wave or continuous wave Doppler).

General Considerations

Choice of Transducer

The choice of a transducer depends on the size of the animal. In general, a 10 or 7.5 MHz transducer is adequate for cats and dogs weighing less than 10 kg, 5 MHz is adequate for medium-size dogs, and 3.5 or 2.25 MHz is adequate for large or giant breeds (Doberman, Great Dane, Bull Mastiff, etc.). Most current transducers are multifrequency. The transducer must be covered in gel and, if necessary, the animal's skin should be shaved to ensure contact without any kind of air interference, which could block the ultrasounds.

Positioning the Animal

There are two possible positions for the animal: lying down or standing against a support. In the first option, the animal is placed in a lateral position on a table with a side hole, which allows for the placement of the transducer against the

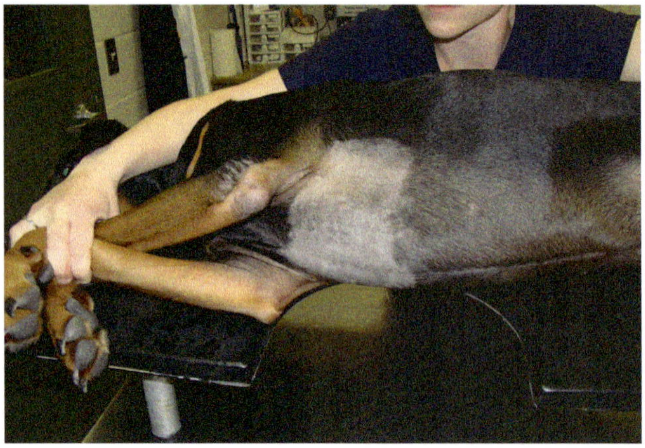

• **Fig. 1-1** Animal positioned on the imaging table to perform an ultrasound. See Video 1-1 for the standing position. (Photo credit: Éric de Madron.)

thorax on the lateral side (Figure 1-1). Right-sided views are thus obtained with the animal in right lateral recumbency and vice versa. The standing position is often better tolerated by very large breed dogs and also by stressed or dyspneic animals (Video 1-1). A trained operator can obtain similar and repeatable measurements from these two positions [8].

Settings

The depth must be set so that the cardiac image occupies the entire screen. The ultrasound beam gradually loses its energy as it progresses through the thorax and reflects off the successive interfaces. Echoes from the deep structures are thus weak whereas those from structures near the transducer are very intense. To compensate for this phenomenon, the proximal echo signals must be attenuated and the distant ones amplified. This compensation can be set in a progressive fashion [2,9]. Also, the ultrasound beam energy is set using total gain so as to clearly visualize all structures, including those with low reflectivity such as the myocardium, while avoiding image saturation by overly bright echoes. There are many settings to choose from, including the focal position, endocardial echo amplification, erythrocyte echo attenuation, beam width, and sweep frequency repetition.

Normal Bidimensional Views

These views have been well described in dogs [10,11] and in cats [12]. Videos 1-2 to 1-7 demonstrate how to obtain these views with the animal in a standing position. Videos 1-9 to 1-15 show views with the animal in a recumbent position.

Right Parasternal Long Axis Views

Long Axis 4 Chambers View: Optimized for Viewing the Atria

The beam is aligned with the long axis of the heart and angulated to view both ventricles and both atria (Figure 1-2, *A;* see also Video 1-8). This is the best view to observe the interatrial septum.

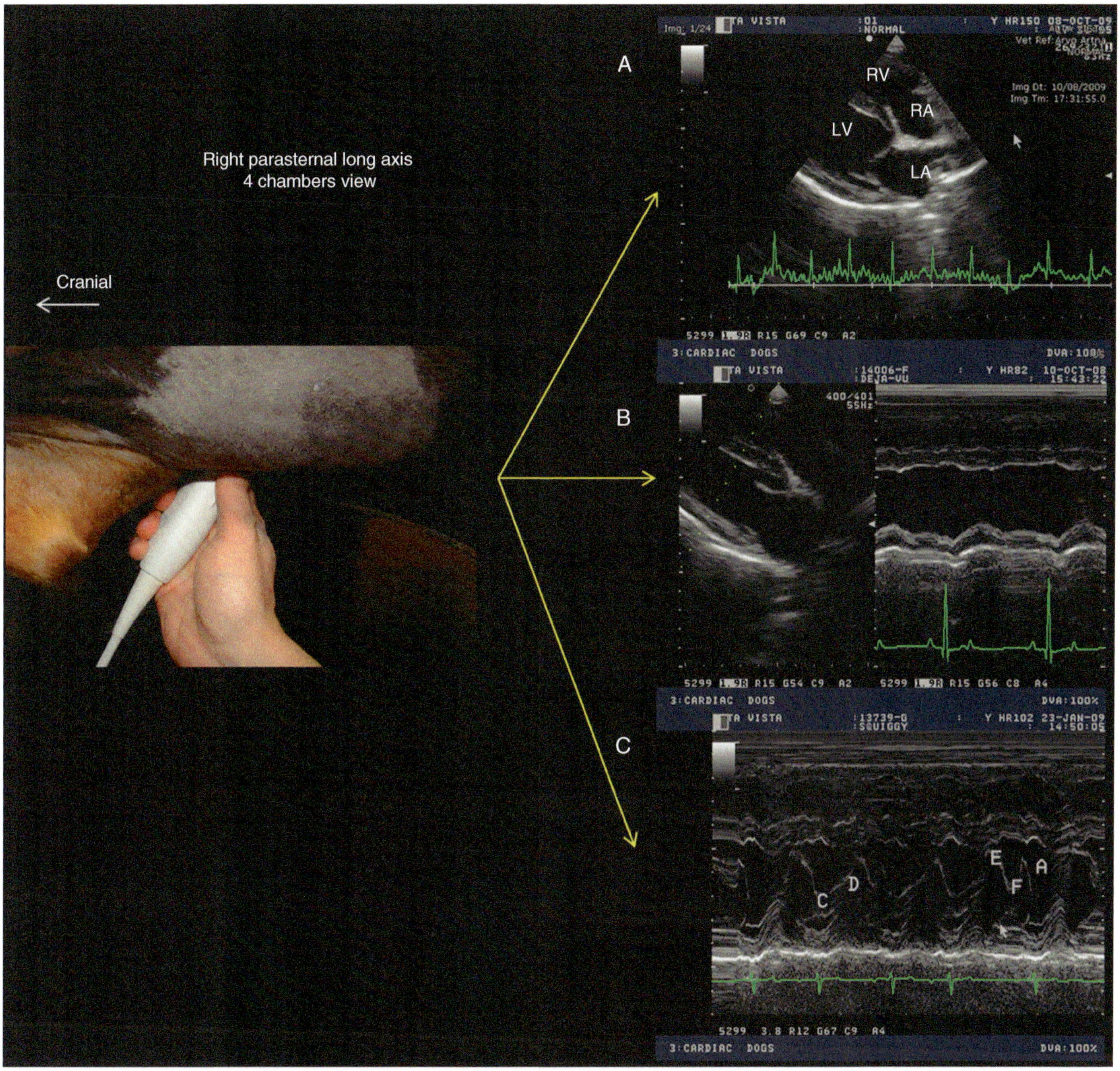

• **Fig. 1-2** Transducer position used to obtain a right parasternal long axis 4 chambers view. The beam must be oblique, pointing toward the spine. A, Bidimensional echocardiogram (right parasternal long axis view, optimized for the atria) in a normal dog. *LA,* Left atrium; *LV,* left ventricle; *RA,* right atrium; *RV,* right ventricle. B, Time-motion (TM) echocardiogram of the left ventricle. The TM cursor perpendicularly transects the left ventricular walls, just downstream of the mitral valve. C, TM echocardiogram of the mitral valve. The mitral valve movements are clearly identifiable with a systolic closure (CD segment), an early-diastolic maximal opening (point E), a mid-diastolic partial closure (point F), and reopening associated with atrial systole (point A). (Photo credit: Éric de Madron.)

Long Axis 5 Chambers View: Optimized for Viewing the Aorta

The beam is placed in the apex–great arteries plane, perpendicular to the interventricular septum. From there both ventricles, a portion of the right atrium and of the tricuspid valve, the aorta with the noncoronary and left aortic cusps, and a portion of the left atrium and its atrial appendage can be viewed (Figure 1-3; see also Videos 1-2 and 1-9).

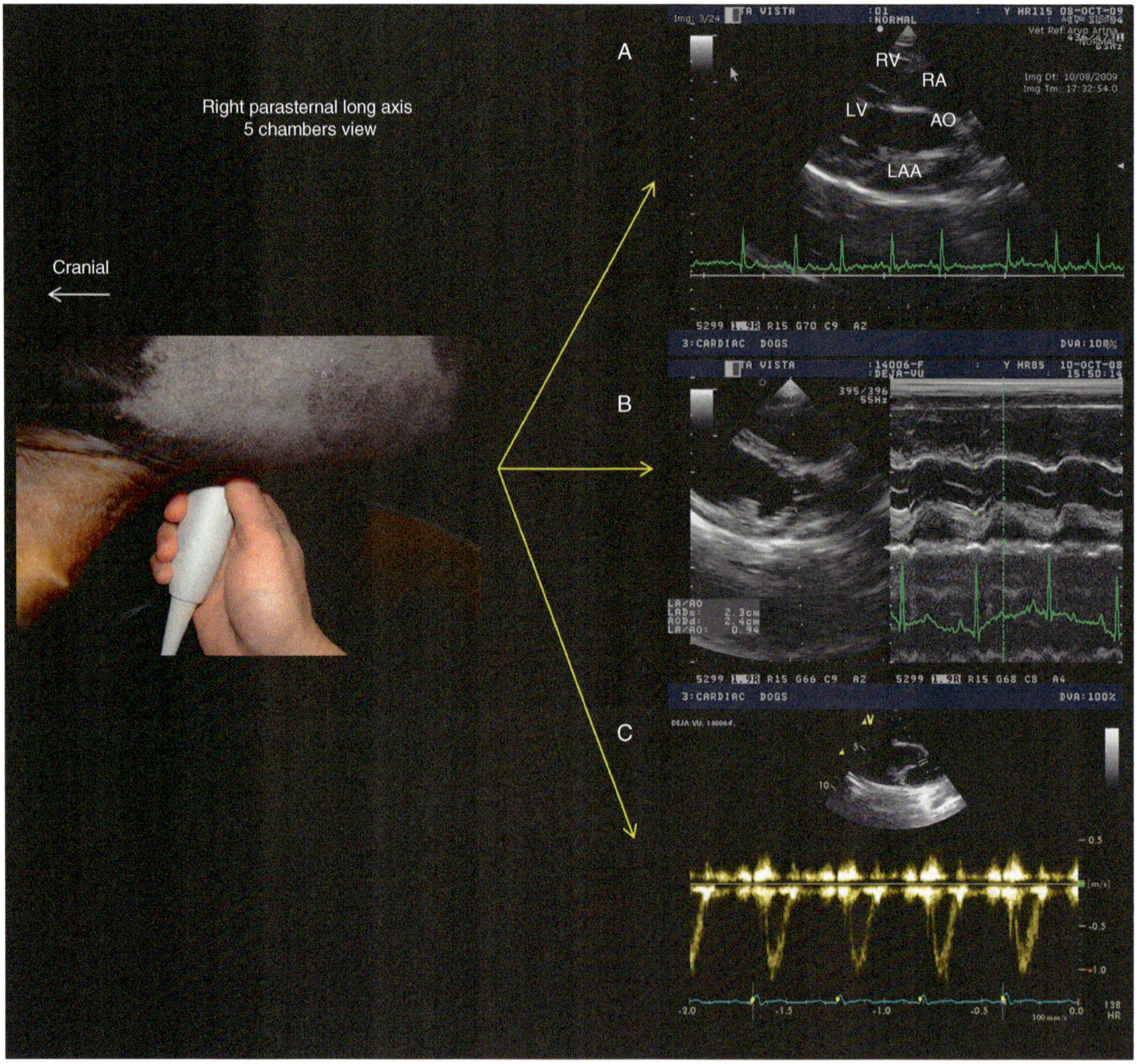

• **Fig. 1-3** Transducer position used to obtain a right parasternal long axis 5 chambers view. The beam orientation is now more vertical. A, Bidimensional echocardiogram (right parasternal long axis 5 chambers view) in a normal dog. The aorta (Ao) is now visible and only the left atrial appendage (LAA) appears. *LV,* Left ventricle; *RA,* right atrium; *RV,* right ventricle. B, Transaortic time-motion (TM) echocardiogram in a normal dog. The TM cursor crosses the commissure of the aortic valve cusps, perpendicular to the aortic walls. C, Pulsed wave spectral Doppler of the transaortic flow obtained from a right parasternal long axis 5 chambers view by placing the recording zone within the descending aorta. The Doppler cursor must be as oblique as possible so as to obtain the best possible alignment with the aortic flow. (Photo credit: Éric de Madron.)

Right Parasternal Short Axis Views

These views can be obtained by rotating the transducer 90 degrees from the previous positions (Figures 1-4 and 1-5; see also Videos 1-3, 1-4, 1-10, 1-11, and 1-12).

Apex Level

On this view (referred to as a transapical view) only the extremity of the left ventricular cavity is visible. It is small in size compared to the predominant myocardium (see Figure 1-4, *A*).

Papillary Muscle Level

The right ventricular cavity becomes visible along with the cranial and caudal papillary muscles (hence the name of this view: short axis transpapillary view) (see Figure 1-4, *B*).

Chordae Tendineae Level

At this level the left ventricular cavity is larger than on the preceding view (hence the name of this view: short axis transventricular view). This is the best view to obtain an equatorial transventricular TM echocardiogram (see Figure 1-4, *C* and Video 1-10).

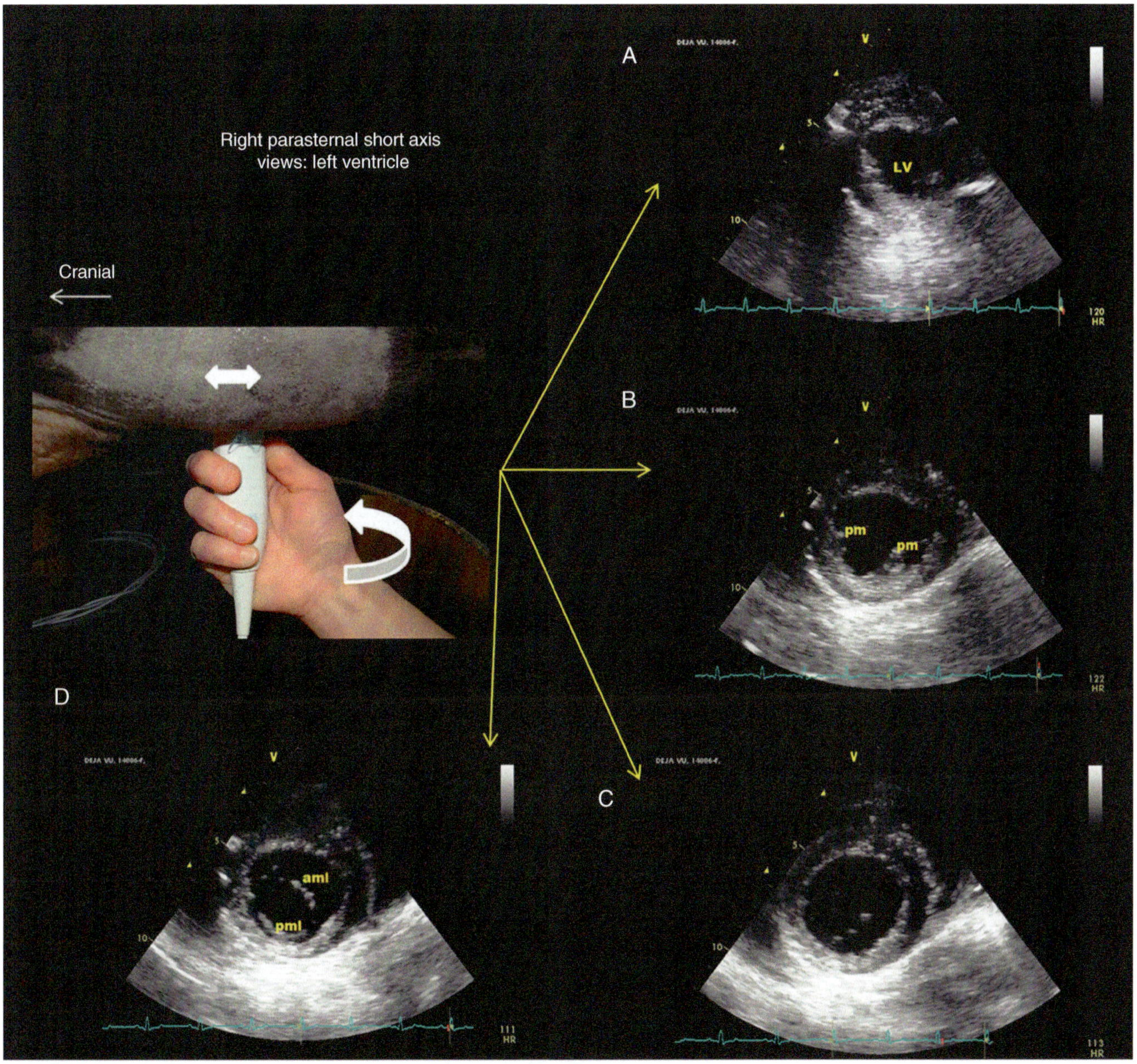

• **Fig. 1-4** Transducer position used to obtain the right parasternal short axis left ventricular views. The transducer is rotated by 90 degrees and the different views are obtained by slightly tilting the transducer toward the base or apex of the heart. **A**, Bidimensional echocardiogram (right parasternal short axis view) at the level of the apex of the left ventricle (LV). **B**, Bidimensional echocardiogram (right parasternal short axis view) at the level of the LV papillary muscles (pm). **C**, Bidimensional echocardiogram (right parasternal short axis view) at the level of the chordae tendineae. **D**, Bidimensional echocardiogram (right parasternal short axis view) at the level of the mitral valve. On this diastolic image, the anterior (aml) and posterior (pml) mitral leaflets are apart, forming a characteristic "fish mouth" shape. (Photo credit: Éric de Madron.)

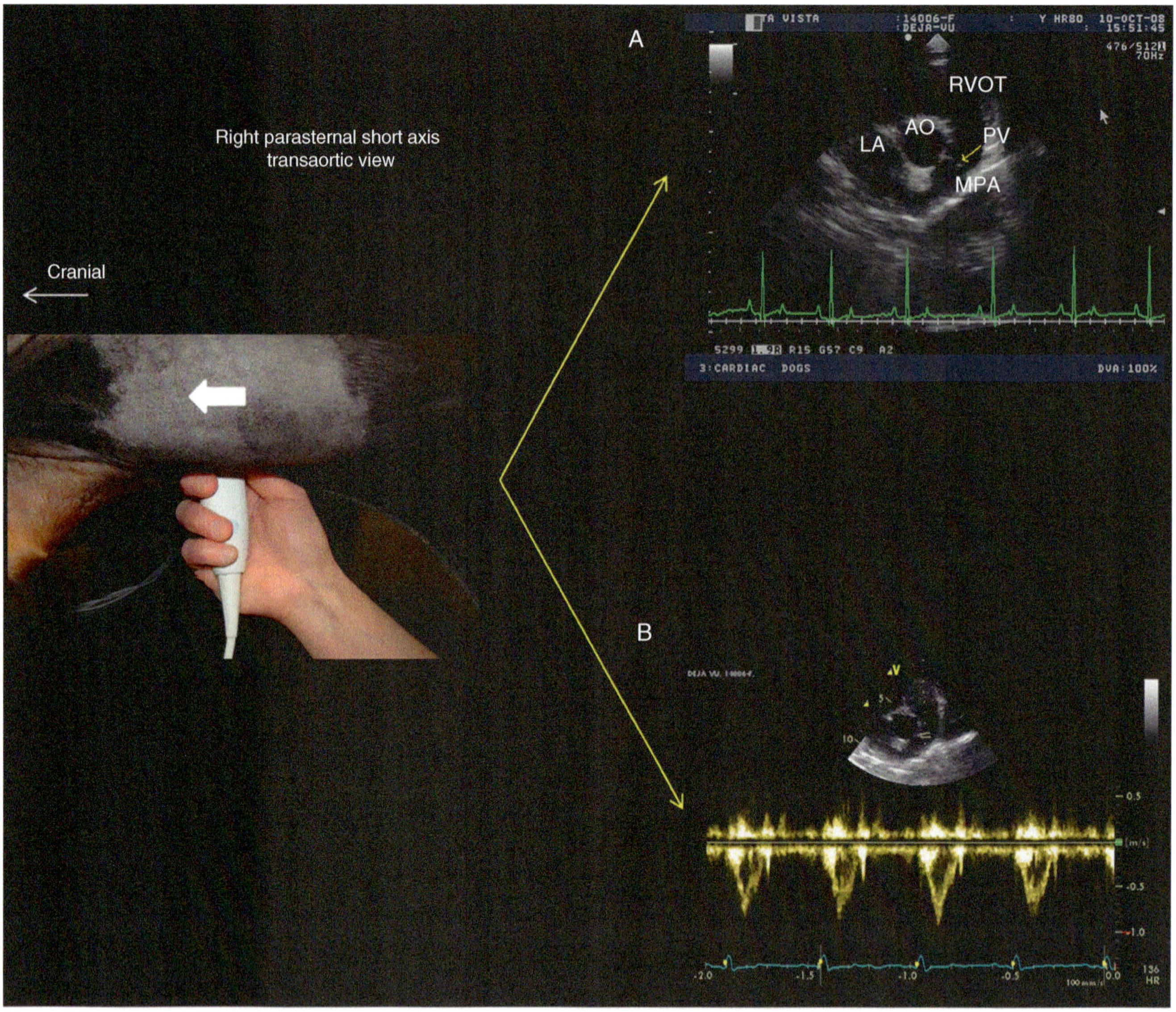

• **Fig. 1-5** Transducer position used to obtain a right parasternal short axis transaortic view. The transducer is either in the same position as in Figure 1-4, but with an oblique inclination toward the heart base, or moved cranially by one intercostal space. A, Bidimensional echocardiogram (right parasternal short axis transaortic view) in a normal dog. The different structures that can be viewed are the aorta (AO) in the center, the left atrium (LA) beneath and slightly to the left of the image, the right ventricular outflow tract (RVOT) above the aorta, the pulmonic valve (PV) to the right of the aorta, and the main pulmonary artery (MPA) below it. B, Pulsed wave spectral Doppler of the transpulmonic flow obtained from a right parasternal short axis transaortic view. The recording zone is placed at the level of the pulmonic valve. (Photo credit: Éric de Madron.)

Mitral Valve Level

At this level the mitral valve appears as a "fish mouth," opening in diastole and closing in systole (hence the name of this view: transmitral short axis). The left ventricular cavity is now perfectly circular. The right ventricular outflow tract is visible (see Figure 1-4, *D* and Video 1-11).

Aorta–Main Pulmonary Artery Level

The aortic root occupies the center of the image with its three cusps (hence the name of this view: short axis transaortic view). In dogs as in cats, only one or two of the cusps are usually visible. The right ventricular outflow tract is wrapped around the aortic root (see Figure 1-5, *A* and Video 1-12). The pulmonic valve and the main pulmonary artery are visible. The left atrium and its appendage appear beneath the aorta, bordered by the right atrium on the left of the screen. The tricuspid valve forms a circular structure.

Left Parasternal, Caudal, or Apical Projections

The transducer is placed on the left hemithorax, where the precordial thump is felt best (Figures 1-6 to 1-8). The beam cuts the heart from the apex to the base along the interventricular septum axis (see Videos 1-5, 1-6, 1-13, 1-14, 1-15).

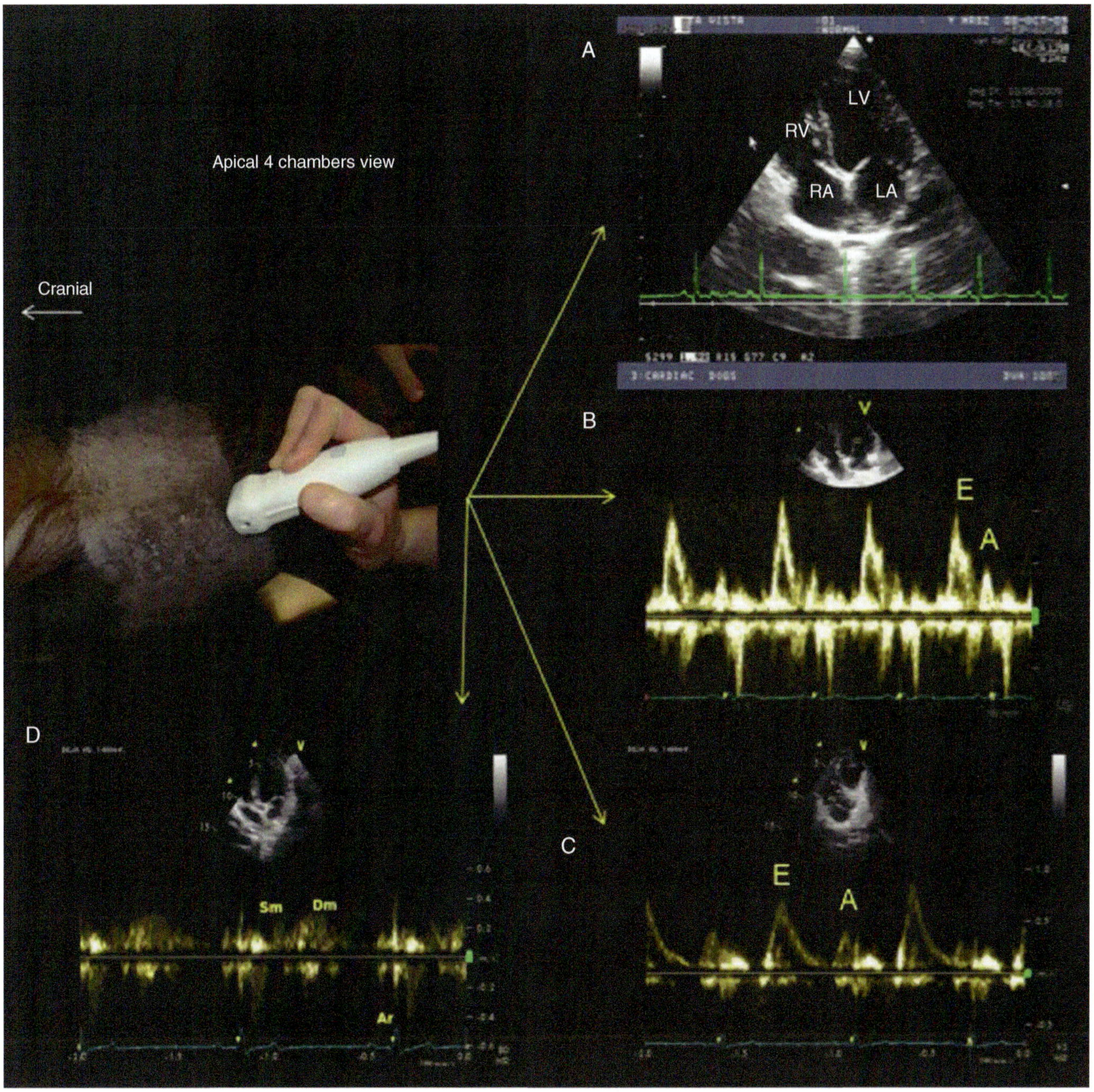

• **Fig. 1-6** Transducer position for obtaining an apical 4 chambers view. The transducer is placed at the level of the cardiac apex. A, Bidimensional echocardiogram (left apical 4 chambers view) showing the four cardiac cavities. *LA,* Left atrium; *LV,* left ventricle; *RA,* right atrium; *RV,* right ventricle. B, Pulsed wave spectral Doppler of the transmitral flow obtained by placing the recording zone at the level of the mitral valve on a left apical 4 chambers view. C, Pulsed wave spectral Doppler of the transtricuspid flow obtained by placing the recording zone at the level of the tricuspid valve on a left apical 4 chambers view. D, Pulmonary venous flow in a normal dog obtained from an apical 4 chambers view, with the sample volume in the medial pulmonary vein. Three waves can be seen: systolic (Sm), diastolic (Dm), and retrograde end-diastolic waves (Ar). (Photo credit: Éric de Madron.)

Apical 4 and 5 Chambers Views

The apical 4 chambers view is characterized by the visualization of both ventricles and both atria (see Figure 1-6, *A* and Video 1-13). By changing the transducer position, the left ventricular outflow tract and the aorta (not visible in the preceding view) appear; this is the apical 5 chambers view (see Figure 1-7, *A* and Video 1-14).

Apical 2 Chambers View

This view is obtained from the apical 4 chambers view by rotating the transducer by 90 degrees. In this way, either the left atrium or ventricle (see Figure 1-8, *A*) or the left ventricular outflow tract and the aorta become visible (see Figure 1-8, *B;* see also Video 1-15).

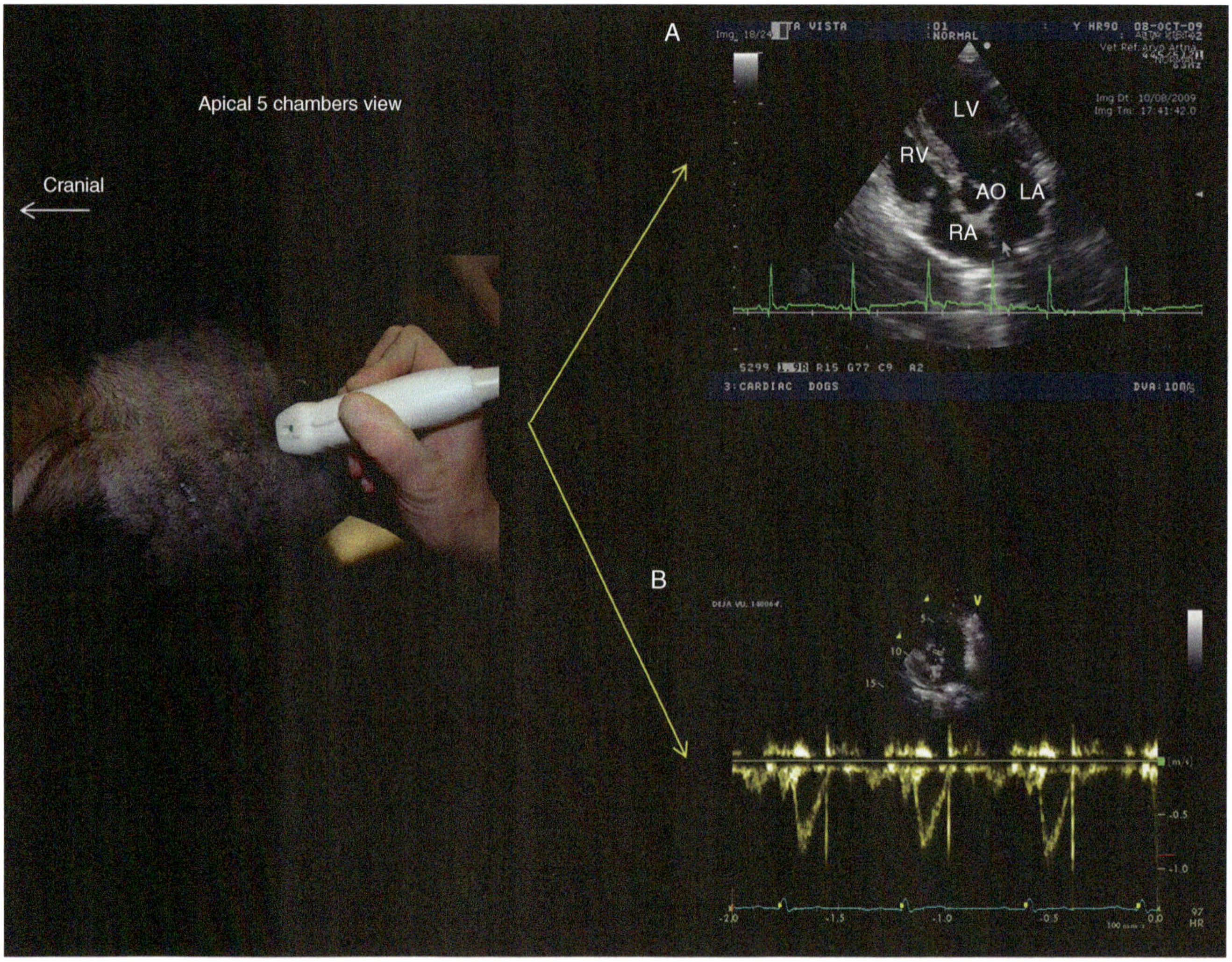

• **Fig. 1-7** Transducer position used to obtain an apical 5 chambers view. The transducer is in the same position as in Figure 1-6 but has been rotated 30 degrees clockwise. A, Bidimensional echocardiogram (left apical 5 chambers view) showing the aorta (AO) and the four cardiac cavities. *LA,* Left atrium; *LV,* left ventricle; *RA,* right atrium; *RV,* right ventricle. B, Pulsed wave spectral Doppler of the transaortic flow obtained by placing the recording zone at the level of the aortic valve on a left apical 5 chambers view. (Photo credit: Éric de Madron.)

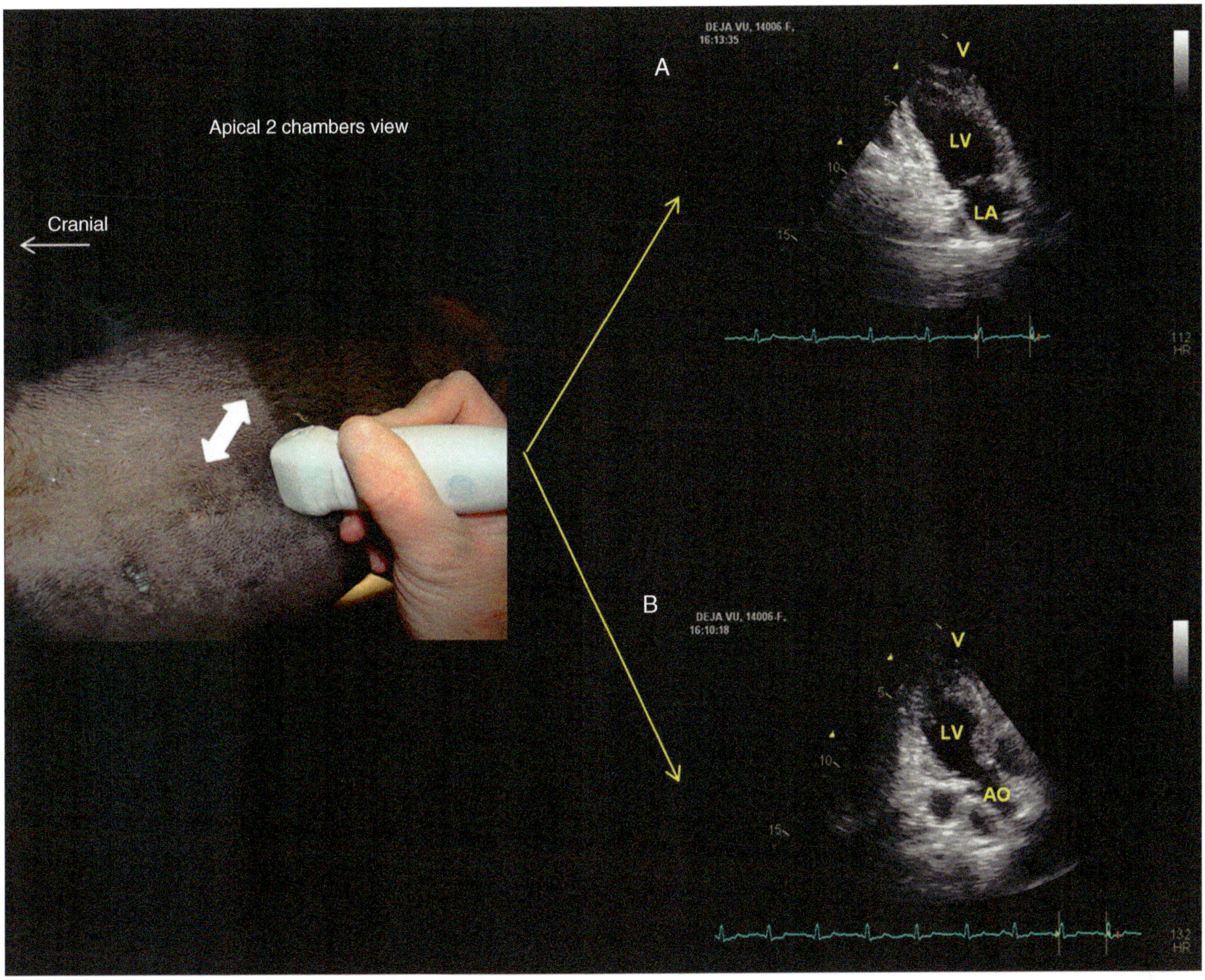

• **Fig. 1-8** Transducer position used to obtain the apical 2 chambers view. The transducer is in the same position as in Figure 1-6 but has been rotated 90 degrees clockwise. A, Bidimensional echocardiogram (left apical 2 chambers view) showing the left ventricle (LV) and the left atrium (LA). B, Bidimensional echocardiogram (left apical "left ventricular outflow tract" view) showing the long axis of the left ventricular outflow tract. *AO,* Aorta. (Photo credit: Éric de Madron.)

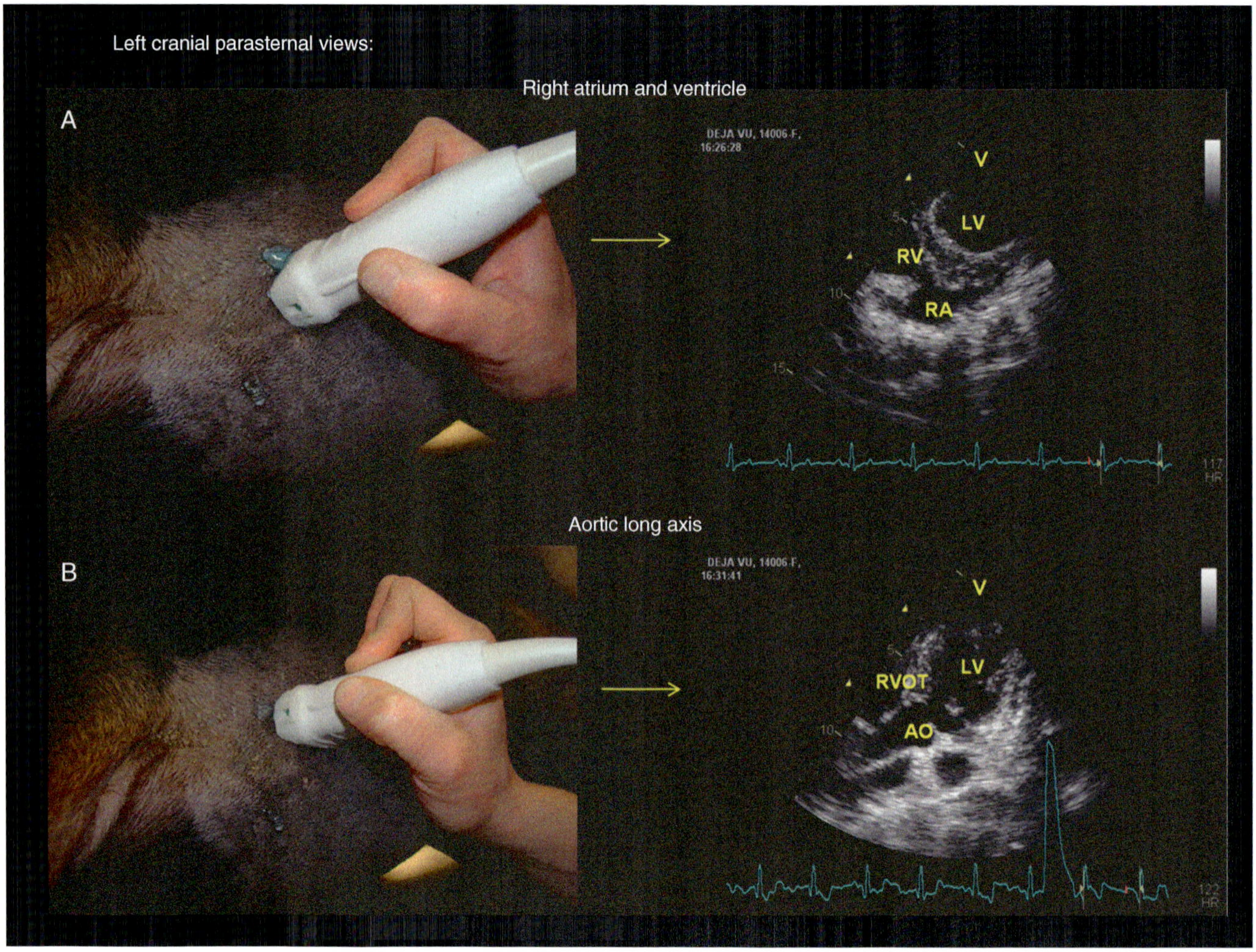

• **Fig. 1-9** Left cranial parasternal views. A, Transducer position used to obtain a left cranial parasternal "right atrium" view. The transducer is placed at the level of the fifth intercostal space. This allows one to obtain the left cranial parasternal "right atrium" view, in which the right atrium (RA) and a portion of the caudal vena cava running along the left ventricle (LV) are visible. *RV,* Right ventricle. B, Transducer position used to obtain a left cranial parasternal "aortic long axis" view. The transducer is placed at the level of the fifth intercostal space and rotated approximately 45 degrees from the position in part A. This allows one to obtain the left cranial parasternal "aortic long axis" view, in which the ascending aorta (AO) and the LV are visible. A portion of the right ventricular outflow tract (RVOT) is also visible. (Photo credit: Éric de Madron.)

Left Cranial Parasternal Projections

The transducer is moved cranially from the fifth intercostal space (Figures 1-9 and 1-10; see also Video 1-7). It is thus possible to see the right atrium with the cranial and/or caudal vena cava (see Figure 1-9, *A*), the descending aorta (see Figure 1-9, *B*), the right ventricular outflow tract, and the pulmonic valve (see Figure 1-10, *A*).

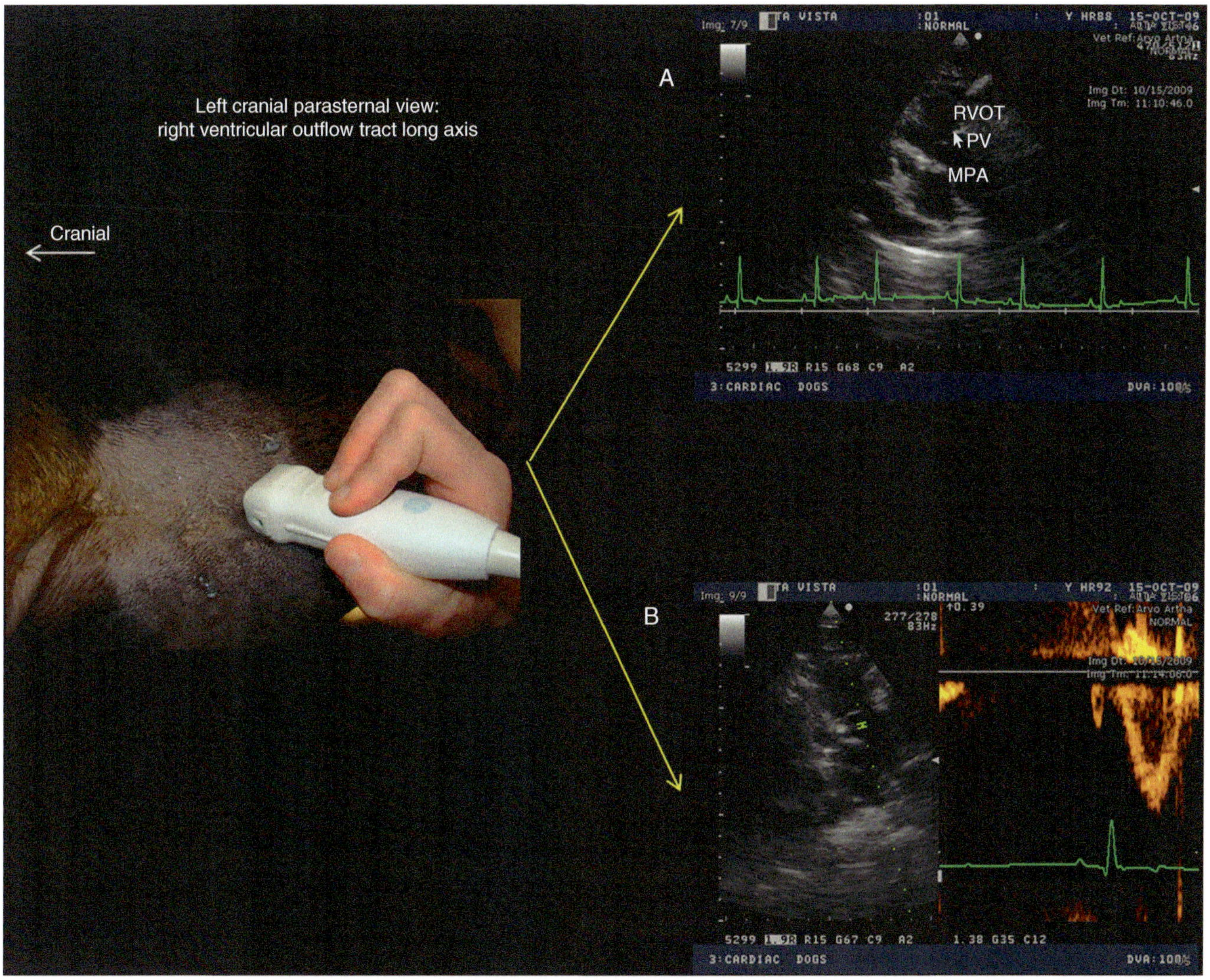

• **Fig. 1-10** Transducer position for obtaining a left cranial parasternal "right ventricular outflow tract" view. The transducer is placed at the level of the fifth intercostal space as shown in Figure 1-9, *A*, and inclined in such a manner as to be more parallel to the left thoracic wall. A, Bidimensional echocardiogram (left cranial parasternal "right ventricular outflow tract" view) displaying the right ventricular outflow tract (RVOT), the pulmonic valve (PV), and the main pulmonary artery (MPA). B, Pulsed spectral Doppler of the transpulmonic flow obtained by placing the recording zone within the pulmonic valve area on a left cranial parasternal "right ventricular outflow tract" view. (Photo credit: Éric de Madron.)

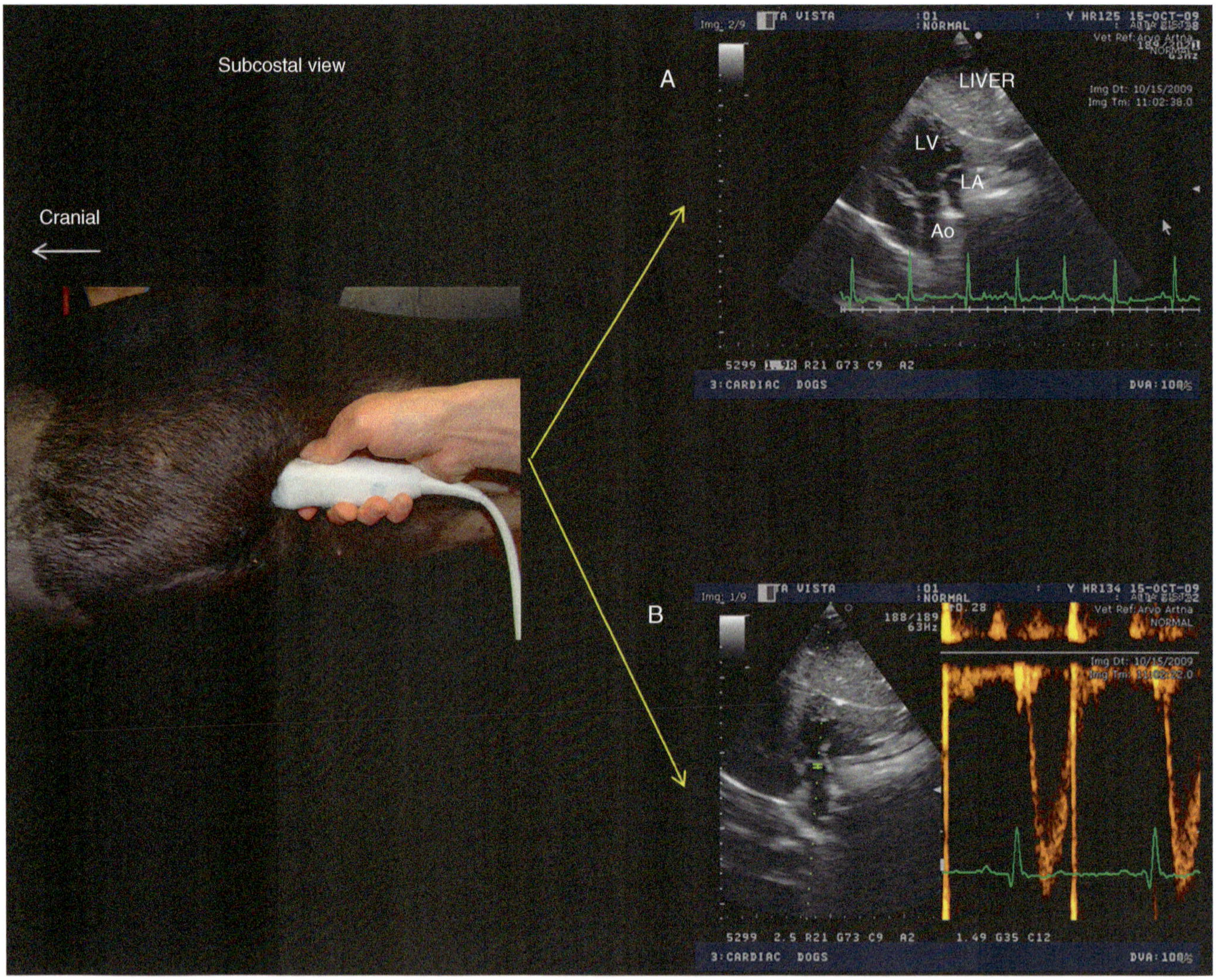

• **Fig. 1-11** Transducer position used to obtain a subcostal or subxiphoid view. The transducer is placed beneath the ribs, right above the xyphoid process. A, Bidimensional echocardiogram (subcostal view) displaying the left ventricle (LV) and the aorta (Ao) through the liver. *LA*, Left atrium. B, Pulsed wave spectral Doppler of the transaortic flow obtained by placing the recording zone within the aortic valve area on a subcostal view. (Photo credit: Éric de Madron.)

Subcostal (or Subxiphoid) Projection

It is possible to obtain a view similar to the left apical 5 chambers view previously described by placing the transducer just behind the ribs so that the ultrasound beam passes through the liver before reaching the heart (Figure 1-11).

Normal TM Views

TM mode is obtained by selecting a line crossing through the cardiac structures on a 2D image. Anatomic M-mode enables, still from the 2D image, one to change the point of origin and orientation of this line. It is used in practice to obtain a better alignment with cardiac structures when this is not possible with classic TM techniques. However, the resolution of the image obtained by anatomic M-mode is inferior to that of standard M-mode. TM projections are obtained using right parasternal long or short axis views.

Three projections are mainly used [2,13,14]. As a rule, using human echocardiography as an analogy, the motion of the structures moving away from the transducer is qualified as "posterior" whereas the motion of those moving toward it is qualified as "anterior."

Transventricular View

The beam transects the left ventricle at the level of the chordae tendineae of the mitral valve. It must intersect the interventricular septum right below its inflection point in order not to cross the left ventricular outflow tract (see Figure 1-2, *B*). In this view the septum and left ventricular free wall move toward each other in systole and away from each other in diastole. This synchronism between the two left ventricle walls is a criterion for good alignment with the left ventricular short axis. However, it must be noted that the amplitude of the septal movement is generally inferior to that of the free wall because the septum moves up toward the transducer prior to the end of systole, due to the displacement of the heart toward the thoracic wall at that time. A small septal posterior dip is also noted in early diastole, probably resulting from the slight desynchronization of the filling of the two ventricles. The ventricular filling resulting from the atrial contraction leads to an increased separation of the ventricular walls in end-diastole [2,15].

Transmitral View

The mitral valve leaflets are visible. Their separation during diastole varies: it reaches its maximum in early diastole (point E), then decreases in mid-diastole (point F), and once again increases during atrial contraction (point A). The two leaflets coapt during systole (segment CD). This segment has a positive slope due to the displacement of the mitral annulus in systole toward the transducer (see Figure 1-2, *C*).

In contrast with the previous view, the ventricular myocardium is thinner and the ventricular cavity is larger. The interventricular septal motion changes. It becomes posterior in diastole and anterior in systole due to the influence of the aortic motion. In moving toward the aorta, the continuity of the anterior mitral leaflets with the aortic wall becomes evident [2,14,15].

Transaortic View

Depending on its position, the beam can cross either the right ventricular inflow tract (visible tricuspid valve, looking like the mitral valve) or the right ventricular outflow tract. It then crosses the aortic root, which is displayed as two parallel lines moving anteriorly in systole and posteriorly in diastole. The noncoronary and left aortic cusps are joined in a line located in the middle third of the aortic root in diastole. They separate in systole, which gives them a boxlike appearance. The beam finally crosses the left atrium, generally at the level of the left atrial appendage. The lateral left atrial wall is animated by the same motion as the aortic root but much more attenuated (see Figure 1-3, *B*). In normal animals the diameters of these three zones (right ventricle, aorta, left atrium) are roughly equal [13,14].

Normal Spectral Doppler Examination

In normal humans as well as in normal cats and dogs, all blood flows are laminar, with a velocity <2 m/s (see Chapter 2). This allows them to be recorded with pulsed wave Doppler by setting the baseline so as to avoid any aliasing artifact [3-5].

Transmitral and Tricuspid Flows

The left apical 4 chambers view is the best view to record these atrioventricular flows. Using pulsed wave Doppler the sample volume is placed at the edge of the valvular funnel, at a place where valve noises are minimal and flow signal is optimal. Both atrioventricular flows are diastolic and characterized by two velocity peaks: a large early diastolic peak (E wave), corresponding to rapid ventricular filling, and a small peak (A wave) accompanying the atrial contraction (see Figure 1-6, *B*). The amplitudes of the transtricuspid flow wave velocities vary with respiration.

Transaortic and Transpulmonic Flows

The ventricular ejection flows are systolic. They move from the left and right ventricles toward the aorta and the main pulmonary artery, respectively. Their Doppler envelopes have a triangular shape. The transaortic flow is asymmetric whereas the transpulmonic flow has the shape of an isosceles triangle [16]. The transaortic flow is recorded from an apical 5 chambers view (see Figure 1-7, *B*) or a subcostal view (see Figure 1-11, *B*). In both cases the sample volume is located at the opening of the aortic cusps [17]. The subxiphoid projection allows a better alignment of the ultrasound beam with the blood flow. One can also obtain a good aortic flow Doppler from a right parasternal long axis view by placing the sample volume in the ascending aorta (see Figure 1-3, *C*) [17]. The transpulmonic flow (see Figure 1-5, *B*) is generally recorded using a right parasternal view (short axis transaortic view), the sample volume being located on the opening of the pulmonic valve. A better alignment is sometimes obtained by using a left cranial parasternal view (see Figure 1-10, *B*).

Pulmonary Venous Flow

The pulmonary venous flow can be obtained by placing the sample volume in the medial pulmonary vein, using the left apical 2, 4, and/or 5 chambers views. Three phases can be observed: the systolic phase associated with an anterograde flow (S or Sm wave), the early diastolic phase associated with an anterograde flow (D or Dm wave), and the end-diastolic phase with a retrograde flow (AR wave) (see Figure 1-6, *D*) [18,19].

Color Doppler

In a normal dog, no color mosaic indicating a turbulent flow should be found (Figures 1-12 to 1-14 and Videos 1-16 to 1-19). In cats it is possible to observe a turbulent flow in the right ventricular outflow tract in the absence of any cardiac anomaly [12,13].

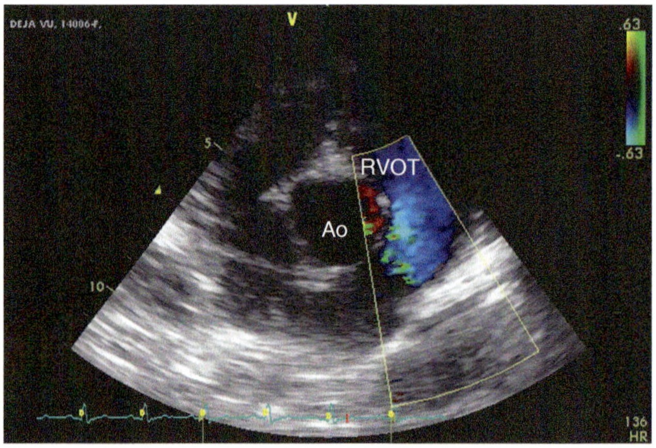

• **Fig. 1-13** Color Doppler echocardiogram of the right ventricular outflow tract showing the transpulmonic flow in systole traveling away from the transducer thus appearing in blue. *Ao,* Aorta; *RVOT,* right ventricular outflow tract. (Photo credit: Éric de Madron.)

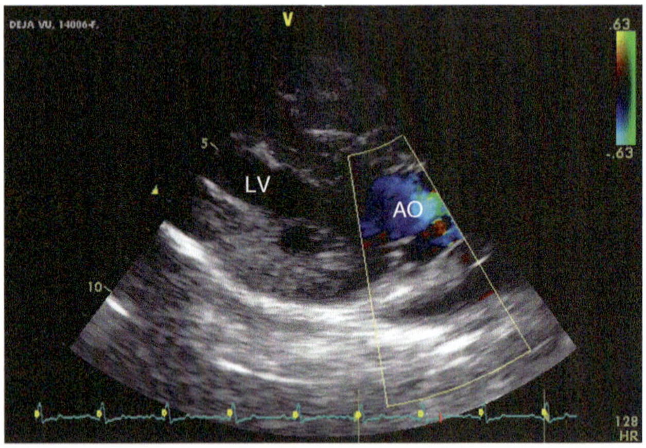

• **Fig. 1-12** Color Doppler echocardiogram (right parasternal long axis view, centered on the left ventricular outflow tract) displaying the transaortic ejection flow in systole. The flow is moving away from the transducer thus appearing in blue. *AO,* Aorta; *LV,* left ventricle. (Photo credit: Éric de Madron.)

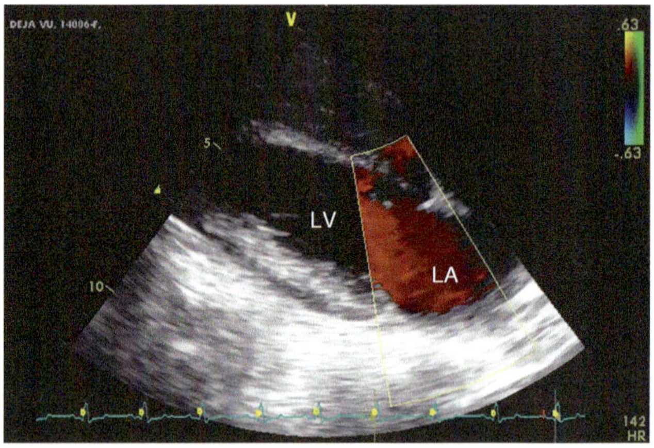

• **Fig. 1-14** Color Doppler echocardiogram (right parasternal long axis 4 chambers view) displaying the flow moving from the left atrium toward the left ventricle in diastole. The flow is moving toward the transducer thus appearing in red. The flow is laminar: no aliasing and no mosaic images are visible. *LA,* Left atrium; *LV,* left ventricle. (Photo credit: Éric de Madron.)

REFERENCES

[1] Mashiro I, Nelson RR, Cohn JN. Ventricular dimensions measured non-invasively by echocardiography in the awake dog. J Appl Physiol 1976;41:953–9.

[2] Feigenbaum H. Echocardiography. In: Baunwald E, editor. Heart disease. A Textbook of cardiovascular diseases. 4th ed. Philadelphia: WB Saunders; 1992, p. 84–115.

[3] Hatle L, Angelsen B. Doppler ultrasound in cardiology. Philadelphia: Lea & Febiger; 1985.

[4] Goldberg SJ, Allen HD, Marx GR, Finn CJ. Doppler echocardiography. Philadelphia: Lea & Febiger; 1985.

[5] De Madron E. Rôle de l'échocardiographie Doppler en mode continu et pulsé dans le diagnostic et l'évaluation de la sévérité des cardiopathies des petits animaux (1re et 2e parties). Prat Med Chir Anim Comp 1991;26:23–42.

[6] Kisslo J, Adams DB, Belkin RN. Doppler color flow imaging. New York: Churchill Livingstone; 1988.

[7] Miller RW, Bonagura JD. Doppler color flow imaging. In: Compte rendu du VIIth Annual Veterinary Medical Forum. San Diego: Calif.; 1989.

[8] Chetboul V, Tidholm A, Nicolle A, et al. Effects of animal position and number of repeated measurements on selected two-dimensional and M-mode echocardiographic variables in healthy dogs. J Am Vet Med Assoc 2005;227:743–7.

[9] Feigenbaum H. In: Echocardiography. 3rd ed. Philadelphia: Lea & Febiger; 1982, p. 1–45.

[10] Thomas WP. Two-dimensional, real time echocardiography in the dog: technique and anatomic validation. Vet Radiol 1984;25:50–64.

[11] Thomas WP, Gaber CE, Jacobs GJ, et al. Recommendations for standards in transthoracic two-dimensional echocardiography in the dog and cat. J Vet Intern Med 1994;7:247–52.

[12] De Madron E, Bonagura JD, Herring DS. Two-dimensional echocardiography in the normal cat. Vet Radiol 1985;26:149–58.

[13] Bonagura JD. M-mode echocardiography: basic principles, cardiopulmonary diagnostic techniques. Vet Clin North Am Small Anim Pract 1983;13:299–319.

[14] De Madron E. L'échocardiographie en mode M chez le chien normal. Maisons-Alfort, France: Thèse Doc Vét 1983.

[15] De Madron E, Bonagura JD, O'Grady MR. Normal and paradoxical septal motion in the dog: an echocardiographic study. Am J Vet Res 1985;46:1832–41.

[16] Brown DJ, Knight DH, King RR. Use of pulsed wave Doppler echocardiography to determine aortic and pulmonary velocity and flow variables in clinically normal dog. Am J Vet Res 1991;52:543–50.

[17] Riesen SC, Doherr MG, Lombard CW. Comparison of Doppler-derived aortic velocities obtained from various transducer sites in healthy dogs and cats. Vet Radiol Ultrasound 2007;48:570–3.

[18] Desai MY, Klein AL. Assessment of diastolic function by echocardiography. In: Otto CM, editor. The practice of clinical echocardiography. 3rd ed. Philadelphia: Saunders Elsevier; 2007, p. 237–61.

[19] Schober KE, Stern JA, DaCunha D.N.Q.T., et al. Estimation of left ventricular filling pressure by Doppler echocardiography in dogs with pacing-induced heart failure. J Vet Intern Med 2008;22:578–85.

2

Normal Echocardiographic Values: TM, 2D, and Doppler Spectral Modes

ÉRIC DE MADRON

Normal TM and 2D Mode Values, 22
Spectral Wave Doppler Normal Values, 32

The normal values for cardiac dimensions in dogs and cats have been the subject of many studies for the last two decades. Due to the considerable phenotypical differences characterizing the canine species, creating a universal model for normal values has remained a challenge for a long time. Recently, several publications have suggested new models that now meet this challenge. Moreover, attempts have finally been made to better evaluate the complex heart cavity anatomy by using not only linear dimensions, but also cross-sectional areas and volumes. Evaluation of ventricular volumes, as well as the systolic and diastolic functions indices, is discussed in Part 3.

Normal values of valvular and venous blood flow in spectral wave Doppler mode are presented in this chapter, along with several composite indices.

Normal TM and 2D Mode Values

Time-motion (TM) mode remains the cornerstone of echocardiography because it is the most accurate method for measuring wall thickness and endocavitary diameters. To achieve reliable measurements, the TM cursor should be perfectly perpendicular to the cardiac structures measured. Technical improvements have improved proper positioning of the cursor considerably. First, all current echocardiographic machines allow the selection of the TM cursor position directly on the bidimensional (2D) image. The most recent improvement is the anatomic TM mode (or "free angle"). This technique enables changing the point of origin and the direction of the TM cursor on the 2D image. It therefore provides better alignment with cardiac structures when standard TM mode is not possible. However, one has to be aware that the modification of the point of origin of the TM cursor will lead to substantial degradation of the resolution of the TM image.

The 2D mode can also be used to measure certain structures with complex geometry, such as the atria. This mode is also used to evaluate the base-to-apex length of the left ventricular cavity as well as cross-sectional areas of the left ventricle and atrium.

General Considerations

The Influence of Phenotype on Normal Values

The phenotype varies considerably from one breed to another in the canine species. Furthermore, weight itself is variable within a given breed. Initial studies demonstrate good correlations between echocardiographic variables and weight or body surface. These relations were either linear [1-3] or curvilinear [4]. However, confidence intervals were very broad, particularly at the extremities of curves. A study then demonstrated that the correlation equations between weight and a given dimension varied according to the breed [5]. This illustrates the difficulties in defining "normalcy" in a species characterized by great phenotypical variety.

Body characteristics are more uniform in the feline species. The echocardiographic normal values are therefore more homogeneous, although influences from breed, weight, and sex have been described (see below).

Allometric Approach

To resolve difficulties resulting from using curves based on weight or body surface area, Cornell et al [6] have recently suggested an allometric analysis of cardiac dimensions. By using dimensions obtained in 494 dogs of different breeds, they have shown that most of these variables were significantly correlated to a body mass index: aM^b, in which the factor *a* and exponent *b* vary according to the echocardiographic variable (see below). This method eliminates the need to use multiple breed-specific reference tables.

"Aortic Ratios" and "Weight Ratios"

Another quantitative method of TM values interpretation in dogs was recently suggested by Brown et al [7]. This method was based on the following principle in dogs, cats, and horses: the ratio between two dimensions, one variable and the other fixed (the typical example being the LA/AO ratio), eliminates the phenotype influence. Two techniques were proposed. The first used the aortic root dimension measured in TM mode (AO_m); this was called the "aortic ratio." The second used an estimate of the aortic root dimension, derived from the weight (AO_p), using the regression equation $AO_p = kW^{1/3}$, where *W* was the weight in kg and *k* was a specific constant in the breed ($k = 0.785$ in dogs and 0.567 in cats) [5]. This was called the "weight ratio." According to these authors, these ratios represent a major advance in quantifying echocardiography in TM mode, particularly in smaller breeds of dogs. These ratios also specify that "weight ratios" give better results than "aortic ratios" in dogs. However, these two ratios provide similar results in cats.

Criteria of the American Society of Echocardiography

TM and 2D measurements are carried out according to the criteria of the American Society of Echocardiography [8,9]. Each acoustic interface produces a line thickness variable. Different dimensions are measured from the leading edge of a given line (closest to the transducer) to the leading edge of the other line. This technique is highly reliable for measurements made in both TM and 2D modes [8-10].

As a rule, the structures nearest to the probe are referred to as anterior while those that are further from the probe are referred to as posterior.

Normal Values of the Left Ventricle

The left ventricle (LV) can be compared to a bullet, with a cylindrical base and a hemispheric apex. The linear dimensions discussed here will be mainly internal diameters and wall thicknesses at its base. The base-to-apex length will also be measured. The left ventricular cross-sectional area will also be used for volume calculation.

Views

The views used for the study of the LV are the right parasternal long axis 4 chambers view and right parasternal short axis transventricular view, at the level of the chordae tendineae.

Right Parasternal Long Axis 4 Chambers View

This view is used to take TM dimensions from the base of the LV and the base-to-apex length (Figure 2-1). For TM measurements, the TM cursor is positioned so as to cross the LV at the level of the chordae tendineae. It should transect the septum perpendicularly and caudal to the inflection point of the septum curve (see Figure 2-1), so as not to be in the left ventricular outflow tract.

Right Parasternal Short Axis Transventricular View, at the Level of the Chordae Tendineae

This view also may be used to take transversal TM measurements of the LV base. The TM cursor is positioned in such a way that it crosses the transversal diameter of the LV, perpendicular to the septum and at equal distance of the extremities of the two left ventricular papillary muscles (Figure 2-2). The left ventricular cross-sectional area can also be measured by planimetry in this view.

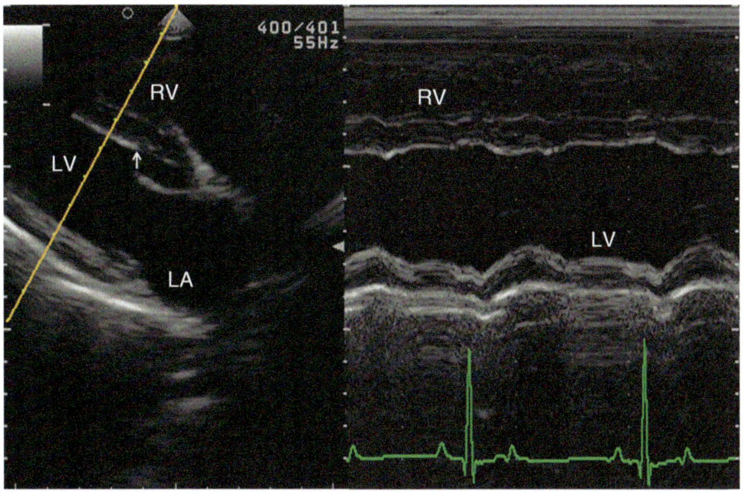

• **Fig. 2-1** Bidimensional echocardiogram (right parasternal long axis 4 chambers view) in a normal dog, showing how to position the TM cursor to take measurements of the right ventricle (RV) and the left ventricle (LV). The cursor should be perpendicular to the septum and to the LV free wall and caudal in relation to the inflection point of the curve of the septum *(arrow)*. Moreover, the walls of the LV (septum and free wall) should be as parallel as possible. *LA,* Left atrium. (Photo credit: Éric de Madron.)

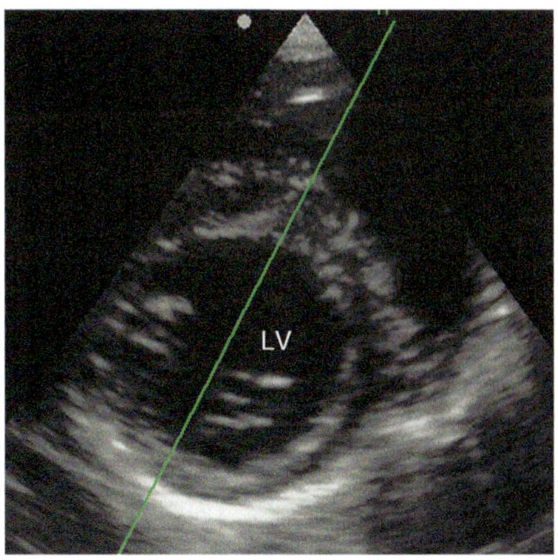

• **Fig. 2-2** Bidimensional echocardiogram (right parasternal short axis view, chordae tendineae level) illustrating how to position the TM cursor to measure ventricular dimensions. *LV,* Left ventricle. (Photo credit: Éric de Madron.)

Linear Dimensions

Measured Parameters

In TM mode, the septum and free wall of the LV move toward each other in systole and away from each other in diastole. This synchrony is a good criterion for adequate alignment between the TM cursor and the ventricular short axis. However, one must remember that the amplitude of septal movement is generally less than that of the free wall, because the septum moves anteriorly at end-systole due to the anterior movement of the heart against the thoracic wall at this precise moment [11]. Moreover, a small posterior dip in the septum is observed at the beginning of diastole because of a slight asynchrony in the filling of the two ventricles. The additional ventricular filling from atrial contraction leads to a discrete increase of the internal diameter of the LV at the end of diastole (Figure 2-3) [11,12].

The most frequently used parameters are the internal end-diastolic and end-systolic left ventricular diameters and the end-diastolic and end-systolic thicknesses of the septum and left ventricular free wall. Diastolic measures are taken at the level of the Q wave on the electrocardiogram (ECG), which corresponds to the maximum filling of ventricles after atrial contraction. Systolic measurements are taken close to the nadir of septum excursion [8]. It is important to note that, at this precise moment, the free wall is not at the end of its anterior excursion (see Figure 2-3) [11]. In case of abnormal septum movement, the end of the T wave on the ECG is a good reference for deciding where to take systolic measures.

Once the internal end-diastolic and end-systolic diameters of the LV have been measured, the percentage of shortening of this diameter in systole can be calculated (shortening fraction, or SF), an indice of systolic function. It is calculated as follows:

$$SF\% = (LVd - LVs)/LVs$$

where *LVd* and *LVs* are the internal end-diastolic and end-systolic left ventricular diameters, respectively. This parameter will be discussed in more depth in Chapter 7.

> **Importance of the Time-Motion (TM) Cursor Angulation Relative to the Ventricular Walls**
>
> A TM cursor transecting obliquely the ventricular walls will produce inaccurate measurements (Figure 2-4). The values of the internal diameters will be artificially increased, which may produce higher or lower shortening fractions.

Normal Values, Aortic and Weight Ratios

In Dogs. The normal theoretical TM values calculated according to the allometric equations of Cornell et al [6] are summarized in Table 2-1. The aortic and weight ratios in dogs [7] are summarized in Tables 2-2 and 2-3.

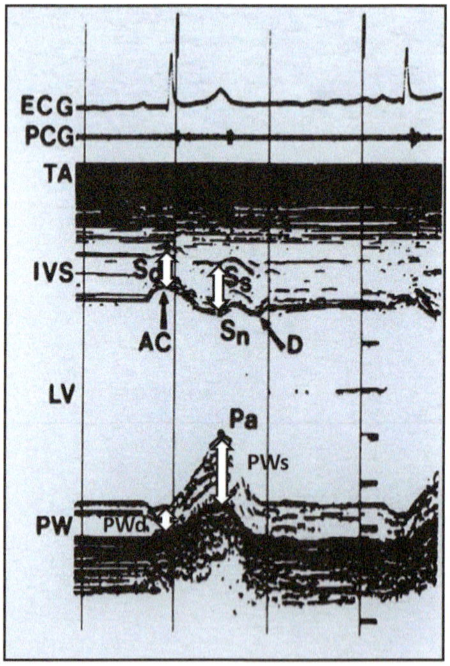

• **Fig. 2-3** Time-motion (TM) echocardiogram of the left ventricle (LV) detailing the characteristics of the interventricular septum (IVS) and the left ventricular posterior wall (PW) motions. The end-diastolic dimensions of these walls are measured at the level of the Q wave on the electrocardiogram (S_d and PWd). The septum reaches its most posterior excursion point (Sp) before the free wall has completed its anterior excursion (Pa). The systolic wall thickness (S_s and PWs) is measured at the S_p level for the septum and at Pa for the posterior wall [11]. *AC,* Atrial contraction; *D,* posterior movement ("dip") of the septum in end-systole; *ECG,* electrocardiogram; *PCG,* phonocardiogram; *TA,* transducer artifact. (Photo credit: Éric de Madron.)

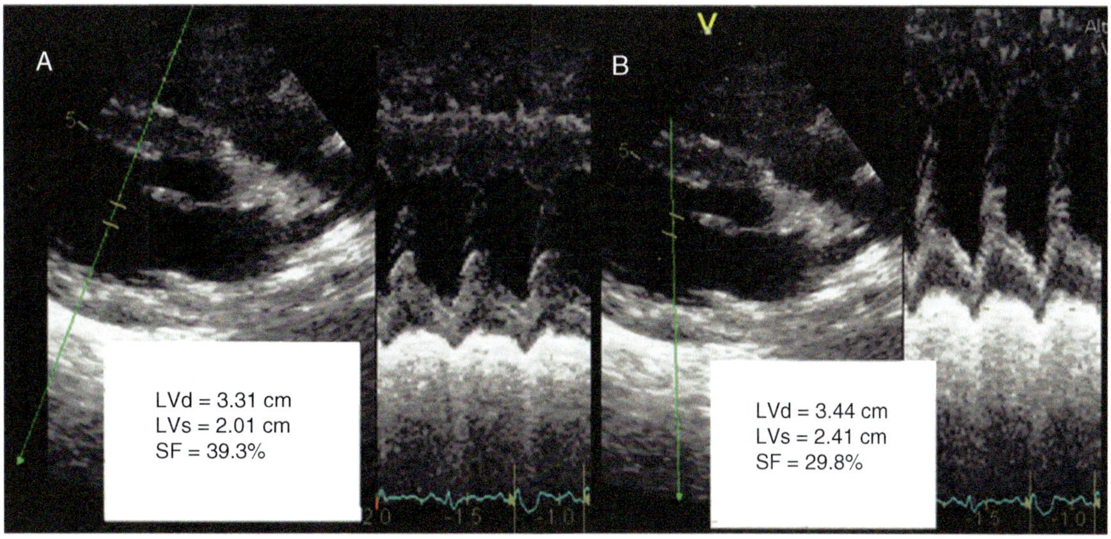

• **Fig. 2-4** Echocardiograms showing the effect of the angulation of the time-motion (TM) cursor on the measurements of the left ventricle. A, The position in this echocardiogram is correct. The TM cursor is completely perpendicular to the ventricular walls. B, The oblique position of the cursor in this echocardiogram results in increased values of the systolic and diastolic left ventricular diameters (LVs and LVd) and a decrease in the shortening fraction (SF). (Photo credit: Éric de Madron.)

TABLE 2-1 Theoretical Normal Allometric Time-Motion (TM) Values (Mean and Minimum-Maximum) in 494 Dogs of Varying Weight [6]

Weight (kg)	LVd (cm)	LVs (cm)	LVFWd (cm)	LVFWs (cm)	IVSd (cm)	IVSs (cm)	Ao (cm)	LA (cm)
$X = aM^b$	$1.53\ (W)^{0.294}$	$0.95\ (W)^{0.315}$	$0.42\ (W)^{0.232}$	$0.64\ (W)^{0.222}$	$0.41\ (W)^{0.241}$	$0.58\ (W)^{0.240}$	$0.78\ (W)^{0.341}$	$0.76\ (W)^{0.345}$
3	2.1 (1.8–2.6)	1.3 (1–1.8)	0.5 (0.4–0.8)	0.8 (0.6–1.1)	0.5 (0.4–0.8)	0.8 (0.6–1)	1.1 (0.9–1.4)	1.1 (0.9–1.4)
4	2.3 (1.9–2.8)	1.5 (1.1–1.9)	0.6 (0.4–0.8)	0.9 (0.7–1.2)	0.6 (0.4–0.8)	0.8 (0.6–1.1)	1.3 (1–1.5)	1.2 (1–1.6)
6	2.6 (2.2–3.1)	1.7 (1.2–2.2)	0.6 (0.4–0.9)	1 (0.7–1.3)	0.6 (0.4–0.9)	0.9 (0.7–1.2)	1.4 (1.2–1.8)	1.4 (1.1–1.8)
9	2.9 (2.4–3.4)	1.9 (1.4–2.5)	0.7 (0.5–1)	1 (0.8–1.4)	0.7 (0.7–1)	1 (0.8–1.4)	1.7 (1.3–2)	1.6 (1.3–2.1)
11	3.1 (2.6–3.7)	2 (1.5–2.7)	0.7 (0.5–1)	1.1 (0.8–1.5)	0.7 (0.5–1.1)	1 (0.8–1.4)	1.8 (1.4–2.2)	1.7 (1.3–2.2)
15	3.4 (2.8–4.1)	2.2 (1.7–3)	0.8 (0.5–1.1)	1.2 (0.9–1.6)	0.8 (0.6–1.1)	1.1 (0.8–1.5)	2 (1.6–2.4)	1.9 (1.6–2.5)
20	3.7 (3.1–4.5)	2.4 (1.8–3.2)	0.8 (0.6–1.2)	1.2 (0.9–1.7)	0.8 (0.6–1.2)	1.2 (0.9–1.6)	2.2 (1.7–2.7)	2.1 (1.7–2.7)
25	3.9 (3.3–4.2)	2.6 (2–3.5)	0.9 (0.6–1.3)	1.3 (1–1.8)	0.9 (0.6–1.3)	1.3 (0.9–1.7)	2.3 (1.9–2.9)	2.3 (1.8–2.9)
30	4.2 (3.5–5)	2.8 (2.1–3.7)	0.9 (0.6–1.3)	1.4 (1–1.9)	0.9 (0.6–1.3)	1.3 (1–1.8)	2.5 (2–3.1)	2.5 (1.9–3.1)
35	4.4 (3.6–5.3)	2.9 (2.2–3.9)	1 (0.7–1.4)	1.4 (1.1–1.9)	1 (0.7–1.4)	1.4 (1–1.9)	2.6 (2.1–3.2)	2.6 (2–3.3)
40	4.5 (3.8–5.5)	3 (2.3–4)	1 (0.7–1.4)	1.5 (1.1–2)	1 (0.7–1.4)	1.4 (1–1.9)	2.7 (2.2–3.4)	2.7 (2.1–3.5)
50	4.8 (4–5.8)	3.3 (2.4–4.3)	1 (0.7–1.5)	1.5 (1.1–2.1)	1.1 (0.7–1.5)	1.5 (1.1–2)	3 (2.4–3.6)	2.9 (2.3–3.7)
60	5.1 (4.2–6.2)	3.5 (2.6–4.6)	1.1 (0.7–1.6)	1.6 (1.2–2.2)	1.1 (0.8–1.6)	1.5 (1.1–2.1)	3.2 (2.5–3.9)	3.1 (2.4–4)
70	5.3 (4.4–6.5)	3.6 (2.7–4.8)	1.1 (0.8–1.6)	1.6 (1.2–2.2)	1.1 (0.8–1.6)	1.6 (1.2–2.2)	3.3 (2.7–4.1)	3.3 (2.6–4.2)

Ao, End-diastolic diameter of the aortic root; *IVSd,* end-diastolic thickness of the interventricular septum; *IVSs,* end-systolic thickness of the interventricular septum; *LA,* end-diastolic TM diameter of the left atrium; *LVd,* end-diastolic diameter of the left ventricle; *LVFWd,* end-diastolic thickness of the left ventricular free wall; *LVFWs,* end-systolic thickness of the left ventricular free wall; *LVs,* end-systolic diameter of the left ventricle; *W,* weight in kilograms.

TABLE 2-2 **Normal Aortic Time-Motion (TM) Ratios in Dogs and Cats using the Real Aortic Dimension (AO_m) [7]**

Parameter	Dogs (n = 53) Mean ± 2 Standard Deviations (Mean Value; Minimum-Maximum)	Cats (n = 32) Mean ± 2 Standard Deviations (Mean Value; Minimum-Maximum)
$IVSd/Ao_m$	0.44 ± 0.077 (0.42; 0.265–0.593)	0.496 ± 0.071 (0.492; 0.347–0.621)
LVd/Ao_m	1.608 ± 0.202 (1.603; 1.117–1.992)	1.589 ± 0.174 (1.615; 1.076–1.883)
$LVFWd/Ao_m$	0.413 ± 0.068 (0.405; 0.284–0.574)	0.489 ± 0.076 (0.5; 0.343–0.634)
$IVSs/Ao_m$	0.598 ± 0.101 (0.591; 0.407–0.831)	0.788 ± 0.105 (0.79; 0.571–1.022)
LVs/Ao_m	1.055 ± 0.171 (1.029; 0.56–1.385)	0.764 ± 0.127 (0.761; 0.495–1.103)
$LVFWd/AO_m$	0.615 ± 0.1 (0.606; 0.434–0.831)	0.813 ± 0.11 (0.838; 0.578–0.989)
LA/Ao_m	1.012 ± 0.139 (1.016; 0.696–1.271)	1.307 ± 0.142 (1.328; 1.036–1.563)
SF (%)	0.344 ± 0.065 (0.336; 0.253–0.499)	0.519 ± 0.063 (0.522; 0.399–0.643)

IVSd, End-diastolic thickness of the interventricular septum; *IVSs,* end-systolic thickness of the interventricular septum; *LA,* end-systolic TM diameter of the left atrium; *LVd,* end-diastolic diameter of the left ventricle; *LVFWd,* end-diastolic thickness of the left ventricular free wall; *LVFWs,* end-systolic thickness of the left ventricular free wall; *LVs,* end-systolic diameter of the left ventricle; *SF,* shortening fraction.

TABLE 2-3 **Normal Aortic Time-Motion (TM) Ratios in Dogs and Cats Obtained by Using the Theoretical Aortic Dimensions (Ao_p) Calculated from the Weight (kg) [7]**

Parameter	Dogs (n = 50) Mean ± 2 Standard Deviations (Mean Value; Minimum-Maximum)	Cats (n = 26) Mean ± 2 Standard Deviations (Mean Value; Minimum-Maximum)
Ao_p	$0.795\ P^{1/3}$	$0.567\ P^{1/3}$
$IVSd/Ao_p$	0.437 ± 0.063 (0.428; 0.279–0.576)	0.489 ± 0.54 (0.498; 0.377–0.591)
LVd/Ao_p	1.601 ± 0.183 (1.62; 1.275–1.946)	1.587 ± 0.179 (1.623; 1.216–1.966)
$PLVGd/Ao_p$	0.408 ± 0.058 (0.407; 0.293–0.574)	0.487 ± 0.068 (0.492; 0.345–0.64)
$IVSs/Ao_p$	0.596 ± 0.088 (0.595; 0.404–0.794)	0.778 ± 0.088 (0.764; 0.607–0.981)
LVs/Ao_p	1.048 ± 0.159 (1.046; 0.786–1.367)	0.773 ± 0.137 (0.781; 0.575–1.018)
$LVFWs/Ao_p$	0.607 ± 0.083 (0.619; 0.429–0.765)	0.813 ± 0.105 (0.82; 0.649–1.036)
LV/Ao_p	1.008 ± 0.107 (1.003; 0.764–1.267)	1.32 ± 0.135 (1.302; 1.144–1.572)
Ao_m/Ao_p	1.003 ± 0.116 (0.986; 0.81–1.433)	1 ± 0.093 (0.981; 0.855–1.194)

Ao_m, Measured end-diastolic diameter of the aorta; *IVSd,* end-diastolic thickness of the interventricular septum; *IVSs,* end-systolic thickness of the interventricular septum; *LA,* end-systolic TM diameter of the left atrium; *LVd,* end-diastolic diameter of the left ventricle; *LVFWd,* end-diastolic thickness of the left ventricular free wall; *LVFWs,* end-systolic thickness of the left ventricular free wall; *LVs,* end-systolic diameter of the left ventricle.

TABLE 2-4 Echocardiographic Time-Motion (TM) Values (Mean ± Standard Deviation) in Cats According to Several Authors

Variable	Jacobs et al [17] (n = 30)	Pipers et al [15] (n = 25)	Moise et al [20] (n = 11)	Soderberg et al [19] (n = 16)	Jacobs et al [18] (n = 30)	Chetboul et al [21] (n = 100)	Chetboul et al [21] (n = 51), breed: Maine coon
LVd (mm)	16 ± 2	15 ± 3	12 ± 2	13 ± 2	14 ± 1	15.9 ± 2.3 (breed, weight)	17.1 ± 1.8 (breed, weight)
LVs (mm)	8 ± 1	9 ± 2	7 ± 0.2	8 ± 1.5	8 ± 2	8.1 ± 1.8	8.8 ± 1.5
LVFWd (mm)	3 ± 1	4 ± 1	5 ± 0.5	3 ± 1	4 ± 0.5	4.3 ± 0.7 (breed, weight)	4.5 ± 0.6 (breed, weight)
IVSd (mm)	3 ± 0.5	4.5 ± 1	5 ± 1	ND	4 ± 1	4.6 ± 0.6 (breed, weight)	4.5 ± 0.7 (breed, weight)
IVSd sub-Ao (mm)	ND	ND	ND	ND	ND	4.1 ± 0.8 (sex)	4.1 ± 0.8 (sex)
LA (mm)	12 ± 1	7 ± 2	12 ± 2	10 ± 2	10 ± 1	ND	ND
Ao (mm)	10 ± 1	7.5 ± 2	10 ± 1.5	9 ± 1	10 ± 1	ND	ND
LA/Ao (TM)	1.3 ± 0.2	ND	1.3 ± 0.2	1.1 ± 0.3	1.1 ± 0.2	0.9 ± 0.1 (2D mode)	0.9 ± 0.1 (2D mode)
SF (%)	49.8 ± 5.3	41.0 ± 7.3	55.0 ± 10.2	34.5 ± 12.6	42.7 ± 8.1	49 ± 7	48 ± 5
HR (bpm)	194 ± 23	167 ± 29	182 ± 22	ND	255 ± 36	184 ± 33	183 ± 35
Weight (kg)	4.1 ± 1.1	4.7 ± 1.2	4.3 ± 0.5	ND	3.9 ± 1.2	4.6 ± 1.2	5.0 ± 1.2

Ao, End-diastolic diameter of the aortic root; *IVSd*, end-diastolic thickness of the interventricular septum; *IVSd sub-Ao*, end-diastolic thickness of the interventricular septum measured in 2D mode in the subaortic region; *HR*, heart rate; *LA*, end-systolic TM diameter of the left atrium; *LVd*, end-diastolic diameter of the left ventricle; *LVFWd*, end-diastolic thickness of the left ventricular free wall; *LVs*, end-systolic diameter of the left ventricle; *ND*, undetermined; *SF*, shortening fraction. Factors that significantly influence these variables ($p < 0.05$) are indicated between parentheses.

Boxers are a special case. Indeed, in this breed the septum and left ventricular free wall tend to be thicker than in other breeds [13]. This trait seems independent of the size of the aorta, velocity of aortic blood flow, and systemic arterial pressure.

In Cats. The normal LV values in cats [14-21] are presented in Table 2-4. Parameters such as the end-diastolic left ventricular internal diameter and the end-diastolic thickness of the left ventricular free wall are influenced by the weight or the breed [21]. This is why it is preferable to use aortic or weight ratios in cats, as in dogs (see Tables 2-2 and 2-3) [7].

Influence of Heart Rate

Besides weight and phenotype, a study showed that the cardiac cycle duration (the RR interval) also has an influence on TM mode measurement, especially on the left ventricular internal end-diastolic (Dd) and end-systolic (Ds) diameters [22]. The authors have suggested regression equations, using the square root of the cardiac cycle duration ($\sqrt{RR}$, *RR* being expressed in seconds) and the weight *W* in kg:

$$Dd = 4.16 + 1.06\,(W) + 18.35(\sqrt{RR})$$

$$Ds = -0.81 + 0.86\,(W) + 10.80(\sqrt{RR})$$

This means that a higher heart rate is associated with smaller internal diameters.

Influence of Hydration Level

The hydration level can have a strong influence on the left ventricular TM dimensions, especially in cats [23]. In fact, dehydration can induce a pseudohypertrophy of the walls of the LV and a quasi-obliteration of the left ventricular cavity in systole. Conversely, the administration of fluids intravenously can dilate the LV.

Length and Sphericity Index

The base-to-apex length (Figure 2-5) has been evaluated in normal dogs [24]. This parameter is rarely used as such but allows the calculation of the sphericity index (SI). This index is obtained by dividing the base-to-apex length by the maximum internal diameter of the LV (SI = L/D) (see Figure 2-5). A study in dogs weighing less than 15 kg established the normal value at 1.43 ± 0.12 [25].

Aorta and Left Atrium

The two atria have a complex geometry, which can be compared to a sphere to which is attached a cone: the atrial appendage. Multiple dimensions are necessary to correctly evaluate this type of structure. The aortic ratio is frequently used to describe the dimensions of the left atrium.

Views

Several views may be used to study the aorta and the left atrium (LA): the right parasternal long axis 5 and 4 chambers and the right parasternal short axis transaortic views.

Right Parasternal Long Axis 5 Chambers View

This view allows the measurements in TM mode of the end-diastolic aortic root and end-systolic left atrial diameters. The TM cursor is positioned so as to be perpendicular to the aorta at the level of its root. The portion of the LA crossed by the cursor is usually the atrial appendage (Figure 2-6).

Right Parasternal Long Axis 4 Chambers View

The TM cursor perpendicularly transects the center of the interatrial septum. This allows the measurement of the septolateral diameter of the LA (LAmax). This measurement is performed in end-systole (Figure 2-7).

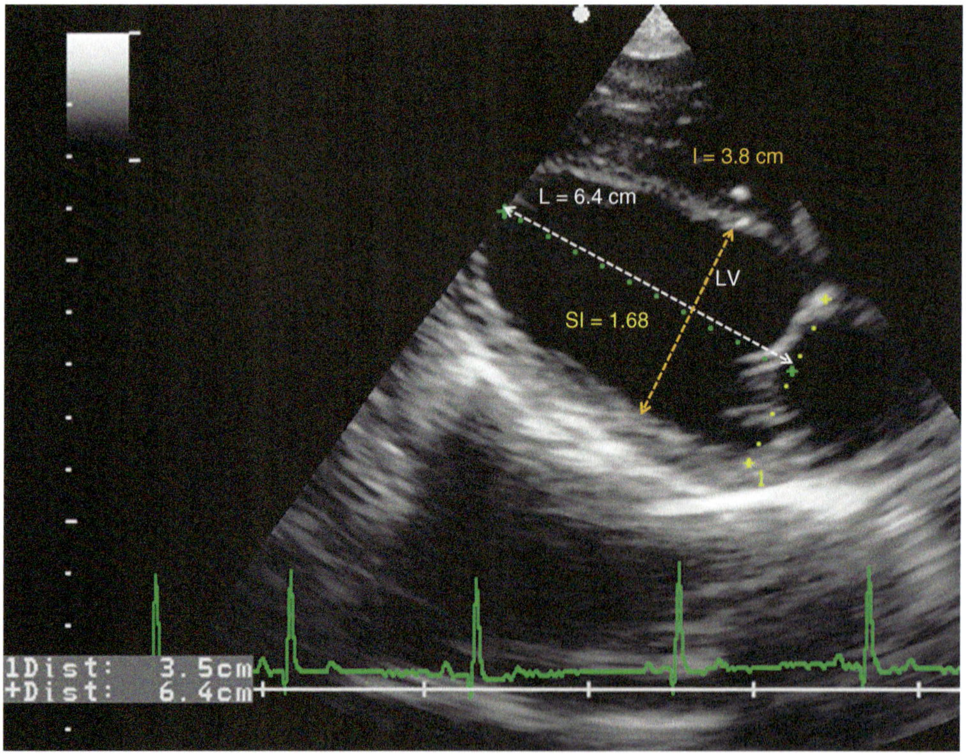

• **Fig. 2-5** Bidimensional echocardiogram (right parasternal long axis view) showing how to measure the length (L) of the left ventricle cavity (LV). By dividing the length *L* by the short axis diameter *l*, the sphericity index (SI) is obtained (in this case, 1.68). (Photo credit: Éric de Madron.)

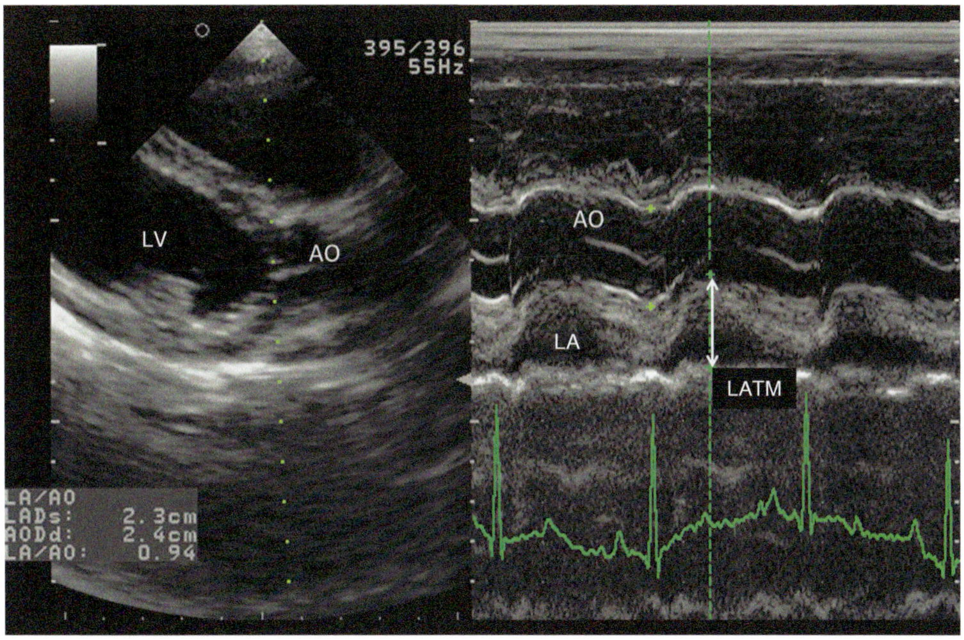

• **Fig. 2-6** Bidimensional echocardiogram (right parasternal long axis 5 chambers view) showing how the time-motion (TM) cursor is positioned to measure the diameter of the aortic root (AO) and the left atrium (LATM). The cursor transects the aorta perpendicularly, going through the point of apposition of the aortic cusps and then the left atrium, usually at the level of the left atrial appendage. On the TM image *(right),* the aortic root has an anterior movement in systole and a posterior movement in diastole. The opening of the cusps in systole has the appearance of a "box." *LA,* Left atrium; *LV,* left ventricle. (Photo credit: Éric de Madron.)

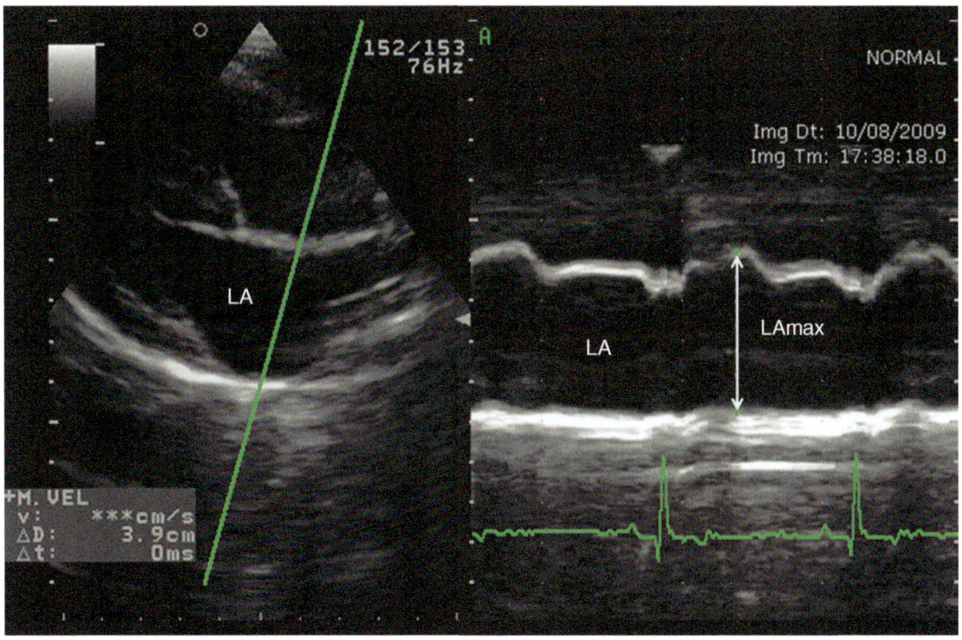

• **Fig. 2-7** Bidimensional echocardiogram (right parasternal long axis 4 chambers view) showing how to position the TM cursor to measure the septolateral diameter of the left atrium (LAmax). The time-motion (TM) cursor perpendicularly transects the interatrial septum and the lateral wall of the left atrium (LA) in their centers. The measurement of the septolateral atrial diameter is taken in end-systole. (Photo credit: Éric de Madron.)

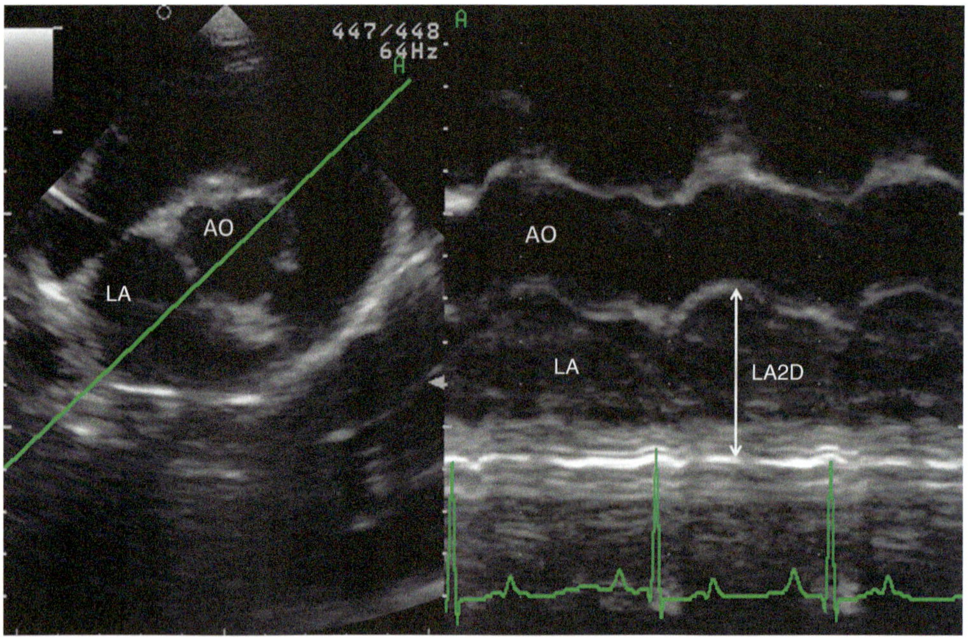

• **Fig. 2-8** Bidimensional echocardiogram (right parasternal short axis transaortic view) showing how to place the time-motion (TM) cursor (here in "free-angle" mode) to measure the aortolateral diameter (LA2D) of the left atrium (LA). This diameter will be greater than the one obtained using the right parasternal long axis view (see Figure 2-6). The aortolateral diameter measurement is done in early or end-diastole. *AO,* Aorta. (Photo credit: Éric de Madron.)

Right Parasternal Short Axis Transaortic View

This view allows the measurement of the aortolateral diameter of the spherical part of the LA as well as its cross-sectional area (Figure 2-8).

Normal Values

TM measurements taken using the right parasternal long axis 5 chambers view are the most reliable for measuring the diameter of the aortic root but tend to give left atrial appendage rather than left atrial dimensions. Therefore 2D echocardiography is now recommended to evaluate LA size in dogs [26,27] as well as in cats [21,28].

In dogs, four measurements of the LA have been evaluated:

- Bidimensional (or aortolateral) diameter (right parasternal short axis transaortic view) (LA2D): the first image following the closure of the aortic valve is selected. The internal diameter of the LA is the distance between the commissure separating the noncoronary and left coronary cusps, and the lateral wall of the LA (see Figure 2-8) [26]. Other authors have recommended taking this measurement in end-diastole rather than in early diastole because the contours are better defined and there is less risk of confusion with the nearby vascular structures, such as the right pulmonary artery or pulmonary veins [27].
- Maximum 2D or septolateral diameter (right parasternal long axis 4 chambers view) (LAmax): this is the maximum septolateral diameter of the LA, measured between the median section of the interatrial septum and the lateral wall of the LA in end-systole (see Figure 2-7) [26].
- Aortic and atrial circumferences (AoCirc and LACirc) (right parasternal short axis transaortic view): they are measured with the same view used for measuring LA2D (Figure 2-9) [26].
- Aortic and atrial areas (AoArea and LAArea) (right parasternal short axis transaortic view): these areas are measured at the same time as AoCirc and LACirc (see Figure 2-9) [26].

In cats, LA2D, AoCirc, LACirc, and AoArea are obtained in a similar fashion [21,28].

As for the LV, hydration can significantly modify the left atrial dimensions [23].

The normal values of these various measurements and ratios are presented in Tables 2-1 to 2-5.

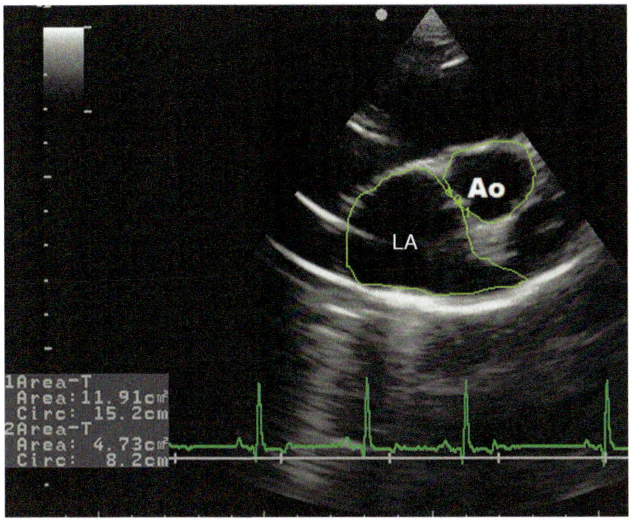

• **Fig. 2-9** Bidimensional echocardiogram (right parasternal short axis transaortic view) showing how to measure by planimetry the aortic and left atrial circumferences and areas (AoCirc, LACirc, AoArea, LAArea). Measurements are taken in early-diastole. *Ao,* Aorta; *LA,* left atrium. (Photo credit: Éric de Madron.)

TABLE 2-5 Normal Values of Different LA/Ao Ratios Obtained in Bidimensional Mode [21,26-28]

LA/Ao	Maximum Value in Normal Dogs [26] (n = 36)	Normal Value in Normal Dogs [27] Mean ± Standard Deviation (Minimum-Maximum) (n = 100)	Normal Value in Cats [28] Mean ± Standard Deviation (n = 17)	Normal Value in Cats [21] Mean ± Standard Deviation (Minimum-Maximum) (n = 100)
LA2D/Ao (early diastolic)	1.59		1.18 ± 0.11	
LA2D/Ao (end-diastolic)		0.9 ± 0.11 (0.52–1.13)		0.9 ± 0.1 (0.5–1.2)
LAmax/Ao (end-systolic)	2.04		ND	
LACirc/AoCirc (early diastolic)	2.45		1.82 ± 0.23	
LAArea/ AoArea (early diastolic)	3.85		2.36 ± 0.53	

Ao, Diameter of the aorta measured in 2D mode; *AoArea,* aortic area; *AoCirc,* aortic circumference; *LA,* left atrium; *LA2D,* aortolateral diameter of the left atrium measured in 2D mode; *LAArea,* left atrial area; *LACirc,* left atrial circumference; *LAmax,* maximum septolateral diameter of the left atrium; *ND,* undetermined.

Right Ventricle and Atrium

The geometry of the right ventricle is complex. Its cavity can be compared to a conical section enveloping the left ventricle. Its base is wide and its apex is straight. There is no easy way to measure such a structure. Only a few linear measurements of the anteroposterior diameter of the right ventricular base have been proposed.

There is no reference value for the right atrium. Its mediolateral or anteroposterior diameters are usually compared to those of the left atrium.

Views

Right Parasternal Long Axis 4 Chambers View

This view measures the diameter of the right ventricular base. The TM cursor position is the same as the one used to measure the LV (see Figure 2-1). The lateroseptal diameter of the right atrium (RA) also may be measured in this view.

Left Apical 4 Chambers View

This view measures the mediolateral diameter of the RA.

Normal Values

In dogs, the diastolic diameter of the base of the right ventricle (RV) has been correlated with weight [4,29]. Normal aortic ratios have been evaluated (see Tables 2-2 and 2-3). The ratio of the diastolic left and right ventricular internal diameters (LVd/RVd) has also been studied [29]. Correlation equations as well as the LVd/RVd ratio are reported in Table 2-6.

In cats, some publications mention the normal diastolic diameter of the RV as well as the systolic thickness of the right ventricular free wall (Table 2-7) [17,18,21]. Influences of weight, size, and sex have been shown in this species [21].

TABLE 2-6 Normal Dimensions and Indices of the Right Ventricle in Dogs Related to Weight (kg)

	De Madron [4] (n = 24)	Lombard et al [29] (n = 25)
RVd (mm)	4.93 $(W)^{0.391}$	0.087 (W) + 6.1
LVd/RVd	ND	3.82 ± 0.65

LVd/RVd, Ratio of the end-diastolic left and right ventricular diameters; *ND,* undetermined; *RVd,* end-diastolic diameter of the right ventricle; *W,* weight.

TABLE 2-7 Normal Values of the Right Ventricle in Cats According to Several Authors

	Jacobs et al [17] (n = 30)	Jacobs et al [18] (n = 30)	Chetboul et al [21] (n = 100), all Breeds	Chetboul et al [21] (n = 51), Breed: Maine Coon
RVd (mm)	6 ± 2	5 ± 2	3 ± 1.4 (breed, weight, and sex)	2.8 ± 1.2 (breed, weight, and sex)
RVWTs (mm)	ND	ND	2.7 ± 0.8	2.8 ± 0.9

ND, Undetermined; *RVd,* internal diameter of the right ventricle in diastole; *RVWTs,* right ventricular wall thickness in systole.
The factors that significantly influence these variables ($p < 0.05$) are indicated in parentheses.

Spectral Wave Doppler Normal Values

General Considerations

Alignment with Blood Flow

The Doppler velocities are proportional to the velocity of the blood flow and the cosine of the angle (referred to as θ) formed by the ultrasonic beam and the direction of the blood flow (see Chapter 1) [30,31]. To avoid underestimating true blood flow velocity, the θ angle should be as close as possible to 0 degrees. Consequently, the ultrasound beam should be as aligned as possible with the blood flow being studied.

The acoustic signal can be very useful since its audio signal helps the operator to improve the alignment. A better alignment will lead to greater audio signal intensity. When the direction of the beam and the blood flow become divergent, the intensity of the audio signal decreases.

Pressure Gradients and Stroke Volumes

Blood flow velocity measurements provide noninvasive quantification of pressure gradients between site 1 and site 2, using the modified Bernoulli equation:

$$P_1 - P_2 = 4 \times \left(V_2^2 - V_1^2\right)$$

where P_1 and P_2 (in mm Hg) represent the pressures and V_1 and V_2 (in m/s) represent the blood velocities in sites 1 and 2, respectively. In practice, [30,31] V_1 can be considered negligible when compared to V_2 and the equation can be simplified as follows:

$$P_1 - P_2 = 4 \times V_2^2$$

The Doppler examination also allows the calculation of the stroke volumes through valves and orifices. These are obtained by measuring the area under the curve of the spectral Doppler envelope (velocity-time integral, or VTI) of the transvalvular or transorifice flow and then multiplying it by the valvular or orifice area.

Laminar or Turbulent Flow

The spectral Doppler signal will display the relative prevalence of the velocity of red blood cells in the sample volume. With a normal transvalvular flow, the majority of these cells transit in the same direction, at the same speed. Therefore dispersion of spectral velocities is minimal and the flow is then qualified as laminar (Figure 2-10). In the opposite situation—as in the case of valvular regurgitation or stenosis, for instance—the red blood cells are propelled in various directions at different speeds due to turbulences, which creates a spectral dispersion. These abnormal flows are called turbulent [30,31].

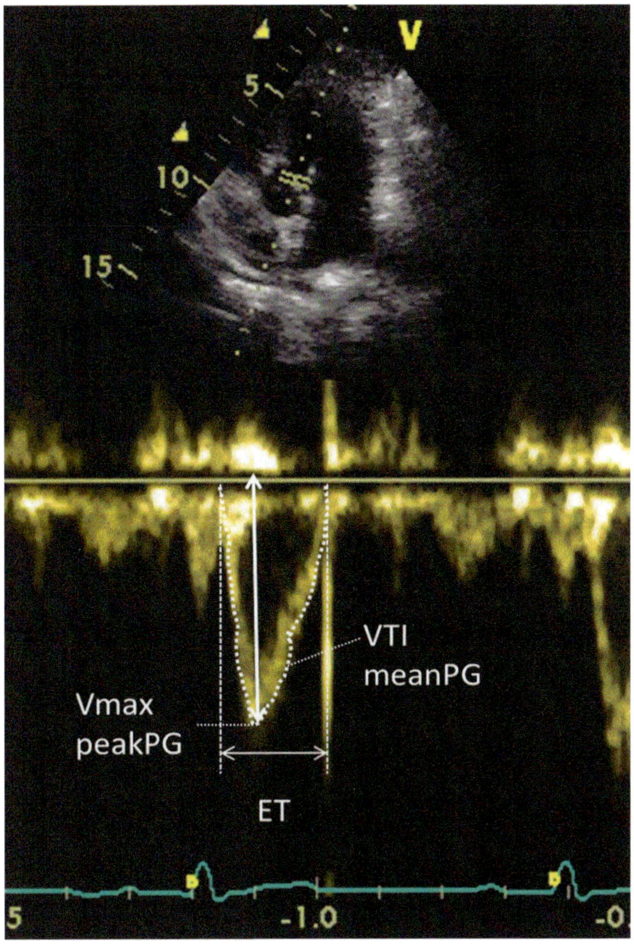

• **Fig. 2-10** Spectral pulsed wave Doppler of the transaortic blood flow obtained from a left apical 5 chambers view by placing the sample volume at the level of the aortic valve. Note the asymmetry of the flow with a short acceleration time. Measurements include the maximal flow velocity (Vmax); the maximal (peak) pressure gradient (peakPG); the area under the curve, or the velocity-time integral (VTI), allowing the calculation of the mean pressure gradient (meanPG); and ejection time (ET). (Photo credit: Éric de Madron.)

In humans, as in normal dogs and cats, all of the intracardiac blood flows are laminar and usually have velocities <2.2m/s [27,30-36]. This allows one to record them in pulsed wave Doppler mode, with baseline adjustments to avoid artifact aliasing [30,31].

Valvular Flow

Views and Techniques

Aortic and Pulmonic Flows

The aortic flow can be obtained from several views (see Chapter 1). The most commonly used views are the left apical 5 chambers and subxiphoid (subcostal) views [32,35]. The latter often provides better alignment between the ultrasound beam and the aortic flow. It is also possible to make a good recording of the aortic blood flow from a right parasternal long axis 5 chambers view by placing the sample volume in the ascending aorta so as to obtain the best alignment between the ultrasound beam and the blood flow [32,35].

The pulmonic flow is generally recorded from the right parasternal short axis transaortic view [32]. Sometimes a better alignment with the pulmonic flow is obtained by using a left cranial parasternal view (see Chapter 1).

Tricuspid and Mitral Flows

The left apical 4 chambers view is best for recording these atrioventricular flows. In spectral Doppler mode, the sample volume is placed at the end of the valvular funnel so as to minimize valvular noise and optimize the recording of blood flow.

Normal Values and Measurements

For the aortic and pulmonic flows, measurements usually include the maximal systolic velocity and peak pressure gradient, the mean systolic velocity and gradient, the velocity-time integral, the ejection time, and the acceleration time/ejection time ratio (AT/ET). The aortic flow (see Figure 2-10) is typically asymmetric, with an AT/ET lower than 0.3 [33]. The pulmonic flow (Figure 2-11) has a more symmetric shape, with an AT/ET greater than 0.43 [33].

The measurements on the diastolic transmitral and transtricuspid flows include the maximum velocities of the E and A waves, E/A ratio, deceleration time and deceleration slope of the E wave, and the duration of the E and A waves (Figure 2-12).

The normal velocities and durations of the transvalvular flows in dogs [27,32-35] and cats [21,36] are presented in Tables 2-8 and 2-9.

Maximum Velocity and Normal Flow

In certain young, active dogs the maximum velocity of the aortic blood flow can sometimes reach 2.5 m/s. However, the flow remains laminar, which is a fundamental difference from the turbulent flow seen with aortic stenosis. Therefore it is important to take into account both the maximum velocity and the laminar or nonlaminar behavior of a flow before calling it normal or abnormal.

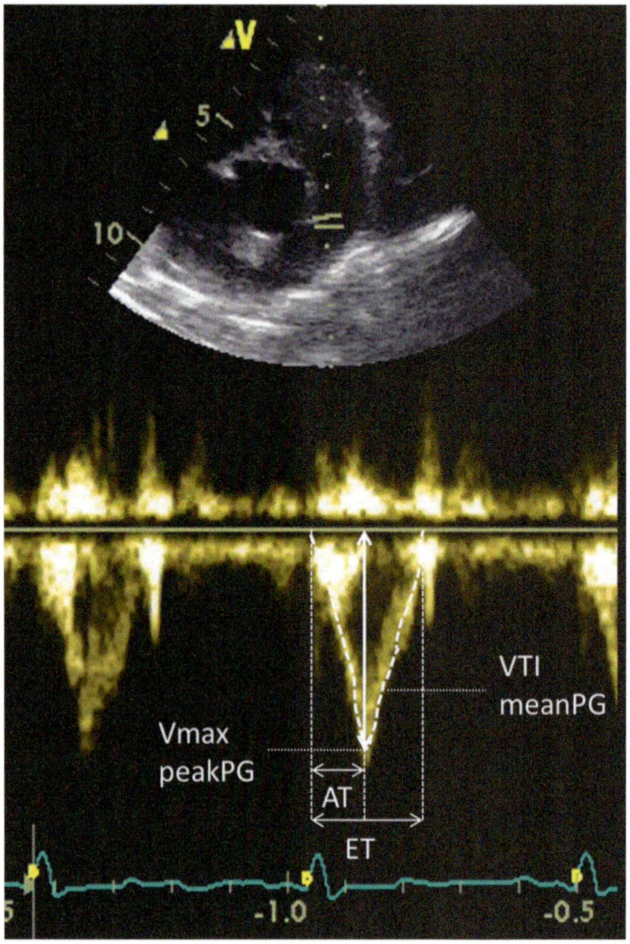

• **Fig. 2-11** Spectral pulsed wave Doppler of the transpulmonic flow obtained from the right parasternal short axis transaortic view. Note that the pulmonic flow is more symmetric than the aortic flow. Measurements include maximal velocity (Vmax); maximal pressure gradient (peakPG); the area under the curve, or velocity-time integral (TVI), allowing the calculation of the mean pressure gradient (meanPG); and the ejection (ET) and acceleration (AT) times, from which the AT/ET ratio is derived. (Photo credit: Éric de Madron.)

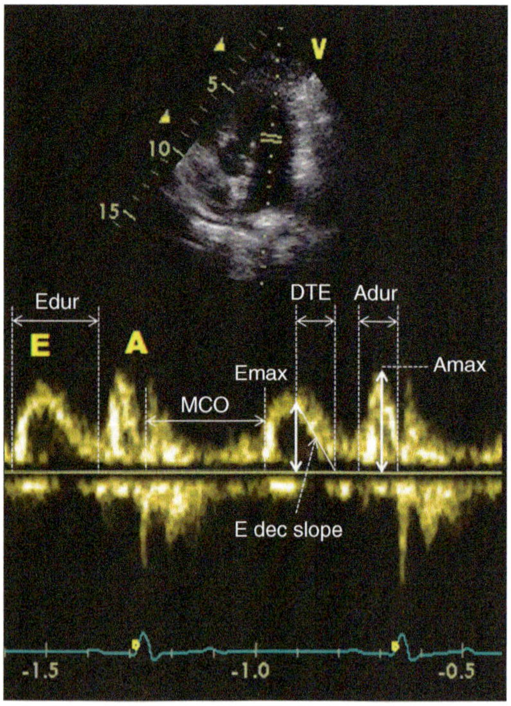

• **Fig. 2-12** Diastolic transmitral blood flow in normal dogs. Measurements include the maximum E and A wave velocities (Emax, Amax) and the E/A ratio, the deceleration time of the E wave (DTE) as well as its slope (E dec slope), and the duration of the E and A waves (Edur, Adur). The time interval between the closure (end of A wave) and the opening of the mitral valve (beginning of E wave) is also measured (MCO). (Photo credit: Éric de Madron.)

TABLE 2-8 **Normal Intracardiac Flow Velocities in Dogs According to Different Authors**

Flow Studied	Maximum Velocity [27] Mean ± Standard Deviation (Minimum-Maximum) (n = 100)	Maximum Velocity [32] Mean ± Standard Deviation (Minimum-Maximum) (n = 50)
Aortic flow (m/s)	1.29 ± 0.22 (0.92–1.88)	1.57 ± 3.3 (1.0–2.29)
Pulmonary flow (m/s)	1.05 ± 0.19 (0.50–1.50)	1.20 ± 2.0 (0.88–1.61)
Mitral E wave (m/s)	0.87 ± 0.13 (0.58–1.17)	0.91 ± 0.15 (0.59–1.18)
Mitral A wave (m/s)	0.61 ± 0.12 (0.39–0.86)	0.63 ± 0.13 (0.33–0.93)
Mitral E/A ratio	1.46 ± 0.35 (0.92–2.72)	1.48 ± 0.31 (1.04–2.42)
Tricuspid E wave (m/s)	0.72 ± 0.11 (0.50–0.98)	0.86 ± 0.2 (0.49–1.31)
Tricuspid A wave (m/s)	0.43 ± 0.09 (0.29–0.70)	0.58 ± 0.163 (0.32–0.94)
Tricuspid E/A ratio	1.75 ± 0.34 (1.09–2.80)	1.60 ± 0.56 (0.69–3.08)

Pulmonary Venous Flow

Views

The pulmonary venous flow can be obtained by placing the sample volume in the pulmonary medial vein, from a left apical 2, 4, or 5 chambers view (see Chapter 1).

Normal Values

The main measurements include the maximum velocities of the Sm, Dm, and AR waves, the Sm/Dm ratio, and the duration of the AR wave (ARdur) (Figure 2-13) [36-41]. The systolic fraction (area under the curve of the Sm wave/sum of the areas under the curve of the Sm, Dm, and AR waves) has also been reported [36]. It is important to note that these values are influenced by the age of the dogs [41] (see Chapter 8). Of note, Doberman Pinschers seem to have values specific to their breed.

Normal velocities and durations of pulmonary venous flow are presented in Table 2-10.

TABLE 2-9 Normal Velocities (Mean ± Standard Deviation) of the Intracardiac Flows in Cats [21]

Flow Studied	All Breeds Included (n = 100)	Maine Coon Cats (n = 51)	European Cats (n = 31)
Aortic flow (m/s)	1.1 ± 0.2	1.1 ± 0.2	1.1 ± 0.2
Pulmonary flow (m/s)	0.9 ± 0.2	1.0 ± 0.2	0.8 ± 0.2
Mitral E wave (m/s)	0.7 ± 0.1	0.7 ± 0.1	0.7 ± 0.1
Mitral A wave (m/s)	0.5 ± 0.1	0.5 ± 0.1	0.5 ± 0.1
E/A ratio	1.5 ± 0.3	1.5 ± 0.4	1.4 ± 0.3
Fused E and A waves (m/s)	0.9 ± 0.1	0.8 ± 0.1	1.0 ± 0.1

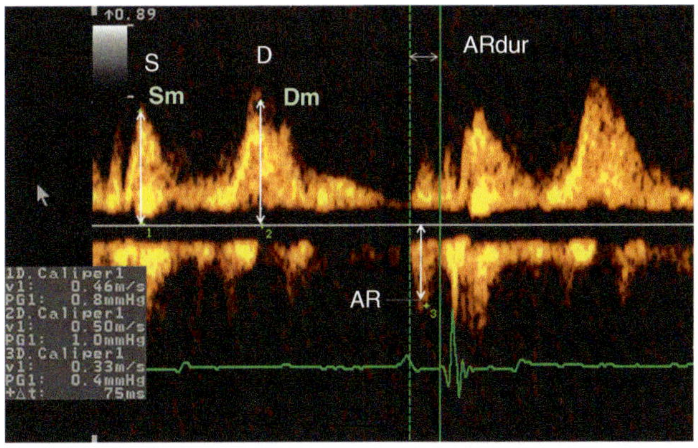

• **Fig. 2-13** Pulmonary venous flow in a normal dog. Three waves are visible: the systolic wave (S), the diastolic wave (D), and the retrograde end-diastolic flow (AR). Maximum velocities of the S (Sm), D (Dm) and AR waves, as well as the AR wave duration (ARdur) are measured. (Photo credit: Éric de Madron.)

TABLE 2-10 Normal Values of Pulmonary Venous Blood Flow in Dogs and Cats According to Multiple Authors

Variable	Dogs (6–10 Years) [41] (n = 11) (Mean 10th–90th Percentiles)	Doberman [37] (n = 10) (Mean ± Standard Deviation)	Cats [40] (n = 87) (Mean ± Standard Deviation)	Cats [36] (n = 20) (Mean ± Standard Deviation)
Sm max (m/s)	0.34 (0.24–0.70)	0.506 ± 0.059	0.48 ± 0.14	0.39 ± 0.12
Dm max (m/s)	0.50 (0.36–0.75)	0.494 ± 0.042	0.47 ± 0.10	0.44 ± 0.09
Sm/Dm	0.79 (0.47–1.12)	1.0 ± 0.1	ND	0.90 ± 0.29
AR max (m/s)	0.24 (0.19–0.30)	0.278 ± 0.044	0.23 ± 0.06	0.22 ± 0.07
ARdur (ms)	67 (57–80)	58 ± 9	53.5 ± 10.3	ND
Systolic fraction (%)	ND	ND	ND	62.55 ± 11.54

ARdur, Duration of the AR wave of the pulmonary venous flow; *AR max,* maximum velocity of the AR wave of the pulmonary venous flow; *Dm max,* maximum velocity of the Dm wave of the pulmonary venous flow; *ND,* undetermined; *Sm max,* maximum velocity of the Sm wave of the pulmonary venous flow.

REFERENCES

[1] Mashiro I, Nelson RR, Cohn JN. Ventricular dimensions measured non-invasively by echocardiography in the awake dog. J Appl Physiol 1976;41:953–9.

[2] Boon J, Wingfield WE, Miller CW. Echocardiographic indices in the normal dog. Vet Radiol 1983;24:214–21.

[3] Lombard CW. Normal values of the canine M-mode echocardiogram. Am J Vet Res 1984;45:2015–8.

[4] De Madron E. L'échocardiographie en mode M chez le chien normal. Thèse Doc Vét, Maisons-Alfort, France; 1983.

[5] Morrison SA, Moise NS, Scarlett J, et al. Effect of breed and body weight on echocardiographic values in four breeds of dogs of different somatotype. J Vet Intern Med 1992;6:220–4.

[6] Cornell CC, Kittleson MD, Della Torre P, et al. Allometric scaling of M-mode cardiac measurements in normal adult dogs. J Vet Intern Med 2004;18:1–311.

[7] Brown DJ, Rush JE, Mac Gregor J, et al. M-mode echocardiographic ratio indices in normal dogs, cats, and horses: a novel quantitative method. J Vet Intern Med 2003;17:2–653.

[8] Sahn DJ, DeMaria A, Kisslo J, Weyman A. Recommendations regarding quantitation in M-mode echocardiography: results of a survey of echocardiographic measurements. Circulation 1980;58:1072–83.

[9] Henry WL, DeMaria A, Gramiak R, et al. Report of the American Society of Echocardiography Committee on nomenclature and standards in two-dimensional echocardiography. Circulation 1980;62:212–7.

[10] Wyatt HL, Hoendchen RV, Meerbaum S, Corday E. Assessment of quantitative methods for two-dimensional echocardiography. Am J Cardiol 1983;52:396–401.

[11] De Madron E, Bonagura JD, O'Grady MR. Normal and paradoxical septal motion in the dog: an echocardiographic study. Am J Vet Res 1985;46:1832–41.

[12] Feigenbaum H. Echocardiography. In: Baunwald E, editor. Heart disease. A Textbook of cardiovascular diseases. 4th ed. Philadelphia: WB Saunders; 1992, p. 84–115.

[13] Cunningham SM, Rush JE, Freeman LM, et al. Echocardiographic ratio indices in overtly healthy boxer dogs screened for heart disease. J Vet Intern Med 2008;22:924–30.

[14] Moise NS. Echocardiography. In: Fox PR, Sisson D, Moïse NS, editors. Canine and feline cardiology. New York: Churchill Livingstone; 1988, p. 113–56.

[15] Pipers FS, Hamlin RL. Clinical use of echocardiography in the domestic cat. J Am Vet Med Assoc 1980;176:57–61.

[16] Fox PR, Bond BR, Peterson ME. Echocardiographic reference values in healthy cats sedated with ketamine hydrochloride. Am J Vet Res 1985;46:1479–84.

[17] Jacobs G, Knight DH. M-mode echocardiographic measurements in non-anesthetized healthy cats: effects of body weight, heart rate, and other variables. Am J Vet Res 1985;46:1705–11.

[18] Jacobs G, Knight DH. Change in M-mode echocardiography in cats given ketamine. Am J Vet Res 1985;46:1712–3.

[19] Soderberg SF, Boon JA, Wingfield WE, Miller CW. M-mode echocardiography as a diagnostic aid for feline cardiomyopathy. Vet Radiol 1983;24:66–73.

[20] Moise NS, Dietze AE, Mezza LE, et al. Echocardiography, electrocardiography, and radiography in cats with dilatation cardiomyopathy, hypertrophic cardiomyopathy, and hyperthyroidism. Am J Vet Res 1986;47:1476–86.

[21] Chetboul V, Carlos Sampedrano C, Tissier R, et al. Quantitative assessment of velocities of the annulus of the left atrio-ventricular valve and left ventricular free wall in healthy cats by use of two-dimensional color tissue Doppler imaging. Am J Vet Res 2006;67:250–8.

[22] Jacobs G, Mahjoob K. Multiple regression analysis, using body size and cardiac cycle length, in predicting echocardiographic variables in dogs. Am J Vet Res 1988;49:1290–4.

[23] Campbell FE, Kittleson MD. The effect of hydration status on the echocardiographic measurements of normal cats. J Vet Intern Med 2007;21:1008–15.

[24] O'Grady MR, Bonagura JD, Powers JD, Herring DS. Quantitative cross-sectional echocardiography in the normal dog. Vet Radiol 1986;27:34–49.

[25] Serres F, Chetboul V, Tissier R, et al. Comparison of 3 ultrasound methods for quantifying left ventricular systolic function: correlation with disease severity and prognostic value in dogs with mitral valve disease. J Vet Intern Med 2008;22:566–77.

[26] Rishniw M, Erb HN. Evaluation of four 2-dimensional echocardiographic methods of assessing left atrial size in dogs. J Vet Intern Med 2000;14:429–35.

[27] Chetboul V, Carlos Sampedrano C, Concordet D, et al. Use of quantitative two-dimensional color tissue Doppler imaging for assessment of left ventricular radial and longitudinal myocardial velocities in dogs. Am J Vet Res 2005;66:953–61.

[28] Abbott JA, McLean HN. Two-dimensional echocardiographic assessment of the feline left atrium. J Vet Intern Med 2006;20:111–9.

[29] Lombard CW, Ackerman N. Right heart enlargement in heartworm-infected dogs: a radiographic, electrocardiographic, and echocardiographic correlation. Vet Radiol 1984;25:210–27.

[30] Hatle L, Angelsen B. Doppler ultrasound in cardiology. Philadelphia: Lea & Febiger; 1985.

[31] Goldberg SJ, Allen HD, Marx GR, Finn CJ. Doppler echocardiography. Philadelphia: Lea & Febiger; 1985.
[32] Kirberger RM, Bland-van der Berg P, Darazs B. Doppler echocardiography in the normal dog. Part I. Velocity finding and flow patterns. Vet Radiol Ultrasound 1992;33:370–9.
[33] Kirberger RM, Bland-van der Berg P, Grimbeek RJ. Doppler echocardiography in the normal dog. Part II. Factors influencing blood flow velocities and a comparison between left and right heart blood flow. Vet Radiol Ultrasound 1992;33:380–6.
[34] Brown DJ, Knight DH, King RR. Use of pulsed-wave Doppler echocardiography to determine aortic and pulmonary velocity and flow variables in clinically normal dog. Am J Vet Res 1991;52:543–50.
[35] Riesen SC, Doherr MG, Lombard CW. Comparison of Doppler-derived aortic velocities obtained from various transducer sites in healthy dogs and cats. Vet Radiol Ultrasound 2007;48:570–3.
[36] Santilli RA, Bussadori C. Doppler echocardiographic study of the left ventricular diastole in non-anesthetized healthy cats. Vet J 1998;156:203–15.
[37] O'Sullivan ML, O'Grady MR, Minors SL. Assessment of diastolic function by Doppler echocardiography in normal Doberman Pinschers and Doberman Pinschers with dilated cardiomyopathy. J Vet Intern Med 2007;21:81–91.
[38] Desai MY, Klein AL. Assessment of diastolic function by echocardiography. In: Otto CM, editor. The practice of clinical echocardiography. 3rd ed. Philadelphia: Saunders Elsevier; 2007, p. 237–61.
[39] Schober KE, Stern JA, DaCunha DNQT, et al. Estimation of left ventricular filling pressure by Doppler echocardiography in dogs with pacing-induced heart failure. J Vet Intern Med 2008;22:578–85.
[40] Disatian S, Bright JM, Boon J. Association of age and heart rate with pulsed-wave Doppler measurements in healthy, nonsedated cats. J Vet Intern Med 2008;22:351–6.
[41] Schober KE, Luis Fuentes V. Effects of age, body weight, and heart rate on transmitral and pulmonary venous flow in clinically normal dogs. Am J Vet Res 2001;62:1447–54.

3

Intra- and Interoperator Variability

VALÉRIE CHETBOUL

Repeatability, Reproducibility, and Operators, 40
Operator's Effect on the Variability of Echocardiographic Measurements, 40
Practical Consequences, 41
Conclusion, 43

Echocardiography is an ultrasound technique that allows quantitative analysis of cardiac morphology and kinetics. Used in practice for diagnostic purposes, this imaging tool is also used effectively in longitudinal tracking of heart disease. This facilitates the study of regression, stability, or aggravation of lesions evaluated by different quantitative variables at the time of diagnosis. Clinical, pharmacologic, or dietetic trials may even use repeated echocardiographic measurements over a specific period (varying from a few weeks to a year) in order to detect differences after initiation of a specific treatment or diet [1-7]. A prerequisite to this practice of repeated use of echocardiography is to have the knowledge of the metrologic characteristics of this technique. This is critical to research, according to the *Guideline on Statistical Principles for Veterinary Clinical Trials*, published by the European Medicines Agency (EMA) [8]. It clearly stipulates that variables used as "primary endpoints" in a clinical trial must be validated beforehand.

Repeatability, Reproducibility, and Operators

Definitions

The use of echocardiography for follow-ups (whether in a clinical or research capacity) is based on comparisons in measurements and therefore on repetition of the latter. The operator's ability to repeat these measurements with exactitude is quantified by the statistical notions of repeatability and reproducibility. *Repeatability* measures *intraday variability*, which is the range of values obtained by a given operator during one examination day. *Reproducibility* measures *interday variability*, which is the range of values obtained by a given operator over several days of examination. Usually these inter- and intraday ranges are expressed as coefficients of variation (CV in %). It is important to point out that the validation of a method must take into account the needs of its clinical application. For example, if one wishes to study variations of 100% in one parameter, a method displaying a CV of 20% for a given operator may be sufficient. On the other hand, if smaller variations of 10% are to be detected, it is obvious that CVs lower than 10% are required. For quantitative imaging techniques such as echocardiography, repeatability and reproducibility are generally considered to be good for CVs lower than 15%.

History

In veterinary medicine, a first study carried out in 1986 on anesthetized cats focused on the interday variability of echocardiographic measurements done in time-motion (TM) mode by a single operator (once a week for 5 weeks) [9]. The reproducibility of measurements done in TM and bidimensional (2D) modes was then evaluated by the same operator in calves and nonsedated horses [10,11].

It was only later, in 2003, that this metrology issue was again approached in domestic carnivores by our team in collaboration with the National Veterinary College of Toulouse, under normal examination conditions (nonsedated animals) and, for the first time, comparing operators with different skill levels [12-15]. Before this work was completed, interoperator variability of echographic measurements on noncardiac tissues (horse tendon and striated skeletal muscle in sheep) had already been evaluated [16,17]. Note that a study was also published in 2002 on the variability of Doppler examination in dogs. However, it was difficult to determine the interoperator variability in this study because the two echocardiographers had similar experience but did not perform these examinations on the same days [18].

Intra- and Interoperator Notions of Variability

During an echocardiographic follow-up, the repetition of measurements implies taking potential variation factors of the examination into account. More precisely, one can distinguish *biological factors* (such as breed, age, body weight, physical shape, heart rate, anesthetic, or type of heart disease) from *factors that are inherent to technique* (such as the position of the animal: standing or recumbent), the equipment used (echographic machine, probe), and the *operator* (experience, probe positioning, etc.). Appreciation of the problem raised by this last variable, the operator, is fundamental to achieving optimal interpretation of the echocardiographic data.

- When different values are obtained for a given parameter during an echocardiographic follow-up of an animal, how much of the differences are linked to the operator (intraoperator, intraday, or interday variability)? For example, is an increase of 2 mm in the left ventricular diameter in dogs considered significant when taking into account the operator's intra- or interday CV?
- Does the training of the operator guarantee better repeatability and reproducibility? Is it indispensable for an animal to be reimaged by the same operator? These questions also lead to another question: What is the interoperator variability?
- Finally, does this interoperator variability significantly affect the number of animals required to observe differences in measurement (during a clinical trial, for example)?

Operator's Effect on the Variability of Echocardiographic Measurements

Examples of Intra- and Interoperator Variability in Echocardiography

To best study intra- and interoperator variables of a technique, it is best to repeat measurements many times on a small number of animals (in contrast with the usual recommendation when aiming to analyze a biological variability). This has been done in the field of canine and feline echocardiography in two different studies. In the first [12], 96 exams in 2D and TM mode were done on four cats. In the second [13], 192 exams, each done randomly, were performed on six dogs over 4 nonconsecutive days by four operators with different levels of experience (less than 4 months of training to several years for a diplomate of the European College of Veterinary Internal Medicine). In both studies, a *significant effect from the operator was shown.*

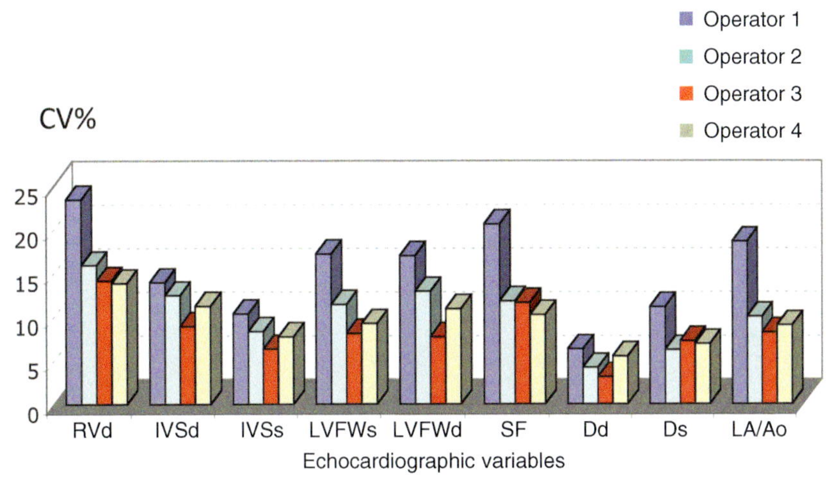

• **Fig. 3-1** Coefficient of variation (CV in %) of the intraobserver, intraday variability (repeatability) for nine echocardiographic variables tested in dogs: diastolic diameter of the right ventricle (RVd), thickness of the interventricular septum in diastole (IVSd) and in systole (IVSs), left ventricular free wall in diastole (LVFWd) and in systole (LVFWs), shortening fraction (SF), diameter of the left ventricle in diastole (Dd) and in systole (Ds), and the left atrium to aorta ratio (LA/Ao). Operators 1 and 2 were the least trained in echocardiography (training period of 2.5 months and 6 months, respectively). Operators 3 and 4 were more experienced (resident at the end of studies and European College of Veterinary Internal Medicine diplomate, respectively). (Findings from Chetboul V, Athanassiadis N, Concordet D, et al. Observer-dependent variability of quantitative clinical endpoints: the example of canine echocardiography. J Vet Pharmacol Ther 2004;27:49–56.)

In the study of dogs [13], all of the lowest intra- and interday CVs were good to very good. Most of them (90%) were obtained by the two most highly trained operators (first-year resident and European College diplomate): respectively, 8.9% and 4.5% for the interventricular septum in diastole (6.3% and 7.0% in systole), 7.7% and 9.4% for the left ventricular free wall in diastole (8.1% and 5.2% in systole), 3.1% and 5.0% for the left ventricular diameter in diastole (6.2% and 7.0% in systole), 10.2% and 10.8% for the shortening fraction, and, finally, 8.2% and 9.8% for the left atrium/aorta ratio (Figure 3-1). All of the highest CVs were recorded for the two least trained operators. Finally, for all but the most experienced operators, a "dog-operator" interaction was shown for some echocardiograph variables (diameters of the left ventricle, free wall of the left ventricle in diastole). Depending on the dog examined, this interaction means that the operator could underestimate or overestimate the measurement.

The reference operators had CVs between 5.5% and 11.2% for repeatability and between 4.0% and 15.7% for reproducibility. The highest CVs for repeatability were obtained with the least trained operator for all variables tested, except one [12].

Practical Consequences

Consequence #1

The intra- and interoperator variability results (see above) show the *unfeasibility of replacing the reference operator with a less trained operator.* For example, Figure 3-2 shows the differences between the mean measurements obtained by each operator and the reference operator for a particular echocardiographic variable, the diastolic thickness of the interventricular septum in cats. A wide range of values exceeding the standard deviation of the reference operator repeatability is observed. Note that this difference may reach nearly 2 mm. This is considerable if this value is compared to the 6-mm cutoff value, above which the myocardial wall is considered hypertrophied in this species [19].

Consequence #2

Based on the preceding variability data, it is also possible to determine *the number of animals required to show a given difference between two groups* for each echocardiographic variable (for example, the treated and control group in a clinical trial). Within the context of the dog study, the minimum number of animals per group (treated and control) needed to demonstrate a difference of 0.2 for the left atrium/aorta (LA/Ao) ratio would be 27 for the beginner echocardiographer, compared to only 5 for the European College diplomate (Figure 3-3). It is important to take such data into consideration when developing protocol that has ethical, financial, and scientific concerns. For a pharmaceutical laboratory that is considering launching a clinical trial, knowledge of the intra- and interday variability of an investigator is essential.

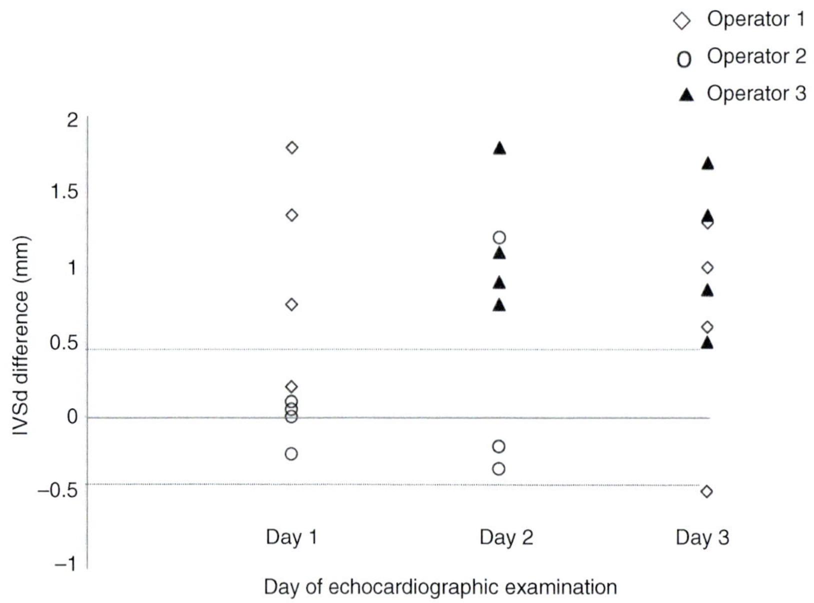

• **Fig. 3-2** Differences in the IVSd parameter (interventricular septum in diastole, in mm) between the averages of the three operators and the reference operator in four cats for the days the reference operator was involved (days 1, 2, and 3). The four cats were scanned by each operator twice a day and the measurement averages were then calculated. The reference operator was a European College of Veterinary Internal Medicine diplomate. Three others were less experienced (a resident, a practitioner with 1 year of experience, and a student, respectively, for operators 1, 2, and 3). The dotted lines represent the intraday standard deviation of the reference operator for the parameter considered. The possibility of switching operators would have been acceptable if the differences in measurements were all located within this interval (± standard deviation). This was not the case for any of the other three operators. (Findings from Chetboul V, Concordet D, Pouchelon JL, et al. Effects of inter- and intra-observer variability on echocardiographic measurements in conscious cats. J Vet Med A Physiol Pathol Clin Med 2003;50:326–31.)

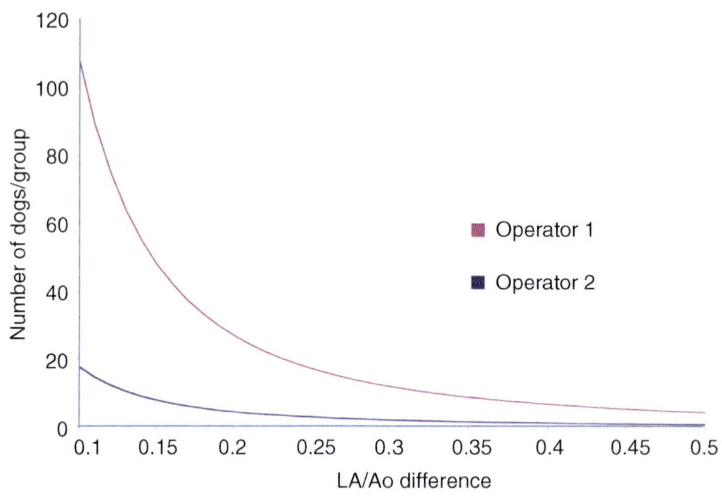

• **Fig. 3-3** Minimum number of dogs per group (treatment and control) required to observe a given difference of the LA/Ao (left atrium/aorta ratio) parameter, depending on whether the investigator is a beginner (Operator 1, pink curve) or a European College diplomate (Operator 2, blue curve). (Findings from Chetboul V, Athanassiadis N, Concordet D, et al. Observer-dependent variability of quantitative clinical endpoints: the example of canine echocardiography. J Vet Pharmacol Ther 2004;27:49–56.)

Consequence #3

Finally, variability studies can also serve to show that one technical modality is comparable—or even superior—to another. For instance, an echocardiographic examination performed by a trained operator on a dog in a standing position is characterized by a similar (and possibly better) variability than an examination performed on a dog in a recumbent position [14]. Therefore it is possible to state objectively that the standing position (particularly useful with nervous or dyspneic animals but rarely used in Anglo-Saxon countries) may be as valid as the recumbent position.

Conclusion

The intra- and interoperator variability studies presented in this chapter confirm that the *echocardiographic examination is a highly operator-dependent procedure.* It is clear that the variability of this technique should be taken into account not only in longitudinal studies that require repeated echocardiographic measurements, but also in clinical practice in order to optimally interpret repeated measures on a given animal. Finally, knowing one's own variability and working to improve it could be used as an objective and innovative learning tool to develop echocardiographic proficiency.

REFERENCES

[1] Allworth MS, Church DB, Maddison JE, et al. Effect of enalapril in dogs with pacing-induced heart failure. Am J Vet Res 1995;56:85–94.

[2] Kittleson MD, Keene B, Pion PD, Loyer CG. Results of the multicenter spaniel trial (MUST): taurine- and carnitine-responsive dilated cardiomyopathy in American cocker spaniels with decreased plasma taurine concentration. J Vet Intern Med 1997;11:204–11.

[3] Rush JE, Freeman LM, Brown DJ, Smith FW. The use of enalapril in the treatment of feline hypertrophic cardiomyopathy. J Am Anim Hosp Assoc 1998;34:38–41.

[4] Amberger CN, Glardon O, Glaus T, et al. Effects of benazepril in the treatment of feline hypertrophic cardiomyopathy: results of a prospective, open-label, multicenter clinical trial. J Vet Cardiol 1999;1:19–26.

[5] Rush JE, Freeman LM, Brown DJ, et al. Clinical, echocardiographic, and neurohormonal effects of a sodium-restricted diet in dogs with heart failure. J Vet Intern Med 2000;14:513–20.

[6] Snyder PS, Sadek D, Jones GL. Effect of amlodipine on echocardiographic variables in cats with systemic hypertension. J Vet Intern Med 2001;15:52–6.

[7] Chetboul V, Lefebvre HP, Carlos Sampedrano C, et al. Comparative adverse cardiac effects of pimobendan and benazepril monotherapy in dogs with mild degenerative mitral valve disease: a prospective, controlled, blinded, and randomized study. J Vet Intern Med 2007;21:742–53.

[8] EMEA. Guideline on Statistical Principles for Veterinary Clinical Trials. EMEA/CVMP/816/00-FINAL, December 5. The European Agency for the Evaluation of Medicinal Products. London, UK: Committee for Veterinary Medicinal Products; 2001.

[9] Moise NS, Horne WA, Flanders JA, Strickland D. Repeatability of the M-mode echocardiogram and the effects of acute changes in heart rate, cardiac contractility, and preload in healthy cats sedated with ketamine hydrochloride and acepromazine. Cornell Vet 1986;76:241–58.

[10] Amory H, Jakovljevic S, Lekeux P. Quantitative M-mode and two-dimensional echocardiography in calves. Vet Rec 1991;128:25–31.

[11] Young LE, Scott GR. Measurement of cardiac function by transthoracic echocardiography: day to day variability and repeatability in normal Thoroughbred horses. Equine Vet J 1998;30:117–22.

[12] Chetboul V, Concordet D, Pouchelon JL, et al. Effects of inter- and intra-observer variability on echocardiographic measurements in awake cats. J Vet Med A Physiol Pathol Clin Med 2003;50:326–31.

[13] Chetboul V, Athanassiadis N, Concordet D, et al. Observer-dependent variability of quantitative clinical endpoints: the example of canine echocardiography. J Vet Pharmacol Ther 2004;27:49–56.

[14] Chetboul V, Tidholm A, Nicolle A, et al. Effects of animal position and number of repeated measurements on selected two-dimensional and M-mode echocardiographic variables in healthy dogs. J Am Vet Med Assoc 2005;227:743–7.

[15] Serres F, Chetboul V, Tissier R, et al. Comparison of 3 ultrasound methods for quantifying left ventricular systolic function: correlation with disease severity and prognostic value in dogs with mitral valve disease. J Vet Intern Med 2008;22:566–77.

[16] Pickersgill CH, Marr CM, Reid SW. Repeatability of diagnostic ultrasonography in the assessment of the equine superficial digital flexor tendon. Equine Vet J 2001;33:33–7.

[17] Ferré PJ, Concordet D, Laroute V, et al. Comparison of ultrasonography and pharmacokinetic analysis of creatine kinase release for quantitative assessment of postinjection muscle damage in sheep. Am J Vet Res 2001;62:1698–705.

[18] Dukes-McEwan J, French AT, Corcoran BM. Doppler echocardiography in the dog: measurement variability and reproducibility. Vet Radiol Ultrasound 2002;43:144–52.

[19] Fox PR, Liu SK, Maron BJ. Echocardiographic assessment of spontaneously occurring feline hypertrophic cardiomyopathy: an animal model of human disease. Circulation 1995;92:2645–51.

PART II

New Cardiac Ultrasound Imaging Techniques

4 Myocardial Tissue Doppler, Derived Techniques, and Speckle Tracking Imaging, 47

5 Transesophageal Echocardiography, 85

6 Veterinary Applications of the Tridimensional Echocardiography, 95

4

Myocardial Tissue Doppler, Derived Techniques, and Speckle Tracking Imaging

VALÉRIE CHETBOUL

Normal Myocardial Kinetics, 48

Myocardial Tissue Doppler or Tissue Doppler Imaging, 50

TDI-Derived Techniques (Tissue Tracking Imaging, Strain Imaging, and Strain Rate Imaging), 62

Speckle Tracking Imaging, 74

Conclusion, 82

Echocardiography, introduced in veterinary medicine about 30 years ago, has become the "core" imaging modality in cardiology, allowing the analysis of cardiac morphology and kinetics. The so-called conventional Doppler mode appeared later. It complements the echocardiographic data by providing valuable hemodynamic information through a precise study of blood flow (duration, velocity, direction, and laminar or turbulent pattern of the latter).

New cardiovascular ultrasound imaging techniques, still mainly used in specialized institutions (mostly for research), were developed at the beginning of the twenty-first century. Resulting from both technological and computer advances, they include (in chronological order) myocardial tissue Doppler or tissue Doppler imaging (TDI), techniques derived from tissue Doppler (tissue tracking imaging, strain imaging, strain rate imaging), and speckle tracking imaging. Novel indices of myocardial function have thus emerged: myocardial wall motion velocity, deformation (strain), deformation velocity (strain rate), rotation and torsion angles, and segmental synchronism. These new imaging tools, which can be combined to various degrees, provide a precise analysis of regional and global myocardial function, complementing the one obtained by conventional ultrasound imaging.

After covering a few reminders on normal myocardial function, this chapter will introduce the principle of these new techniques, their indications, and normal images. The main anomalies associated with cardiopathies are addressed in specific chapters.

Normal Myocardial Kinetics

Myocardial fibers have a relatively complex layout. They wrap around the left ventricle chamber as spirals around the major axis (Figure 4-1) [1-4]. More precisely, fibers are set up in successive layers. Within a layer, fibers are "relatively" parallel. However, their orientation changes gradually from one layer to the next, from a helix layout in the subendocardial layer, to a circular layout in the midwall layer, and then back to a helix layout in the subepicardial layer, but in the opposite direction from the previous one. This layout shows that the innermost and outermost myocardial fibers have a longitudinal layout, unlike the median fibers, whose orientation is mainly radial.

This specific geometry reveals that left ventricular kinetics are complex and include three motions, to which is added a heterogeneity of myocardial velocities within each region:

- A *radial motion* (Figure 4-2) involving localized radial fibers mainly in the median region of the left ventricular free wall. Myocardial velocities increase from the subepicardium to the subendocardium; this radial motion is associated with a *circumferential deformation* of the myocardium.
- A *longitudinal motion* (Figure 4-3) involving localized longitudinal fibers mainly in the subendocardial and subepicardial region of the left ventricular free wall. The flow velocity increases from the apex to the base.
- An *axial rotation* (see Figure 4-1). This rotational motion is carried out in the short axis plane of the heart and in opposite directions for the base and apex (clockwise and counterclockwise, respectively, when the heart is viewed from the apex) [5-10]. The left ventricle undergoes a real torsion in systole and inversely a detorsion (or *recoil*) in early diastole. This untwisting motion plays an important role in the filling of the left ventricle.

To these three intrinsic motions of the myocardium is added a "passive" motion, known as *translation*, corresponding to the motion of the heart within the thoracic cavity, to which is added the one caused by the contraction of the adjacent segments.

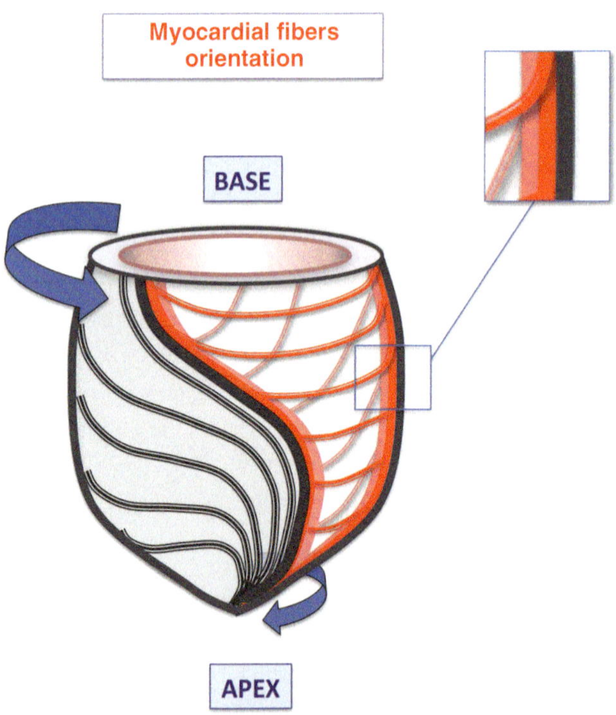

• **Fig. 4-1** Layer arrangement of left ventricular myocardial fibers. Within the same layer, the adjacent fibers are parallel to each other but, from one layer to the next, the angulation is different. Fibers in the midwall have a circular layout around the left ventricle chamber. On the other hand, the innermost and outermost layers have a more longitudinal layout. (Adapted from Streeter DD, Hanna WT. Engineering mechanics for successive states in canine left ventricular myocardium: II. fiber angle and sarcomere length. Circ Res 1973;33:656–64.)

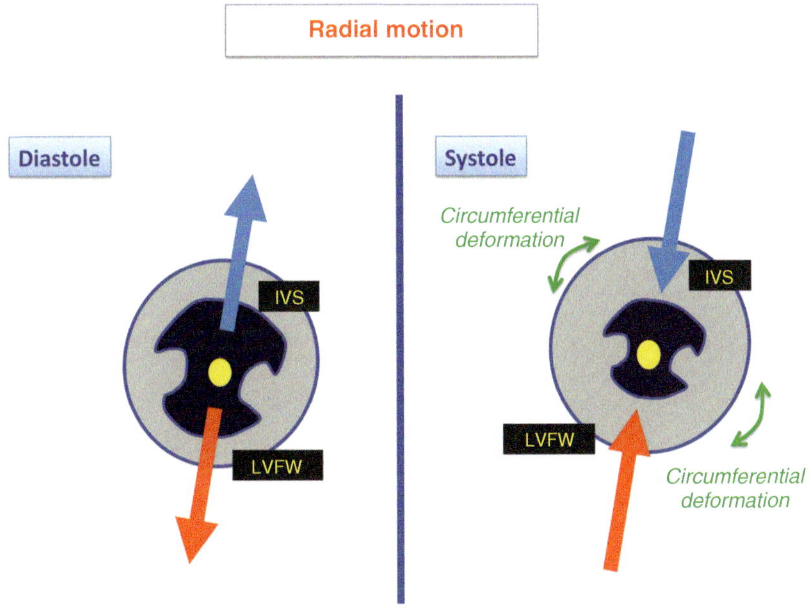

• **Fig. 4-2** Graphic representation of the radial motion. In systole, the left ventricular free wall (LVFW) and the interventricular septum (IVS) converge toward a geometric center *(yellow point)* located within the left ventricular chamber. Conversely, the two walls diverge during diastole. There is also a circumferential deformation with shortening of fibers in systole *(double green arrows)*. (Photo credit: Valérie Chetboul.)

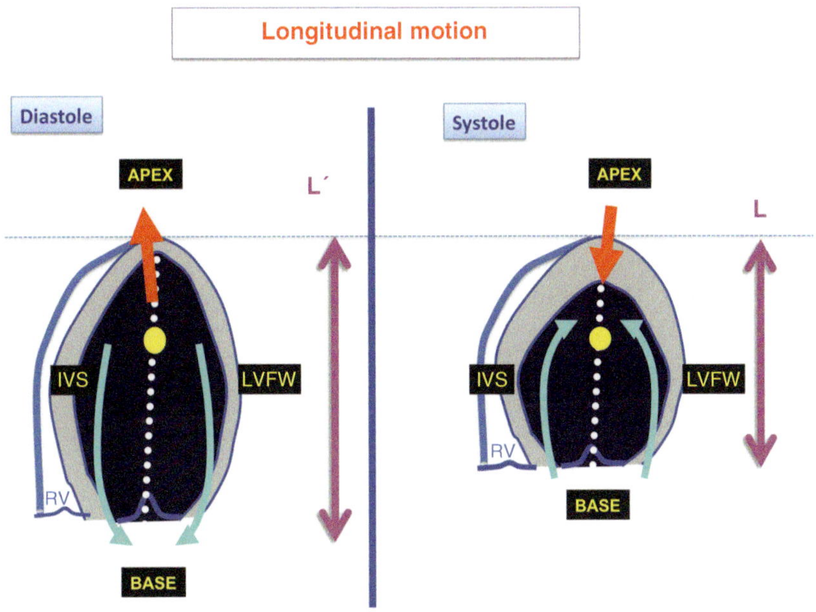

• **Fig. 4-3** Graphic representation of the longitudinal motion. In systole, the length of the heart (L) decreases because the apex, the left ventricular free wall (LVFW), and the interventricular septum (IVS) all converge toward a geometric center *(yellow point)*, located on the long axis of the left ventricular chamber close to the apex (approximately at one third of the base-apex length). Conversely, in diastole, the three myocardial walls move away from this center, the motion of the apex having an opposite direction than that of the other two walls. Thus the length (L′) of the left ventricle increases. *RV,* Right ventricle. (Photo credit: Valérie Chetboul.)

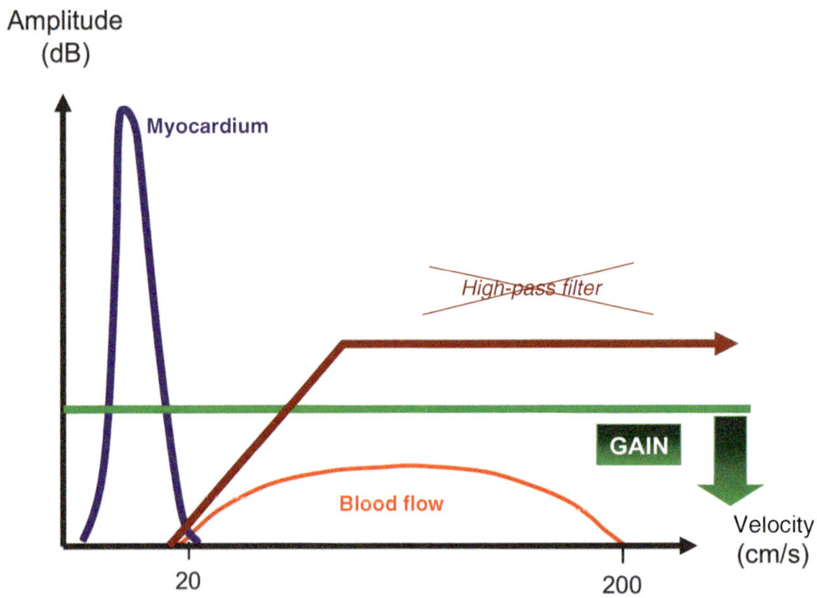

• **Fig. 4-4** Differences in physical and acoustic properties between myocardium and blood flow. Compared to blood flow, the radiofrequency signal reflected from the myocardial interfaces has higher energy. On the other hand, the myocardial motion velocity is much lower than the blood flow velocity. By eliminating the high-pass filter (used in conventional Doppler to reduce tissue signals) and by decreasing the gain, the myocardial signal, analyzed by TDI, is enhanced. (Adapted from Derumeaux G, Jamal F. Myocardial Doppler tissue. In: Abergel E, Cohen A, Gueret P, Roudaut R, editors. Adult clinical echocardiography, volume 1. Issy-les-Moulineaux, France: Estem; 2003. pp. 87–96.)

Myocardial Tissue Doppler or Tissue Doppler Imaging

Definition and History

TDI is a special Doppler technique that consists of measuring the myocardial motion velocities throughout the entire cardiac cycle [11,12].

The first quantitative analysis of myocardial motion was performed in France in 1989 by Karl Isaaz and his collaborators [13]. They had the idea of changing the settings of the conventional pulsed wave Doppler mode to obtain the profile of the left myocardium velocities as a function of time. A few years later, the Scottish team of Sutherland and McDicken developed the first quantification software for myocardial velocities through color TDI [14,15], validated *in vitro* [16] and then *in vivo* against other gold-standard techniques of myocardial function analysis, such as sonomicrometry [17].

Physical Principles

Like the conventional Doppler technique used to analyze blood flows, TDI relies on the Doppler effect principle. However, the motion analyzed by TDI is the myocardial motion and not the red blood cell motion. There are differences in the physical and acoustic properties of blood flows and myocardial tissue (Figure 4-4). The myocardium moves at a slow velocity (<20 cm/s) while blood flow velocity can reach more than 200 cm/s [12]. Conversely, the acoustic reflectivity of the myocardial interfaces is high, hence producing high-amplitude Doppler signals (about 40 dB), while that of the blood cells is much lower, hence generating very low-amplitude Doppler signals [12].

To exclude the Doppler information coming from the blood flows and to focus on low-velocity and high-amplitude myocardial signals, the TDI technique consists of removing high-pass filters (used in traditional Doppler systems), using low-pass filters, and decreasing the gain (see Figure 4-4) [12].

As in conventional Doppler, velocity estimation measured by TDI is much more accurate when the axis of the Doppler beam and the motion of the analyzed structure are parallel. In other words, the angle between the ultrasound beam and the motion vector of the myocardium must be as close to zero as possible to avoid underestimating the real myocardial velocity.

The Three Tissue Doppler Modes

Doppler tissue signals can be acquired using three different modes, each of which has its own advantages and disadvantages: the single-gated pulsed wave TDI, the color time-motion (TM) TDI, and the color bidimensional (2D) TDI modes. Depending on the mode used, the spectral curves of the myocardium motion velocities as a function of time are obtained at a given point on the myocardium (single-gated pulsed wave TDI mode), on an entire wall (color TM TDI mode),

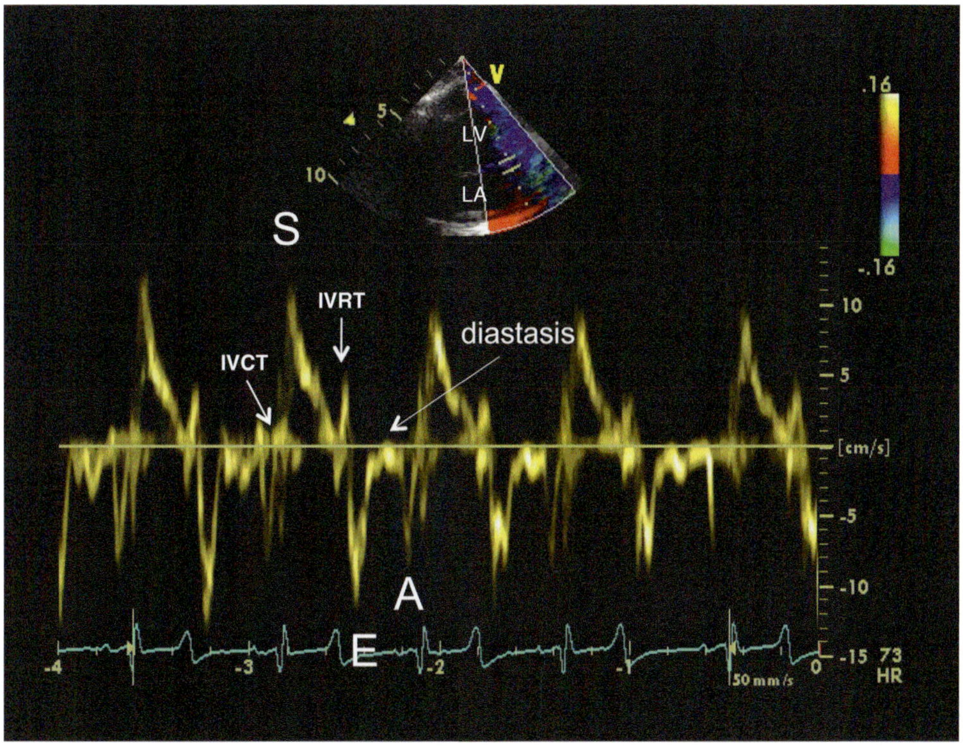

• **Fig. 4-5** Example of a normal single-gated pulsed wave tissue Doppler imaging (TDI) tracing. The sample volume is placed at the level of the mitral valve annulus at the base of the left ventricular free wall (left apical 4 chambers view). Systole begins with a brief isovolumic contraction phase (IVCT), followed by a phase of systolic ejection during which the myocardium moves closer to the probe. Velocity, reaching its maximum at point S, is therefore positive. Diastole consists of four phases. The first phase corresponds to the short isovolumic relaxation period (IVRT). Then the filling phase begins during which the myocardium moves away from the probe at high velocity (negative velocity, reaching its maximum at point E). Then the diastasis phase occurs, characterized by low velocities. Diastole is completed by a second filling phase during which the myocardium is again moving away from the probe at higher velocities than during the diastasis phase but not as high as it did in the beginning of diastole (velocity is still negative, reaching maximum at point A). *LA,* Left atrium; *LV,* left ventricle. (Photo credit: Valérie Chetboul.)

or at several points simultaneously (color 2D TDI mode) [11,12]. Today, the latter mode is widely preferred over the first two because of the ability to simultaneously analyze the motion of multiple myocardial segments belonging to the same or different walls, thus providing an analysis of both intra- and interventricular synchronicity [18].

Pulsed Wave TDI Mode

Like the classical Doppler pulsed wave mode, the pulsed wave TDI mode enables the analysis, in a sample volume or "Doppler gate," of instantaneous myocardial velocities as a function of time [11,12,19]. It is also called single-gated pulsed wave TDI mode. This sample volume is placed in the myocardial wall, either on a right parasternal short axis transventricular view or a left parasternal long axis view, in order to analyze, respectively, the radial or longitudinal myocardial motion [11,19]. A spectral curve of the myocardial motion velocities as a function of time is thus obtained without using any "postprocessing" software (Figure 4-5). Just as in conventional Doppler, the velocities are positive when the myocardium is moving toward the probe and negative when moving away from it.

The pulsed wave TDI mode is characterized by an excellent temporal resolution (<4 ms) [12]. However, it has several limitations:

- As with conventional pulsed wave Doppler mode, there is a maximum measurable velocity (inversely proportional to the frequency of the probe and to the depth of exploration) beyond which an aliasing artifact occurs [11,12].
- The myocardial velocity analysis is performed only in a single sample volume, unlike the color TM TDI and color 2D TDI modes, which allow, respectively, for the study of the entire wall and multiple myocardial segments simultaneously.
- Unlike the color 2D TDI mode (see below), the position of this sample volume cannot be changed during the course of the cardiac cycle in order to

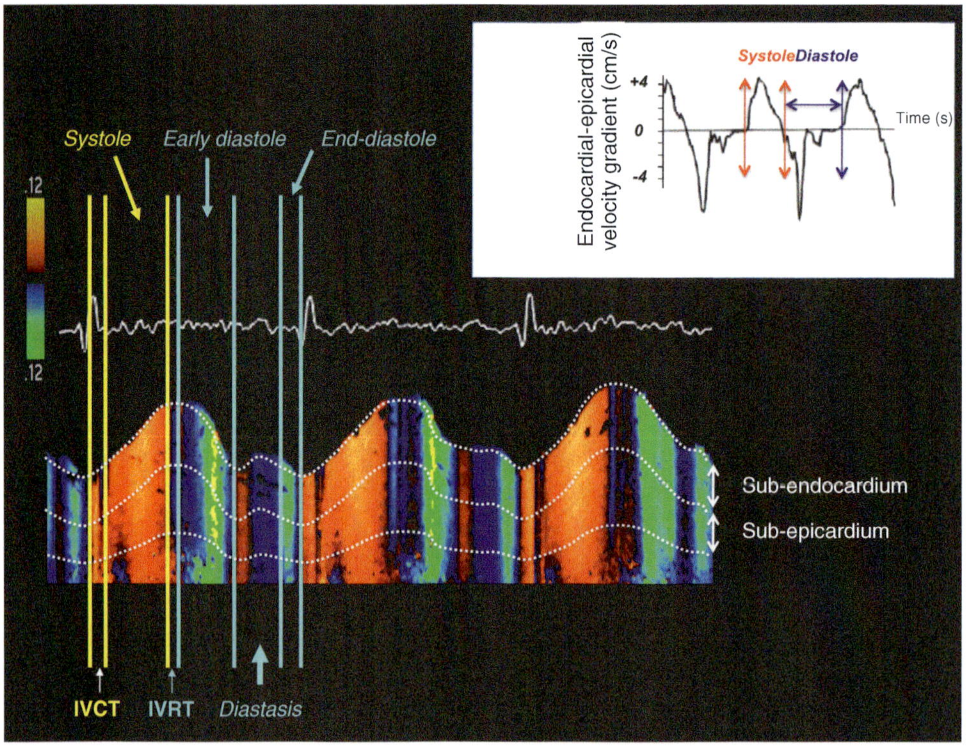

• **Fig. 4-6** Example of radial motion analysis of the left ventricular free wall in a healthy dog using color time-motion (TM) tissue Doppler imaging (TDI) mode. This color TM TDI tracing shows the radial myocardial, systolic, and diastolic velocities throughout the entire left ventricular free wall transected by the TM line. These velocities are color coded. After a short isovolumic contraction period (IVCT), the systolic ejection phase occurs during which the myocardial wall moves toward the probe and is coded in red. Diastole begins with a brief isovolumic relaxation phase (IVRT), followed by an early filling phase (early diastole) during which the myocardial wall moves away from the probe and is coded in blue. Then a diastasis occurs at low velocities (therefore dark colors) and, finally, a late filling phase occurs (end of diastole) during which the myocardium again moves away from the probe and is coded in blue. The quantitative velocity analysis is later performed using a specific "postprocessing" software *(top right)* The trace shown here corresponds to the instantaneous velocity differences between the internal subendocardial layer (faster) and external subepicardial layer (slower). This difference in velocities or endocardium-epicardium gradient corresponds to the velocity of segmental radial deformation. (Photo credit: Valérie Chetboul.)

"track" the region of interest (i.e., follow the motion of the analyzed myocardial wall during the cardiac cycle).

Color TM TDI Mode

Color TM TDI mode is used to analyze, over a given period, the myocardial velocities along an ultrasound line that is positioned on the 2D image [11,12]. The color coding is identical to that of the conventional color Doppler and color 2D TDI modes: red when the myocardium moves toward the probe and blue when it moves away from it. The higher the motion velocity, the clearer the color (Figure 4-6).

The color TM TDI mode is mainly used to analyze the radial myocardial motion of the left ventricular free wall and the interventricular septum from the right parasternal short axis transventricular view (see Figure 4-6). However, the left apical long axis view can also be used to analyze the longitudinal motion of one of these two walls or both simultaneously.

Unlike the single-gated pulsed wave TDI mode, quantification software (on a separate workstation or more often integrated with the echocardiographic machine) is necessary to assign numbers to the colors according to the chosen colorimetric scale (shown on the screen of the ultrasound system; see Figure 4-6). The color TM TDI mode also presents the advantage of being able to calculate the velocities of an entire section of myocardium (the one transected by the TM line) or of multiple sublayers of this wall, thus allowing the calculation of velocity

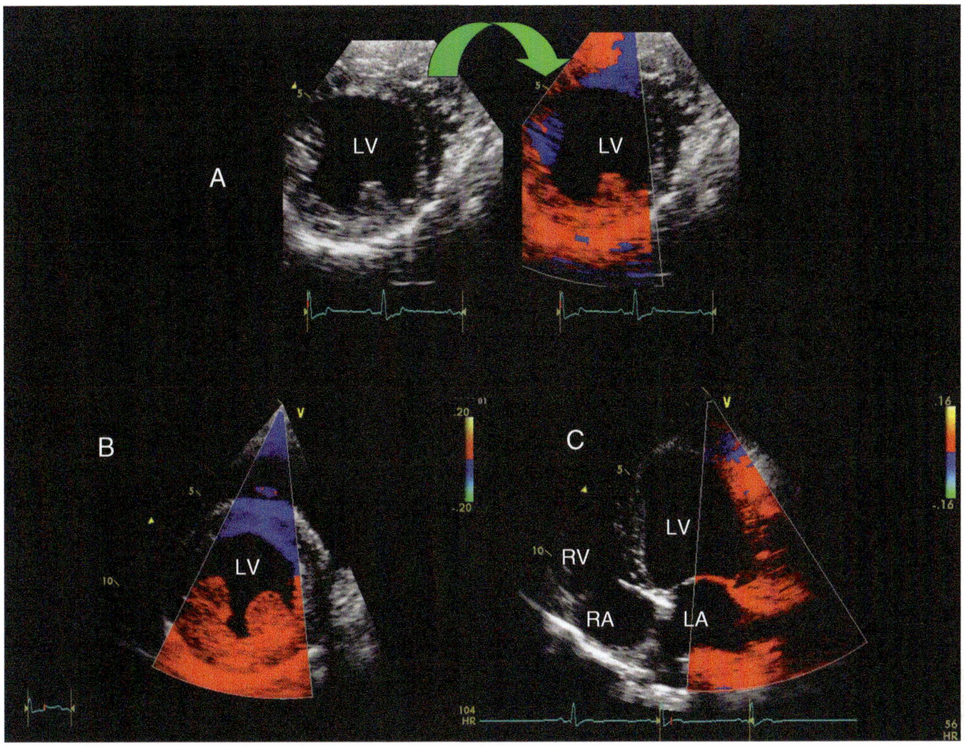

• **Fig. 4-7** Illustration of the color bidimensional (2D) tissue Doppler imaging (TDI) mode principle applied to myocardial radial and longitudinal motion. In color 2D TDI mode, color coding of myocardial velocities is superimposed in real time on the 2D image (**A**) and is similar to the one used in color time-motion (TM) TDI mode (see Figure 4-6). The radial (**B**) and longitudinal (**C**) motion of the myocardium can be analyzed according to the chosen view of study (respectively, right parasternal short axis transventricular and left apical 4 chambers views). Thus on the right parasternal short axis transventricular view, taken at end systole (**B**), the left ventricular free wall is color coded in red because it is moving toward the probe. On the other hand, the interventricular septum, moving in the opposite direction is color coded in blue. *LA,* Left atrium; *LV,* left ventricle; *RA,* right atrium; *RV,* right ventricle. (Photo credit: Valérie Chetboul.)

gradients (see below: "Concepts underlying TDI-derived parameters"), markers of the segmental myocardial deformation rate (see Figure 4-6). Due to its very high imaging rate, color TM TDI mode offers excellent temporal (<4 ms) and spatial axial (1 mm) resolutions, greater than those of the color 2D TDI mode [11,12]. It thus allows the detection of subtle abnormalities of the myocardial function [11,12,20,21]. The limitations of the color TM TDI mode are as follows:

- It is subject to aliasing artifact, as in conventional pulsed wave Doppler and single-gated pulsed wave TDI modes.
- The myocardial velocities are analyzed only for the selected TM ultrasound line.

Color 2D TDI Mode

In color 2D TDI mode, the myocardial motion velocity and direction are color coded. This color coding (identical to that of conventional color Doppler and color TM TDI modes) is superimposed in real time on the 2D grayscale images (Figure 4-7) [11,12,20]. As with the color TM TDI mode, the use of specific software is required in order to obtain myocardial velocities as a function of time. It is thus possible to analyze

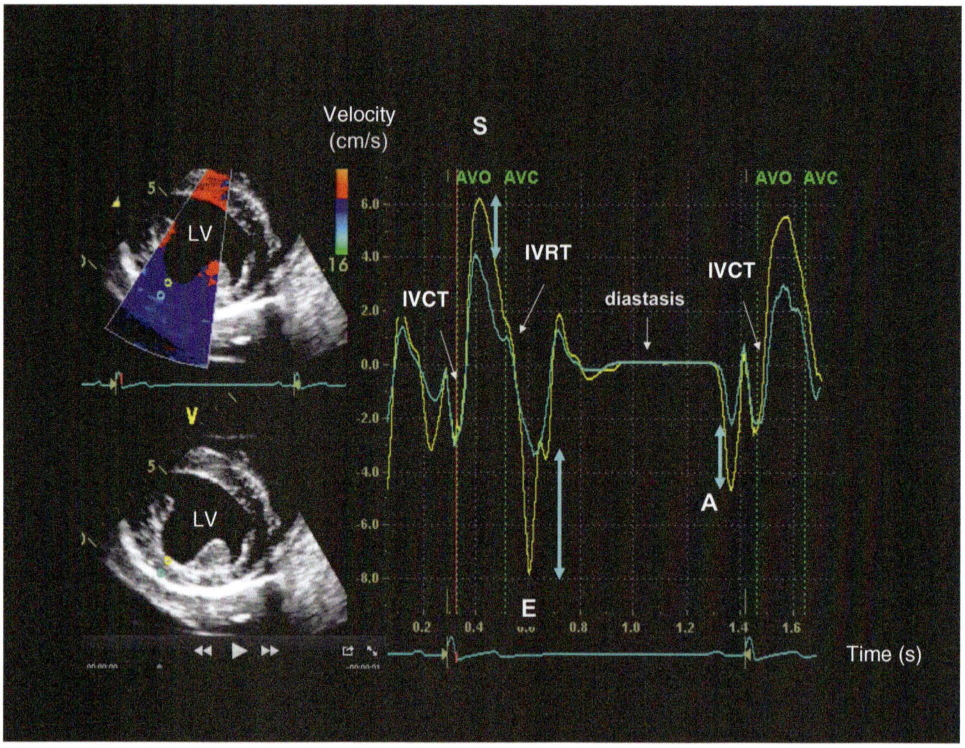

• **Fig. 4-8** Example of radial motion analysis of the left ventricle free wall in color bidimensional (2D) tissue Doppler imaging (TDI) mode in a healthy dog. *(Top left)* The velocity color coding is superimposed in real time on the right parasternal transventricular short axis cross-section. Using specific software, the myocardial velocities are analyzed simultaneously in two circular segments of 2-mm diameter each: a subendocardial segment *(yellow)* and a subepicardial segment *(green)* of the left ventricular free wall. The tracing obtained shows that the subendocardium moves more rapidly *(yellow curve)* than the subepicardium segment *(green curve)* during both systole and diastole, thus defining an intramyocardial velocity gradient throughout the cardiac cycle *(double blue arrows)*. As in pulsed wave TDI mode (see Figure 4-5), the myocardial velocities are positive when the myocardium moves toward the probe and negative when it moves away from it. The different phases of the cardiac cycle are identified, including a positive S wave during systole and negative E (here biphasic) and A waves, concomitant with early and end-diastole, respectively. The wealth of information brought by the color 2D TDI mode is illustrated here, the mechanical events (myocardial velocity and motion at different points) being analyzed concomitantly with electrical (electrocardiographic tracing) and hemodynamic events. *AVC,* Aortic valve closure; *AVO,* aortic valve opening; *IVCT,* isovolumic contraction time; *IVRT,* isovolumic relaxation time; *LV,* left ventricle. (Photo credit: Valérie Chetboul.)

the left myocardial radial motion from the right parasternal short axis transventricular view (Figure 4-8) and the longitudinal left, septal, and right myocardial motions (Figures 4-9 to 4-11) from the left apical long axis view. The color 2D TDI mode was put at a disadvantage for a very long time because of a low temporal resolution with a frame rate that would not exceed 30 frames per second [12]. The development of new modes of ultrasound emission-reception currently allows work with high frame rates, reaching 100 to 200 frames per second with a 30- to 45-degree ultrasound beam angle (corresponding to a <10 ms temporal resolution) [12].

The color 2D TDI mode is widely preferred over the other two modes because of the ability to analyze simultaneously the motion of multiple myocardial segments belonging to the same ventricular wall (see Figures 4-8 to 4-10) or to different walls (see Figure 4-11). This simultaneous analysis allows the study of intra- and interventricular synchronicity [18]. Finally, unlike pulsed wave TDI mode, *tracking* of the region of interest is possible with specific "postprocessing" software (see above). The operator can thus modify the position of the myocardial region being analyzed in order to follow the global motion of the myocardial wall and remain within the latter, in the same area, throughout the cardiac cycle.

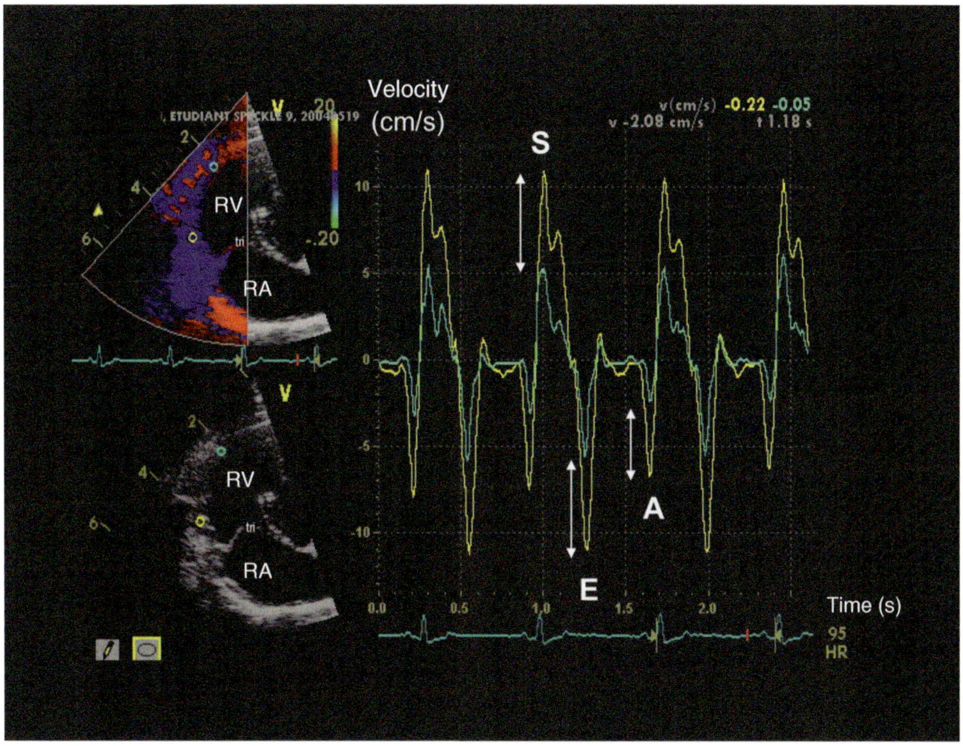

• **Fig. 4-9** Example of radial motion analysis of the left ventricular free wall in a healthy dog by color bidimensional (2D) tissue Doppler imaging (TDI) mode. *(Top left)* Velocity color coding is superimposed in real time on the left apical 4 chambers cross-section. The right myocardial velocities are analyzed simultaneously in two 2-mm diameter circular segments: a basal segment *(yellow)* and an apical segment *(green)* of the right ventricular wall. The tracing obtained shows that the basal segment moves more rapidly *(yellow curve)* than the apical segment *(green curve)* during both systole and diastole, thus defining an intramyocardium velocity gradient throughout the cardiac cycle *(double white arrows)*. As with the radial motion of the left ventricular wall (see Figure 4-8), the right longitudinal motion includes a positive maximum systolic S wave and negative E and A waves, respectively, in early and end-diastole. *RA,* Right atrium; *RV,* right ventricle. (Photo credit: Valérie Chetboul.)

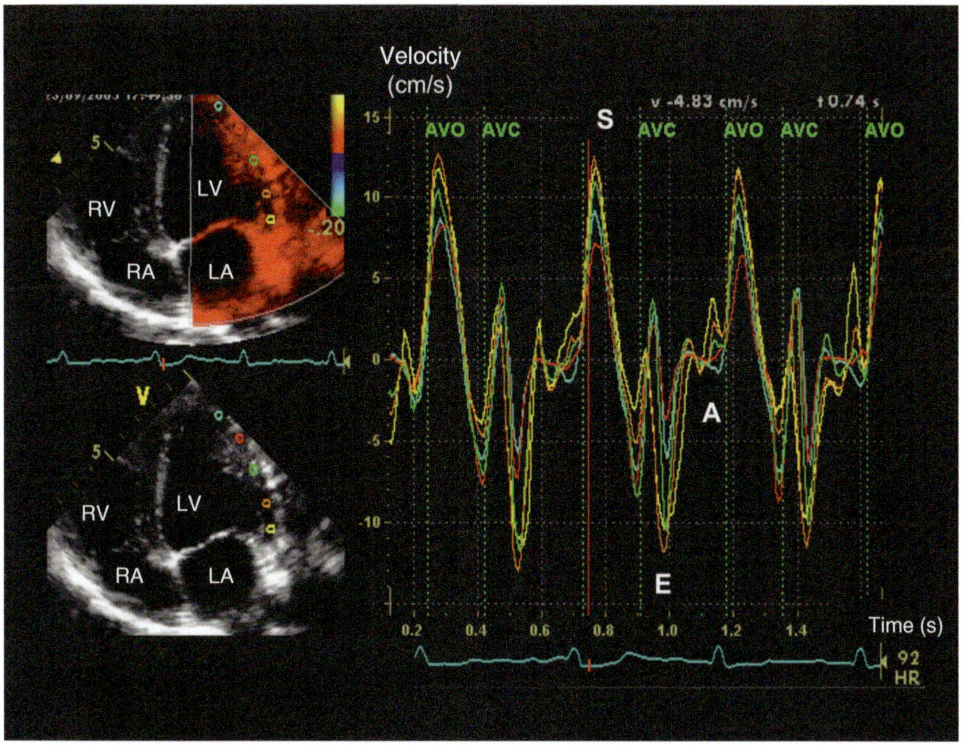

• **Fig. 4-10** Example of longitudinal interventricular synchrony analysis in color bidimensional (2D) tissue Doppler imaging (TDI) mode in a healthy dog. Velocities are recorded in five distinct 2-mm diameter segments, positioned within the left ventricular free wall from the base to the apex. *(Top left)* The velocity color coding is superimposed in real time on the apical 4 chambers cross-section. *(Right)* Five longitudinal velocity curves confirm perfect synchronism between the five segments. During each cardiac cycle, all include a positive systolic wave (S) and two negative waves (E and A) in early and end-diastole, respectively. *AVC,* Aortic valve closure; *AVO,* aortic valve opening; *LA,* left atrium; *LV,* left ventricle; *RA,* right atrium; *RV,* right ventricle. (Photo credit: Valérie Chetboul.)

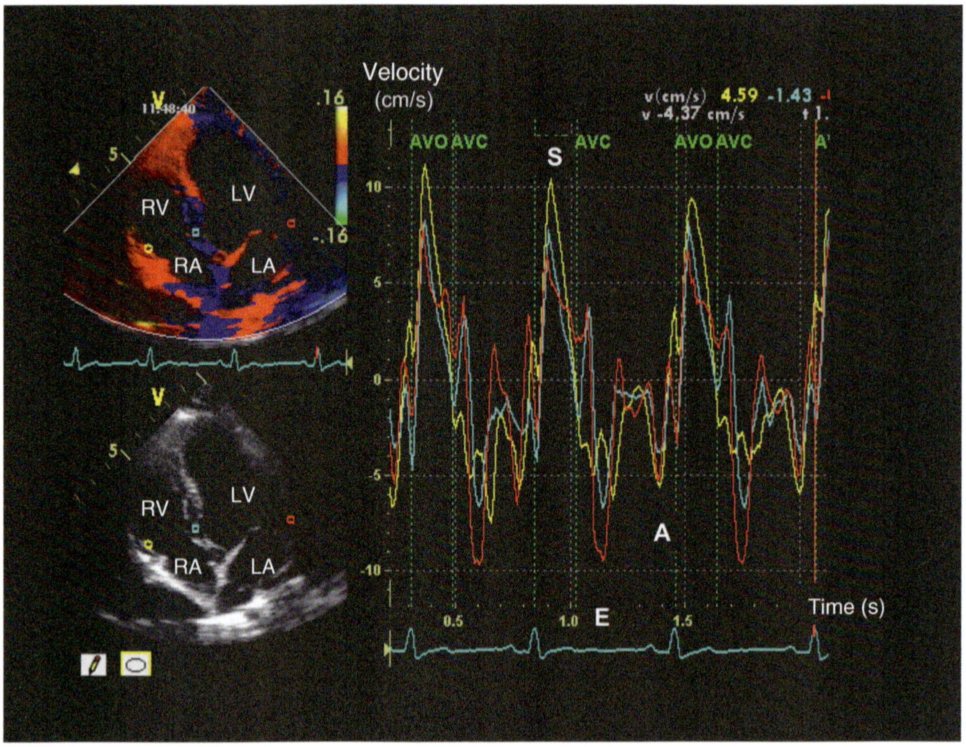

• **Fig. 4-11** Example of a longitudinal interventricular synchrony analysis using color bidimensional (2D) tissue Doppler imaging (TDI) mode in a healthy dog. The velocities are recorded in three distinct 2-mm diameter segments positioned at the base of the three ventricular myocardial walls: red, blue, and yellow segments, which respectively belong to the left ventricular free wall, the interventricular septum, and the right myocardial wall. *(Top left)* The velocity color coding is superimposed in real time to the apical 4 chambers cross-section. *(Right)* The red, blue, and yellow curves respectively represent the longitudinal velocity curves recorded in segments of the left ventricular free wall, the interventricular septum, and the right myocardial wall. They allow the observation of a perfect synchronism between the walls and all include, with each cardiac cycle, a positive systolic wave (S) and two negative waves (E and A) in early and end-diastole, respectively. As often is the case in healthy dogs, the right myocardial wall motion velocities *(yellow curve)* are higher than those of the other two walls *(blue and red curves)*. *AVC,* Aortic valve closure; *AVO,* aortic valve opening; *LA,* left atrium; *LV,* left ventricle; *RA,* right atrium; *RV,* right ventricle. (Photo credit: Valérie Chetboul.)

Normal Velocity Profiles and Variation Factors

Normal Velocity Profiles

Regardless of the TDI mode, the radial and longitudinal velocity profiles of the left ventricular free wall include a brief isovolumic contraction period, then a positive systolic wave with a maximum in S, followed by a short isovolumic relaxation phase, and finally two negative early and end-systolic waves, maximal in E and A, separated by a more or less long diastasis phase (see Figures 4-5, 4-6, 4-8, 4-10, and 4-11; Tables 4-1 to 4-4) [19, 21-26]. The early diastolic E wave as well as the isovolumic phases can be biphasic in dogs (see Figure 4-8) and in cats [22]. In felines, the E and A waves frequently merge

TABLE 4-1 Parameters of the Radial Motion of the Left Ventricular Free Wall (Subendocardium and Subepicardium) Calculated using Tissue Doppler Imaging (TDI) in 100 Healthy Dogs of Different Breeds [26]

TDI Variable		Subendocardium	Subepicardium
Systolic S wave (cm/s)	Mean ± SD	6.4 ± 1.4[a,b]	3.9 ± 1.1
	Min-max	3.1-10.8	1.0-6.5
Early diastolic E wave (cm/s)	Mean ± SD	7.8 ± 2.2[a,c]	4.0 ± 1.6
	Min-max	2.9-14.9	1.4-10.2
End-diastolic A wave (cm/s)	Mean ± SD	4.1 ± 1.4[a,b,c]	1.9 ± 1.2[b,c]
	Min-max	1.4-8.3	0.1-5.6
E/A ratio	Mean ± SD	2.1 ± 0.9	3.2 ± 3.9
	Min-max	1.0-5.1	0.9-36.0
Heart rate during TDI exam (bpm)	Mean ± SD	103 ± 24	
	Min-max	59-171	

Values are expressed in mean ± standard deviation (SD) and minimum-maximum (Min-max). Note: Unpublished data, established with a GE Vivid 5.
[a]Significantly different from the value in the subepicardium ($p < 0.001$).
[b]Significantly different from E in the same segment ($p < 0.001$).
[c]Significantly different from S in the same segment ($p < 0.001$).

TABLE 4-2 Parameters of Longitudinal Motion of the Left Ventricular Free Wall (Base, Middle of Wall, Apex) Calculated Using Tissue Doppler Imaging (TDI) in 100 Healthy Dogs of Different Breeds [26]

TDI Variable		Base	Middle	Apex
Systolic S wave (cm/s)	Mean ± SD	7.6 ± 2.7[a,b,c]	4.7 ± 2.48[a,c]	1.8 ± 1.5[b]
	Min-max	3.0-19.6	1.0-13.5	0.1-6.7
Early diastolic E wave (cm/s)	Mean ± SD	9.0 ± 2.5[a,b]	7.4 ± 2.68[a]	2.1 ± 1.6[b]
	Min-max	3.2-14.7	1.7-14.2	0.1-9.4
End-diastolic A wave (cm/s)	Mean ± SD	5.5 ± 1.9[a,b,c,d]	3.1 ± 1.8[a,c,d]	0.6 ± 0.5[b,c,d]
	Min-max	0.8-10.6	0.2-7.7	0.1-2.5
E/A ratio	Mean ± SD	1.8 ± 0.8	4.1 ± 5.3	4.7 ± 5.0
	Min-max	0.9-5.6	1.0-35.0	0.5-34.0
Heart rate during TDI exam (bpm)	Mean ± SD	97 ± 23		
	Min-max	52-171		

Values are expressed in mean ± standard deviation (SD) and minimum-maximum (Min-max). Note: Unpublished data, established with a GE Vivid 5.
[a]Significantly different from the value at the apex ($p < 0.001$).
[b]Significantly different from the value in the middle of the wall ($p < 0.001$).
[c]Significantly different from E in the same segment ($p < 0.001$).
[d]Significantly different from S in the same segment ($p < 0.001$).

TABLE 4-3 Parameters of the Radial Motion of the Left Ventricular Free Wall (Subendocardium and Subepicardium) Calculated Using Tissue Doppler Imaging (TDI) in 100 Healthy Cats of Different Breeds [24]

	Effect of Breed, Sex, Body Weight, and Age	Values: Mean ± SD	Values: Min-Max
Systolic Velocities and Gradient			
S wave (subendocardium) (cm/s)	Breed and sex ($p < 0.05$)	4.7 ± 1.1	3.0-8.1
S wave (subepicardium) (cm/s)	Breed ($p < 0.05$)	2.5 ± 0.9	1.1-5.6
Systolic gradient between subendocardium and subepicardium (cm/s)	Age ($p < 0.05$)	2.2 ± 0.7	0.8-3.6
Diastolic Velocities and Gradients (for Cats without EA Fusion, n=92)			
E wave (subendocardium) (cm/s)	Breed ($p < 0.001$)	5.7 ± 1.5	3.5-10.8
E wave (subepicardium) (cm/s)	Absent	2.4 ± 1.0	0.5-4.3
A wave (subendocardium) (cm/s)	Absent	3.0 ± 1.0	0.9-5.0
A wave (subepicardium) (cm/s)	Breed ($p < 0.05$)	1.2 ± 0.6	0.2-3.2
E/A (subendocardium)	Breed ($p < 0.01$)	2.1 ± 1.2	1.1-10.2
E/A (subepicardium)	Absent	2.5 ± 1.8	1.0-13.0
Early diastolic gradient between subendocardium and subepicardium	Breed ($p < 0.001$)	3.3 ± 1.3	1.1-8.4
End diastolic gradient between subendocardium and subepicardium (cm/s)	Absent	1.8 ± 0.7	0.2-3.5
TDI Time Intervals			
IVCT (subendocardium) (ms)	Breed ($p < 0.01$)	40 ± 10	24-73
IVCT (subepicardium) (ms)	Breed ($p < 0.01$)	40 ± 10	24-73
IVRT (subendocardium) (ms)	Age ($p < 0.05$)	45 ± 10	21-75
IVRT (subepicardium) (ms)	Absent	45 ± 10	21-75
Heart rate during TDI exam (bpm)	Absent	174 ± 25	122-242

IVCT, Isovolumic contraction time; *IVRT,* isovolumic relaxation time.

Values are expressed in mean ± standard deviation (SD) and minimum-maximum (Min-max). The effects of breed, sex, body weight, and age were studied using a general linear model and are presented with the corresponding p value, when the result is statistically significant. Note: Unpublished data, established with a GE Vivid 5.

TABLE 4-4 Parameters of the Longitudinal Motion of the Left Ventricular Free Wall (Mitral Annular, Base, Apex) Calculated Using Tissue Doppler Imaging (TDI) in 100 Healthy Cats of Different Breeds [26]

	Effect of Breed, Sex, Body Weight, and Age	Values	
		Mean ± SD	Min-Max
Systolic Velocities and Gradient			
S wave (annulus) (cm/s)	Absent	4.4 ± 1.3	2.2-8.4
S wave (base) (cm/s)	Absent	4.5 ± 1.2	2.4-8.4
S wave (apex) (cm/s)	Absent	1.7 ± 0.9	0.2-4.5
Systolic gradient base-apex (cm/s)		2.7 ± 0.8	1.2-5.5
Diastolic Velocities and Gradients (for Cats without EA Fusion, n=90)			
E wave (annulus) (cm/s)	Absent	5.5 ± 1.6	2.6-10.2
E wave (base) (cm/s)	Absent	5.8 ± 1.6	2.8-9.9
E wave (apex) (cm/s)	Weight (p <0.05)	2.7 ± 1.2	0.5-5.6
A wave (annulus) (cm/s)	Absent	2.9 ± 1.3	0.3-5.8
A wave (base) (cm/s)	Absent	2.9 ± 1.0	1.1-5.5
A wave (apex) (cm/s)	Weight (p <0.05)	0.8 ± 0.6	0.2-3.7
E/A (annulus)	Absent	2.2 ± 1.1	1.0-6.6
E/A (base)	Breed (p <0.05)	2.2 ± 0.9	1.1-5.8
E/A (apex)	Breed (p <0.05)	4.3 ± 3.0	1.1-17.5
Early diastolic gradient base-apex (cm/s)	Breed (p <0.05)	3.1 ± 1.4	0.3-7.3
End of diastole gradient base-apex (cm/s)	Absent	2.1 ± 0.9	0.2-4.4
TDI Time Intervals			
IVCT (base) (ms)	Absent	36 ± 9	21-71
IVCT (apex) (ms)	Absent	36 ± 9	21-71
IVRT (base) (ms)	Absent	55 ± 12	28-90
IVRT (apex) (ms)	Absent	55 ± 12	28-90
Heart rate during TDI exam (bpm)	Breed (p <0.01)	173 ± 28	105-253

IVCT, Isovolumic contraction time; *IVRT,* isovolumic relaxation time.
Values are expressed in mean ± standard deviation (SD) and minimum-maximum (Min-max). The effects of breed, sex, body weight, and age were studied using a general linear model and are presented with the corresponding p value, when the result is statistically significant. Note: Unpublished data, established with a GE Vivid 5.

into one negative EA wave of larger amplitude than that of the E wave, because of their elevated heart rates (Figure 4-12) [23,24]. This is a limitation for the TDI technique in analyzing diastolic function in feline species.

In cats [23,24] as in dogs [25,26], the left radial myocardial motion is characterized by its heterogeneity, the subendocardial fibers moving more quickly than the subepicardial fibers throughout the cardiac cycle (see "Normal myocardial kinetics"; see also Tables 4-1 and 4-3), thus defining a systolic and diastolic radial intramyocardial gradient (see Figure 4-8). In a study conducted by our team on 100 healthy dogs of different breeds, the radial intramyocardial gradients, obtained by color 2D TDI mode and defined as the difference between endocardial and epicardial velocities, were (mean ± standard deviation) 2.5 ± 0.8, 3.8 ± 1.5, and 2.3 ± 0.9 cm/s in systole, early diastole, and end-diastole, respectively (Figure 4-13) [26]. In a similar study conducted on 100 healthy cats of different breeds, the endo-epicardial gradients were 2.2 ± 0.7, 3.3 ± 1.3, and 1.8 ± 0.7 cm/s in systole, early diastole, and end-diastole, respectively (see Figure 4-13) [24].

The longitudinal motion of the left ventricular wall is also characterized by its nonuniform aspect (see "Normal

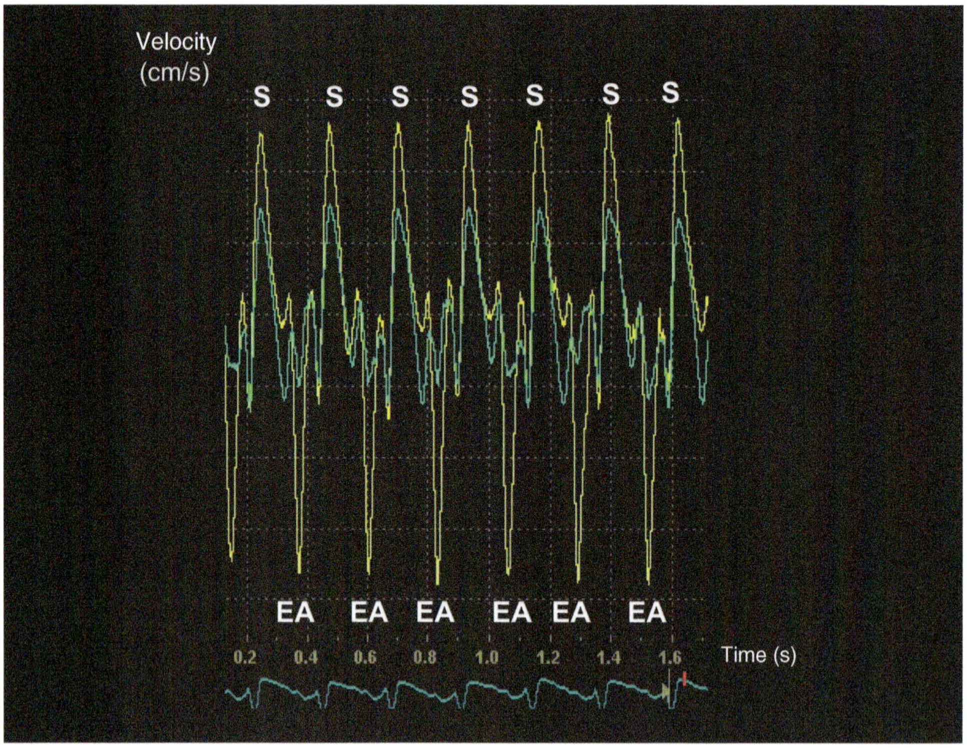

• **Fig. 4-12** Analysis of the radial motion of the left ventricular free wall in a healthy cat (heart rate: 250 beats/min) in color bidimensional (2D) tissue Doppler imaging (TDI) mode. As in Figure 4-8, the myocardial velocities are simultaneously analyzed in two circular segments of the left ventricular free wall (1-mm diameter each): a subendocardial segment *(yellow curve)* and a subepicardial segment *(green curve)*. The two velocity profiles include the positive systolic S wave but only one negative EA wave. Because of tachycardia, the negative E and A waves have merged. (Photo credit: Valérie Chetboul.)

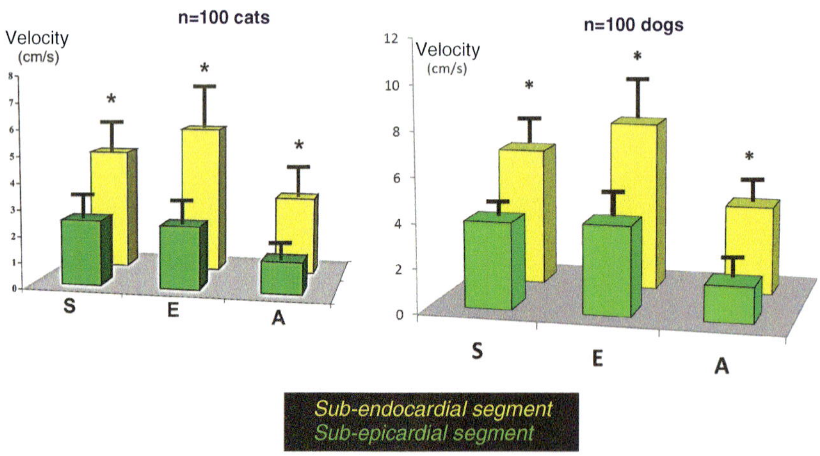

• **Fig. 4-13** Values (mean ± standard deviation) of radial S (systolic), E (early diastolic), and A (end-diastolic) waves obtained in color bidimensional (2D) tissue Doppler imaging (TDI) mode in healthy cats (n=100) [26] and dogs (n=100), [26] awake and in standing position for the radial motion of the left ventricle free wall. Note that subendocardial velocities *(yellow bars)* are significantly higher (* = p <0.01) than subepicardial velocities *(green bars)* in the two species, thus defining an endo-epicardial velocity gradient throughout the cardiac cycle. (Photo credit: Valérie Chetboul.)

myocardial kinetics") because the myocardial velocities decrease from the base to the apex, defining a longitudinal intramyocardial gradient in both systole and diastole (see Tables 4-2 and 4-4). Thus in the study conducted in 100 healthy dogs, the base-apex gradients, calculated using color 2D TDI mode and defined as the difference between basal and apical velocities, were 5.9 ± 2.2, 6.9 ± 2.5, and 4.9 ± 1.7 cm/s in systole, early diastole, and end-diastole, respectively [26]. In a similar fashion, in a study conducted on 100 healthy cats, the values obtained were 2.7 ± 0.8, 3.1 ± 1.4, and 2.1 ± 0.9 cm/s in systole, early diastole, and end-diastole, respectively [24].

A longitudinal base-apex gradient was also demonstrated for the interventricular septum (in a Doberman) and the right ventricular wall (in dogs of different breeds), with higher velocities at the base than at the apex (see Figure 4-9) [27,28]. Thus in a study performed on 64 healthy dogs, the right base-apex gradients calculated in color 2D TDI mode were 7.8 ± 2.8, 6.2 ± 2.6, and 5.1 ± 1.7 cm/s in systole, early diastole, and end-diastole, respectively [28].

To this physiologic heterogeneity within the same wall, one can add a heterogeneity between different walls. In a normal cat, for example, the early diastolic velocities of the interventricular septum are higher than those of the left ventricular free wall [29]. Similarly, in a dog, the right longitudinal velocities are higher than those of the left ventricular free wall, at both the base and the apex [28]. This can be explained by the different load conditions of the two ventricles. A difference in myocardial fibers architecture could also contribute to this, as demonstrated in humans [30].

Variation Factors

Intraday (Repeatability) and Interday (Reproducibility) Variation

For a quantitative imaging technique to be considered repeatable and reproducible, the generally accepted upper limit of coefficients of variation (CV) must be 20% or, ideally, 15% [23,25]. The left and right intraday (repeatability) and interday (reproducibility) variability of color 2D TDI measurements was studied in awake cats and dogs, imaged in a standing position [23,25,28]. It was good for the majority of the tested parameters when the operator was trained (more than 2 years of experience in TDI) [23,25,28]. For example, in dogs, interday CVs of S, E, and A waves of the right longitudinal motion were 15.5%, 3.5%, and 10.2%, respectively. In cats, lower CVs were measured for radial subendocardial motion of the left ventricular free wall (8.2% and 6.5% for the S wave and the E wave, respectively) and for the basal longitudinal motion in early diastole (5.5%).

The greatest variability of TDI measurements in dogs and cats was observed at the left apex [23,25]. This characteristic of apical measurements is also found in humans and can be explained by both low myocardial motion velocity values in this region and the difficulty in clearly visualizing the apex on left apical 4 or 5 chambers views [31].

One of the limitations of the TDI technique is its highly operator-dependent nature, requiring the sonographer to be very experienced to ensure that the exam is repeatable and reproducible (respectively, has the lowest possible intraday and interday measurement variability). Thus in a first study, interday CVs of the left longitudinal waves at the base for an operator with 2 years of experience with this technique were still relatively high (27.0%, 19.0%, and 17.8% for S, E, and A waves, respectively) [25]. After 2 years of additional training, interday CVs for the same operator decreased to less than 15% (10.3%, 5.6%, and 10.9%, for S, E, and A waves, respectively) [28].

Several precautions for the untrained operator should be considered:

- It is crucial that the ultrasound beam is set as parallel as possible to the vector of myocardial motion because of the risk of underestimating the analyzed segment velocity (the TDI technique relies on the Doppler effect principle).
- It is strongly recommended to reduce the width of the ultrasound beam so as to image only the wall being analyzed, if possible, in order to improve the lateral resolution.
- It is important to avoid stationary reverberation artifacts due to interference with the thoracic wall, appearing as hyperechoic zones in the myocardium. These artifacts could lead to falsely diagnosing wall akinesia (see details below in "Strain imaging and strain rate imaging").
- For the TDI curves to be interpretable, it is necessary to adjust the velocity scale precisely (the myocardial motion velocities must be lower than the aliasing velocity).

Other Variation Factors

The S, E, and A waves measured by TDI depend on several factors, mainly including breed, heart rate, and drugs (e.g., anesthetics), thus illustrating the need to carefully interpret the values obtained.

A breed effect was demonstrated for the first time in a study carried out on 100 healthy dogs, on the radial and longitudinal S waves of the left ventricular free wall, respectively measured in the subendocardium and at the base [26]. The subendocardial radial S wave was significantly lower in Beagles (5.4 ± 0.8 cm/s) than in German Shepherds (7.0 + 1.0 cm/s) and Golden Retrievers (7.0 ± 1.3 cm/s). In these three breeds, similar results were obtained for the basal S wave: 6.5 ± 1.6 cm/s, 7.9 ± 1.6 cm/s, and 9.3 ± 4.3 cm/s, respectively.

The heart rate influence varies depending on the studies. In dogs, a positive correlation was demonstrated between the heart rate and the longitudinal S wave at the base of the left ventricular free wall ($r = 0.25$; $p < 0.05$) [26]. A similar correlation was reported in cats ($p < 0.05$) between the heart rate and the subendocardial radial ($r = 0.24$) and subepicardial ($r = 0.21$) systolic S wave as well as the annular longitudinal ($r = 0.23$) and basal ($r = 0.21$) S wave [24].

Finally, the reference intervals reported for awake animals cannot be transposed to tranquilized or anesthetized animals. To support that, a study of healthy dogs showed that general anesthesia (isoflurane and vecuronium) improves the repeatability of TDI measurements (CVs all below 10% and 13% for radial and longitudinal velocity) but significantly decreases left radial and longitudinal myocardial velocities (up to 60% when comparing to values obtained in awake animals) [25].

Main TDI Applications

The first animal TDI studies appeared within a few years of the human ones. Myocardial motions were first described in cats in single-gated pulsed wave TDI mode (1999), [19] then in color 2D TDI mode (2004) in cats and dogs, with repeatability and reproducibility analysis of the technique [23,25]. Demonstrations of the value of TDI, especially regarding its ability to detect early myocardial alterations, then multiplied in the two species.

TDI was already known, in humans, to be a more sensitive technique than classical echocardiography to detect acute myocardial rejection dysfunction after a heart transplant [32], to differentiate the left ventricular physiologic hypertrophy in athletes from pathologic hypertrophy [33], or even to diagnose various cardiomyopathies [34-36].

This TDI sensitivity was demonstrated for the first time by our team in dogs using a special spontaneous model of dilated cardiomyopathy, GRMD (Golden Retriever muscular dystrophy) model [21,37]. This spontaneous dystrophic myopathy, equivalent to Duchenne muscular dystrophy in humans, is hereditary, linked to the X chromosome, and due to a dystrophin coding gene mutation. Color TM TDI mode proved to be better than conventional echocardiography in the early diagnosis of systolic alteration in GRMD puppies. This systolic dysfunction, characterized by a decrease in endo-epicardial systolic radial gradient, was highlighted while conventional ultrasound indications (left ventricular diameters, myocardial thickness, fractional shortening) were still normal [21]. Early radial and longitudinal systolic and diastolic TDI alterations were then demonstrated with this same model in color 2D TDI mode [37]. A greater TDI sensitivity to detect myocardial injury early was then demonstrated in cats with a similar model of hypertrophic cardiomyopathy (linked to a dystrophin coding gene mutation) [38], in cases of spontaneous hypertrophic cardiomyopathy in cats of various breeds and in Maine Coons [39,40], and in the presence of systemic hypertension [39]. TDI was also shown to be more sensitive than the ultrasound exam and conventional Doppler in the diagnosis of systolic pulmonary hypertension in dogs [41].

TDI technique has also been used to study pathophysiologic mechanisms underlying some cardiopathies such as feline hypertrophic cardiomyopathy [39,42,43] or canine dilated cardiomyopathy [44].

Finally, TDI is an extremely powerful, noninvasive research tool that can be used to assess the effect (beneficial or deleterious) of a treatment (e.g., cell grafting) on global or regional myocardial function [45].

TDI-Derived Techniques (Tissue Tracking Imaging, Strain Imaging, and Strain Rate Imaging)

Concepts Underlying TDI-Derived Parameters

The basic TDI variable is the segmental *myocardial motion velocity* (Figure 4-14). The first parameter, which can be calculated from the previous one, is the *velocity gradient*. This gradient is defined as the difference between the velocities of two segments. In practice, the most commonly calculated gradients are the gradient between the endocardium and the epicardium (for the left radial motion) and the gradient between the base and the apex (for left longitudinal motion). The advantage of the gradient, when compared to the calculation of the velocities' absolute values, is twofold:

- Limitation of the effect of the angle between the ultrasound beam and the myocardial motion vector
- Disappearance of the influence of the cardiac translation velocities, which by adding themselves to the intrinsic velocities of myocardial segments "pollute" the value of the latter

Thus in pathologic conditions, velocity gradients often prove to be more discriminating than the velocities' absolute values for analysis of diastolic or systolic dysfunction [12,21,46].

Other parameters derived from velocities can be calculated (see Figure 4-14). *Displacement parameters* and *deformation parameters* have resulted in tissue tracking imaging, strain imaging, and strain rate imaging, three other techniques of ultrasound imaging that are considered to be derived from TDI.

Tissue Tracking Imaging

The instantaneous myocardial velocity (usually expressed in cm/s), calculated by TDI, represents the distance traveled by a myocardial segment per unit of time. The total distance traveled by this segment can be determined by performing

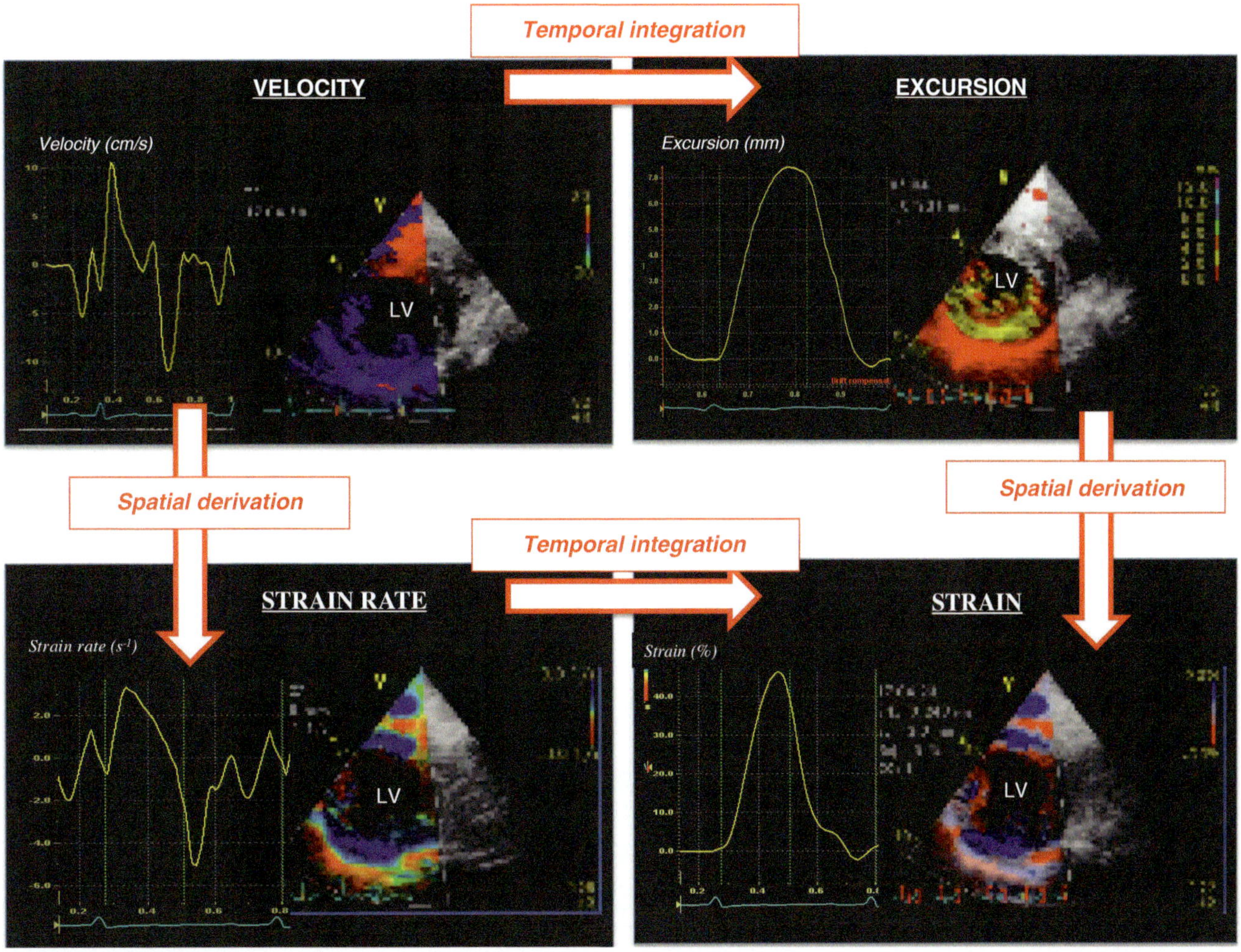

• **Fig. 4-14** Parameters derived from tissue Doppler imaging (TDI). With TDI in color bidimensional (2D) mode *(top left)*, myocardial velocities are color coded in real time. On this color mapping a velocity profile (in cm/s) of a myocardial segment as a function of time can be obtained. The temporal integration of this curve displays this segment motion (in mm) over time, which can also be color coded in real time *(top right)*. This is the principle of tissue tracking imaging. Spatial derivation of the velocities allows one to obtain the velocity profile of myocardial deformation or strain rate (in s^{-1}) as well as its color coding in real time. This is the principle of strain rate imaging *(bottom left)*. Finally, the temporal integration of the strain rate profile and the spatial derivation of the displacement allow the determination of the myocardial deformation or strain (%), the basis of strain imaging (as in previous techniques, color coding and values profile as a function of time). *LV,* Left ventricle. (Photo credit: Valérie Chetboul.)

a velocity-time integral (VTI) of the TDI curve (Figures 4-15 to 4-17). A myocardium displacement curve as a function of time can be obtained, as well as its color coding in real time (see Figures 4-14 to 4-16). This technique is called tissue tracking imaging. A good correlation between displacements obtained by tissue tracking imaging and by sonomicrometry (gold-standard invasive technique using two piezoelectric crystals inserted directly on the myocardial wall) was demonstrated in dogs (see Figure 4-17) [47].

The limitations of tissue tracking imaging are the same as those of TDI:

- Being derived from Doppler TDI technique, the movement measured is dependent on ultrasound angle. A perfect alignment between the segment being analyzed and the myocardial motion is thus necessary to avoid risking underestimating the actual displacement.
- The displacement (as well as the velocities' absolute values) is influenced by the overall heart motion. This includes the contraction of segments adjacent to the ones being analyzed and the displacement of the organ itself within the thorax.

The parameters of local myocardial strain partially alleviate these limitations.

Strain Imaging and Strain Rate Imaging

In addition to the distance traveled, other derived parameters, called deformation parameters, can be calculated from the instantaneous myocardial velocities: the *relative deformation,* or strain, and *deformation velocity,* or strain rate. These parameters represent the basis for techniques of strain imaging and strain rate imaging, respectively [27,48-54].

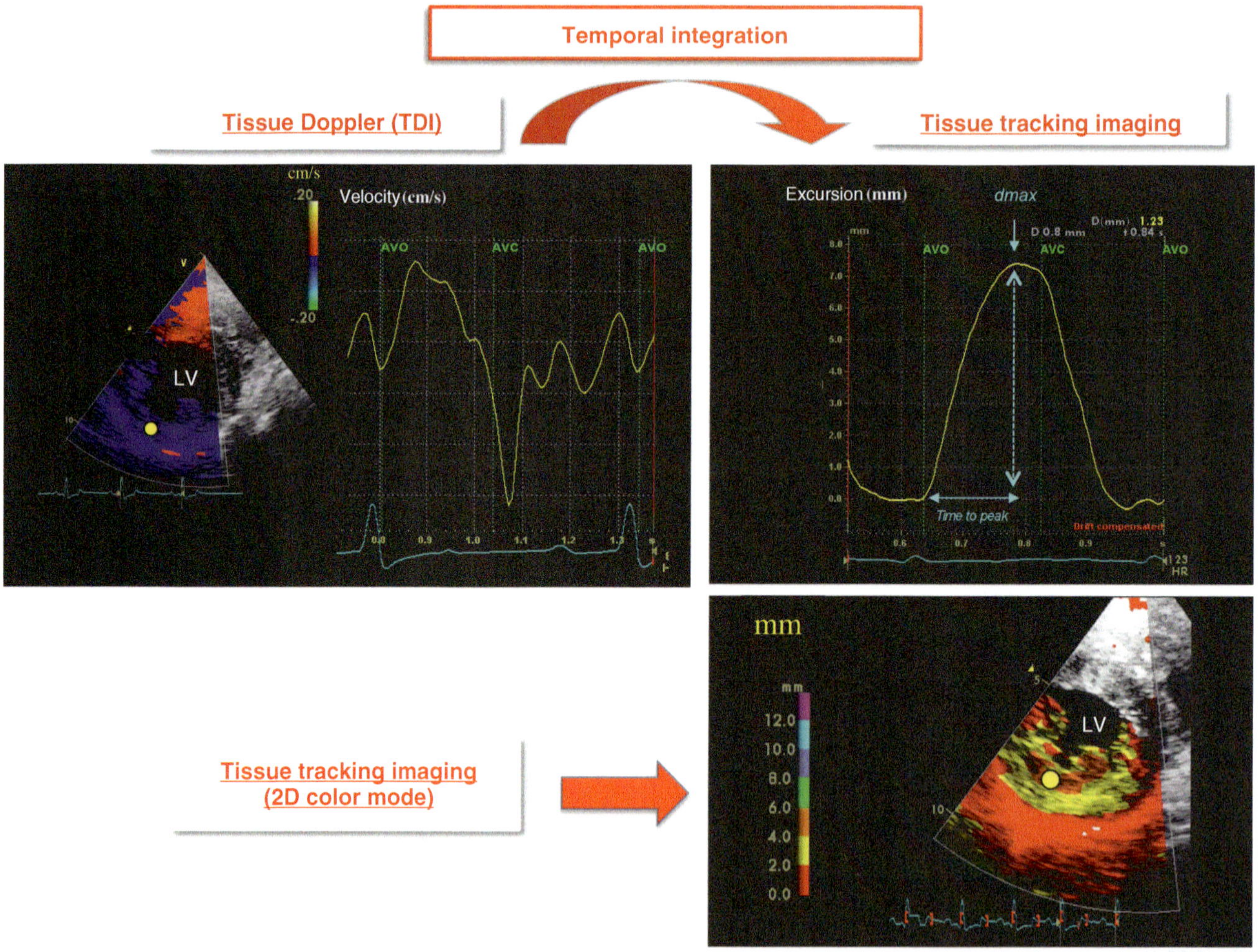

• **Fig. 4-15** Illustration of the tissue tracking imaging principle. Tissue Doppler imaging (TDI) examination allows one to obtain the velocity curve of a myocardial segment (in cm/s) as a function of time *(top left)*. The temporal integration of this curve allows the determination of the distance traveled by this segment over time *(top right)*. This is the principle of tissue tracking imaging, a technique derived from TDI, consisting of quantifying the myocardial displacement (in mm) from its velocity. This technique does not take into account the instantaneous segmental velocity (at a given moment) but rather the variation of this velocity over an entire period. Complementary to TDI, from which it is derived, tissue tracking imaging allows one to calculate the maximal systolic motion (dmax) and the time required to reach dmax (Time to peak). Bidimensional (2D) color coding of the myocardial displacement superimposed in real time on the 2D grayscale image also provides a color displacement map at a given moment *(bottom right)*. *AVC,* Aortic valve closure; *AVO,* aortic valve opening; *LV,* left ventricle. (Photo Credit: Valérie Chetboul.)

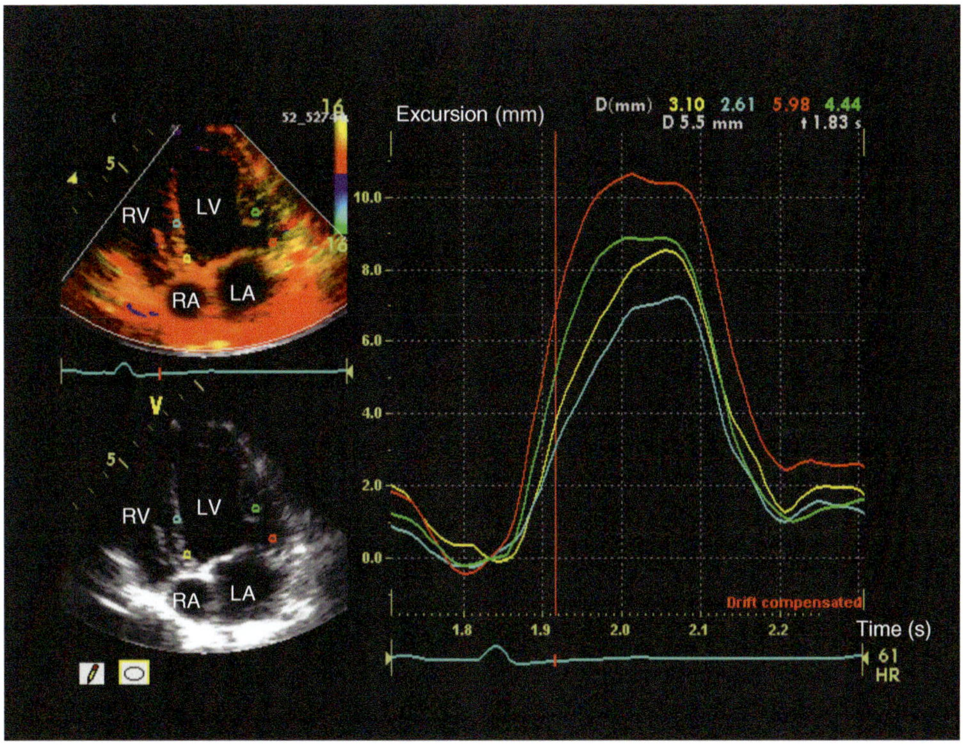

• **Fig. 4-16** Tissue tracking imaging of four myocardial segments. The longitudinal myocardial displacement is simultaneously analyzed in four circular 1-mm diameter segments: a basal *(red curve)* and median *(green curve)* segment of the left ventricular free wall and a basal *(yellow curve)* and median *(blue curve)* segment of the interventricular septum. The displacement of the four segments is synchronous. The color coding of the myocardial velocities (from which the movements are deducted) is superimposed in real time on the bidimensional (2D) image *(top left)*. *LA,* Left atrium; *LV,* left ventricle; *RA,* right atrium; *RV,* right ventricle. (Photo credit: Valérie Chetboul.)

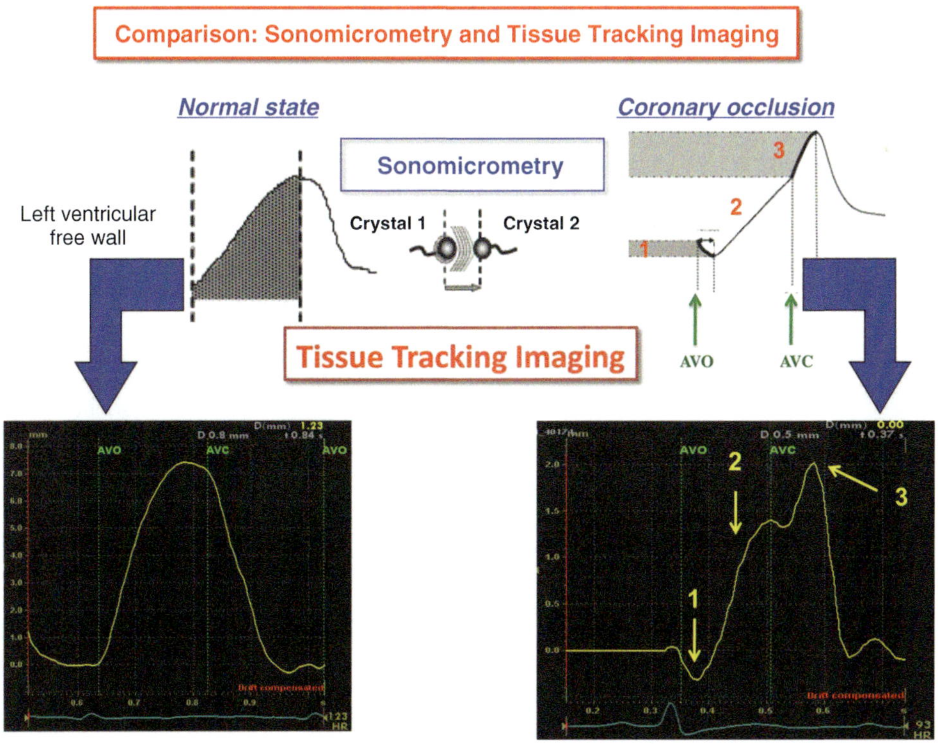

• **Fig. 4-17** Comparison of sonomicrometry and tissue tracking imaging. A good correlation was demonstrated in dogs between tissue tracking imaging *(bottom images)* and sonomicrometry. This was demonstrated for both normal myocardial segments (here, the left ventricular free wall) and postcoronary occlusion (here, the descending anterior coronary artery). Sonomicrometry is the gold-standard invasive technique used to quantify the regional myocardial motion, using two piezoelectric crystals attached to the myocardium *(top traces)*. The ultrasound velocity being constant, the distance that separates the two crystals can be determined by measuring the time taken by the ultrasound beam to cross it. The sonomicrometry trace *(top right)* and the tissue tracking imaging *(bottom right)* show that the coronary occlusion resulted in a myocardial kinetic anomaly known as "myocardial stunning" phase. This anomaly is characterized on two plots by an abnormal early systolic thinning (1), then a systolic thickening (2), and finally a postsystolic thickening (3) (recorded after aortic valve closing). *AVC,* Aortic valve closure; *AVO,* aortic valve opening. (Adapted from Lucats L, Monnet X, Bize A, et al. Regional and temporal heterogeneity of post-systolic wall thickening is associated with left ventricular asynchrony in normal and experimental stunned myocardium. Basic Res Cardiol 2008;103:385–96. Photo credit: Valérie Chetboul.)

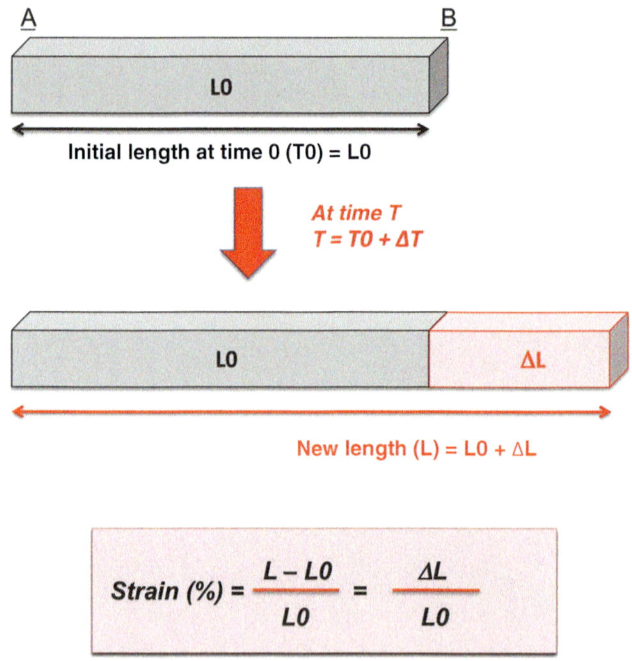

• **Fig. 4-18** Illustration of myocardial strain of a unidimensional segment. The only measurable unidimensional strain is lengthening or shortening. Consider a myocardial segment of L0 length between points A and B at time T0. The velocity of the two points, A and B, can be determined by tissue Doppler imaging (TDI). It is thus possible to deduce the new length (L) of the segment at given time T (T = T0 + ΔT). From this new length, the relative deformation (or strain) of the myocardial segment during the ΔT period can be calculated. It is defined as the percentage of variation of the segment length—i.e., the difference between the two lengths (L – L0) divided by the initial length L0. Thus if the segment undergoes an increase in length (elongation), L is greater than L0 and the strain is positive. Conversely, if the segment undergoes a decrease in length (compression), L is less than L0 and the strain is negative. (Photo credit: Valérie Chetboul.)

Consider a myocardial segment of L0 length delimited by two points, A and B (Figure 4-18). A moment later, the new length of this segment will be L, equal to L0 + ΔL. Relative deformation or strain undergone by this segment during the time interval ΔT is expressed as a percentage and is defined by the following formula:

$$\text{Strain} = \Delta L / L0$$

The strain of a segment thus represents strain undergone by the segment and normalized by its initial dimensions (see Figure 4-18). Strain is therefore the spatial derivative of movement (see Figure 4-14) [48,49].

Strain rate is defined as the velocity at which deformation (or strain) occurs. It is thus equal to the strain divided by ΔT:

$$\text{Strain rate} = \text{Strain}/\Delta T$$

Strain rate is therefore the temporal derivative of the strain (see Figure 4-14) and is expressed in s^{-1}. Conversely, the relative deformation or strain is obtained by the temporal integration of the strain rate.

Strain rate can also be calculated directly from the myocardial velocities of points A and B (see Figure 4-18). In fact, assuming a homogeneous distribution of velocities between the two points, the strain undergone by the segment AB during the time interval ΔT equals:

$$\text{Strain} = \Delta L / L0 = (DB - DA)/L0$$

where *DB* and *DA* are the distances traveled by points B and A, respectively. However, if VB and VA are the velocities of points B and A:

$$DB = VB \times \Delta T \ \textit{and} \ DA = VA \times \Delta T$$

The strain can thus be written as follows:

$$\text{Strain} = (DB - DA)/L0 = (VB \times \Delta T - VA \times \Delta T)/L0$$
$$\textit{or} \ (VB - VA) \times \Delta T / L0$$

Thus strain rate, defined as the strain /ΔT ratio, equals (VB – VA)/L0. In other words, the calculation of strain rate is the difference between the velocities of the two points A and B divided by the distance between them [12]. Like the velocity (measured by TDI) and the motion (measured by tissue tracking imaging), the strain and the myocardial strain rate are two indicators that can be quantitatively analyzed in the form of a curve of values over a time period, or qualitatively by 2D color coding (Figures 4-19 to 4-22). The description of the normal

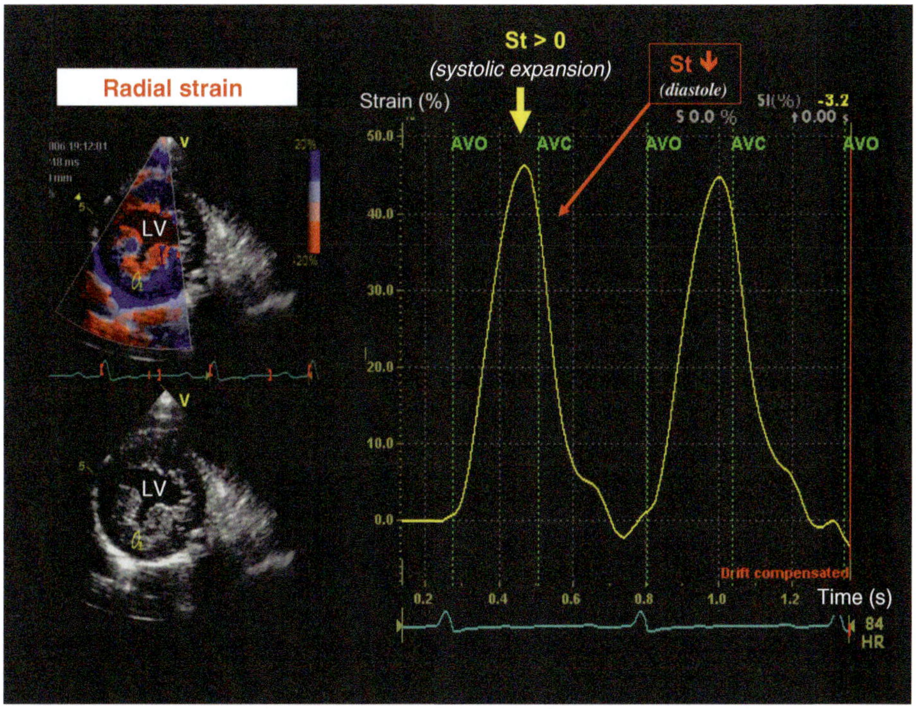

• **Fig. 4-19** Analysis of the radial segmental deformation of the left ventricular free wall in a normal dog by strain imaging from the right parasternal short axis transventricular view (bidimensional [2D] image at *bottom left*). The radial deformation (or strain, St) is positive and maximal in end-systole *(yellow arrow)*, then decreases during diastole *(red arrow)*, which confirms systolic thickening and local diastolic shortening, respectively. The color coding of the deformation is superimposed in real time on the 2D image *(top left)*. Size of the region of interest: 5 mm/3 mm. *AVC,* Aortic valve closing; *AVO,* aortic valve opening; *LV,* left ventricle. (Photo credit: Valérie Chetboul.)

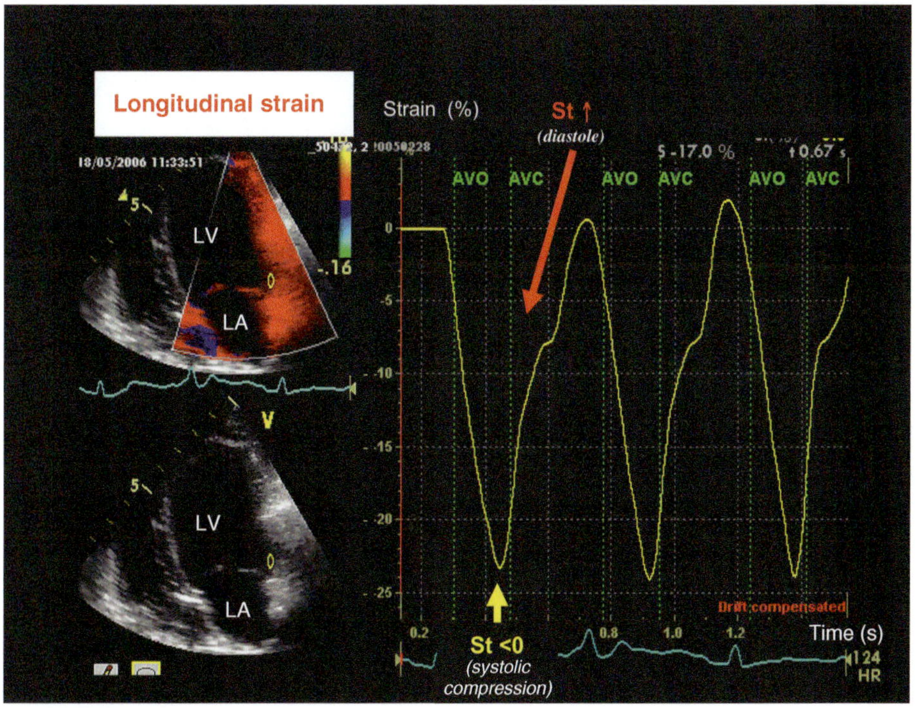

• **Fig. 4-20** Analysis of the longitudinal segmental deformation velocity of the left ventricular free wall in a dog using normal strain imaging from the left apical 4 chambers view (bidimensional [2D] image at *bottom left*). The longitudinal systolic deformation (or strain, St) is the opposite of the one in Figure 4-19, thus negative, and its absolute value is maximal in end-systole *(yellow arrow)*. The trace reaches the baseline during diastole *(red arrow)*, which confirms systolic shortening and local diastolic elongation, respectively. The corresponding velocity color coding is superimposed in real time on the 2D image *(top left)*. Size of the region of interest: 5 mm/3 mm. *AVC,* Aortic valve closing; *AVO,* aortic valve opening; *LA,* left atrium; *LV,* left ventricle. (Photo credit: Valérie Chetboul.)

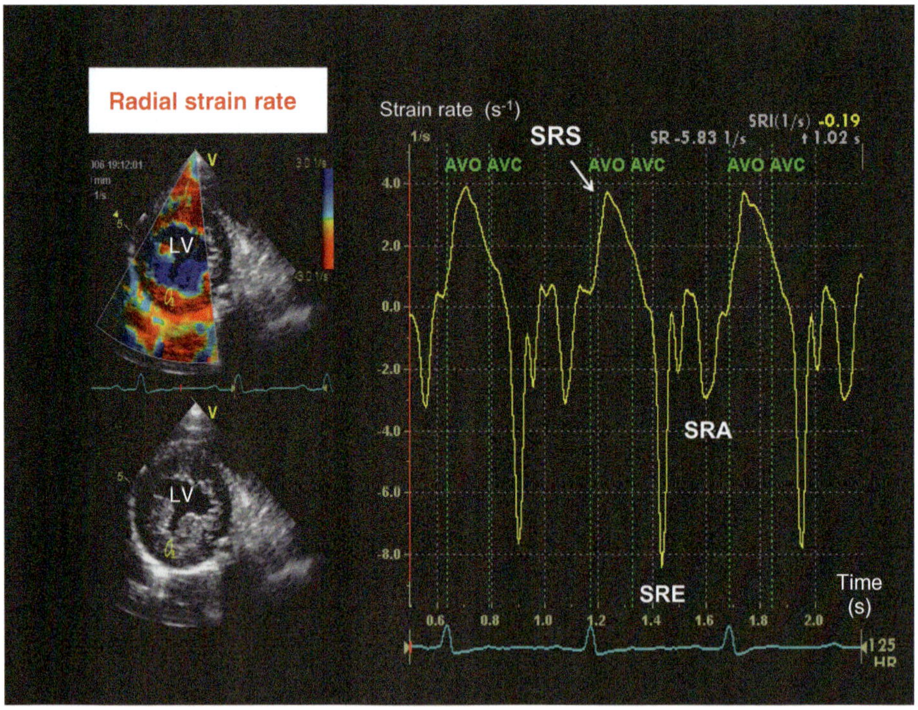

• **Fig. 4-21** Analysis of the longitudinal segmental deformation velocity of the left ventricular free wall in a dog using normal strain rate imaging from the left apical 4 chambers view (bidimensional [2D] image at *bottom left*). The velocity of radial deformation (or strain rate, s^{-1}) is positive during systole (SRS), which indicates local thickening. It is subsequently characterized by two negative diastolic peaks at the beginning of ventricular filling (SRE) and during atrial contraction (SRA), corresponding to a two-stage thinning, faster in early diastole than in end-diastole. The color coding of deformation velocity is superimposed in real time on the 2D image *(top left)*. Size of the region of interest: 5 mm/3 mm. *AVC,* Aortic valve closing; *AVO,* aortic valve opening; *LV,* left ventricle. (Photo credit: Valérie Chetboul.)

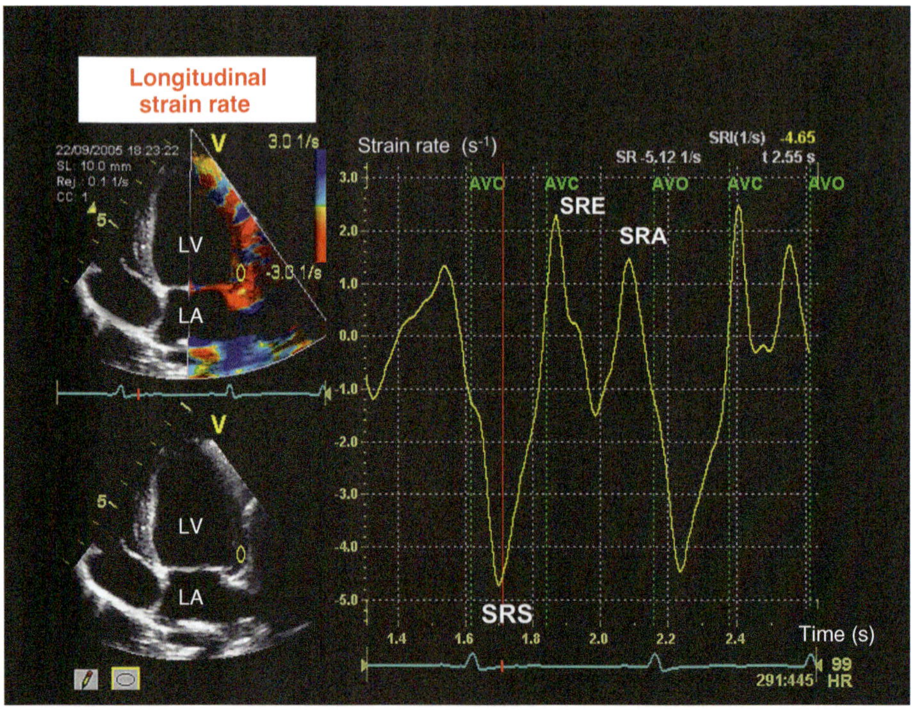

• **Fig. 4-22** Analysis of the longitudinal segmental deformation velocity of the left ventricular free wall in a dog using normal strain rate imaging from the left apical 4 chambers view (bidimensional [2D] image at *bottom left*). The longitudinal deformation velocity (or strain rate, s^{-1}) is inversed compared to the one in Figure 4-21, thus negative during systole (SRS), which indicates a local shortening. It is subsequently characterized by two positive diastolic peaks at the beginning of ventricular filling (SRE) and during atrial contraction (SRA), corresponding to a two-stage elongation, faster in early diastole than in end-diastole. Deformation velocity color coding is superimposed in real time on the 2D image *(top left)*. Size of the region of interest: 5 mm/3 mm. *AVC,* Aortic valve closing; *AVO,* aortic valve opening; *LA,* left atrium; *LV,* left ventricle. (Photo credit: Valérie Chetboul.)

aspect of strain imaging and strain rate imaging curves is shown in Figures 4-19 to 4-22 for the radial and longitudinal motion of the left ventricular free wall. Peak systolic strain is usually end-systolic, occurring just before the end of the aortic valve closing (see Figures 4-19 and 4-20). The peak systolic strain rate usually occurs in mid-systole (see Figures 4-21 and 4-22).

These deformation indices present a major advantage: the process of subtracting one velocity from the other eliminates the translational motions of the heart (Figure 4-23), as does the calculation of the velocity gradients in TDI (see above "Concepts underlying TDI-derived parameters"). Therefore only active or intrinsic motions of the myocardium are considered. In humans as well as in various animal models of myocardial ischemia, these indices (especially peak systolic strain and strain rate) often prove to be more discriminating than classical TDI parameters for the appreciation of myocardial viability after an ischemic accident, the assessment of myocardial function, or walls synchronism [18,50-54].

Among the limitations of these techniques, especially for strain rate, we note that the variability of this parameter directly depends on those of two velocities (VA and VB). This explains that strain rate imaging characterizes itself by a signal/noise report lower than the TDI signal (Figure 4-24). By increasing the size of the region of interest, the signal/noise ratio can nevertheless be improved; the signal is, in fact, higher in this case because the difference between VA and VB increases (due to the underlying radial and longitudinal motion physiologic gradient). For this reason, the size of the chosen regions of interest in strain rate imaging and even in strain imaging is often superior to the one used with the TDI technique.

Just like TDI, strain imaging and strain rate imaging are Doppler techniques and therefore have the drawback of depending on the angle between the ultrasound beam and the motion vector of the myocardium segment under examination.

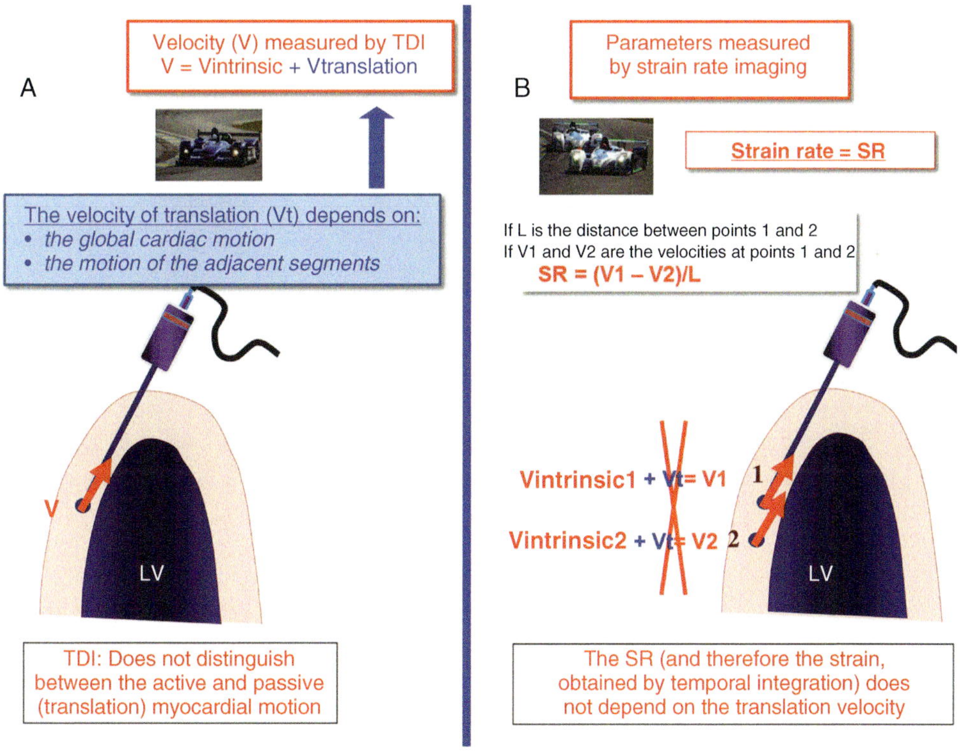

• **Fig. 4-23** Comparison of the principles of tissue Doppler imaging (TDI) and deformation techniques (example of strain rate imaging). A, TDI technique consists of analyzing local myocardial velocity as a function of time. This velocity is the sum of the intrinsic velocity of the analyzed segment (active motion) and the velocity of translation (Vt) associated with passive motions, called myocardial translation (due to the global heart motion in the thorax and stretching by adjacent segments). Therefore TDI does not allow differentiation between active motion associated with the intrinsic function of the myocardium and passive motion. B, On the other hand, strain rate (SR) is defined as the velocities gradient divided by distance. By process of subtraction of the two velocities, the translation passive velocity cancels itself. Therefore strain rate only takes into account active (or intrinsic) motion of the myocardial segments. If these do not have any intrinsic motion, SR equals zero. *LV,* Left ventricle. (Photo credit: Valérie Chetboul.)

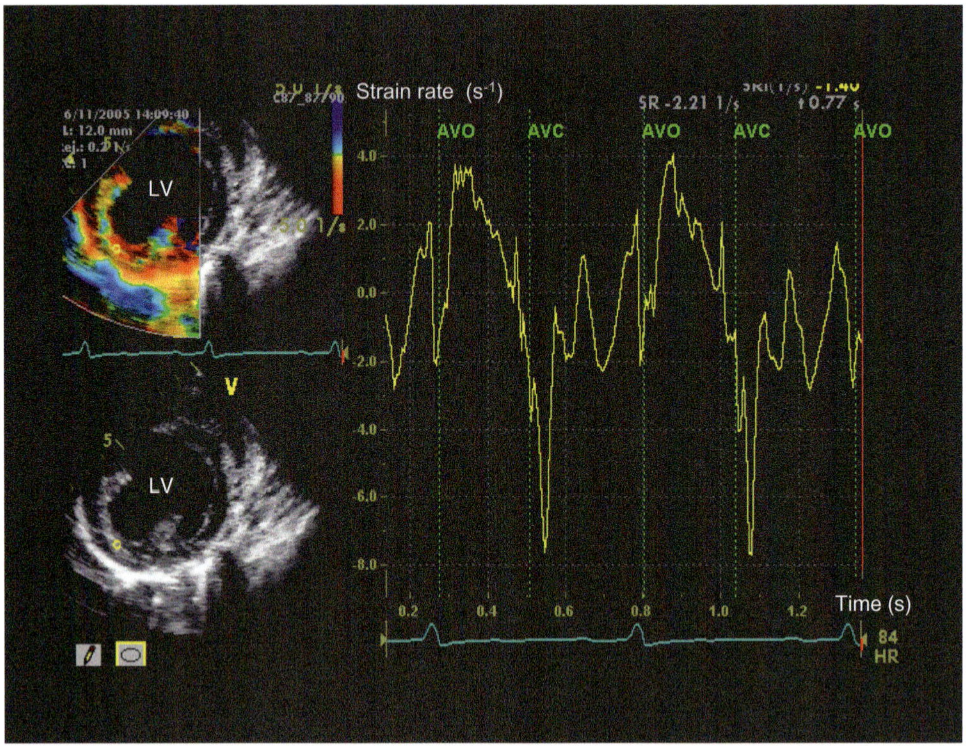

• **Fig. 4-24** Signal/noise ratio of the strain rate imaging. This figure shows the analysis of the radial segmental deformation velocity of the left ventricular free wall in a normal dog by strain rate imaging (left apical 4 chambers view; bidimensional [2D] image at *bottom left*). It is the same animal and same size of the region of interest as in Figure 4-8 (showing the myocardial velocity curve as a function of time). Notice the hatched aspect of the curve obtained in strain rate mode, which is not the case with the tissue Doppler imaging (TDI) technique (characterized by a higher signal/noise ratio). *AVC,* Aortic valve closing; *AVO,* aortic valve opening; *LV,* left ventricle. (Photo credit: Valérie Chetboul.)

Finally, strain imaging and strain rate imaging require the highest caution when interpreting the values obtained. In fact, these techniques are subject to a number of artifacts, especially stationary reverberation artifacts (Figure 4-25), potentially leading to normal myocardial segments that falsely appear akinetic or dyskinetic. The possibility of using the "tracking" function, allowing the region of interest to follow the myocardial wall during its displacement, is particularly useful to prevent its superposition with the reverberation areas.

Because of these limitations, it is easy to understand that strain imaging and strain rate imaging techniques require specialized training for clips acquisition and their postprocessing.

Strain imaging and strain rate imaging are emerging techniques in veterinary cardiology [55-58]. The repeatability (intraday variation) and reproducibility (interday variation) of the systolic strain and strain rate, of both the left and the right ventricular free wall (at the base and apex), were studied in the awake dog for the first time by our team in 2006 [55]. For the trained user, all CVs were satisfactory (less than 15%). A study conducted on 30 healthy dogs allowed us to conclude that, as in humans, the absolute value of the

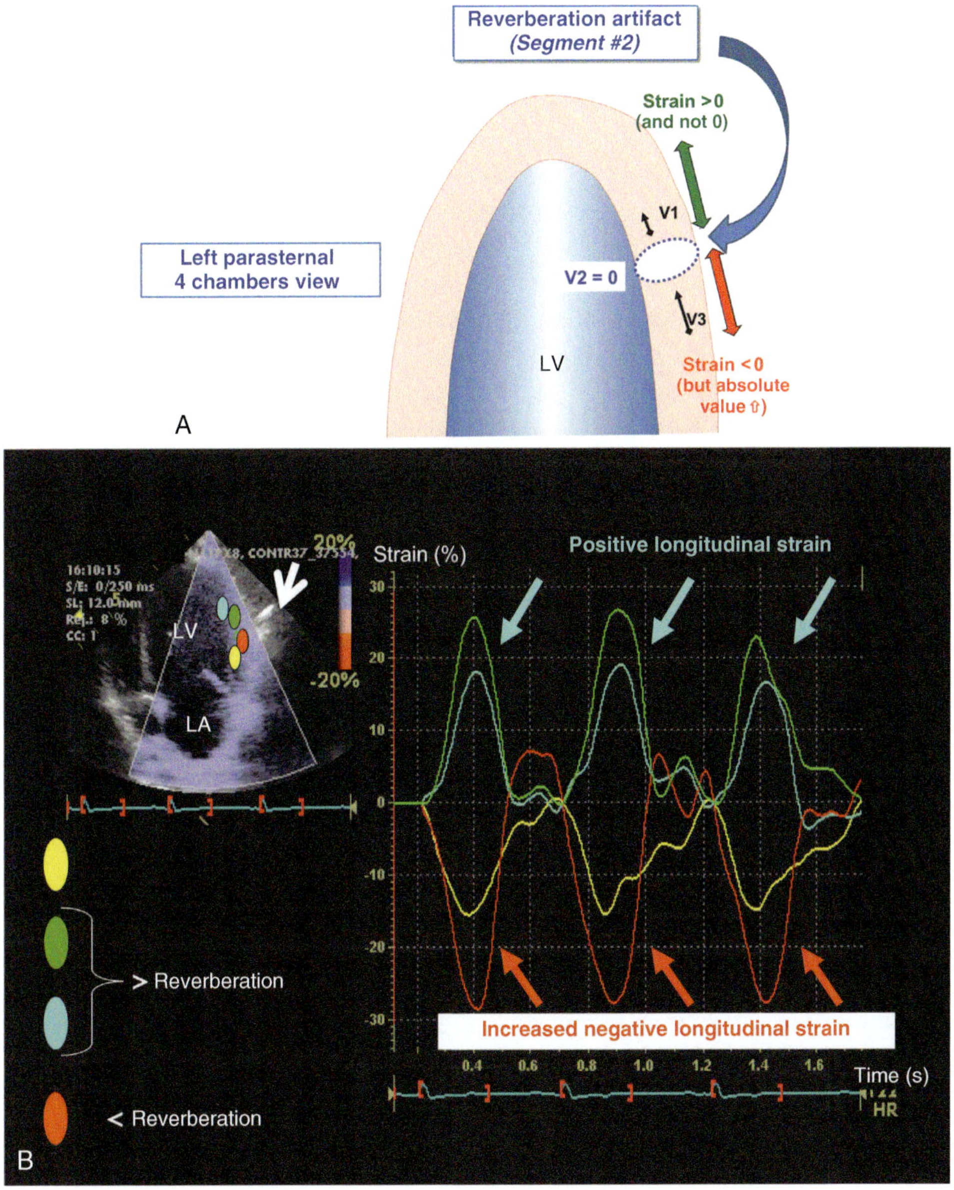

• **Fig. 4-25** Reverberation artifacts and their consequences on deformation techniques (strain and strain rate imaging). The acoustic reverberation artifacts appear on the bidimensional (2D) grayscale image in the form of hyperechoic motionless structures (therefore null intrinsic velocity). They result from one or more back-and-forth reflections of echoes between two interfaces with strong acoustic impedance in the proximal region (most often the thoracic wall). The resulting image thus appears distally. A, Let us assume three myocardial points on the left ventricular free wall (V1, V2, and V3, from the apex to the base). Let us further assume that there is a stationary reverberation artifact at V2 (left apical 4 chambers view). This artifact is characterized by its absence of motion (velocity at V2 therefore equals 0 in an "artifactual" way). The strain rate (SR) directly depends on the difference between two velocities and the velocities are increasing from the apex to the base (base-apex gradient). Therefore above the reverberation (e.g., segment between V1 and V2) the systolic strain rate will be positive and not negative, because of the difference (V1 – V2), with V2 = 0 and V1 positive. Inversely, underneath the reverberation zone (e.g., segment between V3 and V2) the strain rate will be negative and of higher absolute value because it depends on (V2 – V3), with V2 = 0 and V3 positive. The reasoning is similar for the strain values calculated by strain imaging. B, The hyperechoic reverberation artifact is indicated by the white arrow on the left apical 4 chambers view. Above this reverberation area ("anterior" part of the screen), the strain curves (*green* and *blue*) are positive (instead of negative: see Figure 4-20), mimicking parietal dyskinesia. Underneath the reverberation area ("posterior" part of the screen), the strain curves (*yellow* and *red*) are negative (with high absolute values for the *red curve*), mimicking hyperkinesia. *LA, Left atrium; LV, left ventricle*. (Photo credit: Valérie Chetboul.)

longitudinal systolic deformation indices was higher for the right ventricular wall than for the left one. It was also greater for the left radial motion than for the left longitudinal motion (Tables 4-5 and 4-6). Radial and left longitudinal myocardial systolic deformation impairment was shown to be associated with dilated canine cardiomyopathy [56]. As with cats, strain imaging was recently used to show longitudinal function impairment associated with hypertrophic cardiomyopathy [58].

TABLE 4-5 Left Ventricular Wall Systolic Radial Deformation Indices Calculated by Strain Imaging and Strain Rate Imaging in 30 Healthy Dogs of Different Breeds [55]

			Correlations		
	Values	Min-Max	Age (Years)	Heart Rate (bpm)	Shortening Fraction (%)
Peak systolic strain (%)	62.9 ± 10.4	45.3-87.0	NS	NS	0.47 (p = 0.008)
Time to peak systolic strain (ms)	228 ± 41	155-328	NS	−0.42 (p = 0.004)	NS
Peak systolic strain rate (s^{-1})	5.8 ± 1.1	3.5-8.2	NS	NS	0.39 (p = 0.032)

NS, Not statistically significant.

Indices include peak systolic strain (%), time to peak systolic strain (ms), and peak systolic strain rate (s^{-1}), expressed in mean ± standard deviation (SD) and minimum and maximum values (Min-max). The Pearson correlation coefficient is also indicated when the correlation with age, heart rate, and shortening fraction is statistically significant. Note: Unpublished data, established with a GE Vivid 5.

TABLE 4-6 Longitudinal Systolic Deformation Indices Calculated by Strain Imaging and Strain Rate Imaging at the Base and Apex of the Left Ventricular Free Wall, Interventricular Septum, and Right Ventricular Wall in 30 Healthy Dogs of Different Breeds [55]

			Correlations		
	Values	Min-Max	Age	Heart Rate (bpm)	Shortening Fraction (%)
Left Ventricle Free Wall					
Peak systolic strain (base) (%)	−25.5 ± 3.6	−34.8 - −18.8	NS	0.39 (p = 0.032)	NS
Time to peak systolic strain (base) (ms)	234 ± 57	107-374	NS	−0.51 (p = 0.004)	NS
Peak systolic strain rate at (base) (s^{-1})	−3.1 ± 0.7	−4.9 - −2.1	NS	NS	NS
Peak systolic strain (apex) (%)	−23.2 ± 4.0[a]	−36.5 - −17.3	NS	0.43 (p = 0.017)	NS
Time to peak systolic strain (apex) (ms)	192 ± 61	87-313	NS	−0.43 (p = 0.017)	NS
Peak systolic strain rate peak (apex) (s^{-1})	−2.6 ± 0.8[a]	−4.4 - −1.4	NS	NS	NS
Interventricular Septum					
Peak systolic strain (base) (%)	−24.5 ± 3.2	−30.8 - −17.2	NS	NS	NS
Time to peak systolic peak strain (base) (ms)	210 ± 49	118-303	NS	NS	NS
Peak systolic strain rate peak (base) (s^{-1})	−2.6 ± 0.6[b]	−3.7 - −1.7	NS	0.60 (p = 0.001)	NS
Peak systolic strain peak (apex) (%)	−22.9 ± 2.7[a]	−28.8 - −17.5	NS	0.45 (p = 0.017)	NS
Time to peak systolic strain peak (apex) (ms)	219 ± 41	123-303	NS	NS	NS
Peak systolic strain rate peak (apex) (s^{-1})	−2.2 ± 0.6[a]	−3.5 - −1.2	NS	−0.47 (p = 0.013)	NS
Right Ventricular Wall					
Peak systolic strain peak (base) (%)	−39.5 ± 5.5[b,c]	−50.2 - −29.5	NS	NS	NS
Time to peak systolic peak strain (base) (ms)	223 ± 56	126-346	NS	NS	NS
Peak systolic strain rate peak (base) (s^{-1})	−5.2 ± 0.8[b,c]	−7.1 - −4.0	NS	NS	NS
Peak systolic strain (apex) (%)	−36.3 ± 4.3[a,b,c]	−45.7 - −28.4	NS	NS	−0.44 (p = 0.020)
Time to peak systolic strain (apex) (ms)	198 ± 46	67-228	NS	NS	NS
Peak systolic strain rate (apex) (s^{-1})	−4.7 ± 1.1[a,b,c]	−7.1 - −2.7	NS	NS	NS

NS, Not statistically significant.

Indices include peak systolic strain (%), time to peak systolic strain (ms), and peak systolic strain rate (s^{-1}), expressed in mean ± standard deviation (SD) and in minimum and maximum values (Min-max). The Pearson correlation coefficient is indicated when the correlation with age, heart rate, and shortening fraction is statistically significant. Note: Unpublished data, established with a GE Vivid 5.

[a]p <0.01 versus corresponding value at the base.

[b]p <0.001 versus corresponding value in the left ventricle free wall.

[c]p <0.001 versus corresponding value in the interventricular septum.

Speckle Tracking Imaging

"Speckle tracking" echocardiography (speckle tracking imaging, currently marketed as 2D-strain or VVI) is the most recently developed ultrasound technique to simultaneously assess regional myocardial function in multiple segments. This technique identifies and then tracks over a period of time the motion of the "small white spots" or "speckles" visible within the myocardium in classical 2D echocardiography mode (Figures 4-26 and 4-27) [59-63]. These speckles appear as small bright echoes homogeneously distributed throughout the myocardium. They result from reflection, dispersion, and interference between the tissue and the ultrasound beam on the 2D image. In a sense, they represent the natural acoustic signature of the myocardial tissue that can be followed from one frame to another throughout the cardiac cycle. By following these random speckles while completing autocorrelations to take into account the movement of the stable structures, different motion parameters (motion velocity, distance, strain, and strain rate) can be determined simultaneously in different segments, with real-time color coding and graphic representation of values as a function of time (Figures 4-28 to 4-35 and Videos 4-1 and 4-2).

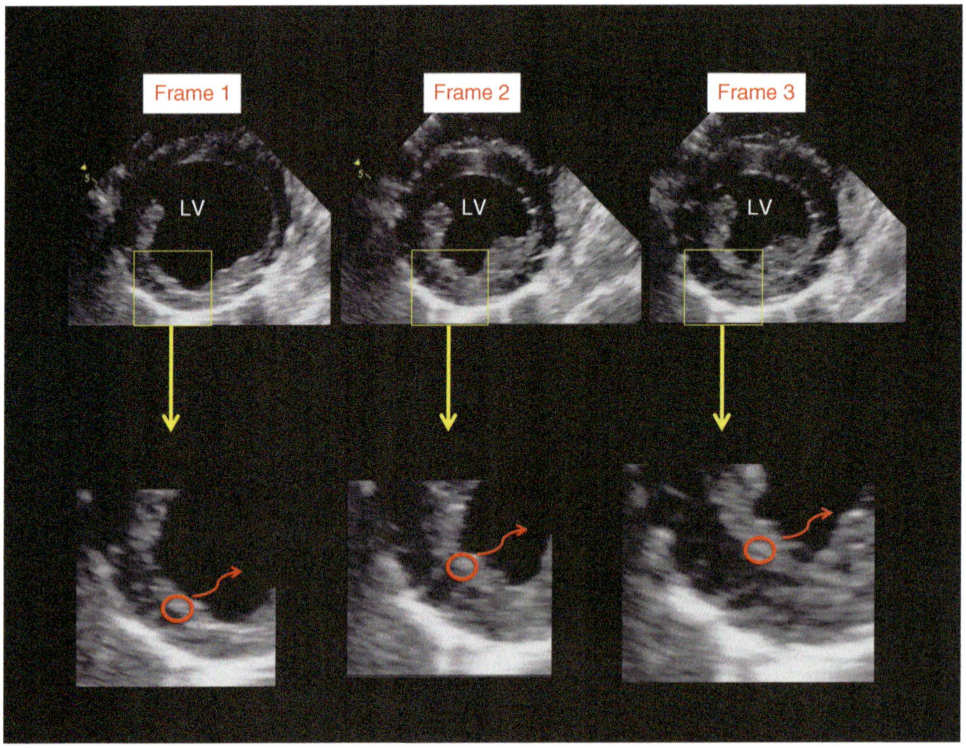

• **Fig. 4-26** Illustration of the principle of speckle tracking imaging. The top three pictures show a right parasternal short axis transventricular view in bidimensional (2D) mode, obtained in end-diastole (Frame 1), mid-systole (Frame 2), and end-systole (Frame 3). As illustrated in the three bottom pictures, the ultrasonic speckle tracking imaging technique consists of following over a period of time ("tracking") the small hyperechoic elements (or "speckles") that constitute the myocardial tissue from the 2D grayscale image. These "speckles" are actual imprints of the myocardium, which can be tracked in their displacements; the latter are then reconstituted using a mathematical model. *LV,* Left ventricle. (Photo credit: Valérie Chetboul.)

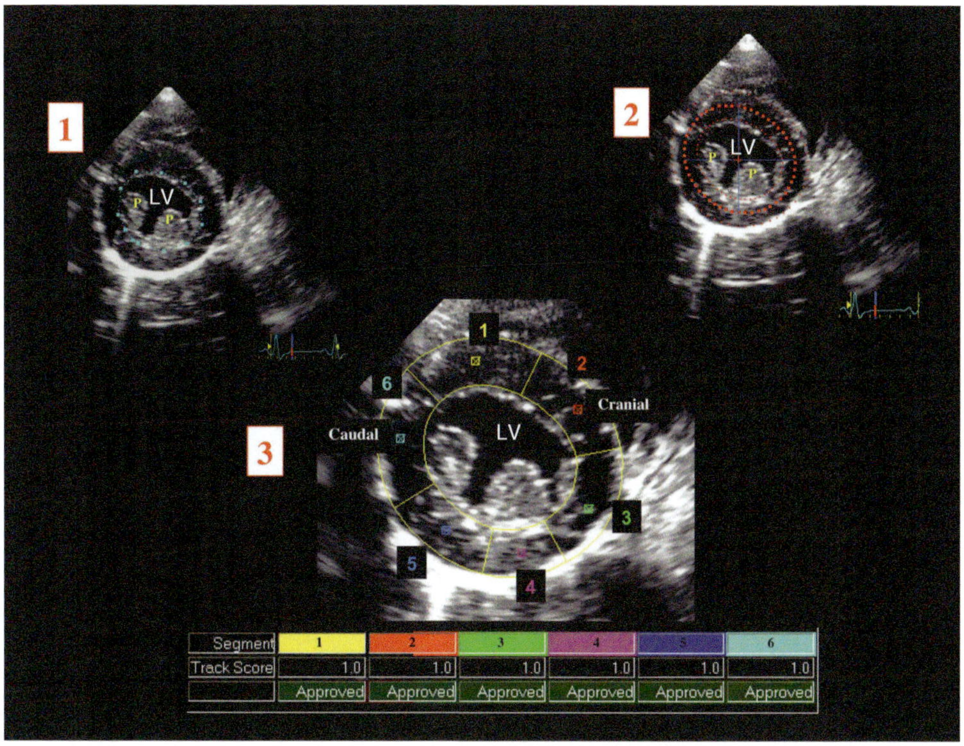

• **Fig. 4-27** The three initial steps necessary to performing speckle tracking imaging: example of analysis of the left ventricular radial motion from the right parasternal short axis transventricular view. The first step (1) consists of delimiting the myocardial outline on the bidimensional (2D) image. Next (2), the software automatically defines the region of interest (ROI), centered on the outline defined in (1), including the interventricular septum and the left ventricular free wall. It is in this ROI that tracking will be performed. The user must set the width so as to include the external myocardial outline. The ROI is then (3) automatically divided into six myocardial segments of equal sizes, numbered 1 to 6, in which tracking analysis will occur independently. *LV,* Left ventricle; *P,* papillary muscles. (Photo credit: Valérie Chetboul.)

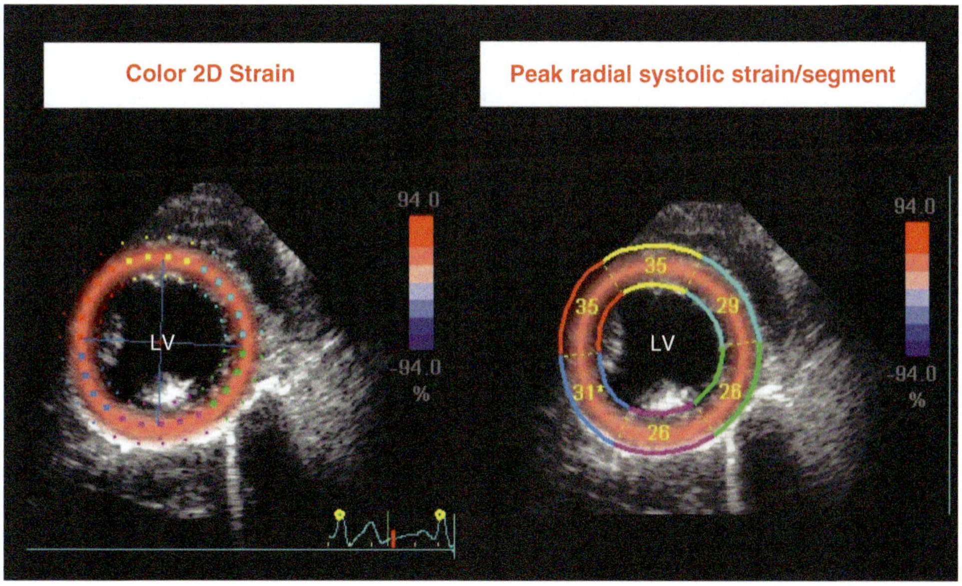

• **Fig. 4-28** Fourth step of speckle tracking imaging: example of analysis of the left ventricular radial strain from the right parasternal short axis transventricular view. During this fourth step, the parameter being analyzed (here, the radial strain, in %) is color coded, this color coding being superimposed on the bidimensional (2D) image *(left)*. The software is also able to obtain, directly on the color 2D mode image, the value of the radial peak systolic strain (here, 26% to 35%) for each of the six segments being examined *(right)*. *LV,* Left ventricle. (Photo credit: Valérie Chetboul.)

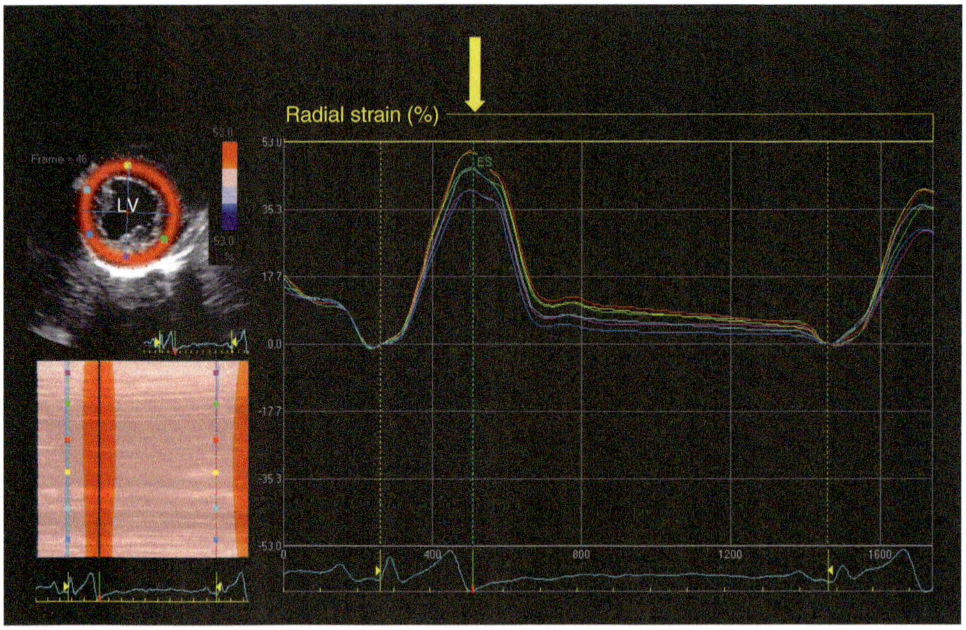

• **Fig. 4-29** Fifth step of speckle tracking imaging: example of analysis of the left ventricular radial strain from the right parasternal short axis transventricular view. This final step consists of obtaining six radial strain tracings (%) as a function of time, recorded in the six myocardial segments defined in Figure 4-27. Note that for this healthy dog the strain of these six segments is homogeneous and synchronized and the peak strain *(yellow arrow)* occurs in end-systole. The color-coded strain is superimposed on the bidimensional (2D) image in real time *(top left)* and displayed as a function of time *(bottom left)*. The aspect of these curves is similar to the one obtained by the method derived from tissue Doppler imaging (see Figure 4-19). *LV,* Left ventricle. (Photo credit: Valérie Chetboul.)

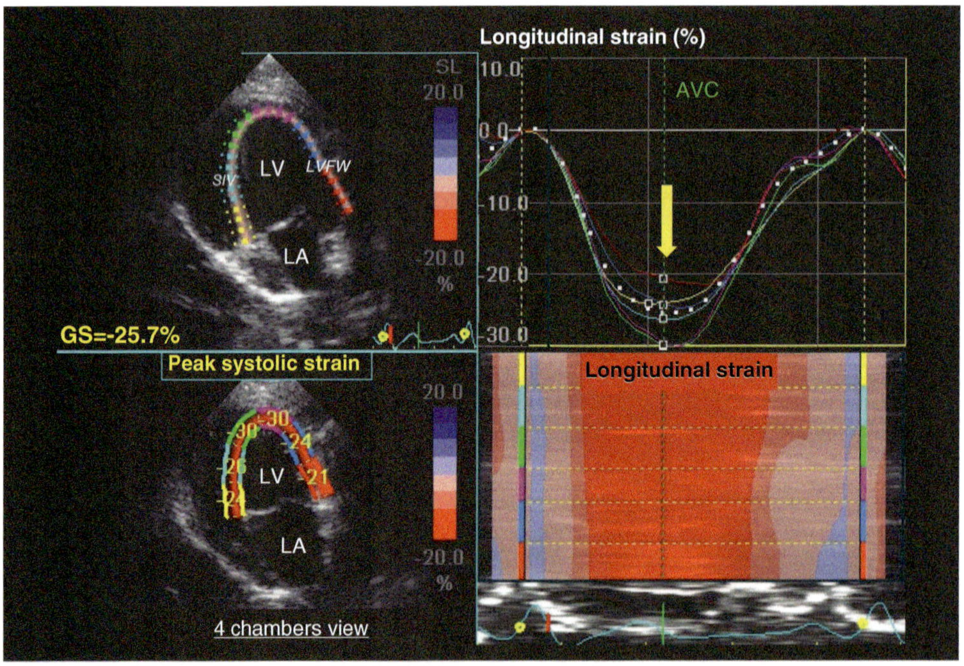

• **Fig. 4-30** Analysis of the left ventricular longitudinal strain from the left apical 4 chambers view. The left ventricular myocardial longitudinal outline was first delimited. This helped to define the region of interest (ROI), including the interventricular septum (IVS) and the left ventricular free wall (LVFW). This ROI was then automatically divided into six myocardial segments of equal size. The color-coded longitudinal strain is superimposed on the bidimensional (2D) image *(top left)* and displayed as a function of time *(bottom right)*. *(Bottom left)* The value of the peak longitudinal systolic strain (here, –21% to –30%) for each of the six segments being examined is superimposed on the color 2D image. The global peak strain (GS), average of the six segment peaks and novel index of global systolic function, is automatically given (–25.7%). Finally, the six curves of longitudinal strain (%) as a function of time are shown *(top right)*. The aspect of these curves is similar to the curve obtained by a method derived from tissue Doppler imaging (see Figure 4-20). The deformation of the six segments is synchronized. For each of them, the nadir—corresponding to the peak of negative deformation *(yellow arrow)*—is obtained in end-systole at the time of the aortic valve closure (AVC). *LA,* Left atrium; *LV,* left ventricle; *LVFW,* left ventricular free wall. (Photo credit: Valérie Chetboul.)

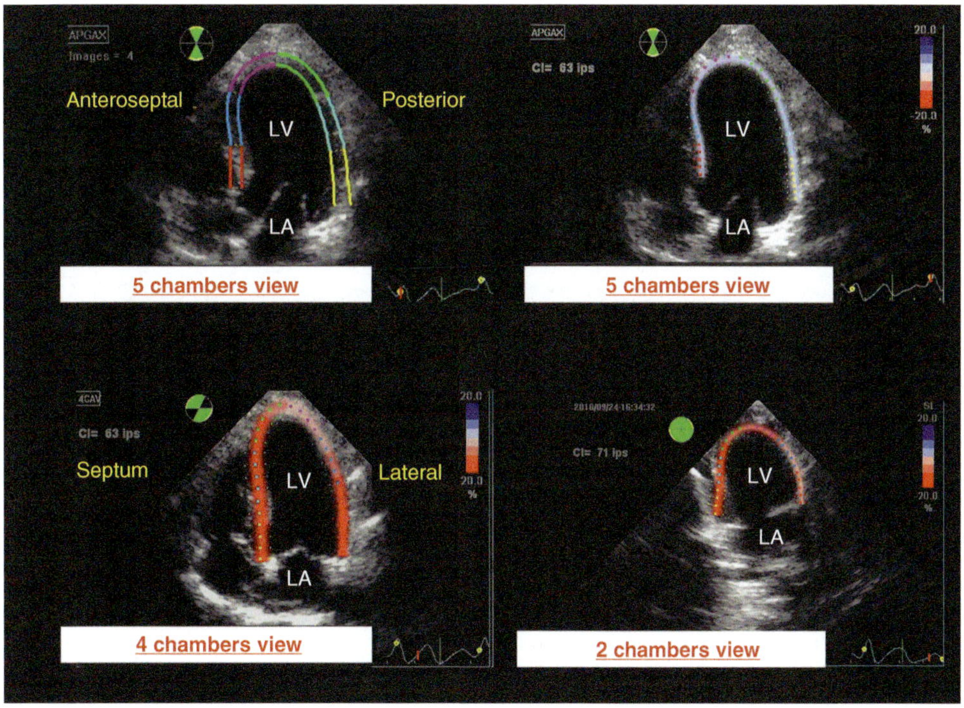

• **Fig. 4-31** Complete analysis of the left ventricular longitudinal strain from the three left apical views, using automated function imaging (AFI). The left ventricular myocardial outline is delimited on the 4 chambers views, as in Figure 4-30. Two additional long axis views are used: the 2 and 5-chambers views. As the *top left* image shows, for each view the region of interest (ROI) is automatically divided into six myocardial segments of equal size. *LA,* Left atrium; *LV*, left ventricle. (Photo credit: Valérie Chetboul.)

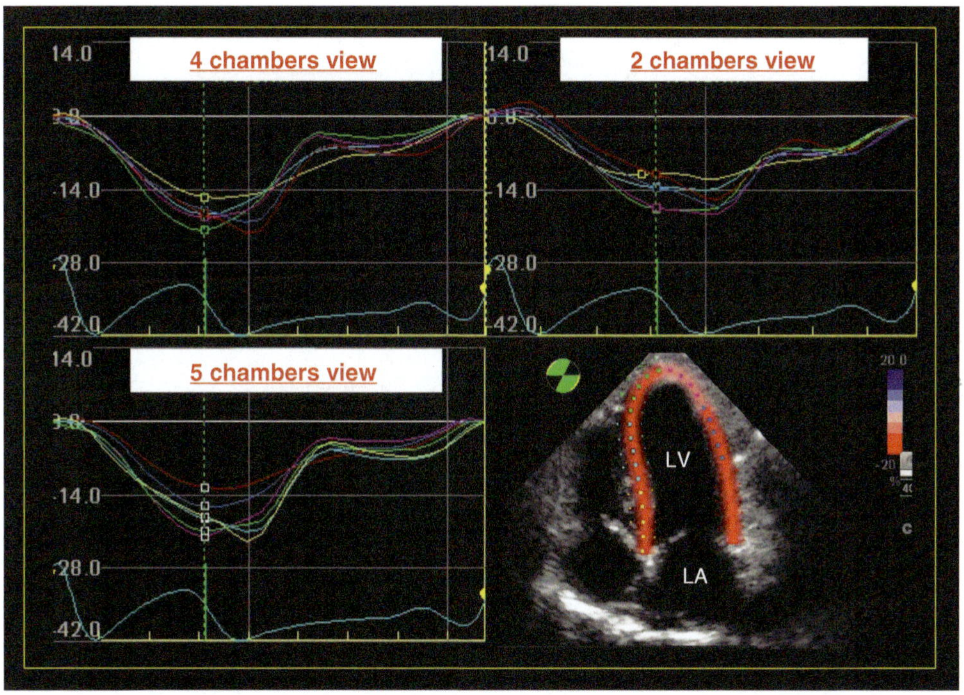

• **Fig. 4-32** Complete analysis of the left ventricular longitudinal strain from the three left apical views defined in Figure 4-31, using automated function imaging (AFI). For each view (2, 4, and 5 chambers), tracings are obtained displaying the longitudinal strain (%) of the six myocardial segments as a function of time. The color-coded strain is superimposed on the bidimensional (2D) 4 chambers view *(bottom right)*. The aspect of the set of curves is similar to the one obtained by a method derived from tissue Doppler imaging (see Figure 4-20). *LA,* Left atrium; *LV,* left ventricle. (Photo credit: Valérie Chetboul.)

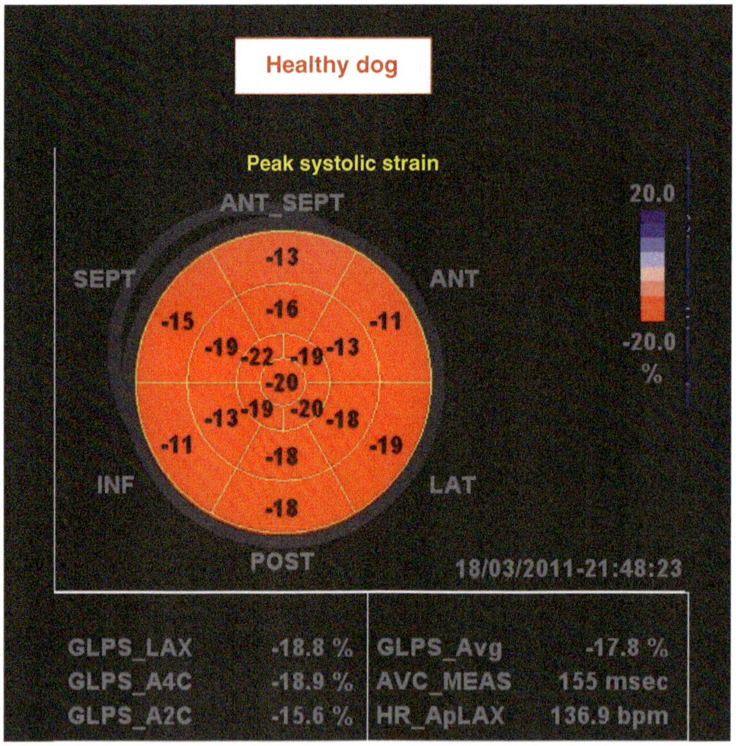

• **Fig. 4-33** Representation of the previous longitudinal left ventricular strain data obtained by automated function imaging (AFI) (see Figures 4-31 and 4-32) with bull's eye mapping. The longitudinal peak strain of the different myocardial segments (18 altogether) is displayed on the same diagram (left ventricle seen from the apex), with color coding of the values. Here, the homogeneous color indicates, at a single glance, perfect longitudinal deformation synchronism. The value of each global strain for the three views being analyzed (2, 4, and 5 chambers) is indicated in the left column (–15.6%, –18.9%, and –18.8%, respectively), the corresponding total global strain (–17.8%) appears in the right column as along with the average heart rate. *ANT*, Anterior segment; *ANT SEPT*, anteroseptal segment; *AP2C*, apical 2 chambers; *AP4C*, apical 4 chambers; *AVC meas,* aortic valve closure measurement; *GLPS*, global peak systolic strain; *HR_ApLAX*, heart rate during the acquisition of the apical long axis view; *INF*, inferior segment; *LAT*, lateral segment; *LAX*, long axis; *POST*, posterior segment; *SEPT*, septal segment. (Photo credit: Valérie Chetboul.)

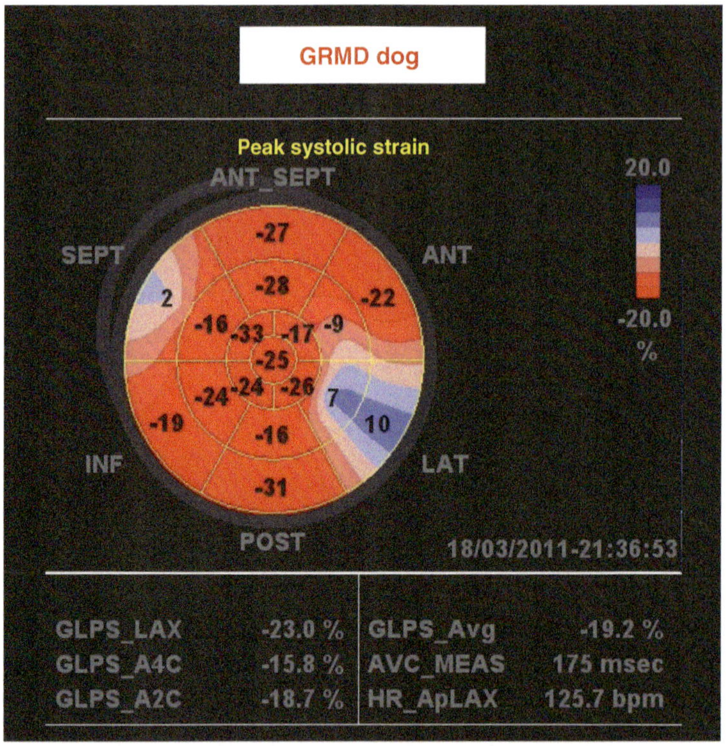

• **Fig. 4-34** Example of asynchronism detected by automated function imaging (AFI) with bull's eye mapping. In this 4-month-old myopathic Golden Retriever with a mutation of the gene coding for dystrophin (GRMD, or Golden Retriever muscular dystrophy), conventional echocardiography still did not reveal any abnormality. However, multiple myocardial segments of the interventricular septum and left ventricular wall appeared coded in blue, already revealing the presence of segmental dyskinesia, their longitudinal strain being positive (and not negative like other normal segments). *ANT*, Anterior segment; *ANT SEPT*, anteroseptal segment; *AP2C*, apical 2 chambers; *AP4C*, apical 4 chambers; *AVC meas,* aortic valve closure measurement; *GLPS*, global peak systolic strain; *HR_ApLAX*, heart rate during the acquisition of the apical long axis view; *INF*, inferior segment; *LAT*, lateral segment; *LAX*, long axis; *POST*, posterior segment; *SEPT*, septal segment. (Photo credit: Valérie Chetboul.)

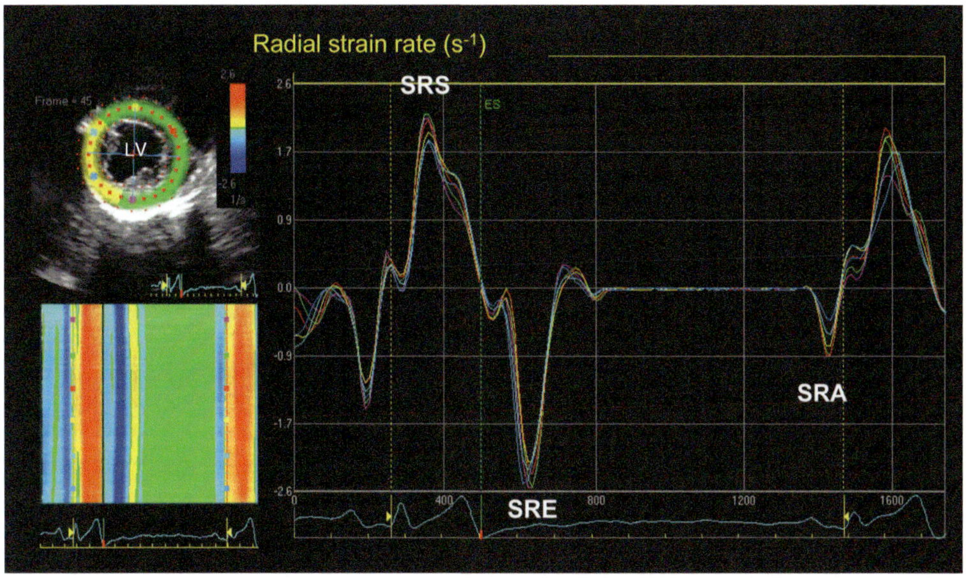

• **Fig. 4-35** Example of analysis of the radial strain rate by speckle tracking imaging in a healthy dog (from the right parasternal short axis transventricular view). For this analysis, the first three steps are the same as the ones described in Figure 4-27, with delimitation of six equidistant myocardial segments in the interventricular septum and the left ventricle free wall. The image on the right shows the six corresponding curves of radial strain rate (in s^{-1}) as a function of time. The aspect of the curve is similar to the one obtained by the method derived from tissue Doppler imaging (see Figure 4-21), including a positive peak during systole (SRS) and two negative diastolic peaks (SRE and SRA). The color-coded strain rate is superimposed in real time on the bidimensional (2D) image *(top left)* and displayed as a function of time *(bottom left)*. *LV,* Left ventricle. (Photo credit: Valérie Chetboul.)

The degree of basal and apical rotation also can be determined from the right parasternal transmitral and transapical short axis views (Table 4-7, Figures 4-36 to 4-38) [5]. Note that the automated function imaging (AFI) system is a tool for semiautomatic analysis based on the speckle tracking imaging technique. AFI allows a complete analysis of the left ventricle longitudinal function, with a bullseye view of segmental systolic strains. To accomplish this, three different views are used: the left apical 2, 4, and 5 chambers views (see Figures 4-31 to 4-34). Each analyzed segment corresponds to a different coronary territory. A global longitudinal strain index can be deduced from it (Video 4-3).

Speckle tracking imaging is based on grayscale imagery. Unlike TDI and its derived techniques, it allows a "non-Doppler" assessment of the local motion of the myocardium. Therefore one of its main advantages is its independence from both the cardiac displacement movement and the ultrasound angle, unlike Doppler techniques.

In 2007 our team showed that speckle tracking imaging is a repeatable and reproducible technique in the awake dog for the radial deformation assessment (strain) and the radial deformation velocity (strain rate) of the left ventricular free wall [63]. In addition, in the healthy dog these measurements are well correlated to the ones obtained by strain imaging and strain rate imaging Doppler techniques [63]. This correlation was also found by other authors in healthy dogs for the interventricular septum longitudinal motion [57]. However, the correlation is not as good for the longitudinal motion of the left ventricular free wall [57]. At this time we still do not know which of these techniques is the most sensitive for the detection of a systolic myocardial dysfunction in animals, diastolic function being probably best assessed by TDI.

Another study performed by our group in 2008, showed that speckle tracking imaging also allowed a noninvasive, repeatable, and reproducible assessment of left ventricular systolic rotation in the awake dog (see Table 4-7 and Figures 4-36 to 4-38) [5]. The basal and apical systolic rotations of the left ventricle and global systolic torsion (defined by the relative rotation of the apex compared to the base) thus represent new parameters of the myocardial function that can be altered in a number of pathologic processes such as dilated cardiomyopathy [5]. Similar alterations of the left ventricular systolic torsion were identified in humans in numerous cardiopathies (cardiomyopathy and myocardial infarction) and could contribute to a certain extent to the reduction of the systolic stroke volume associated with these pathologic conditions [61,62].

Despite its advantages, speckle tracking imaging presents a number of technical limitations, including for example the impossibility of obtaining reliable measurements when reverberation artifacts or shadowed areas are

TABLE 4-7 **Parameters of Left Ventricle Rotation (Base, Apex) Calculated by Speckle Tracking Imaging in 35 Healthy Dogs of Different Breeds [5]**

	Mean ± SD (Min-Max)	
	Beginning of Systole	**End of Systole**
Apical Rotation		
Heart rate during TDI exam (bpm)	107 ± 27 (66-179)	
Peak apical rotation (°)	−1.6 ± 0.8[b] (−3.4 - −0.4)	5.4 ± 3.2[b] (1.0-12.9)
Time to peak apical rotation (ms)	70 ± 22[b] (34-126)	189 ± 36[b] (99-280)
Basal Rotation		
Peak basal rotation (°)	3.9 ± 2.8 (0.2-10.7)	−3.1 ± 1.3 (−5.5 - −1.0)
Time to peak basal rotation (ms)	113 ± 45 (26-177)	261 ± 43 (136-354)
Twist (°)[a] at end-systole		8.4 ± 3.8 (2.5-18)
Heart rate during TDI exam (bpm)		107 ± 29 (68-189)

TDI, Tissue Doppler imaging.
Values are expressed in mean ± standard deviation (SD) and minimum-maximum (Min-max).
[a]Defined as the absolute value of the difference (peak of basal rotation in end-systole – peak of apical rotation in end-systole).
[b]p <0.001 versus the corresponding value at the base.

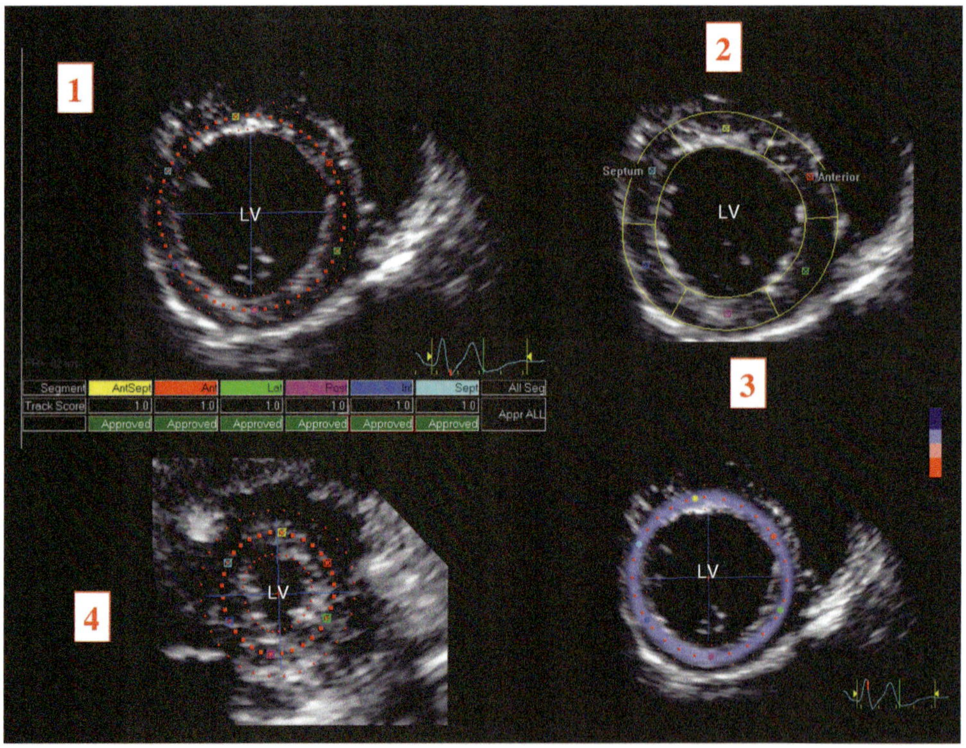

• **Fig. 4-36** Principles of analysis of the left ventricular basal and apical rotation by speckle tracking imaging. For this analysis the first three steps are the same as the ones described in Figure 4-27. The right parasternal transmitral short axis is used to study the rotation of the left ventricular base. After delimitation of the endocardial outline, a region of interest (ROI) is defined, including six equidistant myocardial segments in the septum and the left ventricular free wall (panels 1 and 2). Panel 3 shows the color coding of the rotation (in degrees) superimposed on the bidimensional (2D) image. The same process is applied to the right parasternal transapical short axis view (panel 4) to study the left ventricular apical rotation, going in the opposite direction of that of the base. *LV*, Left ventricle. (Photo credit: Valérie Chetboul.)

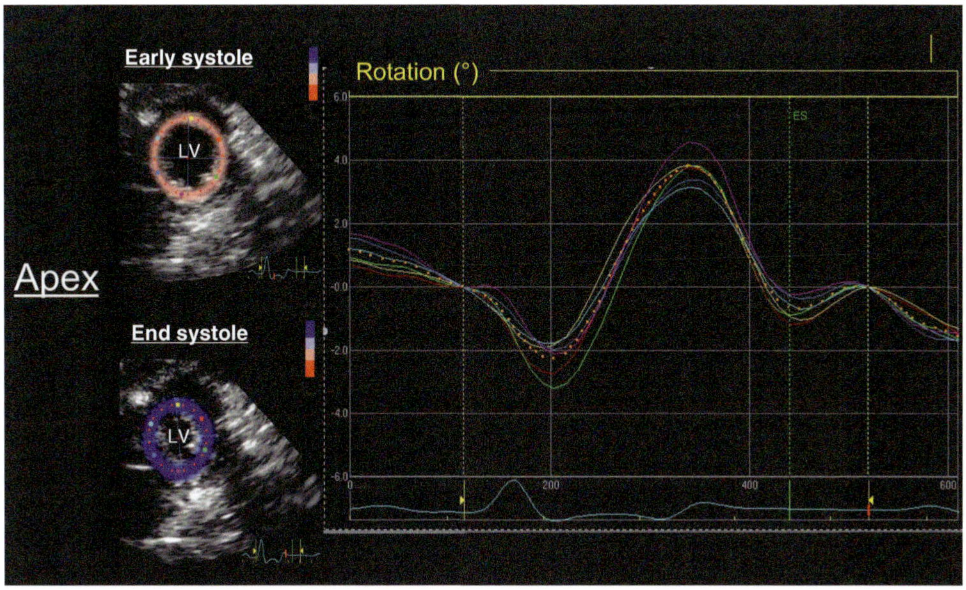

• **Fig. 4-37** Example of analysis of the left ventricular apical rotation by speckle tracking imaging in a healthy dog. The apical rotation is analyzed in six equidistant segments of the interventricular septum and the left ventricular free wall from the right parasternal transapical short axis view. The figure on the right shows the six corresponding curves of rotation as a function of time and the dotted orange line corresponds to the average rotation curve of the six segments as a function of time. Viewed from the apex, the six myocardial segments undergo a homogeneous systolic torsion, starting with a clockwise rotation (negative rotation), followed by a more pronounced counterclockwise rotation (positive rotation). This dual motion is confirmed by color coding of the rotation superimposed in real time on the bidimensional (2D) images *(left)*, showing a clockwise rotation *(red)* at the beginning of systole and a counterclockwise rotation *(blue)* in end-systole. *LV,* Left ventricle. (Photo credit: Valérie Chetboul.)

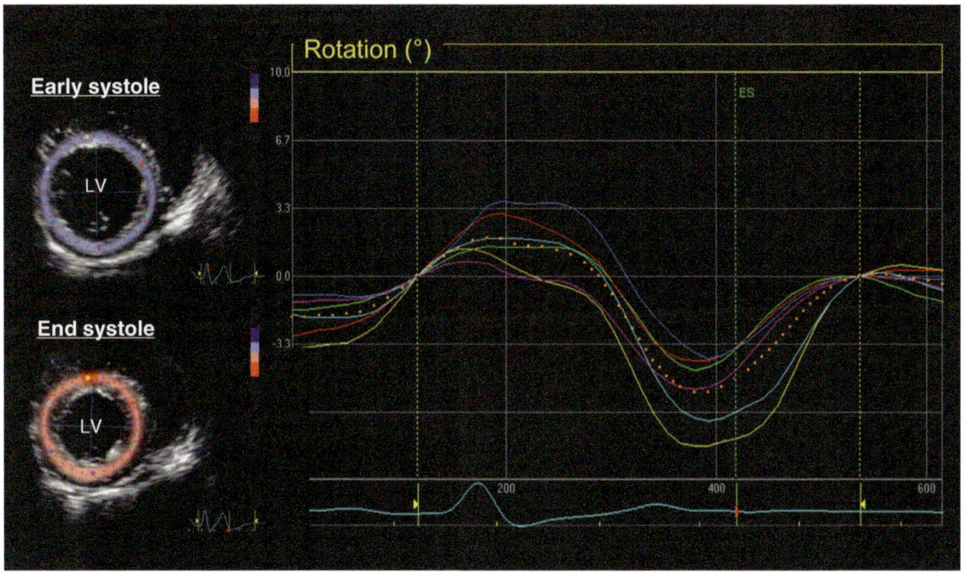

• **Fig. 4-38** Example of analysis of the left ventricular basal rotation by speckle tracking imaging in a healthy dog (same animal as in Figure 4-36). Basal rotation is analyzed in six equidistant segments of the interventricular septum and the left ventricle free wall from the right parasternal transmitral short axis view. The figure on the right shows the six corresponding curves of rotation as a function of time and the dotted orange line corresponds to the average rotation curve of the six segments as a function of time. Viewed from the apex, the six myocardial segments undergo a homogeneous systolic torsion, starting with a rotation in the counterclockwise direction (positive rotation), followed by a more pronounced clockwise rotation (negative rotation). This dual motion, inverse to the apical motion, is confirmed by the color coding of the rotation superimposed in real time on the bidimensional (2D) images *(left)*, showing a counterclockwise rotation *(blue)* at the beginning of systole and a clockwise rotation *(red)* in end-systole. *LV,* Left ventricle. (Photo credit: Valérie Chetboul.)

present on the 2D image used. In addition, when using short axis views, the myocardial longitudinal motion can cause speckles to move into or out of the image plane, thus decreasing the reliability and possibility of their tracking.

Conclusion

One of the most recent and significant advances in cardiac ultrasound imaging has been the emergence of TDI, a noninvasive and precise quantification technique of segmental myocardial kinetics. The superior sensitivity of TDI, compared to conventional echocardiography, in both the prognosis and the diagnosis of local myocardial deterioration can no longer be denied, making TDI a powerful tool for cardiovascular research. One can bet that speckle tracking imaging, an even more recent technique that uses grayscale imaging (independent of the angle between the ultrasound beam and the motion under analysis), will "popularize" myocardial function parameters such as strain and systolic strain rate, which have the advantage of better reflecting intrinsic myocardial function. New studies on large groups of animals with heart disease are necessary to determine the comparative diagnostic benefit of these new imaging techniques and their potential additional value for establishing a prognosis and making therapeutic decisions.

REFERENCES

[1] Sosnovik DE, Wang R, Dai G, et al. Diffusion MR tractography of the heart. J Cardiovasc Magn Reson 2009;11:47.

[2] Streeter DD, Hanna WT. Engineering mechanics for successive states in canine left ventricular myocardium: II. Fiber angle and sarcomere length. Circ Res 1973;33:656–64.

[3] LeGrice IJ, Smaill BH, Chai LZ, et al. Laminar structure of the heart: ventricular myocyte arrangement and connective tissue architecture in the dog. Am J Physiol 1995;269:H571–82.

[4] Lunkenheimer PP, Redmann K, Kling N, et al. Three-dimensional architecture of the left ventricular myocardium. Anat Rec A Discov Mol Cell Evol Biol 2006;288:565–78.

[5] Chetboul V, Serres F, Gouni V, et al. Non-invasive assessment of systolic left ventricular torsion by 2-dimensional speckle tracking imaging in the awake dog: repeatability, reproducibility, and comparison with tissue Doppler imaging variables. J Vet Intern Med 2008;22:342–50.

[6] Rademakers FE, Buchalter MB, Rogers WJ, et al. Dissociation between left ventricular untwisting and filling: accentuation by catecholamines. Circulation 1992;85:1572–81.

[7] Arts T, Meerbaum S, Reneman RS, Corday E. Torsion of the left ventricle during the ejection phase in the intact dog. Cardiovasc Res 1984;18:183–93.

[8] Arts T, Veenstra PC, Reneman RS. Epicardial deformation and left ventricular wall mechanisms during ejection in the dog. Am J Physiol 1982;243:H379–90.

[9] Notomi Y, Martin-Miklovic MG, Oryszak SJ, et al. Enhanced ventricular untwisting during exercise: a mechanistic manifestation of elastic recoil described by Doppler tissue imaging. Circulation 2006;113:2524–33.

[10] Ingels NB, Hansen DE, Daughters GT, et al. Relation between longitudinal, circumferential, and oblique shortening and torsional deformation in the left ventricle of the transplanted human heart. Circ Res 1989;64:915–27.

[11] Chetboul V. Tissue Doppler imaging: a promising technique for quantifying regional myocardial function. J Vet Cardiol 2002;4:7–12.

[12] Derumeaux G, Jamal F. Myocardial tissue Doppler. In: Abergel E, Cohen A, Gueret P, Roudaut R, editors. Clinical echocardiography of the adult 2003, vol. 1: 87–96. Issy-les-Moulineaux, France: Estem.

[13] Isaaz K, Thompson A, Ethevenot G, et al. Doppler echocardiographic measurement of low velocity motion of the left ventricular posterior wall. Am J Cardiol 1989;64:66–75.

[14] McDicken WN, Sutherland GR, Moran CM, Gordon LN. Color Doppler velocity imaging of the myocardium. Ultrasound Med Biol 1992;18:651–4.

[15] Sutherland GR, Stewart MJ, Groundstroem KWE, et al. Color Doppler myocardial imaging: a new technique for assessment of myocardial function. J Am Soc Echocardiogr 1994;7:441–58.

[16] Fleming D, McDicken WN, Sutherland GR, Hoskins PR. Assessment of color Doppler tissue imaging using yest phantoms. Ultrasound Med Biol 1994;20:937–51.

[17] Derumeaux G, Ovize M, Loufoua J, et al. Doppler tissue imaging quantitates regional wall motion during myocardial ischemia and reperfusion. Circulation 1998;97:1970–7.

[18] Estrada A, Chetboul V. Tissue Doppler evaluation of ventricular synchrony. J Vet Cardiol 2006;8:129–37.

[19] Gavaghan BJ, Kittleson MD, Fisher KJ, et al. Quantification of left ventricular diastolic wall motion by Doppler tissue imaging in healthy cats and cats with cardiomyopathy. Am J Vet Res 1999;60:1478–86.

[20] Garot J, Diebold B, Derumeaux G, et al. Comparison of regional myocardial velocities assessed by quantitative 2-dimensional and M-mode color Doppler tissue imaging: influence of signal-to-noise ratio of color Doppler myocardial images on velocity estimators of the Doppler tissue imaging system. J Am Soc Echocardiogr 1998;11:1093–105.

[21] Chetboul V, Escriou C, Tessier D, et al. Tissue Doppler imaging detects early asymptomatic myocardial abnormalities in a dog model of Duchenne's cardiomyopathy. Eur Heart J 2004;25:1934–9.
[22] Koffas H, Dukes-McEwan J, Corcoran BM, et al. Peak mean myocardial velocities and velocity gradients measured by color M-mode tissue Doppler imaging in healthy cats. J Vet Intern Med 2003;17:510–24.
[23] Chetboul V, Athanassiadis N, Carlos C, et al. Quantification, repeatability, and reproducibility of feline radial and longitudinal left ventricular velocities by tissue Doppler imaging. Am J Vet Res 2004;65:566–72.
[24] Chetboul V, Carlos Sampedrano C, Tissier R, et al. Quantitative assessment of velocities of the annulus of the left atrioventricular valve and left ventricular free wall in healthy cats by use of two-dimensional color tissue Doppler imaging. Am J Vet Res 2006;67:250–8.
[25] Chetboul V, Athanassiadis N, Carlos C, et al. Assessment of repeatability, reproducibility, and effect of anesthesia on determination of radial and longitudinal left ventricular velocities via tissue Doppler imaging in dogs. Am J Vet Res 2004;65:909–15.
[26] Chetboul V, Carlos Sampedrano C, Concordet D, et al. Use of quantitative two-dimensional color tissue Doppler imaging for assessment of left ventricular radial and longitudinal myocardial velocities in dogs. Am J Vet Res 2005;66:953–61.
[27] Simak J, Keller L, Killich M, et al. Color-coded longitudinal interventricular septal tissue velocity imaging, strain and strain rate in healthy Doberman Pinschers. J Vet Cardiol 2011;13:1–11.
[28] Chetboul V, Carlos Sampedrano C, Gouni V, et al. Quantitative assessment of regional right ventricular myocardial velocities in awake dogs by Doppler tissue imaging: repeatability, reproducibility, effect of body weight and breed, and comparison with left ventricular myocardial velocities. J Vet Intern Med 2005;19:837–44.
[29] Koffas H, Dukes-McEwan J, Corcoran BM, et al. Pulsed tissue Doppler imaging in normal cats and cats with hypertrophic cardiomyopathy. J Vet Intern Med 2006;20:65–77.
[30] Kukulski T, Hübbert L, Arnold M, et al. Normal regional right ventricular function and its change with age: a Doppler myocardial imaging study. J Am Soc Echocardiogr 2000;13:194–204.
[31] Nikitin NP, Witte KK, Thackray SD, et al. Longitudinal ventricular function: normal values of atrioventricular annular and myocardial velocities measured with quantitative two-dimensional color Doppler tissue imaging. J Am Soc Echocardiogr 2003;16:906–21.
[32] Derumeaux G, Douillet R, Redonnet M, et al. Detection of acute rejection of heart transplantation by Doppler color imaging. Arch Mal Cœur Vaiss 1998;91:1255–62.
[33] Derumeaux G, Douillet R, Troniou A, et al. Distinguishing between physiologic hypertrophy in athletes and primary hypertrophic cardiomyopathies: importance of tissue color Doppler. Arch Mal Cœur Vaiss 1999;92:201–10.
[34] Nagueh SF, Bachinski LL, Meyer D, et al. Tissue Doppler imaging consistently detects myocardial abnormalities in patients with hypertrophic cardiomyopathy and provides a novel means for an early diagnosis before and independently of hypertrophy. Circulation 2001;104:128–30.
[35] Palka P, Lange A, Donnelly JE, et al. Doppler tissue echocardiographic features of cardiac amyloidosis. J Am Soc Echocardiogr 2002;15:1353–60.
[36] Nagueh SF, McFalls J, Meyer D, et al. Tissue Doppler imaging predicts the development of hypertrophic cardiomyopathy in subjects with subclinical disease. Circulation 2003;108:395–8.
[37] Chetboul V, Carlos C, Blot S, et al. Tissue Doppler assessment of diastolic and systolic alterations of radial and longitudinal left ventricular motions in Golden Retrievers during the preclinical phase of cardiomyopathy associated with muscular dystrophy. Am J Vet Res 2004;65:1335–41.
[38] Chetboul V, Blot S, Carlos Sampedrano C, et al. Tissue Doppler imaging for detection of radial and longitudinal myocardial dysfunction in a family of cats affected by dystrophin-deficient hypertrophic muscular dystrophy. J Vet Intern Med 2006;20:640–7.
[39] Carlos Sampedrano C, Chetboul V, Gouni V, et al. Systolic and diastolic myocardial dysfunction in cats with hypertrophic cardiomyopathy or systemic hypertension. J Vet Intern Med 2006;20:1106–15.
[40] MacDonald KA, Kittleson MD, Kass PH, Meurs KM. Tissue Doppler imaging in Maine coon cats with a mutation of myosin binding protein C with or without hypertrophy. J Vet Intern Med 2007;21:232–7.
[41] Serres F, Chetboul V, Gouni V, et al. Diagnostic value of echo-Doppler and tissue Doppler imaging in dogs with pulmonary arterial hypertension. J Vet Intern Med 2007;21:1280–9.
[42] Koffas H, Dukes-McEwan J, Corcoran BM, et al. Colour M-mode tissue Doppler imaging in healthy cats and cats with hypertrophic cardiomyopathy. J Small Anim Pract 2008;49:330–8.
[43] Carlos Sampedrano C, Chetboul V, Mary J, et al. Prospective echocardiographic and tissue Doppler imaging screening of a population of Maine coon cats tested for the A31P mutation in the myosin-binding protein C gene: a specific analysis of the heterozygous status. J Vet Intern Med 2009;23:91–9.

[44] Chetboul V, Gouni V, Carlos Sampedrano C, et al. Assessment of regional systolic and diastolic myocardial function using tissue Doppler and strain imaging in dogs with dilated cardiomyopathy. J Vet Intern Med 2007;21:719–30.
[45] Borenstein N, Chetboul V, Bruneval P, et al. Non-cultured cell transplantation in an ovine model of non-ischemic heart failure. Eur J Cardiothorac Surg 2007;31:444–51.
[46] Uematsu M, Miyatake K, Tanaka N, et al. Myocardial velocity gradient as a new indicator of regional left ventricular contraction: detection by a two-dimensional tissue Doppler imaging technique. J Am Coll Cardiol 1995;26:217–23.
[47] Lucats L, Monnet X, Bizé A, et al. Regional and temporal heterogeneity of postsystolic wall thickening is associated with left ventricular asynchrony in normal and experimental stunned myocardium. Basic Res Cardiol 2008;103:385–96.
[48] D'Hooge J, Heimdal A, Jamal F, et al. Regional strain and strain rate measurements by cardiac ultrasound: principles, implementation and limitations. Eur J Echocardiogr 2000;1:154–70.
[49] Urheim S, Edvardsen T, Torp H, et al. Myocardial strain by Doppler echocardiography: validation of a new method to quantify regional myocardial function. Circulation 2000;102:1158–64.
[50] Thibault H, Derumeaux G. Assessment of myocardial ischemia and viability using tissue Doppler and deformation imaging: the lessons from the experimental studies. Arch Cardiovasc Dis 2008;101: 61–8.
[51] Nesbitt GC, Mankad S. Strain and strain rate imaging in cardiomyopathy. Echocardiography 2009;26: 337–44.
[52] Yip G, Abraham T, Belohlavek M, Khandheria BK. Clinical applications of strain rate imaging. J Am Soc Echocardiogr 2003;16:1334–2.
[53] Greenberg NL, Firstenberg MS, Castro PL, et al. Doppler-derived myocardial systolic strain rate is a strong index of left ventricular contractility. Circulation 2002;105:99–105.
[54] Hoffmann R, Altiok E, Nowak B, et al. Strain rate measurement by Doppler echocardiography allows improved assessment of myocardial viability in patients with depressed left ventricular function. J Am Coll Cardiol 2002;39:443–9.
[55] Chetboul V, Carlos Sampedrano C, Gouni V, et al. Ultrasonographic assessment of regional radial and longitudinal systolic function in healthy awake dogs. J Vet Intern Med 2006;20:885–93.
[56] Chetboul V, Gouni V, Carlos Sampedrano C, et al. Assessment of regional systolic and diastolic myocardial function using tissue Doppler and strain imaging in dogs with dilated cardiomyopathy. J Vet Intern Med 2007;21:719–30.
[57] Wess G, Keller LJ, Klausnitzer M, et al. Comparison of longitudinal myocardial tissue velocity, strain, and strain rate measured by two-dimensional speckle tracking and by color tissue Doppler imaging in healthy dogs. J Vet Cardiol 2011;13:31–43.
[58] Wess G, Sarkar R, Hartmann K. Assessment of left ventricular systolic function by strain imaging echocardiography in various stages of feline hypertrophic cardiomyopathy. J Vet Intern Med 2010;24:1375–82.
[59] Perk G, Tunick PA, Kronzon I. Non-Doppler two-dimensional strain imaging by echocardiography-from technical considerations to clinical applications. J Am Soc Echocardiogr 2007;20:234–43.
[60] Helle-Valle T, Crosby J, Edvardsen T, et al. New non-invasive method for assessment of left ventricular rotation: speckle tracking echocardiography. Circulation 2005;112:3149–56.
[61] Nesser HJ, Winter S. Speckle tracking in the evaluation of left ventricular dyssynchrony. Echocardiography 2009;26:324–36.
[62] Artis NJ, Oxborough DL, Williams G, et al. Two-dimensional strain imaging: a new echocardiographic advance with research and clinical applications. Int J Cardiol 2008;123:240–8.
[63] Chetboul V, Serres F, Gouni V, et al. Radial strain and strain rate by two-dimensional speckle tracking echocardiography and the tissue velocity based technique in the dog. J Vet Cardiol 2007;9:69–81.

5

Transesophageal Echocardiography

CLAUDIO BUSSADORI IN COLLABORATION WITH ORIOL DOMENECH

Introduction and Technical Considerations, 86
Considerations Regarding the Echocardiographer, 86
Complications, 87
TEE Examination Protocol, 87
TEE Indications and Applications, 90
Conclusion, 93

Introduction and Technical Considerations

Multiplane transesophageal echocardiography (TEE) uses a bidimensional phased-array probe, located on the extremity of a flexible device similar to an endoscope, placed in the esophagus and able to provide clear pictures of the cardiac structure through the esophageal wall. This device does not have optic fibers, aspiration, or biopsy channels. However, it contains an ultrasound probe and electrical connections. The connection of the TEE probes to the echocardiographic machine is the same as that of transthoracic echocardiography (TTE) probes. There are two control knobs on the endoscope handle. One of these knobs controls the rotation of the probe from 0 to 180 degrees while the other controls the motions of the extremity of the endoscope from top to bottom (anteroflexion) or from the bottom up (retroflexion). The probe is also equipped with a brake that allows the operator to set the knob to a preselected position of the extremity of the endoscope (locked probe position) (Figure 5-1).

To obtain optimal echocardiographic views, the following movements of the steerable endoscope must be performed during the TEE examination:

- Back and forth motion to check the craniocaudal position
- Clockwise or counterclockwise rotation to guide the ultrasound beam toward the right or the left of the animal, respectively

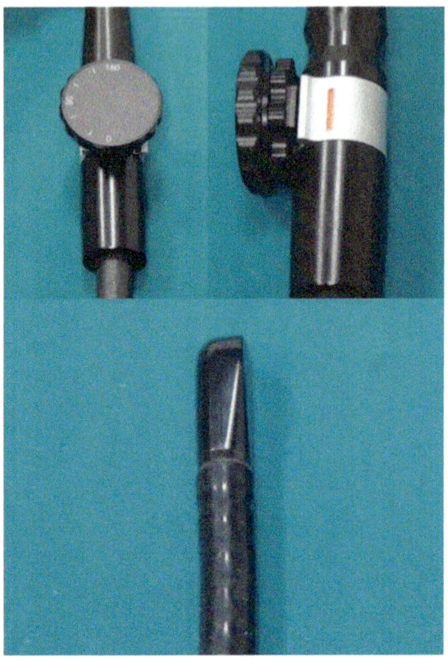

• **Fig. 5-1** Control knobs on the transesophageal probe handle. *(Top images)* The large knobs control the angle of the ultrasound beam and the small knob controls the ventral (retroflexion) or dorsal (anteroflexion) flexion of the extremity of the transducer. *(Bottom image)* View of the extremity of the endoscope containing the transducer. (Photo credit: Claudio Bussadori.)

- Dorsal (upward, retroflexion) or ventral (toward the bottom, anteroflexion) flexions to guide the beam caudally or cranially, respectively

From each of these positions, subtle probe angulation adjustments are necessary to obtain good images. An increase in the multiplane probe angle from 0 to 180 degrees is called a forward rotation while a decrease in angle in the opposite direction is called a backward rotation. This terminology, describing the manipulation of the probe when capturing an image, is taken from the guidelines of the American Society of Echocardiography (ASE) and Society of Cardiovascular Anesthesiologists (SCA) [1]. All of these positions and angulations of the probe provide numerous echocardiographic views. Most manufacturers produce two types of TEE probes: a pediatric probe (tip width of 8 to 10.7 mm) and an adult probe (tip width of 13 to 14 mm). A TEE microprobe with a very small tip width (7.5 mm) was recently manufactured. In human medicine the pediatric probes are used on young children or newborns who weigh more than 2.5 to 5 kg, while the microprobes recently have been used successfully on smaller newborns (1.7 to 5 kg) [2]. In veterinary medicine, the adult and pediatric probes are routinely used on dogs that weigh more than 5 kg and more than 1.5 kg, respectively, without the complications observed in human medicine. This can be explained by the fact that the esophagus in dogs is wider and more extensible than in humans, therefore allowing the use of a wider probe for a given weight. Based on the authors' experience, it is possible to use a pediatric probe in animals that weigh between 1.4 and 3.4 kg, while the probe for adults can be used with caution in dogs that weigh more than 3 to 4 kg.

This echocardiographic technique provides better quality images than TTE, particularly with structures located on or above the atrioventricular junction, in part because of the closer proximity to the heart and also because of the elimination of interference from the thoracic and lungs wall [3-5].

Considerations Regarding the Echocardiographer

It is important to emphasize that any TEE examination should be performed by a TTE echocardiographer who has acquired the necessary knowledge and skills to practice TEE. In 1992 the ASE committee for training physicians in echocardiography published its guidelines on TEE training. These guidelines require that the trainee reach at least the second level of echocardiography training (completing 300 or more supervised TEE examinations) and perform and interpret at least 50 TEE supervised examinations [6]. These guidelines are intended for TEE training for intraoperative and nonoperative purposes. In 2002 a joint ASE and SCA workgroup published similar guidelines regarding perioperative TEE [7]. If we refer to these recommendations in human medicine, TEE in veterinary medicine should always be performed by an echocardiographer trained in TTE. In our institution, TEE is performed only after thorough TTE and TEE training, including at least 150 and 20 supervised examinations, respectively. These examinations must include the complete spectrum of the most frequently encountered perioperative pathologies. Moreover, the perioperative TEE examinations must be performed, interpreted, and documented in a TTE examination report by the trainee in person. Thus properly trained TEE echocardiographers can work independently and supervise beginners. Our experience in performing TEE includes approximately 200 examinations of multiple diseases, including patent ductus arteriosus (PDA), pulmonic valve stenosis (PS), aberrant coronary arteries, ventricular septal defects (VSDs) (muscular, membranous), atrial septal defects (ASDs), aortopulmonary fistulas (AoPFs), cardiac tumors (CTs), and vascular abnormalities such as intrahepatic portosystemic shunts (PSSs).

The TEE echocardiographer must know how to introduce the probe correctly, how to obtain a good-quality image, and how to interpret pictures accurately during the examination. Reviewing video images does not make up for an inadequate examination, especially since this is a semi-invasive method that requires anesthesia and therefore is difficult to repeat. In the majority of cases, a TEE should not be performed before a complete TTE and should not replace an insufficient TTE [3,5].

Complications

TEE is usually a low-risk procedure when performed on correctly screened patients using an appropriate technique. Nevertheless, on rare occasions, serious complications may occur [8,9]. The complete approach of each TEE examination begins by ruling out potential contraindications: symptomatic esophageal stricture, esophageal diverticulum, a recent esophageal surgical intervention, a hiatal hernia, or an esophageal tumor. If an esophageal disease is present, the relative risk of performing a TEE must be considered and weighed against any potential benefit from the procedure. Excessive pressure must never be exerted when inserting and manipulating the probe in the esophagus; in fact, perforations of the esophagus have already been described [10,11]. Additional caution must be exercised when inserting the probe in dogs that weigh less than 5 kg. Studies have shown that TEE can be performed without risk in children and in small anticoagulated animals with an intact mucosa or minimal injuries [12,13], especially if the examinations are performed with appropriate training and caution. The authors have never observed any signs of esophageal trauma in performing 200 examinations. This is in agreement with a previous study, despite the fact that TEE examination durations were particularly long [4]. Other possible complications include anesthetic accidents (especially in seriously ill patients), disease transmission between patients, arrhythmias, and endocarditis secondary to bacteremia induced by the endoscopy [8]. Routine disinfection procedures must be performed on the probe after every examination.

TEE Examination Protocol

To perform a good TEE examination, the probe is inserted in the esophagus after general anesthesia induction and tracheal intubation. The patient is generally positioned in right lateral recumbency. The position of the dog does not seem to influence the quality of the images; it can therefore be dictated by the user's preferences in terms of manipulation of the probe and control knobs [4]. The patient position will also depend on the type of surgical and interventional procedure during which TEE is used. The authors generally perform TEE examinations using the right lateral recumbency position when the procedure is done for diagnostic purposes as well as for interventional cardiology procedures such as PDA occlusions and balloon pulmonary valvuloplasties. Dorsal recumbency is preferred to guide percutaneous occlusions of VSDs or transvenous coil embolization for the treatment of intrahepatic PSS.

The TEE probe must be inserted gently (never use excessive force) with the control knob in the unlocked position. Even if the TEE examination is performed under general anesthesia, a mouth gag must be used as a precaution in order to prevent accidental damage of the probe by the teeth. Resistance may be encountered when entering the thorax of certain patients and gentle manipulation of the probe and the neck may be necessary to pass this zone. Once the TEE probe is inserted, it must be manipulated in order to obtain a sequence of images of the heart and large vessels. Examination of the cardiac structure by TEE starts by moving the probe to the desired zone and then guiding the ultrasound beam in the appropriate direction by manipulating the probe (see the motions described above) to obtain the images listed below. This is best accomplished by observing the images as they change during probe manipulation rather than relying on the depth markings on the probe or the multiplane angle icon on the screen. These markings and direction guides give a general indication of the location of the probe and the direction of the ultrasound beam but the final view selection is always based on the appearance of the displayed images. The view of a cardiac structure can be adjusted by an anterograde or retrograde manipulation of the multiplane angle, while maintaining the structure at the center of the image. It is always preferable to follow the same procedure in every examination. The favored sequence may vary from one person to another but following the same sequence will ensure the assessment of all cardiac structures during each examination. Each structure must be examined from different views and from more than one position of the probe, if possible.

The TEE views are obtained from three positions in the esophagus—cranial, median, and caudal—and from within the stomach (transgastric position). In addition, the images can be obtained from transverse and longitudinal views. The standards for viewing images comply with the ASE/SCA guidelines [1]. The images are displayed with the probe location. The probe's near field appears at the top of the screen and far field appears at the bottom. A multiplane angle of 0 degree provides horizontal or transverse views, with the right side of the patient appearing on the left of the displayed image. A 90-degree clockwise rotation of the multiplane angle allows longitudinal views, with the cranial structures displayed on the left and the apical (or caudal) structures on the right. The longitudinal views display differs from the one described in previous publications [1,4]. However, our display matches the anatomic spatial orientation, which greatly helps during procedures like PDA occlusions. Finally, the 180-degrees rotation of the multiplane angle gives the mirror image of that at 0 degree. The nomenclature of the views used by the authors are based on the location of the probe (cranial, median, caudal, or transgastric) and on the orientation of the cross-section (transverse or short axis and longitudinal or long axis). The main anatomic structure is added to the nomenclature in situations where a given probe location and orientation allow the visualization of two structures by simply turning the probe to the right or to the left. In our laboratory a basic and complete TEE examination includes seven main images:

I. *Cranial transverse view* (Figure 5-2). With this view, it is possible to optimize the image to visualize the pulmonic valve and main pulmonary artery. This view is used to accurately assess the pulmonic valve annulus and to guide percutaneous balloon pulmonic valvuloplasties.

II. *Cranial longitudinal view optimized for the aorta and the PDA* (Figure 5-3). With this view, it is possible to optimize the image to visualize the patent ductus. This view is used for the accurate measurement of the minimal diameter of the ductus

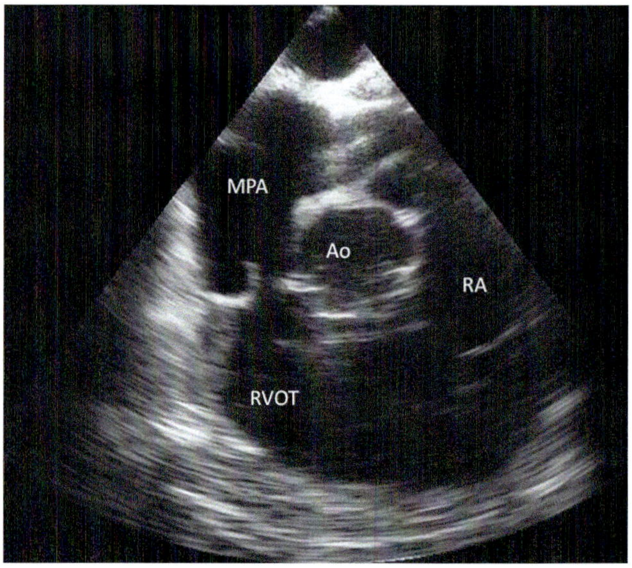

• **Fig. 5-2** Cranial transverse view in a dog (I). The extremity of the transducer is placed on the cranial part of the heart, a slight forward rotation of the ultrasound beam is performed, and the image is optimized through minor adjustments of the transducer tip position and beam. The right and cranial cardiac structures appear on the left and the left and caudal structures appear on the right of the screen. On the left, the long axis of the main pulmonary artery (MPA) is identified, with the closed pulmonic valve cusps (diastolic image). The right ventricular outflow tract (RVOT) and the right ventricle are observed at the bottom of the screen. At the center of the image, the short axis of the aorta (Ao) is shown. The right atrium (RA) is visible on the right of the image. (Photo credit: Claudio Bussadori.)

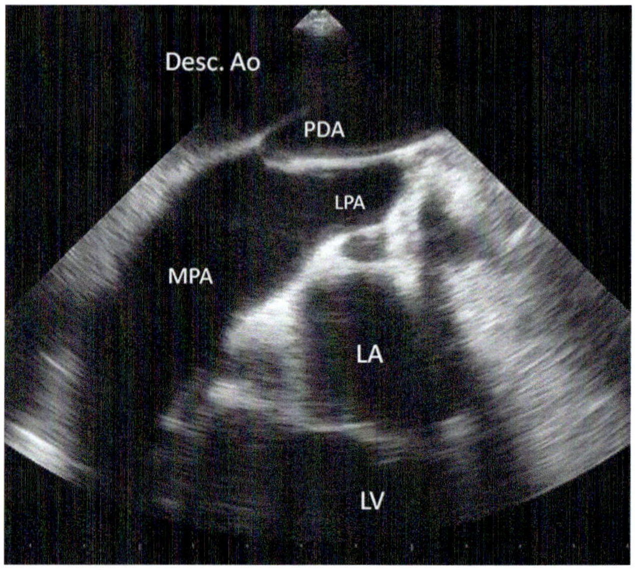

• **Fig. 5-3** Cranial longitudinal view of the aorta and a ductus arteriosus (II). This view is obtained by placing the transducer on the cranial part of the heart with the ultrasound beam angle set to approximately 90 degrees. A slight counterclockwise rotation and an anteroflexion of the endoscope tip may be necessary to obtain a good view of the ascending aorta, while a slight clockwise rotation and a retroflexion will display the long axis of the main pulmonary artery (MPA) and a patent ductus arteriosus (PDA), if present. The PDA is located between the descending aorta (Desc. Ao) and the MPA. The visualization of this structure can be improved by performing small clockwise or counterclockwise rotations of the transducer extremity. *LA,* Left atrium; *LPA,* left pulmonary artery; *LV,* left ventricle. (Photo credit: Claudio Bussadori.)

arteriosus and diameter of the ductal ampulla as well as to guide the occlusion.

III. *Cranial longitudinal view optimized for the main pulmonary artery* (Figure 5-4). With this view, it is possible to optimize the image to visualize the valve and main pulmonary artery. This view is used to accurately measure the dimensions of the pulmonic valve annulus.

IV. *Median transverse view* (Figure 5-5). With this view, the left atrium, the mitral valve, the left ventricle as well as parts of the right atrium and ventricle are visualized.

V. *Median longitudinal view* (Figure 5-6). With this view, it is possible to optimize the image to visualize a membranous VSD.

VI. *Caudal transverse view* (Figure 5-7). With this view, it is possible to optimize the image to visualize the pulmonic valve and main pulmonary artery. This view is used to accurately measure the pulmonic valve annulus and to guide percutaneous balloon pulmonary valvuloplasties.

VII. *Caudal longitudinal view* (Figure 5-8). With this view, it is possible to optimize the image to visualize the anterior extension of a membranous or muscular VSD and to assess the aortic morphology.

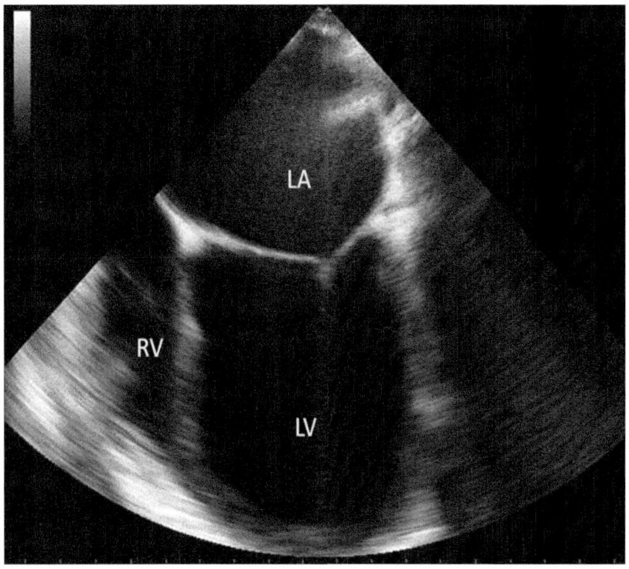

• **Fig. 5-5** Median transverse view (IV). This view is obtained by placing the transducer tip on the median part of the heart. A slight clockwise rotation and a small anteroflexion at the transducer tip were performed. The cranial and right structures appear on the left and the caudal and left structures appear on the right of the screen. The left atrium (LA) can be seen at the top of the screen. The image is centered on the mitral valve and the left ventricle (LV). The mitral valve anterior leaflet and the interventricular septum are visible on the left and the mitral valve posterior leaflet and the left ventricular free wall are visible on the right. It is possible to see a part of the right atrium, the tricuspid valve, and the right ventricle (RV) on the left of the screen. (Photo credit: Claudio Bussadori.)

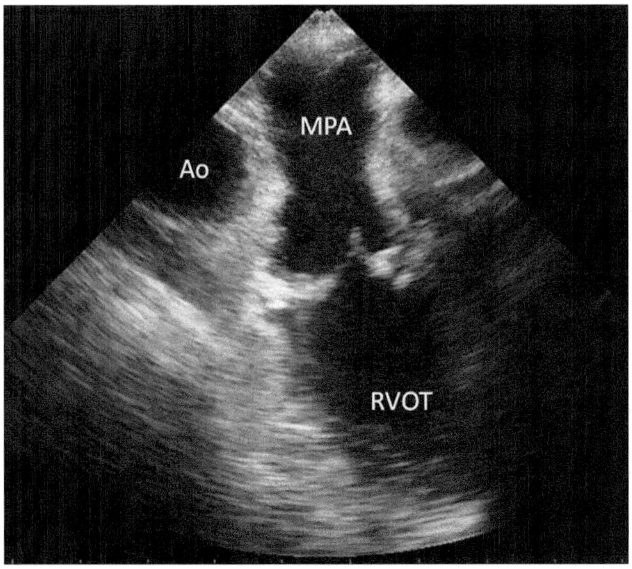

• **Fig. 5-4** Cranial longitudinal view of the main pulmonary artery (III). This view is obtained by placing the transducer tip on the cranial part of the heart with the ultrasound beam angle set to approximately 90 degrees. A slight clockwise rotation of the tip of the transducer has been performed from the position used to obtain the optimized view of the ascending aorta (view II). The cranial structures appear on the left and the caudal structures appear on the right of the screen. The entire main pulmonary artery (MPA) can be visualized at the center of the image, with the pulmonic valve annulus and the right ventricle outflow track (RVOT) at the bottom. To the left of the MPA a portion of the ascending aorta (Ao) is visible. (Photo credit: Claudio Bussadori.)

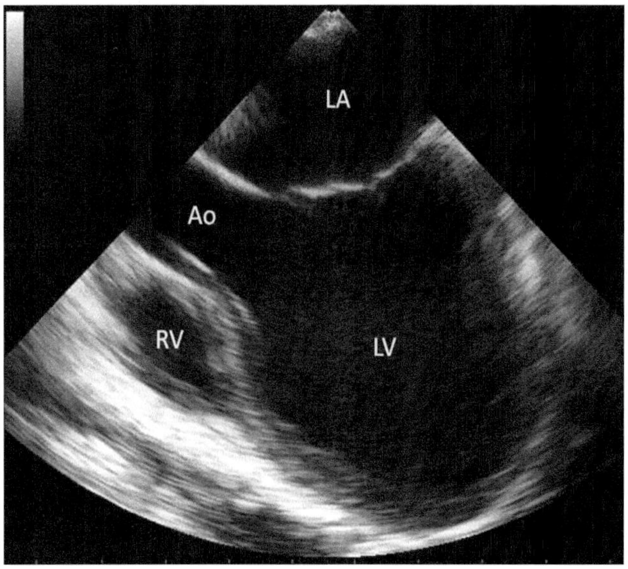

• **Fig. 5-6** Median longitudinal view (V). This view is obtained by placing the transducer tip on the median part of the heart with the ultrasound beam angle set to approximately 90 degrees. An anteroflexion is necessary. The cranial structures appear on the left and the caudal structures appear on the right of the screen. The left atrium (LA) is visible at the top of the image. The picture is centered on the left ventricular outflow tract and the aortic valve annulus (Ao), on the left of the screen. The LA, the mitral valve, and the left ventricle (LV) are visible. A small part of the right ventricle (RV) is also visible on the left of the screen. (Photo credit: Claudio Bussadori.)

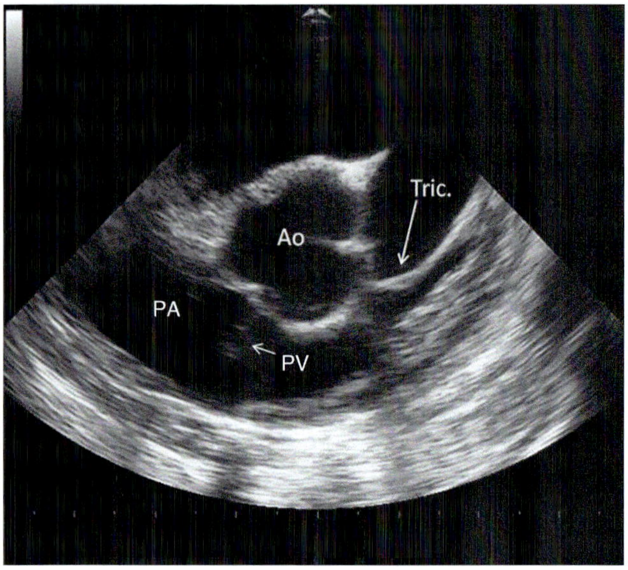

• **Fig. 5-7** Caudal transverse view (VI). This view is obtained by placing the transducer tip on the caudal part of the heart with a pronounced anteroflexion of the transducer tip. The left atrium, sectioned transversely, can be observed in the proximal field. Directly beneath it, parts of the right atrium, the tricuspid valve (Tric.), the right ventricular outflow tract, the pulmonic valve (PV), and the main pulmonary artery (PA) can be seen. This image is centered on the right ventricular outflow tract and filling chamber. *Ao,* Aorta. (Photo credit: Claudio Bussadori.)

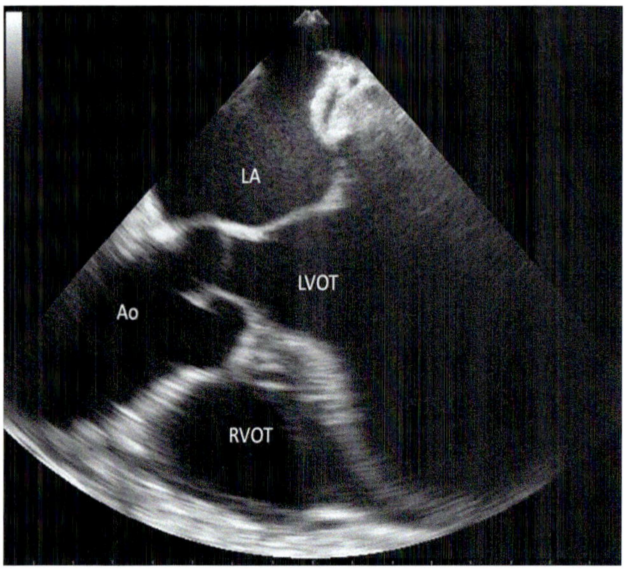

• **Fig. 5-8** Caudal longitudinal view (VII). This view is obtained by placing the transducer tip on the caudal part of the heart with a pronounced anteroflexion of the transducer tip. The cranial structures appear on the left and the caudal structures appear on the right of the screen. The left atrium (LA) can be seen in the proximal field. The mitral valve and particularly the anterior leaflet and the left ventricle on the right can be viewed in the picture. This picture is centered on the left ventricular outflow tract (LVOT), the valve, and the aortic root (Ao) as well as the interventricular septum. In the distal field of the image, the right ventricular outflow tract (RVOT) is visible. (Photo credit: Claudio Bussadori.)

TEE Indications and Applications

There are several indications for performing TEE: a technically inadequate TTE because of a significant thoracic wall abnormality (i.e., a severe pectus excavatum) or a chronic lung disease (i.e., emphysema); identification and assessment of masses, tumors, and sources of embolisms; diagnosis and/or correct assessment of certain congenital cardiomyopathies when the TTE is suboptimal; and assessment of complex congenital malformations [14-16]. We have performed TEE in dogs with VSD (Figure 5-9) and ASD (Figure 5-10), which provided pictures of much higher quality of the malformed anatomy than did TTE and allowed an accurate assessment of the possibility of occluding these septal defects through interventional cardiology. In a dog with a severe pectus excavatum, TEE allowed us to diagnose a double-chambered right ventricle that was not clearly visualized using TTE. TEE also allows a good assessment of the coronary anatomy in PS cases and detection of coronary abnormalities in some of these patients. In one case it proved decisive in identifying a secondary pulmonary dissection from a balloon pulmonic valvuloplasty that was unnoticed by TTE. These vascular abnormalities are even better studied using real-time tridimensional (3D) TEE, which provides more anatomic information and allows a more accurate diagnosis. The TEE also allowed a diagnosis of collateral aortopulmonary arteries in patients assessed for congenital malformations, such as PDA or PS (Figure 5-11). In addition, TEE allows the study of the exact anatomy and dimensions of cardiac malformations such as PDA and PS.

TEE is also used in the operating room to monitor surgical and interventional cardiology procedures. It allows direct visualization of the cardiac performance, thus providing a quick and precise assessment of the cardiac condition during the perioperative period [15]. TEE is used during many interventional cardiology procedures for treatment of congenital cardiomyopathies and significantly reduces fluoroscopy duration and the dose of contrast agent [14,16]. Moreover, it allows continuous assessment of the results and early detection of eventual complications. TEE can be used for ASD, VSD, and PDA occlusions as well as for percutaneous balloon valvuloplasty in human and veterinary medicine [17-24]. In these situations, it was observed that TEE allowed a more in-depth characterization of ASD, VSD, and PDA size and morphology. It is also decisive in the selection of a device of appropriate size and in the supervision of its deployment (position, final check before device release, and assessment of the occlusion effectiveness after release).

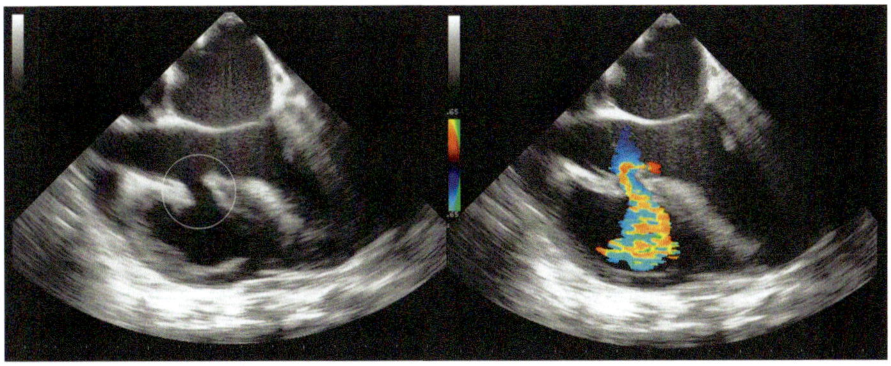

• **Fig. 5-9** Caudal longitudinal view with slight clockwise rotation displaying a significant perimembranous ventricular septal defect *(circle)*. The Doppler color reveals a turbulent flow going from the left ventricular outflow tract toward the right ventricle. (Photo credit: Claudio Bussadori.)

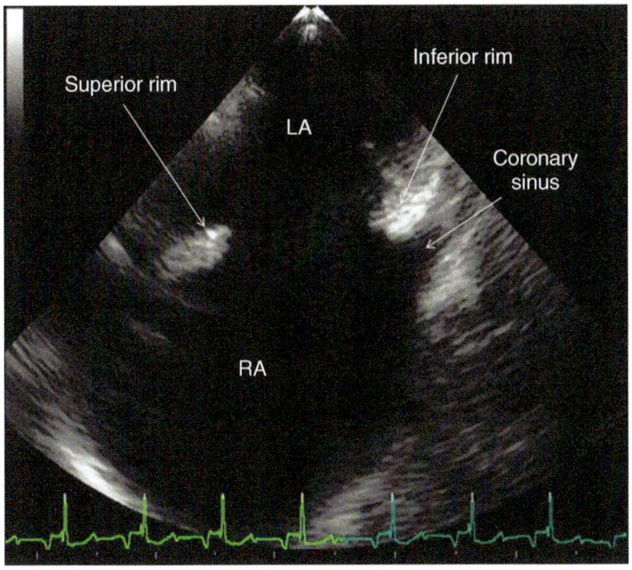

• **Fig. 5-10** Median transverse view with marked anteroflexion of the endoscope extremity allowing assessment of an atrial septal defect. We can see the inferior and superior rims of the septal defect as well as the coronary sinus. *LA*, Left atrium; *RA*, right atrium. (Photo credit: Claudio Bussadori.)

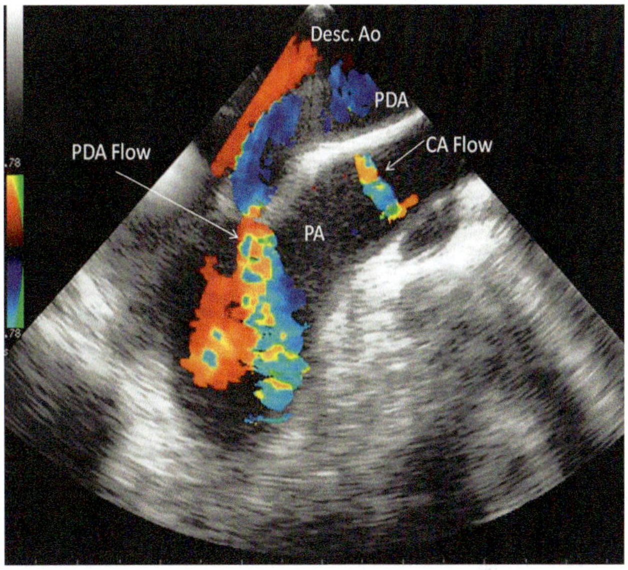

• **Fig. 5-11** Cranial longitudinal view centered on a patent ductus arteriosus (PDA). With this view, one can see the turbulent flow through the patent ductus arteriosus (PDA Flow) as well as other smaller turbulent flows emerging from an aortopulmonary collateral vessel (CA Flow). *Desc. Ao,* Descending aorta; *PA,* patent arteriosus. (Photo credit: Claudio Bussadori.)

In dogs, TEE allows appropriate ductus arteriosus visualization (Figure 5-12) and precise measurement of its dimensions, well correlated with the angiocardiographic measurement—not only for the minimal diameter of the canal, but also for the diameter of the ductal ampulla and its length [23-28]. Moreover, the value of TEE in obtaining anatomic and perioperative information in dogs undergoing PDA occlusion with an Amplatz® canine duct occluder (ACDO) was assessed in a recent study [28]. TEE enables continuous, real-time supervision throughout the procedure: direct visualization of the ACDO release; fitting of the proximal and distal discs to the ductal ampulla and pulmonary ostium, respectively; optimal assessment of the adequate size; stability of the device; and complete ductal occlusion. This represents a relative advantage over fluoroscopy, during which assessment of the position and stability of the occluding device is limited by its back and forth movements and the indirect radiographic appearance of the device and surrounding structures. However, even if the information obtained from TEE during ACDO placement is superior to that obtained by fluoroscopy, this does not mean that fluoroscopy is not necessary in this type of procedure. Furthermore, fluoroscopy is a powerful ally of TEE when performing a catheter-based occlusion because it allows guidance of catheters and guide wires in anatomic regions not accessible by TEE. Besides, even if TEE makes the use of contrasting product unnecessary in the majority of cases, angiocardiography must always remain available.

TEE can be used in cases of PS when performing a balloon pulmonic valvuloplasty. In a recent study, we demonstrated that TEE provides anatomic information about the annulus diameter and the morphologic type of PS, similar to angiography and TEE [29]. However, TEE was shown to be more accurate and more useful than TTE in a minority of cases where the transthoracic acoustic window was very limited. In our experience, TEE offers excellent observation of the right ventricular outflow tract and the pulmonic valve, allowing precise monitoring at all stages of the procedure. This monitoring includes the precise placement of the balloon through the valve, the duration of inflation and deflation of the balloon guided by real-time monitoring of the ventricular function, and the immediate assessment of the results and complications. However, one must admit that the strangulation of the balloon by the stenotic valve, creating a "waist," is best shown through fluoroscopy. The disappearance of this "waist," a marker of effective balloon dilation, is best monitored by fluoroscopy and not by TEE.

TEE also can be used to guide the extraction of adult heartworms using alligator forceps. In fact, it allows visualization of the heartworms in the pulmonary artery (Figure 5-13) and assessment of the feasibility of extraction of the worms, before establishing vascular access through the jugular vein. TEE also allows monitoring of the movements of the flexible alligator forceps, although fluoroscopy is better for this. Finally, TEE allows immediate assessment of the procedure result before the patient wakes up. A study comparing the success rate of worm extraction with flexible alligator forceps using fluoroscopy versus TEE showed similar results with the two procedures [30]. However, the TEE-guided procedure does not require any radiation exposure and facilitates the observation of worms in the cardiac chambers and the pulmonary artery. Therefore the procedure guided by TEE seems useful in this clinical context.

TEE also can facilitate the manipulation of radiofrequency ablation catheters or perforation with laser of valvular atresia, since immediate effects of treatment can be demonstrated [16]. Congenital vascular anomalies such as intrahepatic PSS constitute another noncardiac use of TEE. Transvenous coil embolization is an interventional radiology technique recently described for the treatment of intrahepatic PSS in dogs. In this context, we observed that TEE enables localization and measurement of the shunt and guides the operator during the procedure (Figure 5-14). The injection of physiologic serum is useful to confirm the exact position of the catheters before placing the coils, therefore reducing the volume of contrast product needed. In a previous study, the role of multimodal imaging (scanner, TEE, and fluoroscopy) to guide the intrahepatic PSS treatment procedures by transvenous coil embolization was assessed in dogs. The conclusion was that the combination of information from the scanner and TEE helped to reduce fluoroscopy duration and the volume of contrast product, representing an advantage for both the patient and the operator. Besides, perfect agreement was observed between the shunt measurements obtained by scanner and TEE [31].

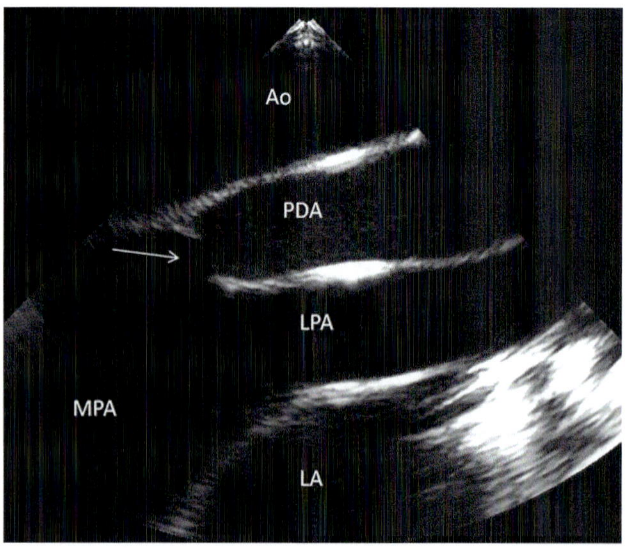

• **Fig. 5-12** Cranial longitudinal view centered on a patent ductus arteriosus (PDA). This zoomed-in image allows the evaluation of the minimal diameter *(arrow)* as well as the entire length and width of the ductus. *Ao,* Descending aorta; *LA,* left atrium; *LPA,* left pulmonary artery; *MPA,* main pulmonary artery. (Photo credit: Claudio Bussadori.)

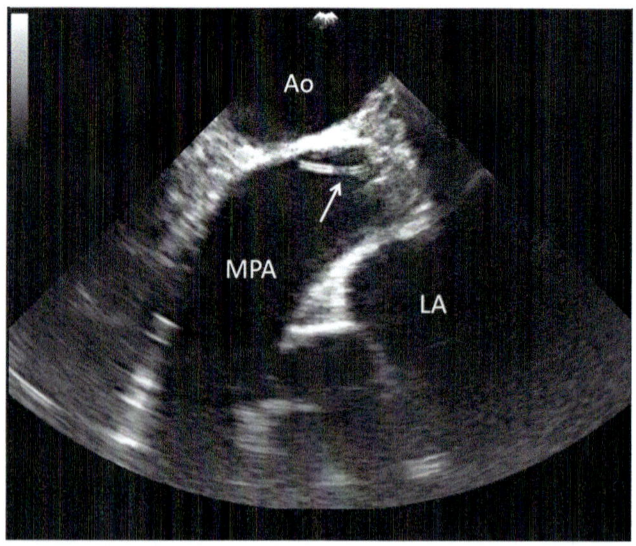

• **Fig. 5-13** Cranial longitudinal view obtained during extraction of heartworms with flexible alligator forceps. Transesophageal echocardiography (TEE) allows visualization of heartworms *(arrow)* in the main pulmonary artery (MPA). The procedure is complete when heartworms are no longer visible. *Ao,* Aorta; *LA,* left atrium. (Photo credit: Claudio Bussadori.)

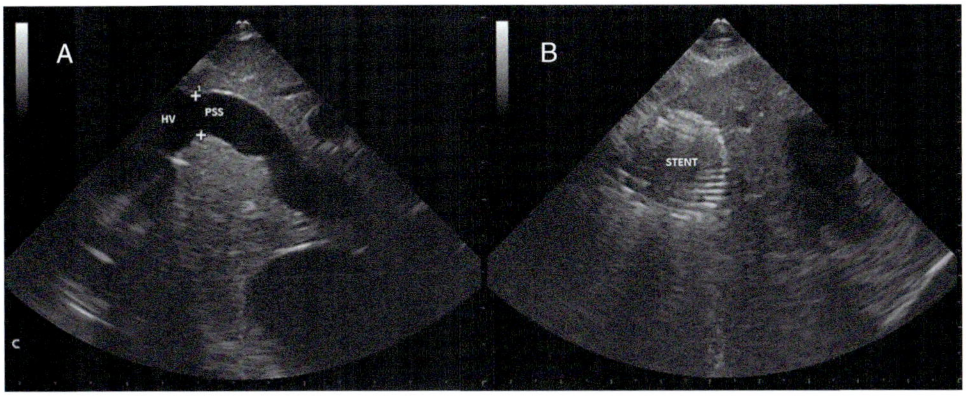

• **Fig. 5-14** A, Transesophageal view of the liver. A left divisional intrahepatic portosystemic shunt (PSS) and a hepatic vein (HV) are observed. B, The stent is observed in the caudal cave vein while using a transverse view. (Photo credit: Claudio Bussadori.)

Conclusion

TEE plays a role both in the diagnosis of cardiopathies and in interventional cardiovascular procedures. In fact, it provides accurate anatomic and functional information and supplements the information provided by TTE. This emphasizes the usefulness of this echocardiographic technique as a powerful diagnostic tool with significant influence on the planning and decision-making processes. During interventional procedures, TEE enables one to monitor the procedure without loss of image quality and increases safety, accuracy, and effectiveness of the interventions.

REFERENCES

[1] Shanewise JS, Cheung AT, Aronson S, et al. ASE/SCA guidelines for performing a comprehensive intraoperative multiplane transesophageal echocardiography examination: recommendations of the American Society of Echocardiography Council for Intraoperative Echocardiography and the Society of Cardiovascular Anesthesiologists Task Force for Certification in Perioperative Transesophageal Echocardiography. J Am Soc Echocardiogr 1999;12:884–900.

[2] Zyblewski S, Shirali G, Forbus G, et al. Initial experience with a miniaturized multiplane transesophageal probe in small infants undergoing cardiac operations. Ann Thorac Surg 2010;89:1990–4.

[3] Armstrong WF, Feigenbaum H. Echocardiography. In: Braunwald E, Zipes DP, Libby P, editors. Heart disease: a textbook of cardiovascular medicine. 6th ed. Philadelphia: WB Saunders; 2001, p. 160–228.

[4] Loyer C, Thomas WP. Biplane transesophageal echocardiography in the dog: technique, anatomy, and imaging planes. Vet Radiol Ultrasound 1995;36:212–26.

[5] Kienle RD, Thomas WP, Rishniw M. Biplane transesophageal echocardiography in the normal cat. Vet Radiol Ultrasound 1997;38:288–98.

[6] Pearlman AS, Gardin JM, Martin RP, et al. Guidelines for physician training in transesophageal echocardiography: recommendations of the American Society of Echocardiography Committee for physician training in echocardiography. J Am Soc Echocardiogr 1992;5:187–94.

[7] Cahalan MK, Abel M, Goldman M, et al. American Society of Echocardiography and Society of Cardiovascular Anesthesiologists task force guidelines for training in perioperative echocardiography. Anesth Analg 2002;94:1384–8.

[8] Daniel WG, Erbel R, Kasper W, et al. Safety of transesophageal echocardiography: a multicenter survey of 10419 examinations. Circulation 1991;83:817–21.

[9] Kallmeyer IJ, Collard CD, Fox JA, et al. The safety of intraoperative transesophageal echocardiography: a case series of 7200 cardiac surgical patients. Anesth Analg 2001;92:1126–30.

[10] Brinkman WT, Shanewise JS, Clements SD, et al. Transesophageal echocardiography: not an innocuous procedure. Ann Thorac Surg 2001;72:1725–6.

[11] Muhiudeen-Russell IA, Miller-Hance WC, Silverman N. Unrecognized esophageal perforation in a neonate during transesophageal echocardiography. J Am Soc Echocardiogr 2001;14:747–9.

[12] Greene MA, Alexander JA, Knauf DG, et al. Endoscopic evaluation of the esophagus in infants and children immediately following intraoperative use of transesophageal echocardiography. Chest 1999;116:1247–50.

[13] O'Shea JP, Southern JF, Ambra MN, et al. Effects of prolonged transesophageal echocardiographic imaging and probe manipulation on the esophagus: an echocardiographic-pathologic study. J Am Coll Cardiol 1991;17:1426–9.

[14] Schiller NB, Maurer G, Ritter SB, et al. Transesophageal echocardiography. J Am Soc Echocardiograph 1989;2:354–7.

[15] Ayres NA, Miller-Hance W, Fyfe DA, et al. Indications and guidelines for performance of transesophageal echocardiography in the patient with pediatric acquired or congenital heart disease: a report from task force of the pediatric council of the American Society of Echocardiography. J Am Soc Echocardiogr 2005;18:91–8.

[16] Cheitlin MD, Armstrong WF, Aurigemma GP, et al. ACC/AHA/ASE 2003 guideline update for the clinical application of echocardiography. Summary article. A report of the American College of Cardiology/American Heart Association Task Force on Practice Guidelines (ACC/AHA/ASE Committee to Update the 1997 Guidelines for the Clinical Application of Echocardiography). Circulation 2003;108:1146–62.

[17] Elzenga NJ. The role of echocardiography in transcatheter closure of atrial septal defects. Cardiol Young 2000;10:474–83.

[18] Van der Velde ME, Sanders SP, Keane JF, et al. Transesophageal echocardiographic guidance of transcatheter ventricular septal defect closure. J Am Coll Cardiol 1994;23:1660–5.

[19] Masani ND. Transesophageal echocardiography in adult congenital heart disease. Heart 2001;86:1130–40.

[20] Tumbarello R, Sanna A, Cardu G, et al. Usefulness of transesophageal echocardiography in the pediatric catheterization laboratory. Am J Cardiol 1993;71:1321–5.

[21] Gordon S, Miller M, Roland M, et al. Transcatheter atrial septal defect closure with the Amplatzer atrial septal occluder in 13 dogs: short- and mid-term outcome. J Vet Intern Med 2009;23:995–1002.

[22] Bussadori C, Carminati M, Domenech O, et al. Transcatheter closure of a perimembranous ventricular septal defect in a dog. J Vet Intern Med 2007;21:1396–400.

[23] Domenech O, Laynez E, Oliveira P, Bussadori C. Echocardiographic and angiographic comparison of patent ductus arteriosus measurements and their role on device size selection in 46 dogs. In: ECVIM-CA Congress. Porto, Portugal; 2009.

[24] Domenech O, Bussadori C, Sancho J, et al. Utilidad de la ecocardiografía transesofágica para el estudio de la morfología del conducto arterioso persistente en perros y su comparación con la angiocardiografía. Clin Vet Peq Anim 2009;29:110–4.

[25] Domenech O, et al. Patent ductus arteriosus measurements obtained by transthoracic (TTE) and transesophageal echocardiography (TEE) compared with angiography. In: ACVIM Congress. Seattle; 2007.

[26] Pariaut R, Sydney Moise N, Kraus MS, et al. Use of transesophageal echocardiography for visualization of the patent ductus arteriosus during transcatheter coil embolization. J Vet Cardiol 2004;6:32–9.

[27] Saunders AB, Miller MW, Gordon SG, Bahr A. Echocardiographic and angiographic comparison of ductal dimensions in dogs with patent ductus arteriosus. J Vet Intern Med 2007;21:68–75.

[28] Saunders AB, Achen SE, Gordon SG, Miller MW. Utility of transesophageal echocardiography for transcatheter occlusion of patent ductus arteriosus in dogs: influence on the decision-making process. J Vet Intern Med 2010;24:1407–13.

[29] Locatelli C, Domenech O, Oliveira P, et al. Transesophageal echocardiography in dogs with pulmonic stenosis. In: Proceedings ECVIM-CA Congress. Seville, Spain; 2011.

[30] Arita N, Yamane I, Takemura N. Comparison of canine heartworm removal rates using flexible alligator forceps guided by transesophageal echocardiography and fluoroscopy. J Vet Med Sci 2003;65:259–61.

[31] Rossi F, Domenech O, Bussadori R, Bussadori C. Role of multi-modality imaging to guide procedures of transveous coil embolisation for the treatment of canine intrahepatic portosystemic shunt. Rio de Janeiro: IVRA (International Veterinary Radiology Association); 2009.

6

Veterinary Applications of the Tridimensional Echocardiography

CLAUDIO BUSSADORI IN COLLABORATION WITH ANTONIA MAVROPOULOU AND JOEL SILVA

3D Echocardiography Technology, 96

The Different 3D Echocardiography Methods, 96

3D Echocardiography in Veterinary Medicine, 98

3D Transesophageal Echocardiography, 102

Tridimensional (3D) echocardiography is a diagnostic method that supplements the other echocardiographic methods (time-motion [TM] mode, bidimensional [2D] mode, and Doppler echocardiography). It allows a 3D observation of the cardiac structures and large vessels. This facilitates an intuitive assessment of the cardiac anatomy, ventricular function, and valvular pathologies. This technique has the potential to improve and extend the diagnostic possibilities [1-5]. The main advantage of 3D echocardiography is the possibility of obtaining a global view of the volume of the cardiac structures being studied and views from any orientation inside this volume.

As with any technology, 3D echocardiography requires a training period for the operator, particularly in data processing. Paradoxically, although the device is more complex than the traditional 2D echocardiograph, 3D data acquisition is simpler and even faster than 2D data acquisition. The acquisition of a few recordings from the right and left parasternal views may be sufficient to gather all data necessary for a complete 3D examination, including most of the 2D classical views. This is done by cropping and selecting views from the raw data. Therefore this acquisition method could eventually be performed by minimally trained operators. The accuracy of traditional echocardiographic measurement depends greatly on the operator's ability to acquire good views. With 3D echocardiography the acquisition process is simpler and the operator learning curve shifts toward postacquisition image processing.

3D Echocardiography Technology

Over the last years, different 3D image acquisition systems have been used. They were essentially based on independent 2D images being reconstructed into a 3D image. With these systems, using a method called "reconstruction," a series of 2D echocardiographic images is obtained. These 2D images are then aligned according to their location to form a final 3D image. This process can be performed using a "random," "hands-free," or "sequential" technique. The "random" and "hands-free" techniques depend on the spatial location of the 2D images. Reconstruction is accomplished by tracking the position of the transducer, then grouping and aligning the images according to their initial positions by means of a computerized process. To accomplish this, several mechanisms were developed: a mechanical arm allowing the transducer position tracking required for image reconstruction and an acoustic or magnetic locator tracking the transducer [1-3,5,6].

The "sequential" technique is based on scanning the region of interest with a preset motion: fanlike, linear, or rotational. The latter was developed so that the system providing the rotation would be included in the transducer itself, thus avoiding the use of other mechanical systems. This was also incorporated into transesophageal transducers [1,2,5]. The "reconstruction" techniques were abandoned because of their complexity and because they did not allow real-time visualization of 3D images, being "offline" techniques. Therefore, with these methods, the spatial angular resolution between two 2D views was often unsatisfactory. The spatial and temporal interpolation of these views in the three directions of the cartesian axes made the data analysis long and difficult and negatively affected the quality of the final images [1,3-5,7].

Technological advances over these last years have led to the development of a new transducer using a compound matrix made up of numerous elements (3000 to 6000). This technology allows a 3D volume scan, using a phased-array system. The matrix arrangement of the elements allows the orientation (electronic direction) of the ultrasound beam in two planes instead of only one, as with phased-array 2D systems. Consequently the acquisition of a 3D volume is based on rapid recording of several lines along three perpendicular axes: X (depth), Y (lateral or azimuthal deviation), and Z (elevation) [1,4,5,7,8].

With each echocardiographic system, the spatial and temporal resolutions are limited by the time taken by the ultrasound wave to cross the tissue and the speed of computerized data analysis. With the 3D system, this limit creates an even more acute problem because of the larger quantity of tissue scanned per unit of time and the amount of data to analyze in order to create a 3D image. For a long time, this constituted the main limitation for clinical use of 3D echocardiography. New techniques allow transmission and simultaneous reception of a larger number of ultrasound impulses, the use of a higher repetition frequency (pulse repetition frequency, or PRF), and a deeper penetration of the ultrasound beam. The result is a pyramid-shaped 3D volume containing all echocardiographic data of the structure being studied. From this data set, contained in a solid virtual body shaped as a truncated pyramid, we can obtain views with any spatial orientation, using cropping and cutting, and assess specific regions in this 3D volume. Once the region to be examined is selected (with appropriately adjusted gain, depth, and 3D viewing planes), the 3D image in motion and in real time becomes visible. The captured volume can also be handled offline with a special software [1,4,5].

The Different 3D Echocardiography Methods

Several modes of 3D scanning are available in the most recent 3D echocardiographs: real-time 3D, 3D zoom, 3D full volume, and 3D color Doppler.

Real-Time 3D Mode

Real-time 3D images are obtained by using "narrow angle" scanning. This corresponds to a pyramid with a 60-degree angle on the Y-axis and a 30-degree angle on the Z-axis (Figure 6-1). The advantage of a "narrow angle" is the ability to perform a rapid and clear scan of the region of interest and to obtain a real-time 3D visualization. Using the trackball, the picture can be pivoted and a "point of view" can be selected in order to show sections or the surface of the structures being studied. The atrioventricular valves can be observed from the ventricle or atrium and the ostium of interventricular or atrial septal defects can be seen using "frontal" views of the surfaces of the right and left interventricular or interatrial septums. However, this technique is limited to relatively small regions [1,2,4,5].

3D Zoom Mode

The volume in this mode is narrower than that in the real-time 3D mode, with a pyramid with Y- and Z-axes angulated at 30 degrees. It yields better spatial and temporal resolution (Figure 6-2). This mode improves the temporal resolution to the detriment of the scanned region size.

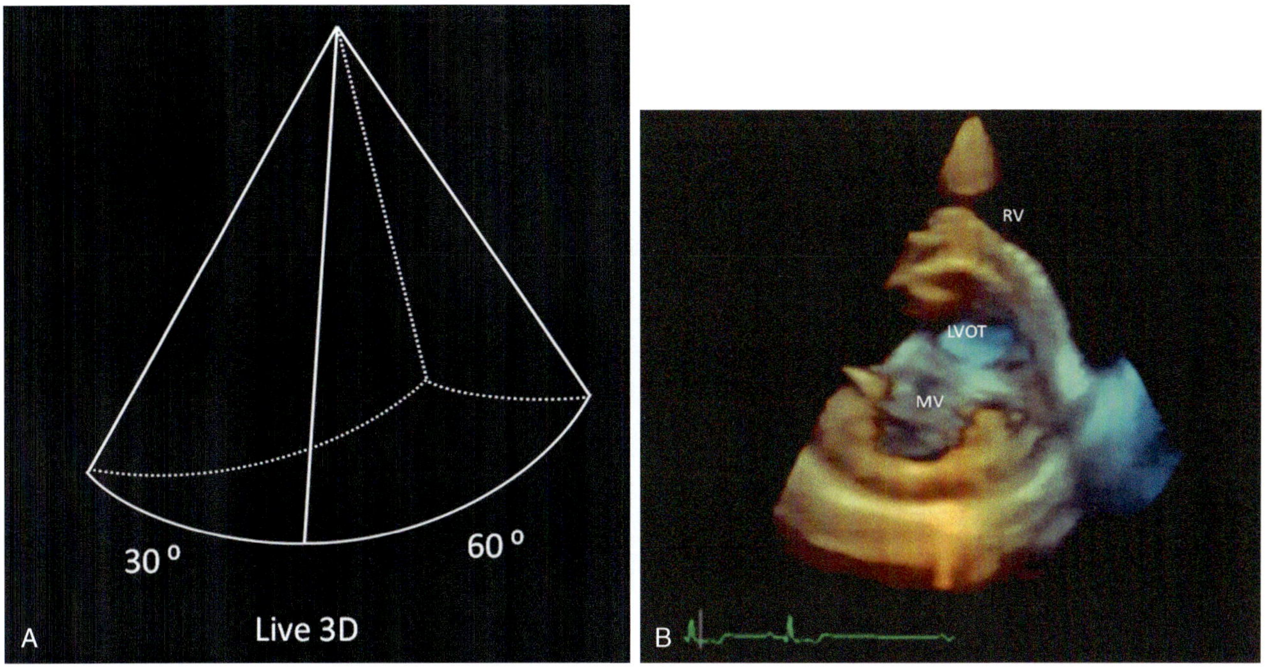

• **Fig. 6-1** A, A "narrow angle" sweep results in a pyramid with a 60-degree angle on the Y-axis (azimuthal deviation) and a 30-degree angle on the Z-axis (elevation degree). B, Real-time tridimensional (3D) pyramid before cropping or selection of the view, containing a part of the left ventricle, right ventricle (RV), mitral valve (MV), and left ventricular outflow tract (LVOT). (Photo credit: Claudio Bussadori.)

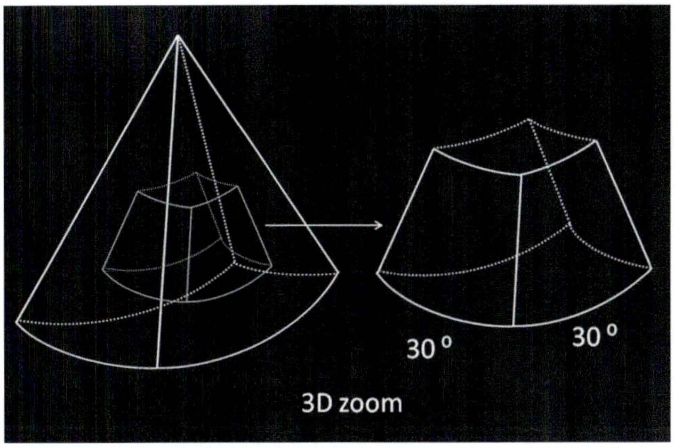

• **Fig. 6-2** Tridimensional (3D) zoom: pyramid with angles of 30 degrees for the Y- and Z-axes. A smaller volume improves the spatial and temporal resolutions of the region of interest. (Photo credit: Claudio Bussadori.)

3D Full Volume Mode

The increased calculation power and greater performance of the new matrix transducers allow the use of the "3D full volume" mode. This mode allows one to obtain a wider volume by using a wide-angle technique for scanning a large pyramid-shaped volume with angles up to 90 degrees × 90 degrees (Figure 6-3). The pyramid is constructed from several scanned segments using electrocardiographic synchronization and then superimposed. As in the case of real-time 3D and 3D zoom, the pyramid can be cropped and pivoted to display the region of interest (Figure 6-4). The quality of acquisition, and consequently the image quality obtained by computerized analysis, is influenced by R-R interval variability. The best results are obtained with a regular rhythm. Irregular cardiac rhythms and respiratory movements are sources of artifacts limiting the quality of the acquired images [1,2,4,5]. The use of this method in veterinary medicine is therefore limited by the frequent presence of a sinus arrhythmia and the inability to ask animals to control their breathing.

3D Color Doppler Echocardiography

With this technique, the Doppler information is displayed in the three Cartesian axes, forming a 3D image of the blood flow. Information on the direction, aliasing speed, and potential turbulences can be obtained. The image can later be pivoted by selecting different cross-sectional planes to show the flow from different angles, including a transversal cross-section (Figure 6-5) [9,10].

Multiplane Reconstruction

Each volume obtained through 3D echocardiography contains information along the X-, Y-, and Z-axes. Consequently, a 2D cross-section can be obtained from any angle inside the acquired volume, regardless of the position of the transducer (Figure 6-6) [1,2,4,5].

The new modes, which are simpler (especially real-time 3D), eliminate a great number of limitations associated

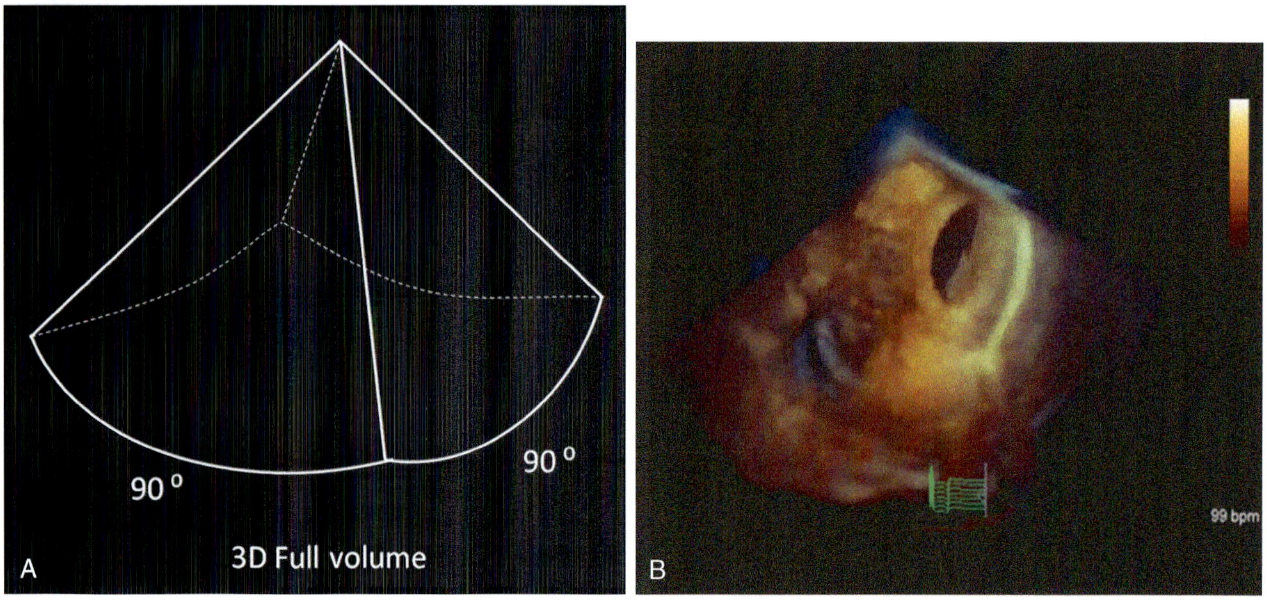

• **Fig. 6-3** A, A "narrow angle" sweep results in a pyramid with angles up to 90 degrees for the Y-axis (azimuthal deviation) and the Z-axis (degree of elevation). B, Tridimensional (3D) full volume view before cropping or selecting the view, including the entire heart. (Photo credit: Claudio Bussadori.)

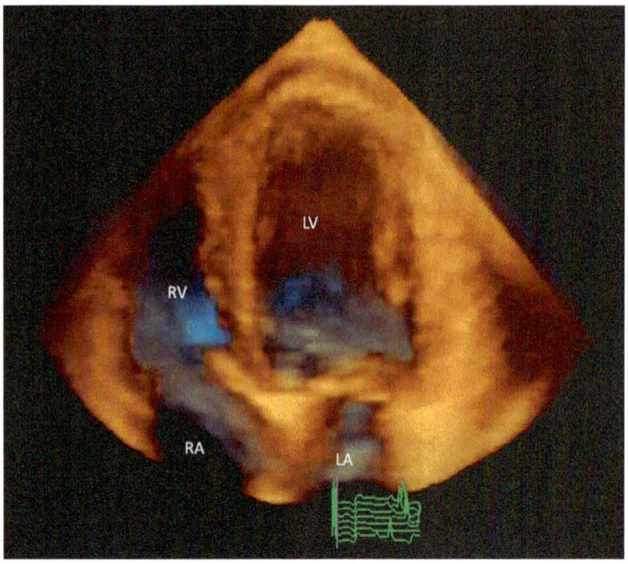

• **Fig. 6-4** Four chambers view after cropping the previously captured full volume view. *LA,* Left atrium; *LV,* left ventricle; *RA,* right atrium; *RV,* right ventricle. (Photo credit: Claudio Bussadori.)

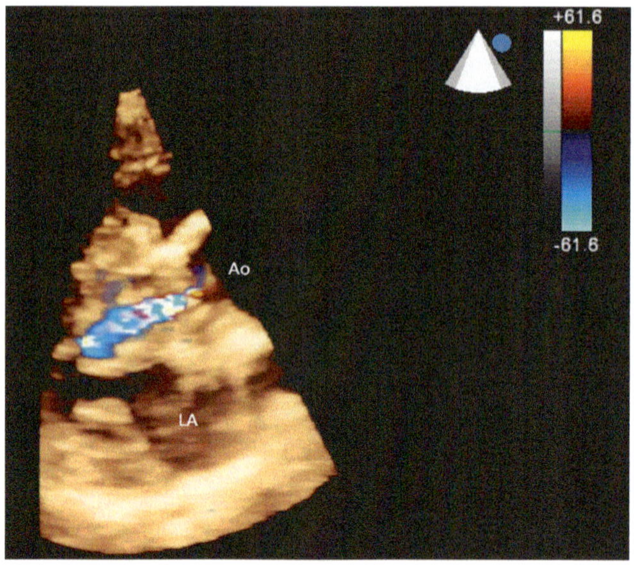

• **Fig. 6-5** Tridimensional (3D) color Doppler of an aortic regurgitant jet. *Ao,* Aorta; *LA,* left atrium. (Photo credit: Claudio Bussadori.)

with the older techniques. The necessity for a patient to hold his or her breath during information acquisition has been eliminated (this had seriously limited the usefulness of the 3D echocardiography in adult humans and prevented its use in human pediatric cardiology and veterinary cardiology, disciplines that are characterized by little patient cooperation). Currently, several high-frequency transducers of reduced size are available, providing excellent imaging even if used in 2D mode. These innovations can lead to the regular use of 3D echocardiography in veterinary cardiology.

3D Echocardiography in Veterinary Medicine

The first experiences with 3D echocardiography in veterinary medicine have shown that 3D transthoracic and transesophageal echocardiographic examinations were feasible and interesting, especially for valvular pathologies and monitoring of percutaneous interventional procedures. In most dogs, with the exception of the giant breeds or situations associated with extreme cardiac dilation, a volume containing the whole heart can be acquired using full volume mode or a specific region can

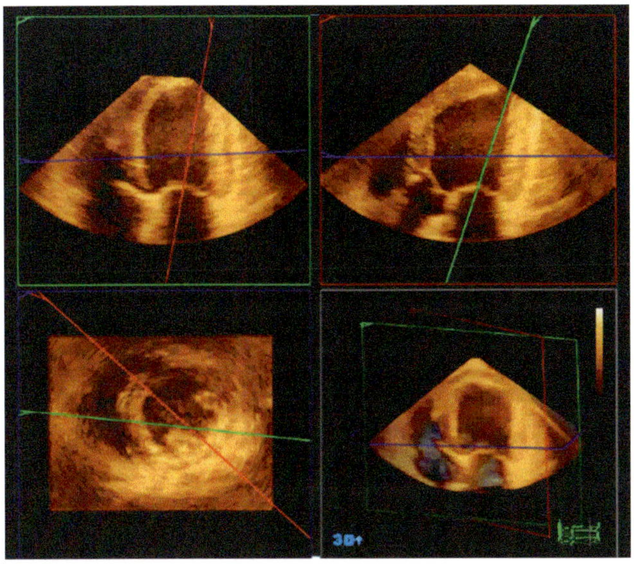

• **Fig. 6-6** From the multiplane reconstruction of the entire cardiac volume, a cross-section can be selected simply by moving the color-coded planes. On this image, the planes were selected in order to obtain the left apical 4 chambers view *(top left, green plane)*, the apical view of the left ventricular outflow tract *(top right, red plane)*, and the right parasternal transventricular short axis view at the level of the papillary muscles *(bottom left, blue plane)*. On each selected plane, the other planes are visible in the form of colored lines, as well as in the tridimensional (3D) reconstruction *(bottom right)*, in order to facilitate alignment with the studied structures. (Photo credit: Claudio Bussadori.)

be examined in real time with the use of real-time 3D mode.

Data Acquisition

The acquisition of three volumes is sufficient to obtain the necessary information for an adequate study of all cardiac structures. The first acquisition is performed using a "right parasternal" position while the other two are performed in "left parasternal" positions: apical to obtain the apical 4 chambers view and cranial and dorsal for study of the large vessels and the base of heart. The quality of volume acquisition for a 3D study depends less on operator skill than in 2D echocardiography. In fact, it is not necessary to change the transducer's position to assess various cardiac structures. A complete volume can be scanned or specific regions can be visualized by selecting proper views with the trackball.

It is recommended to begin the examination in real-time 3D mode because the images on the screen resemble the 2D classical views. From the "right parasternal" projection, the view can be shifted from the long axis (Figure 6-7) to the short axis (Figure 6-8) without changing the transducer's position. 3D acquisition allows the simultaneous visualization of different cross-sections as well as a frontal view of the details of the structures (Figures 6-9 to 6-11). The cross-section planes can be changed easily to assess each anatomic structure from angles that would

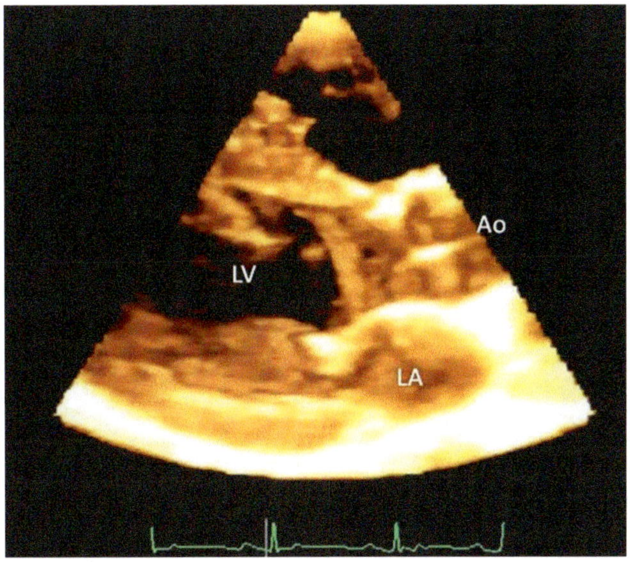

• **Fig. 6-7** Real-time tridimensional (3D) image obtained from a right parasternal cross-section corresponding to a right parasternal long axis view of the left ventricular outflow tract. *Ao,* Aorta; *LA,* left atrium; *LV,* left ventricle. (Photo credit: Claudio Bussadori.)

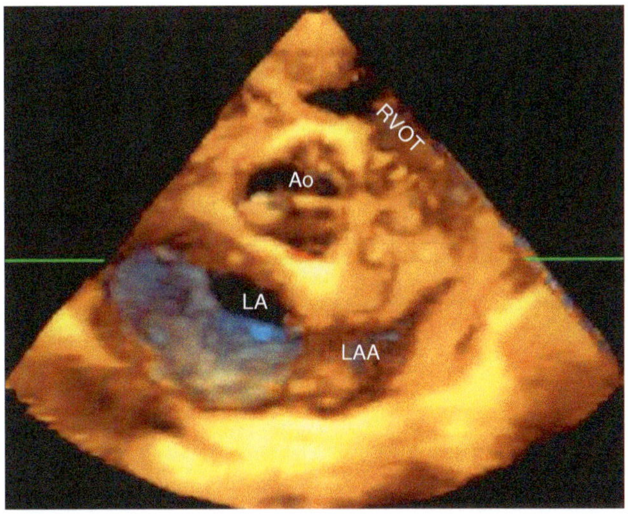

• **Fig. 6-8** Real-time tridimensional (3D) image obtained from a right parasternal cross-section corresponding to a right parasternal transaortic short axis view. *Ao,* Aorta; *LA,* left atrium; *LAA,* left atrial appendage; *RVOT,* right ventricular outflow tract. (Photo credit: Claudio Bussadori.)

be impossible to obtain using standard 2D echocardiography. Most anatomic characteristics of congenital and acquired cardiomyopathies become intuitively identifiable. Using offline analysis, the structures can be shown from various angles during the same event.

Measurement of the Left Ventricular Volume

The quantitative assessment of the left ventricular volume using 2D echocardiography is delicate and traditionally based on geometric hypotheses. This can lead to erroneous values, especially when the ventricular geometry is

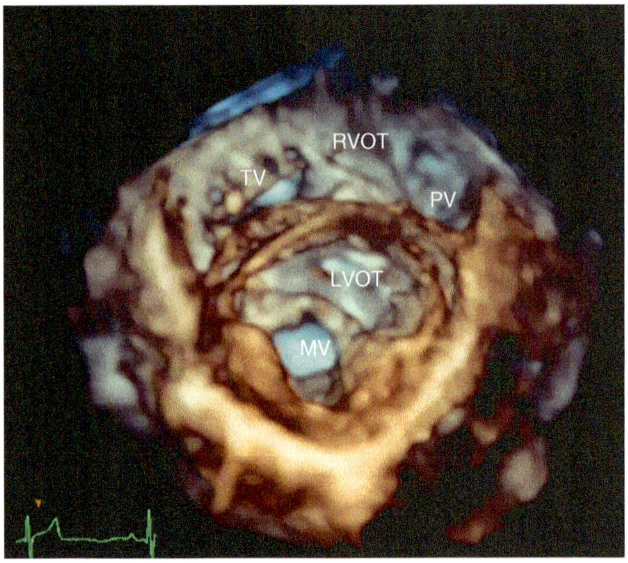

• **Fig. 6-9** Short axis view of the heart at the level of the papillary muscles. This tridimensional (3D) image displays the left ventricular outflow tract (LVOT), part of the mitral structure (MV), the tricuspid valve (TV), the right ventricular outflow tract (RVOT), and part of the pulmonic valve (PV). (Photo credit: Claudio Bussadori.)

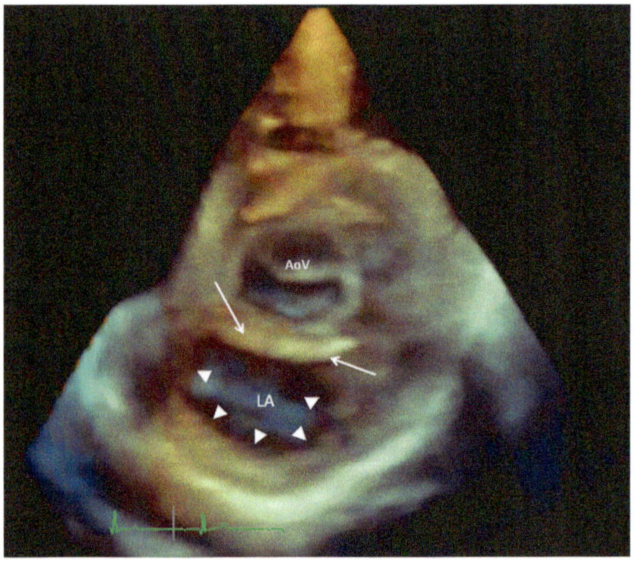

• **Fig. 6-11** Real-time tridimensional (3D) view of the left ventricle in diastole. The anterior mitral leaflet is wide open *(arrows)* and the outlines of the mitral valvular annulus can be seen *(arrowheads)*, with the left atrium (LA) in the background. *AoV,* Aortic valve. (Photo credit: Claudio Bussadori.)

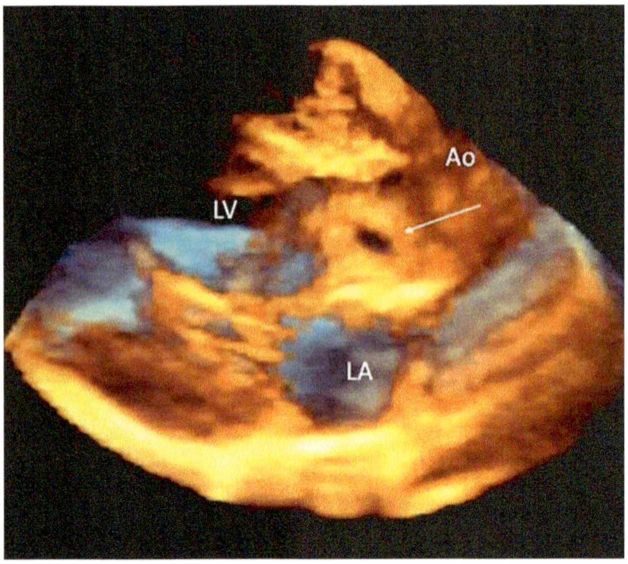

• **Fig. 6-10** Right parasternal long axis view, centered on the left ventricular outflow tract. The aortic root tridimensional (3D) view allows the observation of the right coronary ostium *(arrow)*. *Ao,* Aorta; *LA,* left atrium; *LV,* left ventricle. (Photo credit: Claudio Bussadori.)

modified [11,12]. The addition of a third dimension improves the reliability of volume measurements and decreases the errors due to oblique views [13]. The left chambers volume measurements using 3D echocardiography proved to be well correlated to the ones obtained through magnetic resonance [14-17]. In dogs, with or without cardiac pathology, the volumes obtained through 3D echocardiography are in agreement with those obtained by methods based on 2D echocardiography [18].

The left ventricular volume is obtained by placing the transducer in the same position as the one used to obtain the classic apical 4 chambers view, so as to include the entire left ventricular chamber in the obtained volume. Using special offline software, it is divided into three orthogonal planes corresponding to the apical 4 and 2 chambers views as well as the short axis view. These planes are set in order to obtain the true length and diameter of the left ventricle. Then the mitral valve insertion points on the annulus and the apex are identified on the long axis views and the ventricular wall at the level of the papillary muscles is identified on the short axis view in order to trace the outline of the ventricular endocardium. Finally, automatic detection of the edges allows the measurement of the systolic and diastolic volumes (Figure 6-12).

3D Cardiac Valve Evaluation

The mitral valvular apparatus is a complex 3D structure and the assessment of structural changes of a valvular pathology using 2D echocardiography can prove to be incomplete. 3D echocardiography improves the assessment of the mitral valve morphology and its function [19,20]. The frontal (atrial) (Figure 6-13), ventral (ventricular) (Figure 6-14), and oblique (Figure 6-15) views of the mitral valve display the entirety of the mitral leaflets as well as their degree of apposition, allowing a better evaluation of the structural changes and severity of the valvulopathy (Video 6-1). Moreover, an optimum alignment with the mitral valve plane allows an exact measurement of the dimensions of the mitral annulus,

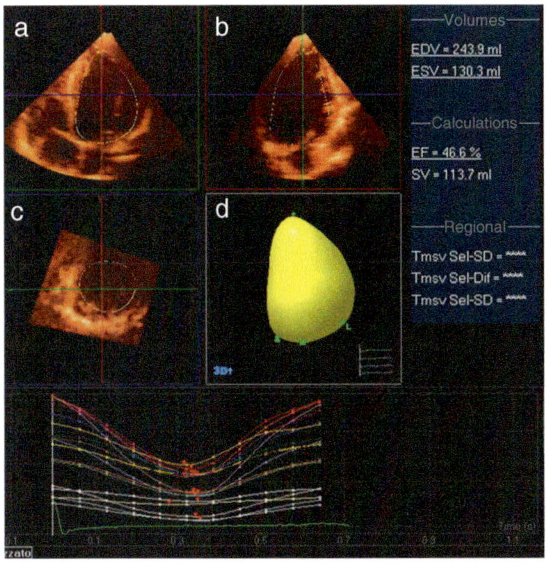

• **Fig. 6-12** Measurement of the left ventricular volume from the tridimensional (3D) echocardiogram. Three simultaneous orthogonal planes corresponding to the (a) apical 4 chambers, (b) apical 2 chambers, and (c) short axis views are used. The 3D representation of the left ventricular volume appears in (d). (Photo credit: Claudio Bussadori.)

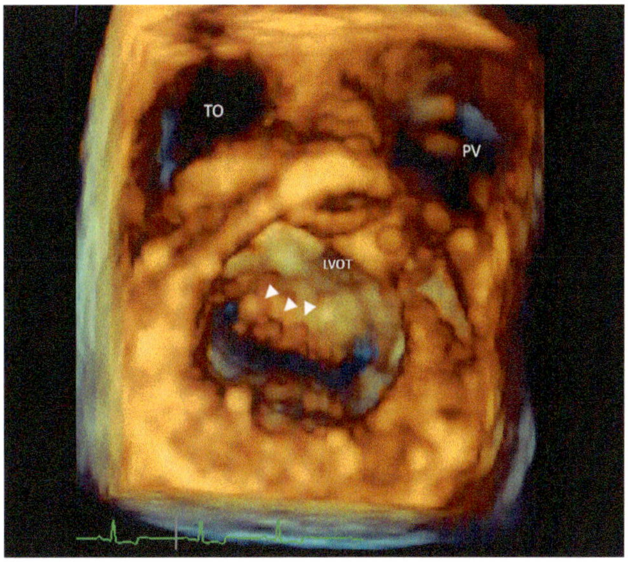

• **Fig. 6-14** Real-time tridimensional (3D) image of the left ventricle in diastole. The mitral leaflets are irregular and thickened. Larger nodules are visible on the anterior leaflet *(arrowheads)* and indentations are present on the edge of the leaflet. *LVOT,* Left ventricular outflow tract; *PV,* pulmonic valve; *TO,* tricuspid ostium. (Photo credit: Claudio Bussadori.)

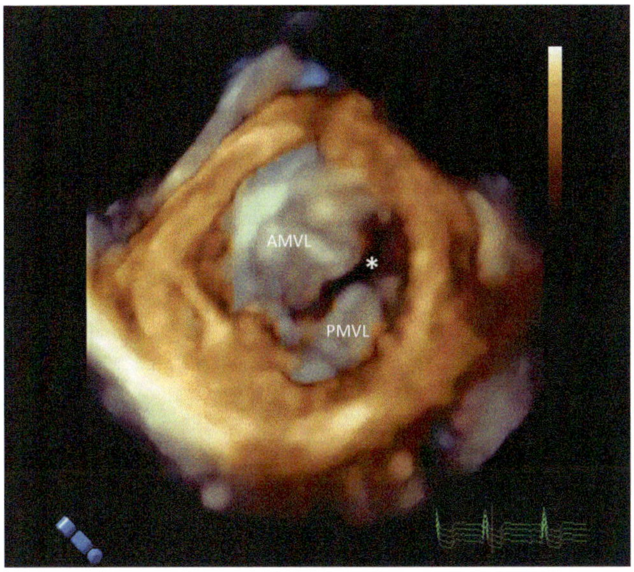

• **Fig. 6-13** Tridimensional (3D) full volume view of the mitral valve region in systole. The mitral leaflets are irregular and thickened. Interstices (*) resulting from inadequate apposition are visible between the leaflets. *AMVL,* Anterior mitral valve leaflet; *PMVL,* posterior mitral valve leaflet. (Photo credit: Claudio Bussadori.)

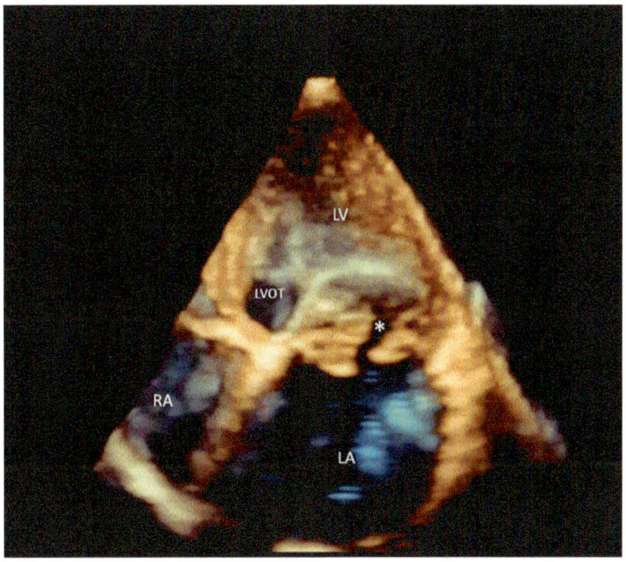

• **Fig. 6-15** Real-time apical view in systole. The mitral leaflets are very irregular and cannot coapt (*). *LA,* Left atrium; *LV,* left ventricle; *LVOT,* left ventricular outflow tract; *RA,* right atrium. (Photo credit: Claudio Bussadori.)

which is used to calculate the regurgitant volume. 3D color Doppler can also be used to more accurately measure the vena contracta (see Chapter 11) [19,20]. The 3D echocardiographic measurement of the left ventricular and atrial volumes is reliable and potentially may allow early detection of mitral disease [18,21,22].

Bacterial endocarditis is a rare disease in dogs and frequently leads to the appearance of vegetation and a variable degree of valvular destruction. The mitral and aortic valves are most often affected [23]. 3D transesophageal echocardiography allows a good assessment of the range and progression of the valvular lesions, using several planes (Figure 6-16). With rapid acquisition of the volume of the valvular region, complete assessment of the lesion is possible while minimizing contention and stress in a potentially unstable patient.

Accurate assessment of congenital cardiopathies strongly depends on diagnostic imaging. The mental reconstruction

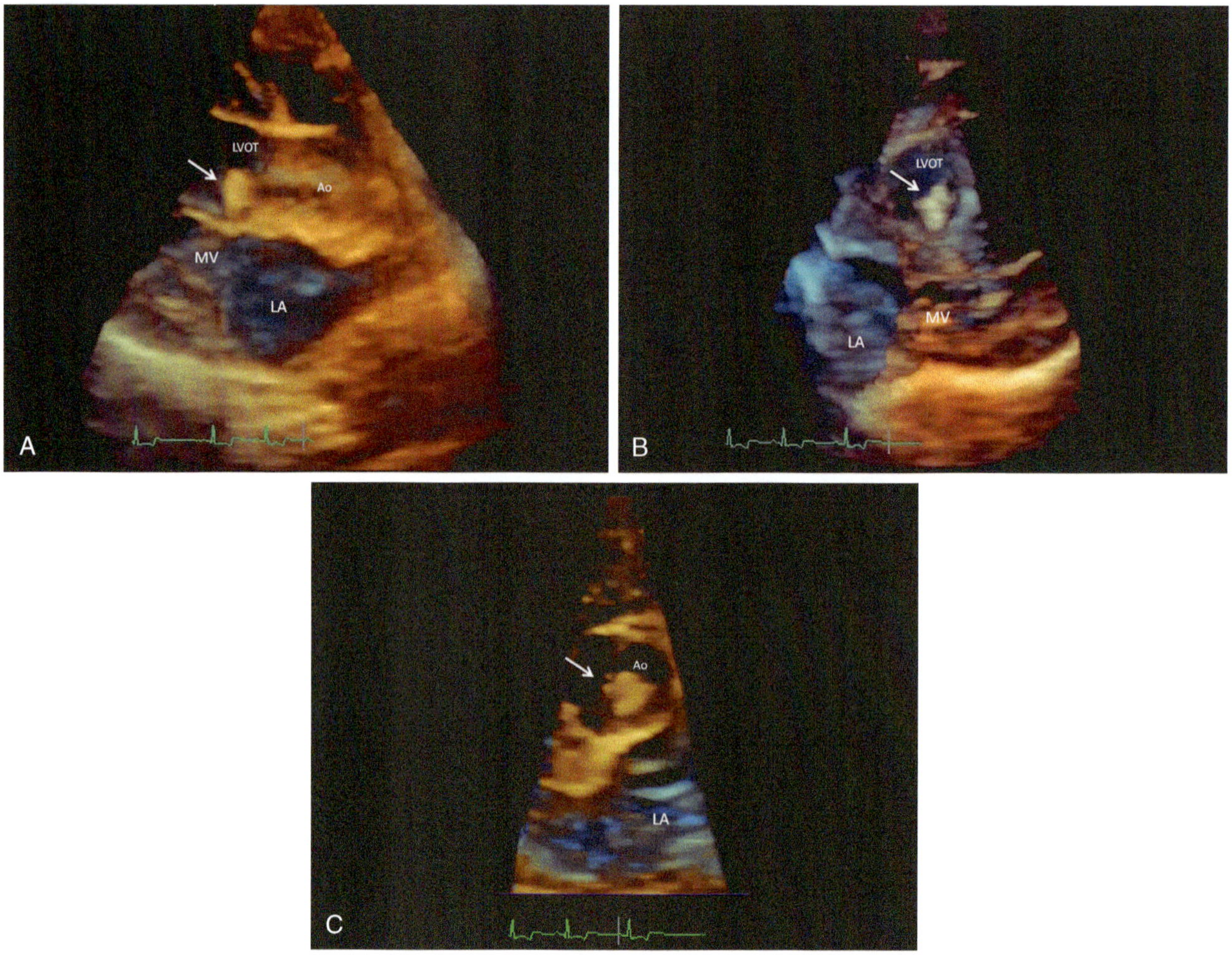

• **Fig. 6-16** Real-time tridimensional (3D) images obtained from a right parasternal view in a dog with a bacterial endocarditis of the aortic valve. The vegetation *(arrow)* herniates into the outflow tract and can be viewed from several angles. A, Long axis of the left ventricular outflow tract (LVOT). B, View from the left ventricle. C, Dorsal view from the aorta (Ao). The affected aortic valve in this dog was associated with a severe aortic regurgitation (not shown). *LA,* Left atrium; *MV,* mitral valve. (Photo credit: Claudio Bussadori.)

of the complex 3D anatomy of the congenital malformations using 2D echocardiography is difficult and depends greatly on the operator. The capability of using 3D echocardiography to choose the best planes, inaccessible with 2D echocardiography, improves the accuracy of the echocardiographic diagnosis (Figures 6-17 and 6-18).

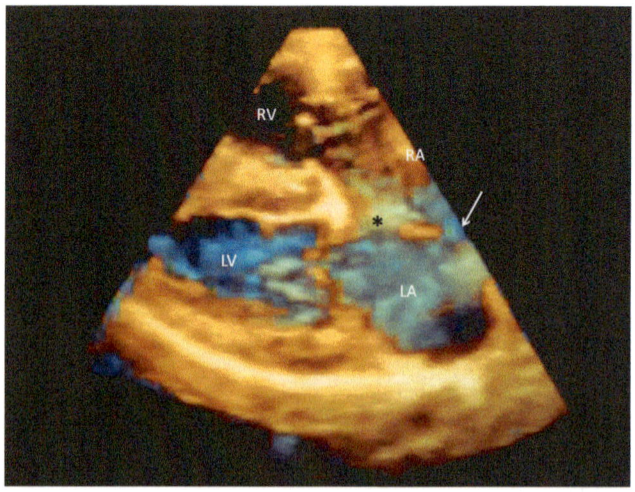

• **Fig. 6-17** Real-time tridimensional (3D) image and multiplane reconstruction in a dog with an incomplete atrioventricular canal. The view corresponds to the right parasternal long axis view. Two atrial septal defects are visible: an ostium secundum defect *(arrow)* in the dorsal part of the interatrial septum and a large ostium primum defect in the ventral portion (*). *LA,* Left atrium; *LV,* left ventricle; *RA,* right atrium; *RV,* right ventricle. (Photo credit: Claudio Bussadori.)

3D Transesophageal Echocardiography

3D Transesophageal Echocardiography in Human Interventional Cardiology

The use of 2D transesophageal echocardiography (TEE) is now widely accepted in human interventional cardiology laboratories. The ability to view endovascular instruments and to determine their position in relation to soft tissues in real time is an advantage over angiography. In veterinary medicine, TEE is also used to monitor certain percutaneous interventions, such as the percutaneous occlusion of patent ductus arteriosus (PDA) and

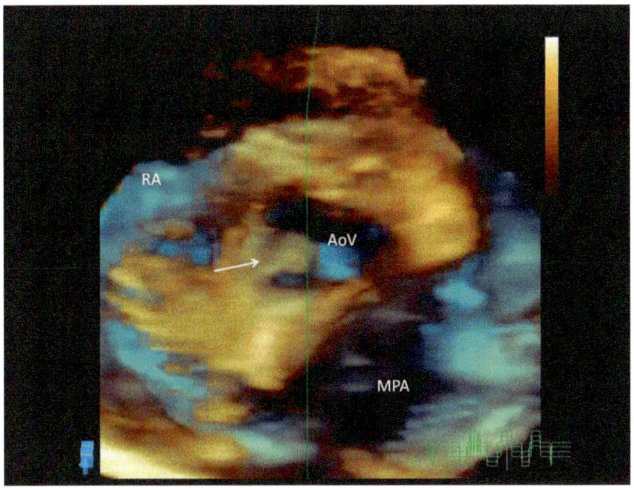

• **Fig. 6-18** Tridimensional (3D) transesophageal echocardiogram in a dog with valvular aortic stenosis. A nodule is visible between the left coronary and noncoronary cusps *(arrow)*. The cusps are also fused. *AoV,* Aortic valve; *MPA,* main pulmonary artery; *RA,* right atrium. (Photo credit: Claudio Bussadori.)

ventricular septal defects, or valvuloplasties of dysplasic pulmonic valves [24-27] (see Chapters 5 and 18).

The images obtained through 2D TEE are somewhat insufficient to track the catheters, guide wires, and occlusion devices because these must be aligned with the ultrasound beam to be visible. Continuous tracking of the endovascular instruments is not always possible because of the movements and the need to assess the neighboring structures. 3D technology allows the visualization of the cardiac structures and endovascular instruments in real time, thus alleviating the limitations of 2D TEE [28]. In human medicine, acceptance of 3D TEE was slow due to the skepticism of certain interventional cardiologists, the long training period needed, and the insufficient quality of the images obtained by the first machines. Currently, this technique is widely used in many interventional cardiology laboratories. It plays a major role in guiding interventions such as:

- Percutaneous occlusion of atrial septal defects, patent foramen ovale [29-37], ventricular defects [29,38-41], and the left atrial appendage for the prevention of thromboembolisms in patients with an atrial fibrillation and mitral disease [29,42-44]
- Percutaneous treatment of functional mitral regurgitation with a mitral clip [29,45,46] (Figure 6-19)
- Mitral stenosis balloon valvuloplasties [29,47,49]
- Percutaneous aortic valve replacement
- Electrophysiologic interventions guidance [29]

For all of these indications, 3D TEE proves to be superior to 2D TEE in the assessment of the real size and morphology of the septal defects, in the selection of patients and the choice of devices, and in guiding the correct placement of the chosen devices.

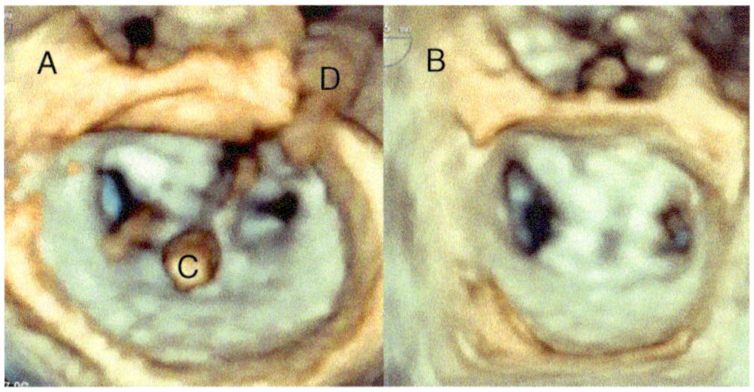

• **Fig. 6-19** Positioning of a mitral clip in a case of severe functional mitral regurgitation in a human. A, The transseptal catheter (D) containing the clip is visible, with the mitral clip (C) in position. B, Repaired mitral valve. (Photo credit: Gianni La Canna.)

Currently, several small transesophageal transducers are available. They are useful in pediatric cardiology and significantly reduce discomfort in adult patients. In veterinary medicine, the small size of these transducers allows their use in dogs of all sizes and in cats.

3D Transesophageal Echocardiography in Veterinary Interventional Cardiology

Over the last 20 years the technological evolution of 2D TEE has improved the assessment of certain congenital cardiomyopathies [50-53] and the monitoring of percutaneous interventions [24-27]. The quality of the echocardiographic images is often better than those obtained by transthoracic echocardiography because of the high resolution of the transducers, the proximity of the structures being studied, and the reduction in interference from other structures [51].

3D TEE (using a Philips iE33 system with the X7-2t TEE transducer) combined with 2D TEE and angiography were used in our interventional cardiology laboratory for interventions such as PDA occlusion and balloon catheter valvuloplasties of the pulmonic valve.

Patent Ductus Arteriosus

The percutaneous occlusion of PDA requires selection of the type and size of the occlusion device based on assessment of the morphology and size of the PDA. The success of this procedure strongly depends on the information obtained by the different diagnostic imaging methods. 3D and 2D TEE are able to show soft tissue in real time as well as the endovascular instruments (guide wires, catheters, and occlusion devices), allowing intraoperative monitoring without requiring contrast agent. Moreover, 3D TEE allows the easy identification as well as good characterization of the PDA through cross-sections that cannot be obtained via 2D echocardiography such as the frontal view of the ductal ostium (Figures 6-20 to 6-22 and Video 6-2). The region of

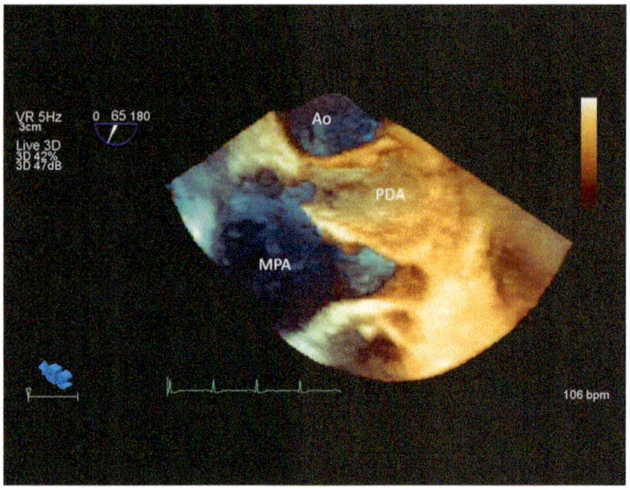

• **Fig. 6-20** Real-time tridimensional (3D) transesophageal echocardiogram in a dog with a patent ductus arteriosus (PDA). Lateral and longitudinal views obtained from a cranial position. *Ao,* Descending aorta; *MPA,* main pulmonary artery. (Photo credit: Claudio Bussadori.)

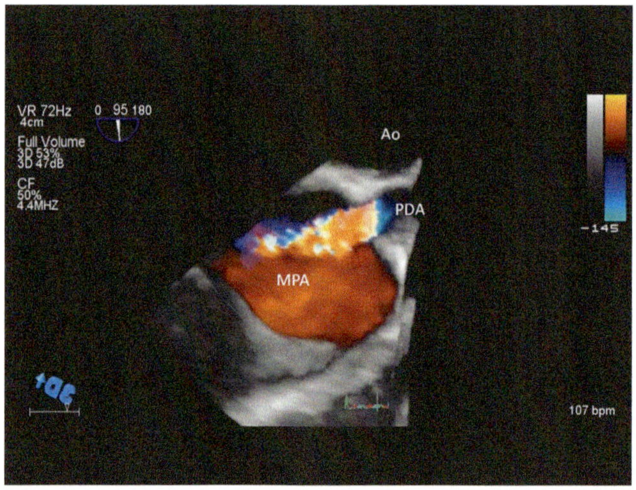

• **Fig. 6-21** Tridimensional (3D) color Doppler transesophageal echocardiogram in a dog with a patent ductus arteriosus (PDA). The turbulent flow through the ductus arteriosus is clearly visible. *Ao,* Descending aorta; *MPA,* main pulmonary artery. (Photo credit: Claudio Bussadori.)

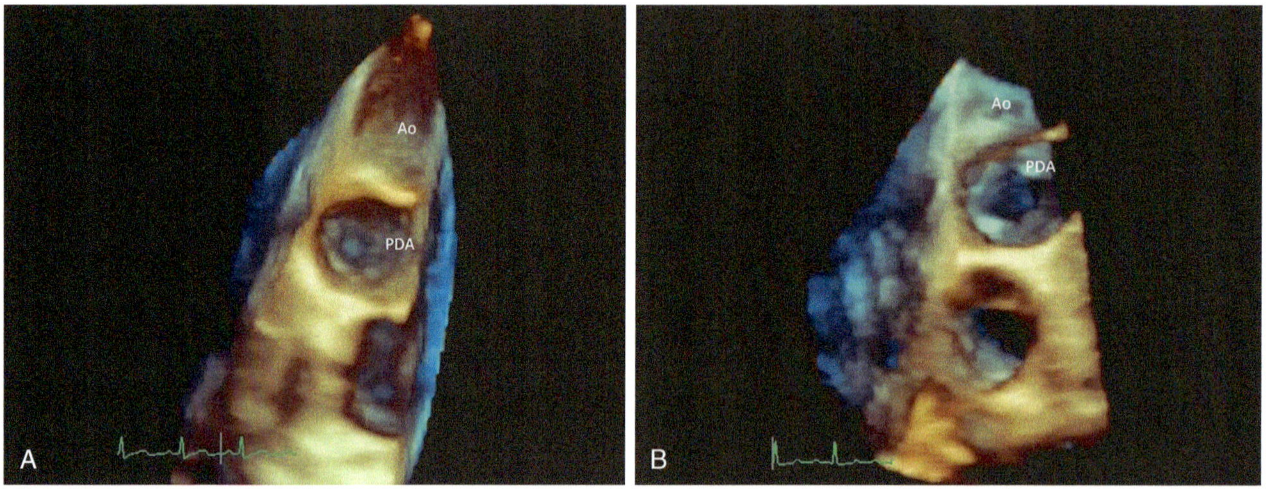

• **Fig. 6-22** Real-time tridimensional (3D) transesophageal echocardiogram in a dog with a patent ductus arteriosus (PDA). Dorsal view obtained from a cranial position. The frontal view of the pulmonary ostium shows several ostium shapes: circular (A) and elliptic (B). This allows better understanding of the ductal morphology and prevents ostium diameter underestimation when selecting the occlusion device. *Ao,* Descending aorta. (Photo credit: Claudio Bussadori.)

the ductal ostium is easily imaged before and after the occlusion, allowing good assessment of the device position and stability in real time and from different angles (Figures 6-23 and 6-24).

Pulmonic Valvuloplasty

During a valvuloplasty, 3D TEE can simultaneously display two orthogonal longitudinal views of the pulmonic valve, facilitating the assessment of the valvular morphology before and after the procedure (Figure 6-25). The "frontal view" allows precise assessment of the valvular apparatus from either the pulmonary artery or the right ventricular outflow tract, with visualization of the valvular orifice.

This study of valvular anatomy plays a potential role in the preoperative assessment of arterial valvular stenoses. The 3D reconstruction of the right ventricular outflow tract and aortic root allows visualization of the coronary arteries. Cases of pulmonic stenosis secondary to an abnormal R2A type coronary artery can be identified clearly by 3D TEE, which represents an advantageous alternative to coronarography, which is often necessary to document the presence of this abnormality (Figure 6-26).

The 3D TEE allows the visualization of the balloon and its position in relation to the valvular and vascular structures and assists in the subjective assessment of the degree of commissurotomy obtained after dilation (Figure 6-27).

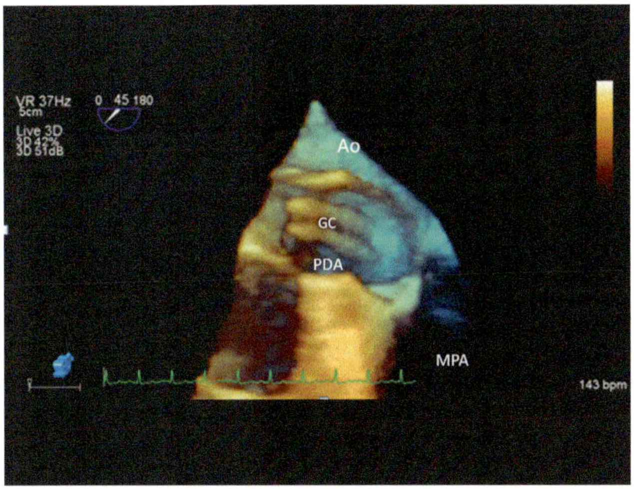

• **Fig. 6-23** Monitoring of a patent ductus arteriosus (PDA) occlusion procedure. The guiding catheter containing the Amplatz® occlusion device (GC) is in the ductus arteriosus. Its spatial relation to the neighboring structures is clearly visible. *Ao,* Descending aorta; *MPA,* main pulmonary artery. (Photo credit: Claudio Bussadori.)

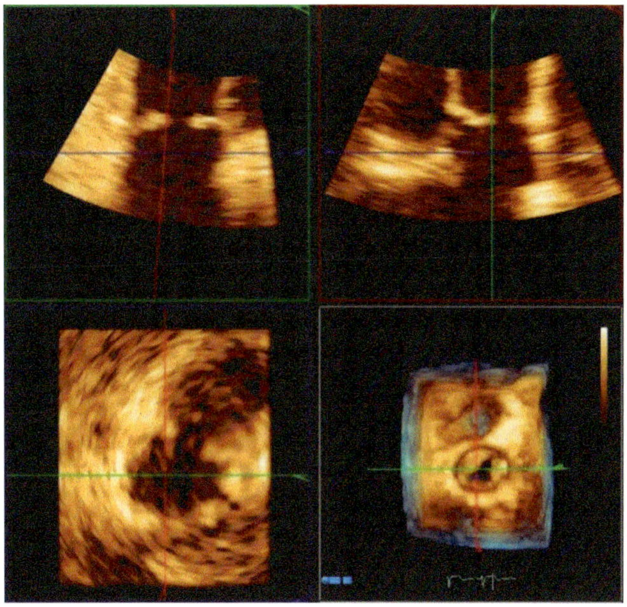

• **Fig. 6-25** Multiplane reconstruction and tridimensional (3D) view of a pulmonic stenosis in a dog. Longitudinal orthogonal views of the pulmonic valve *(top, green and red views);* transverse view of the subvalvular region *(bottom left, blue plane);* "frontal" view of the pulmonic valve from the pulmonary artery *(bottom right)*. (Photo credit: Claudio Bussadori.)

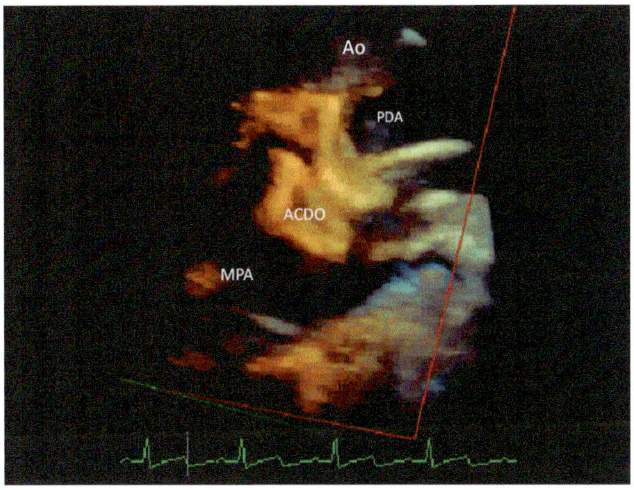

• **Fig. 6-24** Monitoring of a patent ductus arteriosus (PDA) occlusion procedure. Complete deployment of the occlusion device, the Amplatz® canine duct occluder (ACDO). *Ao,* Descending aorta; *MPA,* main pulmonary artery. (Photo credit: Claudio Bussadori.)

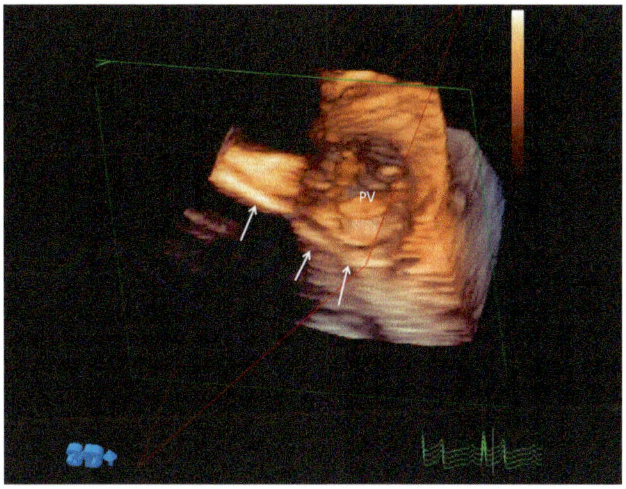

• **Fig. 6-26** Tridimensional (3D) transesophageal echocardiogram of an R2A type coronary anomaly with pulmonic stenosis in a bulldog. The abnormal coronary artery wraps around the right ventricle outflow tract *(arrows)*. *PV,* Pulmonary valve. (Photo credit: Claudio Bussadori.)

Finally, 3D TEE can be useful to detect potential postoperative complications. In a case of pulmonic stenosis treated by valvuloplasty, 3D TEE allowed the detection of a dissection of the proximal pulmonary artery (Figure 6-28). The use of 3D TEE during an intervention does not significantly increase its duration. However, adjusting the luminosity and contrast, selecting the planes, and rotating the images in real time requires more manipulation of the equipment compared to 2D TEE.

Acknowledgments

The authors would like to thank Antonino Bonanno and Andrea Laghi of Philips Healthcare for their technical support.

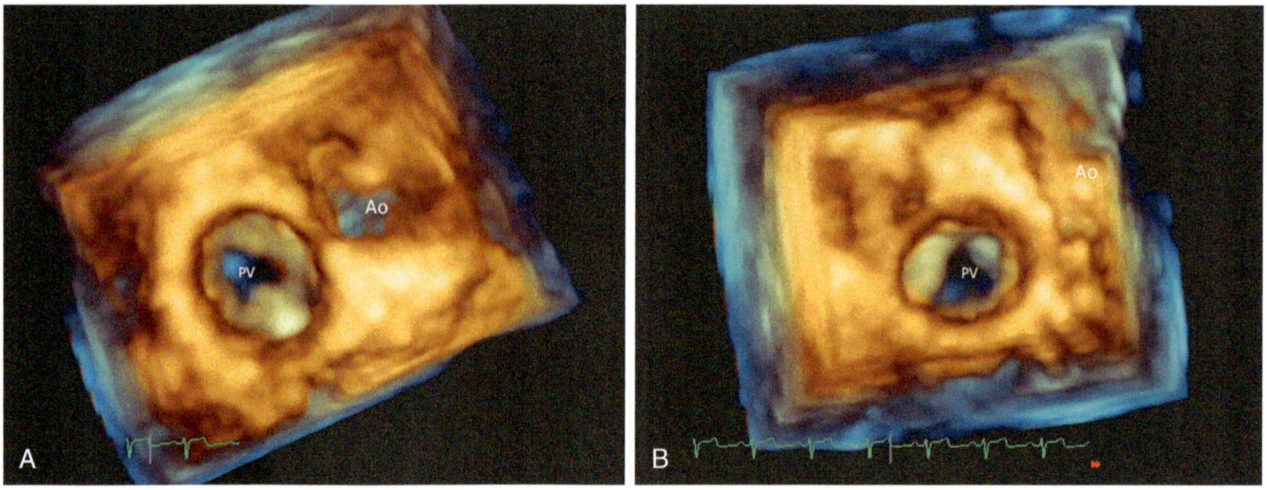

• **Fig. 6-27** Real-time tridimensional (3D) transesophageal echocardiograms in a dog with pulmonic stenosis, obtained from a cranial position, in end-systole. A, "Frontal" view of the pulmonic valve (PV) from the main pulmonary artery. The cusps are fused and the valvular opening is reduced. B, Increased mobility of the leaflets and opening of the PV after balloon valvuloplasty. *Ao,* Aorta. (Photo credit: Claudio Bussadori.)

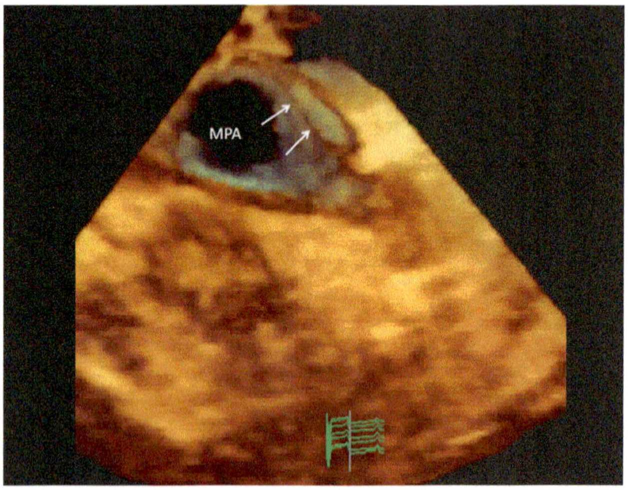

• **Fig. 6-28** Tridimensional (3D) full volume transesophageal echocardiogram of the main pulmonary artery (MPA) in a dog after balloon valvuloplasty. A tissue flap, separated from the arterial wall, is visible (*arrows*). (Photo credit: Claudio Bussadori.)

REFERENCES

[1] Chuang H, Gunasegaran K. Evolution of technology and machine basics. In: Takashiro S, editor. 3D echocardiography. London: Informa UK Ltd; 2007, p. 1–9.

[2] Pandian NG, Roelandt J, Nanda NC, et al. Dynamic three-dimensional echocardiography: methods and clinical potential. Echocardiography 1994;11:237–59.

[3] King DL, King Jr DL, Shao MY. Three-dimensional spatial registration and interactive display of position and orientation of real-time ultrasound images. J Ultrasound Med 1990;9:525–32.

[4] Wang XF, Deng YB, Nanda NC, et al. Live three-dimensional echocardiography: imaging principles and clinical application. Echocardiography 2003;20: 593–604.

[5] Houck RC, Cooke JE, Gill EA. Live 3D echocardiography: a replacement for traditional 2D echocardiography? Am J Roentgenol 2006;187:1092–106.

[6] Hung J, Lang R, Flachskampf F, et al. 3D echocardiography: a review of the current status and future directions. J Am Soc Echocardiogr 2007;20:213–33.

[7] Wang XF. Real time three-dimensional echocardiography: new breakthrough in the field of ultrasonic technique. Chin J Ultrasonogr 2003;12:71–5.

[8] Ahmad M. Real-time three-dimensional echocardiography in assessment of heart disease. Echocardiography 2001;18:73–7.

[9] De Simone R, Glombitza G, Vahl CF, et al. Three-dimensional color Doppler reconstruction of intracardiac blood flow in patients with different heart valve diseases. Am J Cardiol 2000;86:1343–8.

[10] Zhou ZW, Xu YW, Ashraf M, Sahn DJ. Three-dimensional echocardiography of colour Doppler flow. Arch Cardiovasc Dis 2010;103:333–9.

[11] Lang RM, Bierig M, Devereux RB, et al. Chamber Quantification Writing Group, American Society of Echocardiography's Guidelines and Standards Committee, European Association of Echocardiography. Recommendations for chamber quantification: a report from the American Society of Echocardiography's Guidelines and Standards Committee and the Chamber Quantification Writing Group, developed in conjunction with the European Association of Echocardiography, a branch of the European Society of Cardiology. J Am Soc Echocardiogr 2005;18:1440–63.

[12] Kupferwasser I, Mohr-Kahaly S, Stähr P, et al. Transthoracic three-dimensional echocardiographic volumetry of distorted left ventricles using rotational scanning. J Am Soc Echocardiogr 1997;10:840–52.
[13] Lang RM, Mor-Avi V, Sugeng L, et al. Three-dimensional echocardiography: the benefits of the additional dimension. J Am Coll Cardiol 2006;48: 2053–69.
[14] Hozumi T, Yoshikawa J. Left ventricle. In: Takashiro S, editor. 3D echocardiography. London: Informa UK Ltd; 2007, p. 11–25.
[15] Stoylen A. Strain echocardiography. In: Takashiro S, editor. 3D echocardiography. London: Informa UK Ltd; 2007, p. 141–51.
[16] Chang SA, Lee SC, Kim EY, et al. Feasibility of single-beat full-volume capture real-time three-dimensional echocardiography and auto-contouring algorithm for quantification of left ventricular volume: validation with cardiac magnetic resonance imaging. J Am Soc Echocardiogr 2011;24:853–9.
[17] Shimada YJ, Shiota T. A meta-analysis and investigation for the source of bias of left ventricular volumes and function by three-dimensional echocardiography in comparison with magnetic resonance imaging. Am J Cardiol 2011;107:126–38.
[18] Tidholm A, Westling AB, Höglund K, et al. Comparisons of 3-, 2-dimensional, and M-mode echocardiographical methods for estimation of left chamber volumes in dogs with and without acquired heart disease. J Vet Intern Med 2010;24:1414–20.
[19] Bhave NM, Lang RM. Quantitative echocardiographic assessment of native mitral regurgitation: two- and three-dimensional techniques. J Heart Valve Dis 2011;20:483–92.
[20] Zeng X, Levine RA, Hua L, et al. Diagnostic value of vena contracta area in the quantification of mitral regurgitation severity by color Doppler 3D echocardiography. Circ Cardiovasc Imaging 2011;4: 506–13.
[21] Ljungvall I, Höglund K, Carnabuci C, et al. Assessment of global and regional left ventricular volume and shape by real-time 3-dimensional echocardiography in dogs with myxomatous mitral valve disease. J Vet Intern Med 2011;25:1036–43.
[22] Tidholm A, Bodegård-Westling A, Höglund K, et al. Comparisons of 2- and 3-dimensional echocardiographic methods for estimation of left atrial size in dogs with and without myxomatous mitral valve disease. J Vet Intern Med 2011;25:1320–7.
[23] Sykes JE, Kittleson MD, Chomel BB, et al. Clinicopathologic findings and outcome in dogs with infective endocarditis: 71 cases (1992-2005). J Am Vet Med Assoc 2006;228:1735–47.
[24] Saunders AB, Achen SE, Gordon SG, Miller MW. Utility of transesophageal echocardiography for transcatheter occlusion of patent ductus arteriosus in dogs: influence on the decision-making process. J Vet Intern Med 2010;24:1407–13.
[25] Pariaut R, Sydney Moïse N, Kraus MS, et al. Use of transesophageal echocardiography for visualization of the patent ductus arteriosus during transcatheter coil embolization. J Vet Cardiol 2004;6:32–9.
[26] Saunders AB, Miller MW, Gordon SG, Bahr A. Echocardiographic and angiographic comparison of ductal dimensions in dogs with patent ductus arteriosus. J Vet Intern Med 2007;21:68–75.
[27] Bussadori C, Carminati M, Domenech O. Transcatheter closure of a perimembranous ventricular septal defect in a dog. J Vet Intern Med 2007;21:1396–400.
[28] Tsang W, Lang RM, Kronzon I. Role of real-time three dimensional echocardiography in cardiovascular interventions. Heart 2011;97:850–7.
[29] Perk G, Lang RM, Garcia-Fernandez MA, et al. Use of real time three-dimensional transesophageal echocardiography in intracardiac catheter based interventions. J Am Soc Echocardiogr 2009;22:865–82.
[30] Oto MA, Aytemir K, Ozkutlu S, et al. Percutaneous closure of interatrial septal defects: mid-term follow-up results. Turk Kardiyol Dern Ars 2011;39:385–95.
[31] Acar P, Aggoun Y, Le Bret E, et al. 3D-transthoracic echocardiography: a selection method prior to percutaneous closure of atrial septal defects. Arch Mal Cœur Vaiss 2002;95:405–10.
[32] Acar P, Bonhoeffer P, Saliba Z, et al. Three-dimensional reconstruction by transesophageal echocardiography of Amplatzer and CardioSEAL prosthetic devices after percutaneous closure and atrial septal defects. Arch Mal Cœur Vaiss 2000;93:539–45.
[33] Saric M, Perk G, Purgess JR, Kronzon I. Imaging atrial septal defects by real-time three-dimensional transesophageal echocardiography: step-by-step approach. J Am Soc Echocardiogr 2010;23:1128–35.
[34] Podnar T, Martanovic P, Gavora P, Masura J. Morphological variations of secundum-type atrial septal defects: feasibility for percutaneous closure using Amplatzer septal occluders. Catheter Cardiovasc Interv 2001;53:386–91.
[35] Martin-Reyes R, López-Fernández T, Moreno-Yangüela M, et al. Role of real-time three-dimensional transoesophageal echocardiography for guiding transcatheter patent foramen ovale closure. Eur J Echocardiogr 2009;10:148–50.
[36] Nasis A, Harper RW, Mottram PM. Real-time three-dimensional transoesophageal echocardiography for guidance of transcatheter closure of a complex multifenestrated atrial septal defect. Heart Lung Circ 2011;20:343–4.

[37] Mehmood F, Vengala S, Nanda NC, et al. Usefulness of live three-dimensional transthoracic echocardiography in the characterization of atrial septal defects in adults. Echocardiography 2004;21:707–13.
[38] Acar P, Abdel-Massih T, Douste-Blazy MY, et al. Assessment of muscular ventricular septal defect closure by transcatheter or surgical approach: a three-dimensional echocardiographic study. Eur J Echocardiogr 2002;3:185–91.
[39] Wei Y, Wang X, Zhang S, et al. Transcatheter closure of perimembranous ventricular septal defects (VSD) with VSD occluder: early and mid-term results. Heart Vessels 2011. E-pub ahead of print.
[40] Halpern DG, Perk G, Ruiz C, et al. Percutaneous closure of a post-myocardial infarction ventricular septal defect guided by real-time three-dimensional echocardiography. Eur J Echocardiogr 2009;10:569–71.
[41] Chen FL, Hsiung MC, Nanda N, et al. Real time three-dimensional echocardiography in assessing ventricular septal defects: an echocardiographic-surgical correlative study. Echocardiography 2006;23:562–8.
[42] Hara H, Matthews R, Virmani R, et al. Percutaneous left atrial appendage obliteration. JACC Cardiovasc Imaging 2008;1:92–3.
[43] Bayard YL, Omran H, Neuzil P, et al. PLAATO (percutaneous left atrial appendage transcatheter occlusion) for prevention of cardioembolic stroke in non-anticoagulation eligible atrial fibrillation patients: results from the European PLAATO study. EuroIntervention 2010;6:220–6.
[44] García-Fernández MA, Pérez-David E, Quiles J, et al. Role of left atrial appendage obliteration in stroke reduction in patients with mitral valve prosthesis: a transesophageal echocardiographic study. J Am Coll Cardiol 2003;42:1253–8.
[45] Biner S, Perk G, Kar S, et al. Utility of combined two-dimensional and three-dimensional transesophageal imaging for catheter-based mitral valve clip repair of mitral regurgitation. J Am Soc Echocardiogr 2011;24:611–7.
[46] Altiok E, Becker M, Hamada S, et al. Optimized guidance of percutaneous edge-to edge repair of the mitral valve using real-time 3-D transesophageal echocardiography. Clin Res Cardiol 2011;100:675–81.
[47] Eng MH, Salcedo EE, Quaife RA, Carroll JD. Implementation of real time three-dimensional transesophageal echocardiography in percutaneous mitral balloon valvuloplasty and structural heart disease interventions. Echocardiography 2009;26:958–66.
[48] Applebaum RM, Kasliwal RR, Kanojia A, et al. Utility of three-dimensional echocardiography during balloon mitral valvuloplasty. J Am Coll Cardiol 1998;32:1405–9.
[49] Korkmaz S, Demirkan B, Güray Y, et al. Acute and long-term follow-up results of percutaneous mitral balloon valvuloplasty: a single-center study. Anadolu Kardiyol Derg 2011;11:515–20.
[50] Loyer C, Thomas WP. Biplane transesophageal echocardiography in the dog: technique, anatomy and imaging planes. Vet Radiol Ultrasound 1995;36:212–26.
[51] Quintavalla C, Pradelli D, Domenech O, Bussadori C. Transesophageal echocardiography of the left ventricular outflow tract, aortic valve and ascending aorta in Boxer dogs with heart murmurs. Vet Radiol Ultrasound 2006;47:307–12.
[52] Shively BK. Transesophageal echocardiographic (TEE) evaluation of the aortic valve, left ventricular outflow tract, and pulmonic valve. Cardiol Clin 2000;18:711–29.
[53] Miller-Hance WC, Silverman NH. Transesophageal echocardiography (TEE) in congenital heart disease with focus on the adult. Cardiol Clin 2000;18:861–92.

PART III

Hemodynamic Evaluation

7 Global Left Ventricular Systolic Function Assessment, 111

8 Assessment of Diastolic Function, 127

9 Echocardiographic Evaluation of the Left Ventricle Filling Pressure, 139

10 Evaluation of the Right Ventricular Global Systolic Function, 151

7

Global Left Ventricular Systolic Function Assessment

ÉRIC DE MADRON

Left Ventricular Anatomy, 112

Radial Systolic Function: Shortening Fraction, 112

Systolic Indices Derived from Ventricular Volumes, 115

Assessment of the Longitudinal Systolic Function, 118

Systolic Indices Obtained by Spectral Wave Doppler: Systolic Time Intervals and Index of Myocardial Performance (Tei Index), 120

Speckle Tracking–Derived Indices, 121

Conclusion, 122

Global left ventricular systolic function assessment is one of the major goals of an echocardiographic examination. Many echocardiographic indices have been proposed to assess function. The list keeps getting longer due to technologic developments. These indices are obtained from the time-motion (TM), bidimensional (2D), spectral wave Doppler, tissue Doppler, and, finally, speckle tracking methods. A multimodal approach proves to be increasingly necessary to take into account the complexity of the ventricular geometry during systole and the influence of preload and afterload and to detect preclinical systolic dysfunctions.

This chapter discusses the measurement of global left ventricular systolic function indices. The indices of regional contraction obtained by tissue Doppler or speckle tracking, as well as the measurement of ventricular torsion by speckle tracking, are discussed in Chapter 4.

Left Ventricular Anatomy

Left ventricle (LV) anatomic studies in humans [1], as in dogs [2], reveal the coexistence of myocardial fibers oriented in a radial and longitudinal manner. A clear predominance of radially oriented fibers compared to longitudinal fibers is noted at the base of the LV. This predominance decreases toward the apex (Figure 7-1).

Moreover, radial fibers mainly occupy the middle layer of the ventricular wall while the longitudinal fibers are found in the subendocardial and subepicardial regions [2]. The radial dimensions of the LV shorten by 25% to 40% during systole while a sarcomere in normal load conditions only shortens by 10% to 12% [1]. This remarkable thickening of the ventricular walls therefore can be explained only by the combination of radial fiber shortening and transverse longitudinal fiber thickening [1]. Furthermore, the angulation of the longitudinal fibers increases from the base toward the apex, resulting in a helicoidal layout. These subendocardial and subepicardial helices have opposite directions and the subendocardial fibers contract faster than the subepicardial ones. This results in ventricular torsion with a basal clockwise rotation, and an apical counterclockwise rotation when the heart is viewed from the apex [2] (Figure 7-2).

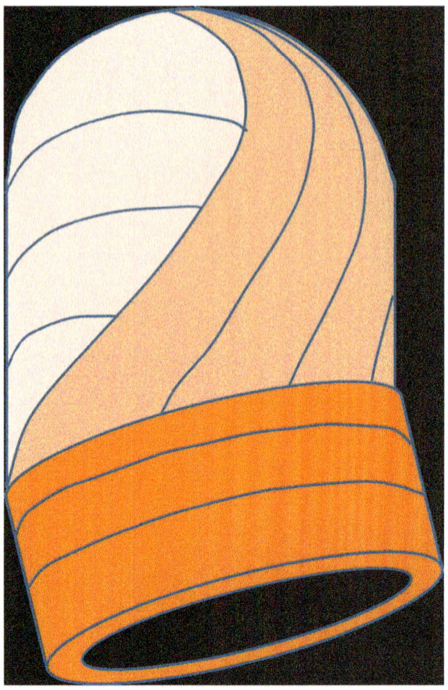

• **Fig. 7-1** Schematic illustration of the orientation of the myocardial fibers in the left ventricle. (Adapted from Henein MY, Gibson DG. Normal long axis function. Heart 1999;81:111–3.)

Conversely, the early diastolic "detorsion" (recoil) of the heart plays an important role in ventricular filling (see also Chapter 4, "Normal Myocardial Kinetics").

Therefore the study of the systolic function will need to consider all of these phenomena.

Radial Systolic Function: Shortening Fraction

Endocardial Shortening Fraction

The shortening fraction (SF) was one of the first echocardiographic systolic function indices developed [3]. It is easy to measure and is one of the most frequently used indices. It is obtained using a TM mode echocardiogram of the LV (right parasternal short axis transventricular view) and measures the LV short axis internal diameter systolic shortening (radial contraction). It is calculated as follows:

$$SF(\%) = [(LVd - LVs)/LVd] \times 100$$

where *LVd* and *LVs* represent the LV end-diastolic and end-systolic internal diameters, respectively. Because these diameters are measured from the septal endocardium to the left ventricular free wall endocardium (Figure 7-3), this index is sometimes called endocardial SF (eSF), compared to mid-wall SF discussed later.

As discussed in Chapter 2, eSF is affected by the angle between the TM cursor and the left ventricular walls. For eSF to be measured correctly, this angle must be as close as possible to 90 degrees.

A systolic dysfunction will be associated with a decrease in value of the eSF. This index has numerous limits, though. First, eSF measures only the radial contractility. However, in many cases, longitudinal systolic function anomalies appear before radial function anomalies [4].

Second, eSF must be interpreted in view of the hemodynamic situation. Indeed, it is affected not only by the state of myocardial contractility but also by preload and afterload conditions. For example, decreased myocardial contractility, hypovolemia, and vasoconstriction can all lead to a decrease in eSF [5,6]. Under conditions of significantly decreased afterload, as in mitral regurgitation, eSF can appear normal or increased, even if systolic dysfunction is present (see Chapter 11).

Moreover, eSF is negatively correlated to the heart rate: it decreases when the ventricle has less time to fill [7].

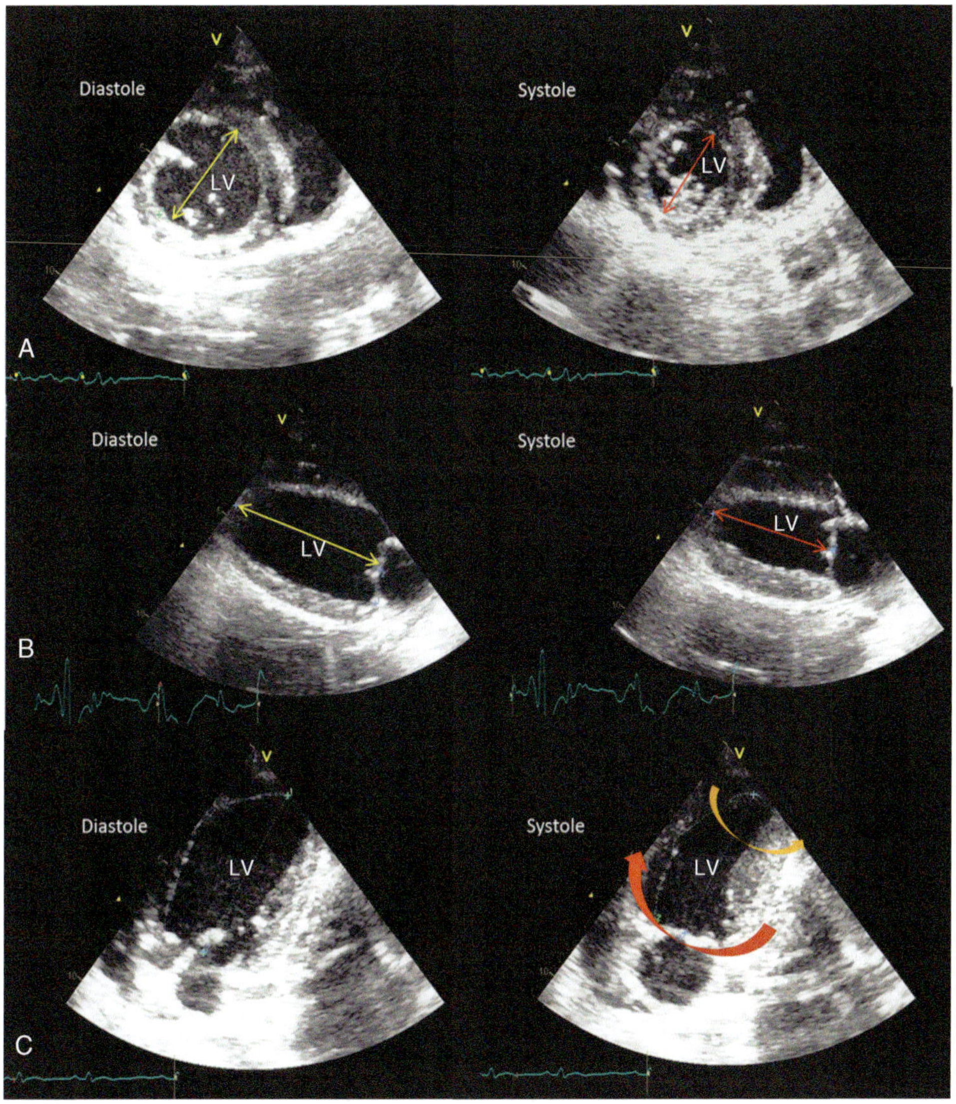

• **Fig. 7-2** Bidimensional (2D) echocardiograms illustrating the geometric changes during ventricular systole. We see (A) a radial contraction of the short axis, (B) a longitudinal contraction of the long axis, and (C) a counterclockwise torsion of the apex and the base of the left ventricle (LV). (Photo credit: Éric de Madron.)

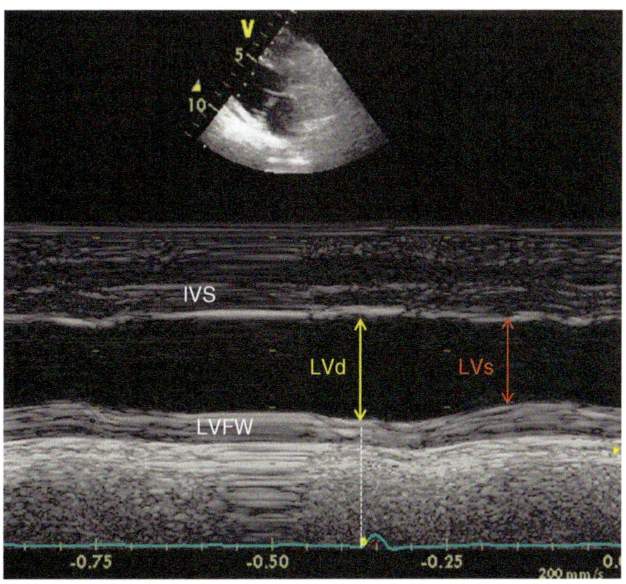

• **Fig. 7-3** Time-motion (TM) echocardiogram of the left ventricle in a dog demonstrating endocardial shortening fraction calculation. *IVS,* Interventricular septum; *LVd,* end-diastolic internal diameter of the left ventricle; *LVFW,* left ventricle free wall; *LVs,* end-systolic internal diameter of the left ventricle. (Photo credit: Éric de Madron.)

TABLE 7-1 Normal Endocardial Shortening Fraction (eSF) in Dogs and Cats [8]

Parameter	Dogs (n = 53) Average ±2 Standard Deviations (Median Value; Minimum-Maximum)	Cats (n = 32) Average ±2 Standard Deviations (Median Value; Minimum-Maximum)
eSF (%)	34.4 ± 6.5 (33.6; 25.3-49.9)	51.9 ± 6.3 (52.2; 39.9-64.3)

Normal eSF values in dogs and cats are presented in Table 7-1 [8]. It is important to note that the breed can have a significant influence on eSF, as noted in the Doberman Pinscher, in which the normal eSF values are lower than those in other breeds: 24 ± 7.2% [9].

Mid-Wall Shortening Fraction

As mentioned above, the myocardial fibers that make up the left ventricular wall are longitudinal in the subendocardial and subepicardial regions and radial in the central region ("mid-wall"). In the event of systolic dysfunction, the loss of contractility of the longitudinal fibers leads to an exaggerated movement of the epicardium [10] that will amplify the endocardial excursion, resulting in an eSF pseudonormalization. Therefore many studies in humans use an index known as mid-wall SF (SFmw) to assess the SF of the central zone of the LV walls, thus eliminating the influence of the epicardial movement [4,11-13].

SFmw is calculated as follows: [11]

$$\mathrm{SFmw} = \{[(\mathrm{LVd} + \mathrm{LVFWd}/2 + \mathrm{IVSd}/2) - (\mathrm{LVs} + \mathrm{IVSs}/2 + \mathrm{LVFWs}/2)]/(\mathrm{LVd} + \mathrm{LVFWd}/2 + \mathrm{IVSd}/2)\} \times 100$$

where *LVd* and *LVs* are the internal end-diastolic and end-systolic diameters of the LV, respectively; *LVFWd* and *LVFWs* are the end-diastolic and end-systolic thicknesses of the LV free wall, respectively; and *IVSd* and *IVSs* are the end-diastolic and end-systolic thicknesses of the interventricular septum, respectively.

For instance, let us consider a 20-kg normal dog with the following left ventricular dimensions (taken from Table 2-1 in Chapter 2): LVd = 3.7 cm, LVs = 2.4 cm, LVFWd = IVSd = 0.8 cm, LVFWs = IVSs = 1.2 cm.

The eSF will be:

$$\mathrm{eSF} = [(3.7-2.4)/3.7] \times 100 = 35\%$$

The SFmw will be:

$$\mathrm{SFmw} = \{[(3.7 + 0.4 + 0.4) - (2.4 + 0.6 + 0.6)]/(3.7 + 0.4 + 0.4)\} \times 100 = 20\%$$

This example illustrates the influence of the longitudinal fibers on the global radial shortening.

SFmw may prove to be more sensitive than eSF in the detection of the systolic dysfunctions [14].

Assessment of End-Systolic Wall Stress

The study of the relationship between the SF and systolic wall stress is another way of assessing systolic function [5,6]. In fact, there is a negative correlation between the SF and the afterload [15]. Wall stress is an indicator of afterload. It is important to know whether a given value is normal for the afterload level (or wall stress) at that moment in order to interpret the significance of any the SF values correctly. This notion is particularly important when afterload is increased, as in systemic arterial hypertension, or significantly decreased, as in mitral regurgitation.

An echocardiographic method to calculate end-systolic wall stress (ESWS) was proposed in 1982 by Reichek et al:[15]

$$\mathrm{ESWS}\ (\text{in dyn/cm}^2) = 0.334\ \mathrm{P}\ (\mathrm{LVs})/[\mathrm{LVFWs}\ (1 + \mathrm{LVFWs}/\mathrm{LVS})]$$

where *P* is the systolic blood pressure, *LVs* is the end-systolic internal diameter of the left ventricle, and *LVFWs* is the end-systolic left ventricular free wall thickness. The echocardiographic ESWS values obtained using this method correlated well with the invasively measured wall stress (by micromanometry). Normal values ranged from 36 to 213 × 10^3 dyn/cm^2. Wall stress was increased in patients with reduced ejection fraction [15].

If we take the same example used above (see "Mid-wall shortening fraction"), the ESWS of a normal 20-kg dog with a systolic blood pressure of 140 mm Hg would be:

$$\mathrm{ESWS} = 0.334 \times 140 \times 2.4/[1.2\,(1 + 1.2/2.4)] = 62.34 \times 10^3\,\text{dyn/cm}^2$$

More recently, another method of calculation of the peak circumferential end-systolic wall stress (PSS, in g/cm^2) from systemic arterial blood pressure and echocardiographic LV dimensions has been proposed, using the cylinder model as a mathematical hypothesis: [16]

$$\mathrm{PSS} = \mathrm{P} \times a^2\,[1 + (b^2/r^2)]\,/\,(b^2 - a^2)$$

where *P* is the systolic arterial blood pressure, *a* is the internal radius (endocardial), *b* is the external radius (epicardial), and *r* is the LV mid-wall radius.

If we apply this formula to the same example used above, the PSS would be:

$$PSS = 140 \times (2.4/2)^2[1 + ((2.4 + 1.2 + 1.2)/2)^2 \\ ((2.4 + 0.6 + 0.6)/2)^2]/[(2.4 + 1.2 + 1.2)/2]^2 - \\ (2.4/2)^2 = 129.73\ g/cm^2 (\text{or } 127.19 \times 10^3 dyn/cm^2)$$

From this point, the SF can be normalized for the wall stress by using the SF/PSS ratio [4,12,13,16].

The role of these indices (SFmw and SF/PSS) remains to be established in veterinary cardiology but they may have value in the detection of systolic dysfunction in cases of afterload reduction such as mitral regurgitation.

Systolic Indices Derived from Ventricular Volumes

Several LV global systolic function indices can be derived from the calculation of the end-diastolic and end-systolic ventricular volumes.

Ventricular Volume Estimation

The methods used to estimate the LV volume are either geometric or planimetric.

Geometric Methods

The LV volume (V) can be obtained from the transverse internal diameter (D), based on several ventricular geometry approximations. Several formulas have been suggested based on one or several LV dimensions [17-24]. In dogs, the most frequently used formulas based on a single dimension are:

$$V = D^3$$

$$V = D^3 \times 7(2.4 + D)$$

$$V_{diastole} = 0.85 \times LVd^3; V_{systole} = 1.20 \times LVs^3$$

$$V = D^{3.16}$$

Other formulas use the short axis diameter and the length, as in the area-length method of Wyatt et al:[18, 22]

$$V = (\pi/6) \times D^2 \times L$$

where *L* is the length of the LV.

Among these equations, the Teichholz formula [20] [$V = D^3 \times 7/(2.4 + D)$] is still used regularly. It is important to recognize the limitations of this particular formula in dogs. Indeed, it has two components: one giving the volume (D^3) and the other describing a geometric shape [$7/(2.4 + D)$]. The second component is derived from a regression equation based on angiograms performed on human patients. In these patients it was found that the length/diameter (L/D) ratio could be calculated using the following formula: $L/D = 13.33/(2.4 + D)$ [20]. Consequently, in a normal human with a left ventricular end-diastolic diameter of approximately 5 cm, the L/D ratio is $13.33/(2.4 + 5) = 1.8$. Using these conditions, the formula $V = (\pi/6) \times D^2 \times L$ gives an acceptable estimation of the ventricular volume. In dogs and cats, this formula is no longer valid. Indeed, in the case of a cat with an end-diastolic left ventricular diameter of 1.5 cm, the L/D ratio would be equal to $13.33/(2.4 + 1.5) = 3.5$ if the above formula was used. This would mean a significantly elongated LV. In this case, a volume calculated with the Teichholz formula would be overestimated by a factor of 2. One way to overcome this would be to replace the D in the Teichholz formula with a dimension that is independent of size—for example, a weight-indexed dimension. The resulting formula could be $L/D = 13.33/(2.4 + k \times LV_{weight})$.

LV_{weight} has a normal diastolic value of 1.6 (see Chapter 2). If we accept a normal L/D ratio of 1.6 for dogs and cats, the diastolic k value would be 3.7.

LV_{weight} has a normal systolic value of 1 in dogs and 0.8 in cats (see Chapter 2). Considering that the L/D ratio does not change in systole, the value of systolic k becomes 5.9 in dogs and 7.4 in cats [25].

The "veterinary" version of the Teichholz formula therefore can be summarized as indicated in Table 7-2 (but this remains to be validated).

TABLE 7-2 "Veterinary" Teichholz Method Formulas [25]

	Dog	Cat
Diastolic volume	$LVd^3 \times 7/[2.4 + 3.7 \times LVd/(0.795 \times W^{1/3})]$	$LVd^3 \times 7/[2.4 + 3.7 \times LVd/(0.567 \times W^{1/3})]$
Systolic volume	$LVs^3 \times 7/[2.4 + 5.9 \times LVs/(0.795 \times W^{1/3})]$	$LVs^3 \times 7/[2.4 + 7.4 \times LVs/(0.567 \times W^{1/3})]$

LVd, Left ventricle end-diastolic diameter (in cm); *LVs*, left ventricle end-systolic diameter (in cm); *W*, weight in kilograms.

Normal end-systolic and end-diastolic volume indices (ESVI and EDVI, respectively) derived from these "veterinary" formulas are proposed in Table 7-3. One can see that these indices increase with the weight. This should be taken into account when attempting to interpret ESVI and EDVI values (see below). These normal values remain to be validated in veterinary medicine.

TABLE 7-3 Proposed Normal Values for the End-Systolic and End-Diastolic Volume Indices (ESVI and EDVI, Respectively, in mL/m²) in Dogs, Calculated Using the Formulas Outlined in Table 7-2 and Using the Normal Theoretic Left Ventricular Values of Cornell et al [25] (See Table 2-1 in Chapter 2)

Weight (kg)	ESVI Mean (Min-Max)	EDVI Mean (Min-Max)
3	8.05 (0.21-16.7)	33.63 (23.7-54.3)
4	9.86 (0.25-16.7)	36.60 (23.7-56.9)
6	11.04 (0.33-19.6)	40.72 (27.8-60.5)
9	11.97 (0.44-22.1)	43.95 (28.5-62.9)
11	12.35 (0.5-24.2)	46.97 (31.4-70.0)
15	13.45 (0.61-26.9)	50.80 (32.6-77.5)
20	14.51 (0.74-27.6)	54.49 (36.3-84.7)
25	15.83 (0.86-30.8)	55.86 (38.1-66.1)
30	17.34 (0.98-32.35)	61.19 (40.3-90.7)
35	17.59 (1.08-34.2)	63.71 (40.2-97)
40	17.96 (1.18-34.2)	63.35 (43.0-99.7)
50	20.28 (1.37-36.7)	66.72 (43.9-102.4)
60	21.46 (1.55-39.6)	70.88 (45.3-110.3)
70	21.43 (1.72-40.9)	72.45 (47.20-115.1)

Planimetric Methods

Planimetric methods do not require any geometric approximations. The ventricular volume is derived from the trace of the endocardial outline of the LV on a 2D image (right parasternal long axis or left apical 2 or 4 chambers views). Several methods have been evaluated in dogs: the Simpson method and two different area-length methods [17,26]. In these three methods, two left apical 4 chambers frames are selected, one at end-diastole and the other at end-systole. The internal area of the LV (closed at the level of the mitral annulus) is obtained by drawing the endocardial contour. The Simpson method divides this area into multiple disks of the same thickness (Figure 7-4).

The two area-length methods use the following equations:

$$V = 0.85\ A^2/L$$

where *V* is the LV volume, *A* is its internal surface, and *L* is its length, [17] or:

$$V = 5/6\ A \times L$$

(the so-called "bullet" method) [27] (Figure 7-5).

The geometric method using the classic formula of Teichholz and the planimetric methods using the Simpson method and the formula $V = 0.85 \times A^2/L$ were compared in dogs [17]. With a trained operator, repeatability and reproducibility of the measurements were good, regardless of the method used. However, the Teichholz method tended to overestimate the ventricular volumes in a nonlinear fashion and is therefore no longer recommended in

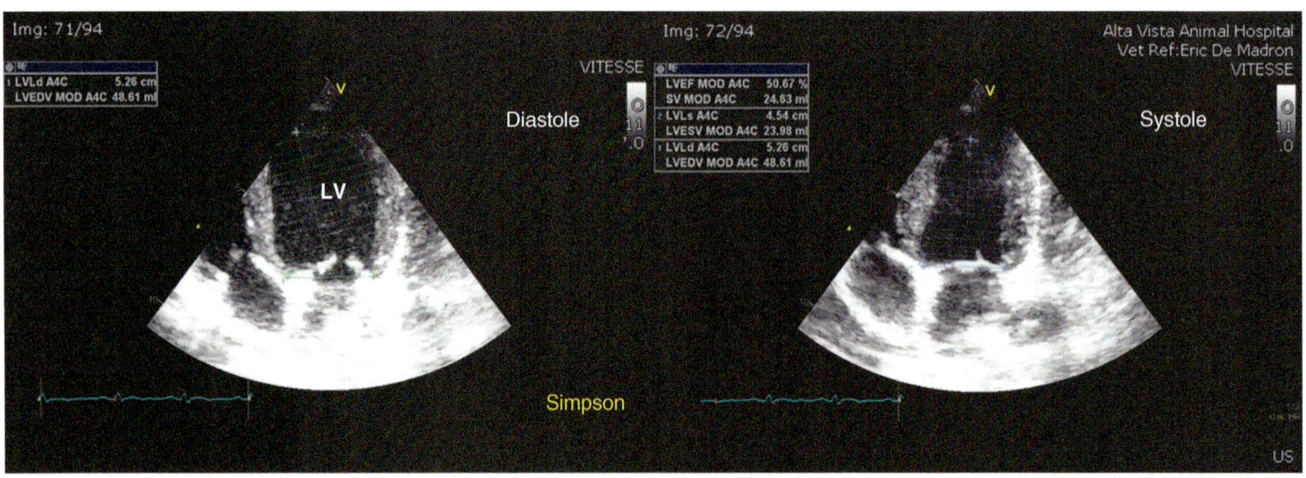

• **Fig. 7-4** Measurements of left ventricular diastolic and systolic volumes using the Simpson method from an apical 4 chambers view. The contour of the left ventricular endocardium is traced on an end-diastolic frame for the calculation of the end-diastolic volume and on an end-systolic frame for the end-systolic volume. Then this area is automatically split into disks of equal thickness. The left ventricular volume is equal to the sum of the volume of each of these disks. *LV*, Left ventricle. (Photo credit: Éric de Madron.)

animals. This is because, unlike the planimetric methods, the geometric method does not use the LV length but only its transversal diameter.

The LV volumes can be indexed to the body surface area in order to normalize them. The normal values of these indexed volumes depend on the method used to calculate the volumes. They are summarized in Table 7-4. Compare these values to the ones proposed in Table 7-3.

Indexed End-Systolic Volume

The indexed end-systolic volume (ESVI) is a useful parameter for assessing the systolic function. Two situations must be considered: normal and reduced afterload.

Systolic Dysfunction in the Absence of Significant Mitral Regurgitation

This is the case of dilated cardiomyopathies. ESVI values higher than 55 mL/m^2 indicate a systolic dysfunction with a sensitivity of 94.4% and a specificity of 97.4% in the Doberman Pinscher (see Chapter 12).

Systolic Dysfunction in the Presence of Significant Mitral Regurgitation

The shortening of left ventricular dimensions is facilitated by the decreased afterload (see Chapter 11), which may hide a systolic dysfunction. The use of the ESVI could help to reveal this dysfunction, which is not the case with SF. In humans, values of less than 30 mL/m^2 indicate preserved systolic function while values exceeding 90 mL/m^2 indicate marked systolic dysfunction, not revealed by the SF value [28]. This approach, based on the Teichholz method, was also used in dogs with mitral regurgitation [29]. However, as discussed above, this method is not ideal because of the overestimation of volumes in small dogs. Planimetric methods are more suitable for dogs but ESVI cutoff values that clearly indicate systolic dysfunction remain to be determined (see Chapter 11) [17].

Ejection Fraction

The ejection fraction (EF) is one of the most frequently used LV systolic function parameters in human medicine. It can be measured by angiography, nuclear

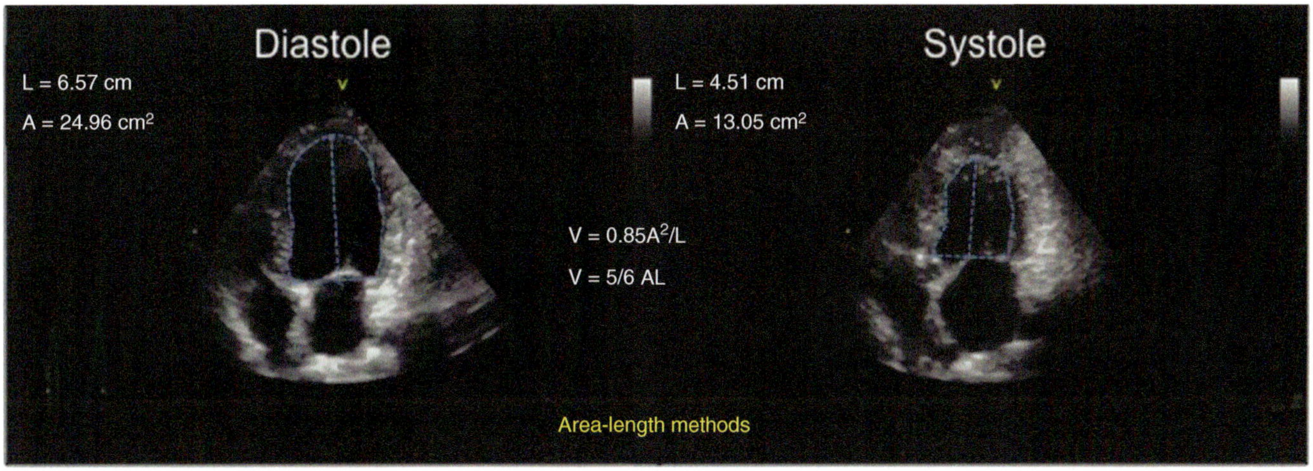

• **Fig. 7-5** Measurement of the diastolic and systolic left ventricular volumes using the area-length methods from a left apical 4 chambers view. The area (A) is obtained by planimetry, by tracing the contour of the left ventricular endocardium on an end-diastolic frame for the end-diastolic volume and on an end-systolic frame for the end-systolic volume calculations. Then the internal base-apex length (L) of the left ventricle is measured. The left ventricular volume (V) is obtained using one of the following formulas: $V = 0.85 \times A^2/L$ or $V = 5/6\ A \times L$. (Photo credit: Éric de Madron.)

TABLE 7-4 Indexed End-Diastolic and End-Systolic Volumes and Ejection Fractions in Healthy Dogs (Mean ± Standard Deviation), Calculated Using Different Methods [17]

Method	Simpson	Area-Length $V = 0.85\ A^2/L$	Teichholz $V = D^3 \times 7/(2.4 + D)$
EDVI (mL/m^2)	47.6 ± 8.4	49.5 ± 10.3	80.4 ± 18.6
ESVI (mL/m^2)	15.9 ± 3.9	16.9 ± 4.3	23.4 ± 7.3
EF (%)	66.5 ± 6.4	65.5 ± 6.7	70.9 ± 6.0

EDVI, Indexed end-diastolic volume; *EF,* ejection fraction; *ESVI,* indexed end-systolic volume.
These volumes were calculated in 24 dogs weighing 2 to 14 kg (8.1 ± 2.8 kg).

ventriculography (NV), and echocardiography. It is an index derived from the LV volumes, calculated as follows:

$$EF(\%) = [(\text{LV end} - \text{diastolic volume} - \text{LV end} - \text{systolic volume}) / (\text{LV end} - \text{diastolic volume})] \times 100$$

EF therefore gives a more comprehensive view of LV systolic performance than SF by better accounting for radial and longitudinal dimension changes. Ventricular volume measurements are necessary to perform the calculation. Therefore the values obtained depend on the method of volume estimation as summarized in Table 7-4 [17].

It is generally accepted that an EF <40% indicates a systolic dysfunction in dogs (see Chapter 12).

The different methods of EF calculation were compared in humans and dogs [27,30,31], In the two species, EF calculated using a planimetric method correlated better with EF measured by NV than with EF calculated using the Teichholz method. The degree of agreement between EF calculated by the Simpson method and EF obtained by NV is ±18% [31]. In dogs, the correlation coefficients between EF calculated by NV and EF calculated by echocardiography vary between 0.79 and 0.88. The correlations are better when 2D rather than TM measurements are used [27].

The limitations of EF as a criterion for systolic function are technical in nature (the need for a 4 chambers view truly passing through the apex with good visualization of the ventricular endocardium) and hemodynamic (influence of the preload, afterload, and heart rate, as with the SF). A study conducted in dogs has shown that the indices using volumes based on a TM dimension proved to be disappointing in the case of systolic dysfunction, due to individual variations [32].

Assessment of the Longitudinal Systolic Function

Several methods are available for analyzing the longitudinal systolic function, which can be affected before the radial function [4,10]. These methods are based on the analysis of mitral valve annulus movement using either the TM or the tissue Doppler modes.

Mitral Annulus Movement

Longitudinal fibers shortening during systole results in a displacement of the atrioventricular plane toward the apex. This "descent" of the mitral annulus begins during the isovolumic period and precedes the shortening of the short axis by about 25 ms. This movement toward the apex continues until the end of ventricular ejection, thereby contributing to the expansion of the left atrial chamber and to a reduction of the left ventricular chamber. At the beginning of diastole, the atrioventricular plane rises quickly toward the left atrium. Atrial systole causes an additional upward movement [33]. The apex remains stationary during the entire ventricular contraction [33]. The left ventricle undergoes a slight counterclockwise torsion during systole [34,35].

In humans, the measurement of the amplitude of the mitral annulus movement (MAM) is correlated with EF [36,37]. In addition, a decrease in longitudinal contractility may precede in a nonlinear fashion a decrease in radial contractility [4,13]. However, there are discrepancies between MAM and EF because MAM is affected not only by the systolic function but also by the diastolic function [38].

The MAM has also been evaluated in dogs [33].

The MAM is measured on the TM echocardiogram of the mitral annulus plane obtained from an apical 4 chambers view, with the TM cursor transecting the septal rim of the mitral annulus. The cursor must be as vertical as possible. The total excursion of the mitral annulus septal rim is measured (Figure 7-6).

The MAM can be indexed to body surface area. The relative contribution of MAM (MAM %) to the total radial and longitudinal LV shortening can be assessed using the following formula:

$$\text{MAM } \% = \text{MAM} / [(\text{LVd} - \text{LVs}) + \text{MAM}] \times 100$$

where *LVd* and *LVs* are the LV end-diastolic and end-systolic diameters, respectively, obtained by right parasternal short axis transventricular TM.

The normal MAM and MAM % values in dogs are listed in Table 7-5 [33].

Using MAM threshold values of 0.45 cm (dogs <15 kg), 0.80 cm (dogs 15 to 40 kg), and 1.20 cm (dogs >40 kg), Schober et al [33] observed that the MAM was preserved, or even increased, in dogs with mitral regurgitation or aortic stenosis whereas the MAM in 81% of dogs with dilated cardiomyopathy was lower than the threshold values, indicating a diminished longitudinal systolic function. The eSF was not correlated to the MAM but was correlated negatively to the MAM %.

Tissue Doppler of the Mitral Annulus

Velocity of the Mitral Annulus S′ Wave

The maximal systolic S′ wave velocity of the mitral annulus, obtained by pulsed wave tissue Doppler imaging (TDI), is correlated to the EF in humans, in the absence of significant regional dyskinesia [39]. This velocity was also found to be decreased in patients with congestive heart failure who have a very low EF, with or without mitral insufficiency [40]. The maximum velocity of the mitral annulus S′ can be affected by

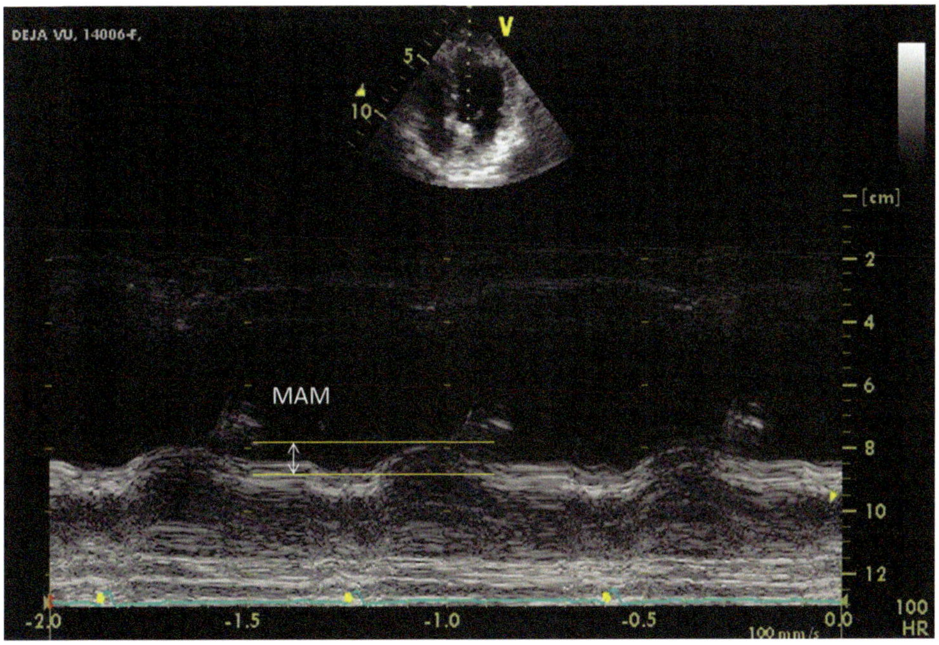

• **Fig. 7-6** Mitral annulus movement (MAM) measurement from a left apical 4 chambers view. The time-motion (TM) cursor must transect the septal rim of the mitral annulus as vertically as possible. (Photo credit: Éric de Madron.)

TABLE 7-5 Normal Mitral Annulus Movement Values in Dogs (95% Average and Confidence Interval [33])

	<15 kg (n = 44)	≥15 kg to ≤40 kg (n = 55)	>40 kg (n = 4)
MAM (cm)	0.70 (0.65-0.75)	1.08 (1.03-1.13)	1.51 (1.21-1.81)
Indexed MAM (cm/m^2)	1.65 (1.47-1.83)	1.11 (1.04-1.18)	1.03 (0.89-1.17)
MAM % (%)	40 (38-42)	42 (40-44)	44 (39-49)
SF (%)	38 (36-40)	33 (31-55)	33 (29-37)

MAM, Mitral annulus movement; *MAM %,* MAM contribution to the axial and longitudinal shortening of the left ventricle in systole; *SF,* shortening fraction.

a reduction in preload [41]. A longitudinal systolic dysfunction with evident reduction in the mitral annulus S′ wave in a dog with systemic arterial hypertension and arteriosclerosis has been reported. The SF in this dog was normal [42]. This illustrates the fact that the longitudinal systolic function can be affected independent of the radial function.

The anomalies of S′ in systolic dysfunctions in dogs is discussed in more detail in Chapter 12. The normal values of S′ in dogs and cats are presented in Chapter 4.

Timing of Left Heart Base Descent

Recently, several TDI temporal indices of global systolic function, measured at the base of the ventricular myocardium, have been evaluated in dogs. These are the left heart base descent time intervals [43]. To obtain these time intervals, the S′ wave of the base of the interventricular septum or left ventricular free wall must be recorded using TDI. The following durations are then measured: Q-beginning of S′, Q-peak of S′, Q-end of S′, and duration of S′ (Figure 7-7).

The normal values of these time intervals are presented in Table 7-6.

In this same study, the authors compared the time intervals of normal dogs and dogs with dilated cardiomyopathy. They observed that the intervals Q-beginning of S′, Q-end of S′ were extended and the maximum velocity of S′ was reduced in dogs with dilated cardiomyopathy. The S′ duration was not affected by the systolic dysfunction [43].

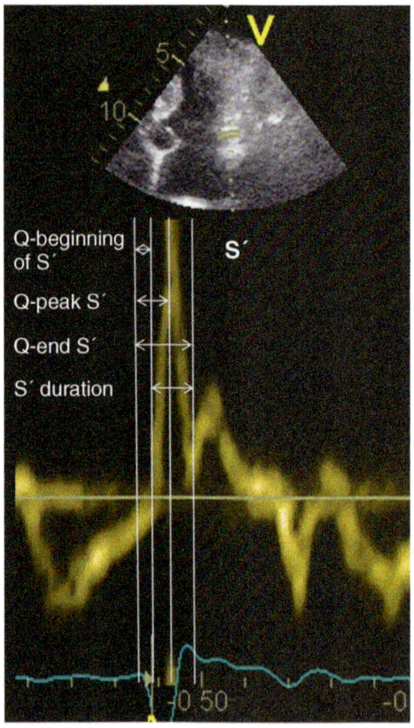

• **Fig. 7-7** Timing of left heart base descent measured by tissue Doppler imaging (TDI). Here, the systolic myocardial velocity (S′) of the base of the left ventricular free wall is recorded. The following durations were measured: Q-beginning of S′, Q-peak of S′, Q-end of S′, and duration of S′. (Photo credit: Éric de Madron.)

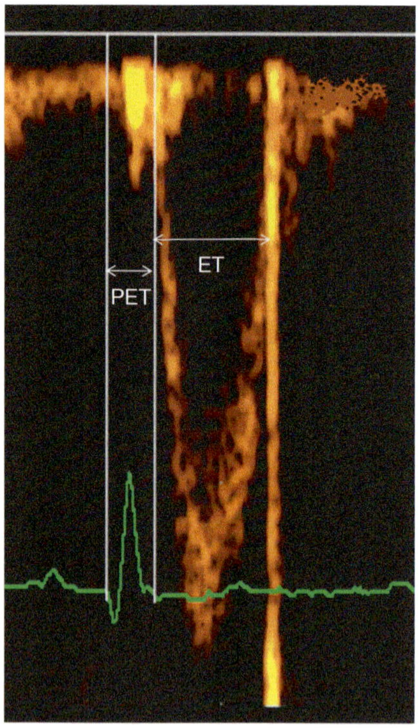

• **Fig. 7-8** Measurement of systolic time intervals from a spectral wave Doppler of the aortic flow. *ET,* Ejection time (duration of the aortic flow); *PEP,* pre-ejection period duration (Q-beginning of aortic flow). (Photo credit: Éric de Madron.)

TABLE 7-6 Time Intervals of Left Heart Base Descent in a Normal Dog, Normalized for the Heart Rate (i.e., Divided by √ R-R, R-R Measured in Seconds [43])

	Base of the Septum	Base of the Left Ventricular Free Wall
Q-beginning S′ (s)	0.085 ± 0.018	0.085 ± 0.028
Q-peak S′ (s)	0.128 ± 0.021	0.124 ± 0.028
Q-end S′ (s)	0.2865 ± 0.030	0.283 ± 0.039
S′ duration (s)	0.201 ± 0.018	0.199 ± 0.029
S′ peak (cm/s)	8.113 ± 1.726	10.363 ± 2.190

TABLE 7-7 Systolic Time Intervals and Left Ventricle (LV) Index of Myocardial Performance (IMP) in Normal Dogs [47]

	3 to 15 kg (n = 15) (Mean ± Standard Deviation)	15.1 to 35 kg (n = 15) (Mean ± Standard Deviation)	35.1 to 55 kg (n = 15) (Mean ± Standard Deviation)
LV IMP	0.380 ± 0.104	0.414 ± 0.102	0.445 ± 0.104
LV PEP (ms)	43.6 ± 8.70	59.6 ± 11.8	66 ± 10.12
LV ET (ms)	172 ± 18	173 ± 16	170 ± 17
LV PEP/ET	0.267 ± 0.055	0.350 ± 0.662	0.377 ± 0.075

ET, Ejection time; *PEP,* pre-ejection period duration.

Systolic Indices Obtained by Spectral Wave Doppler: Systolic Time Intervals and Index of Myocardial Performance (Tei Index)

Systolic Time Intervals

A systolic dysfunction leads to an increase in the pre-ejection period (PEP, or the time interval between the Q wave and the beginning of ventricular ejection), a decrease in the ventricular ejection duration (ejection time, or ET), and therefore an increase in the PEP/ET ratio [44,45].

These systolic time intervals can be obtained from a right parasternal short axis transaortic TM view with good visualization of the aortic valvular leaflets movement [46] or from a spectral wave Doppler of the aortic flow [47] (Figure 7-8).

The normal systolic time interval values in dogs are presented in Table 7-7. A PEP/ET ratio greater than 0.4 is considered an indication of systolic dysfunction (see Chapter 12).

Index of Myocardial Performance

The index of myocardial performance (IMP) is an overall Doppler composite index of both systolic and diastolic ventricular functions. It was developed by Tei [48], who thought that such an index could be more sensitive than the strictly systolic or diastolic indices in patients with dilated cardiomyopathy. In fact, this index is well correlated with the parameters obtained by catheterization such as the dP/dt and the *tau* relaxation constant. It has a prognostic value in dilated cardiomyopathies [49].

The LV IMP is equal to the sum of the LV ejection and isovolumic relaxation times divided by the ejection time. To perform this calculation, the duration between the end of the A wave and the beginning of the E wave must be measured on a mitral flow Doppler signal (time a). Next, the LV ejection time must be measured (time b). The IMP is equal to the ratio (a – b)/b (Figure 7-9). The normal LV IMP values in dogs are presented in Table 7-7 [47].

In a study carried out in Newfoundland dogs, either normal or with dilated cardiomyopathy, IMP proved to be independent of age, sex, and body surface area as well as heart rate [50]. This index is correlated to the severity of the systolic dysfunction but is not superior to other parameters such as PEP/ET ratio. Neither of these two indices appeared to be sensitive enough to detect cases of early systolic dysfunction unequivocally [50].

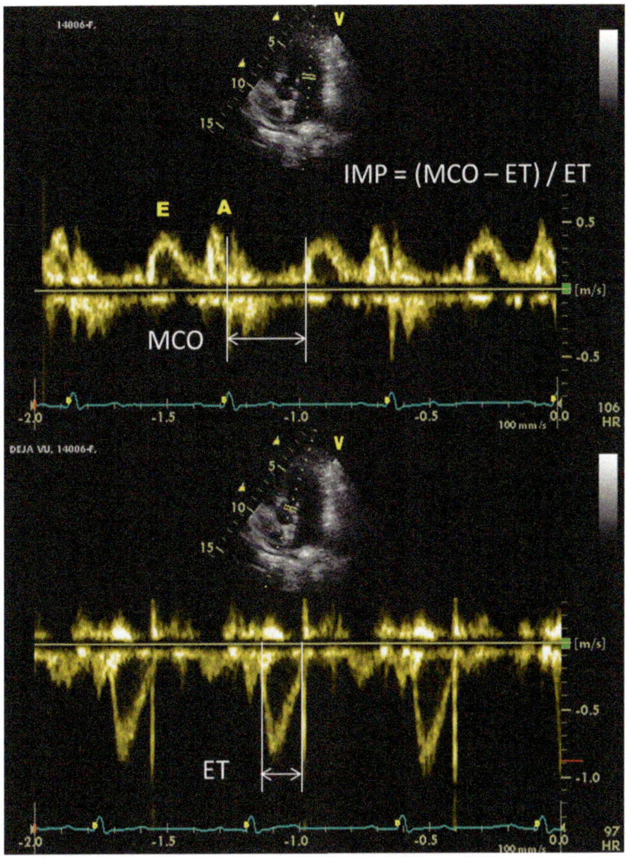

• **Fig. 7-9** Left ventricular index of myocardial performance (IMP) measurement. The time between the closure and the following mitral valve opening (MCO) and the left ventricular ejection time (ET) are measured. The IMP is equal to (MCO – ET)/ET. (Photo credit: Éric de Madron.)

Speckle Tracking–Derived Indices

Speckle tracking–derived indices based on left ventricle strain and strain rate measurements are discussed in detail in Chapters 4 and 12. Global indices include global strain and torsion (see Chapter 4).

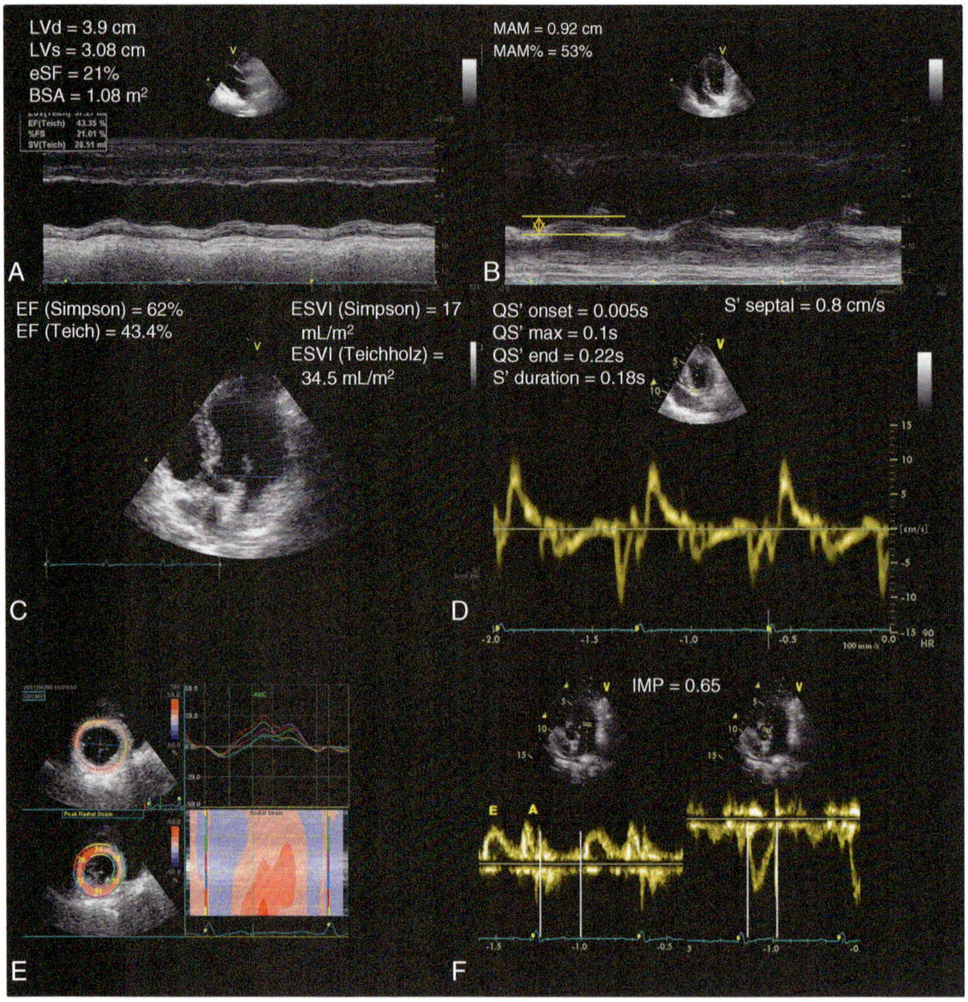

• **Fig. 7-10** Multimodal echocardiographic systolic function assessment in a 35-kg Doberman Pinscher female. A, Transventricular time-motion (TM) mode: the endocardial shortening fraction (eSF) is lower than normal (21%). This indicates equivocal radial systolic function. B, Mitral annulus TM: the mitral annulus movement (MAM) value and the relative contribution of MAM (MAM %) are normal for a dog of this weight. C, Volume and ejection fraction (EF) assessment. This EF is normal according to the Simpson method. D, Tissue Doppler imaging of the mitral annulus. S′ velocity and the time intervals of the left heart base descent, after normalization for heart rate, are normal. The MAM is normal. This indicates good longitudinal systolic function. E, Left ventricular radial strain obtained by speckle tracking. The values are normal. F, Left ventricular index of myocardial performance (IMP): its value is at the upper limit of normal. Therefore four of the six systolic function indices are clearly normal in this female dog and two are equivocal. The conclusion is that the systolic function is still normal but needs to be monitored. (Photo credit: Éric de Madron.)

Conclusion

The echocardiographer has at his or her disposal a growing number of global systolic function indices. The importance of the longitudinal systolic function evaluation is becoming more and more obvious. Nevertheless, all of these indices have their limits, especially in the presence of an early or mild systolic dysfunction. Therefore a multimodal approach to assessing systolic function is necessary in order to reduce the incidence of false positives and false negatives as much as possible (Figures 7-10 and 7-11 and Table 7-8).

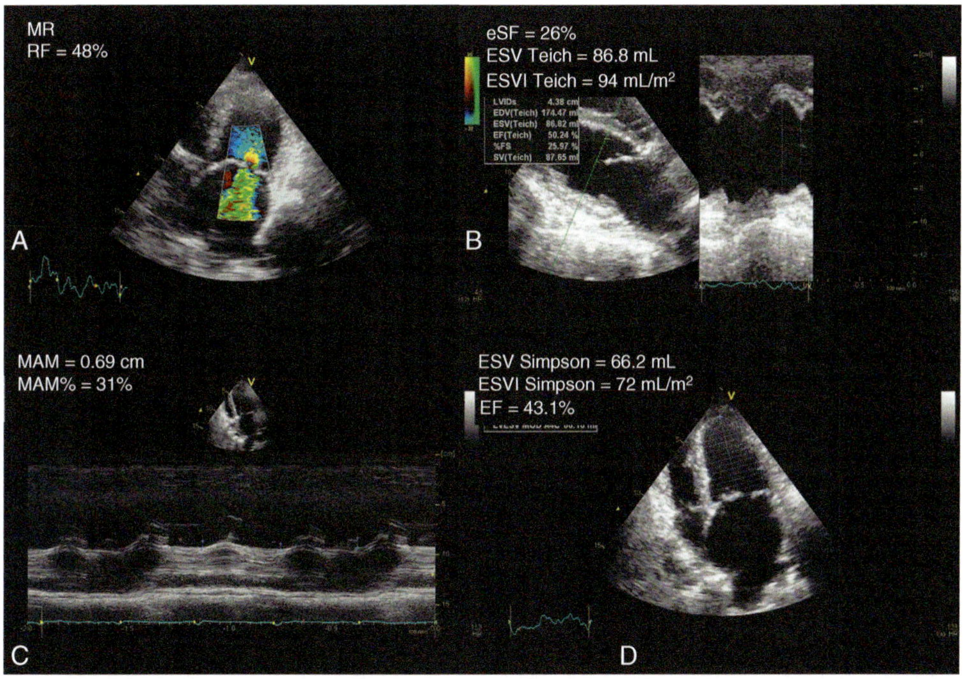

• **Fig. 7-11** Multimodal echocardiographic systolic function assessment in a 27-kg Border Collie with mitral regurgitation. A, A quantification of the amount of mitral regurgitation using spectral and pulsed wave Doppler reveals a moderate regurgitant fraction (RF) of 48%. B, Time-motion (TM) transventricular mode: the endocardial shortening fraction (eSF) is at a limit lower than normal (25%), which is abnormal in a context of decreased afterload. The indexed end-systolic volume (ESVI) calculated by the Teichholz method is significantly increased. C, Mitral annulus TM: the mitral annulus movement (MAM) and relative contribution of MAM (MAM %) are reduced for a dog of this weight, which indicates a longitudinal systolic dysfunction. D, Volume and ejection fraction (EF) evaluation. EF calculated by the Simpson method is low. The ESVI calculated by the Simpson method is greatly above normal. A systolic dysfunction is therefore documented. (Photo credit: Éric de Madron.)

TABLE 7-8 Impact of a Systolic Dysfunction on Different Echocardiographic Parameters

Parameter	Trend in Cases of Systolic Dysfunction
eSF (%)	↓
EF (%)	↓
ESVI	↑
MAM	↓
MAM %	↓
PEP	↑
ET	↓
PEP/ET	↑
IMP	↑
Q-beginning S′	↑
Q-peak S′	↑
Q-end S′	↑
Duration of S′	Unchanged
S′ V_{max}	↓

EF, Ejection fraction; *eSF,* endocardial shortening fraction; *ESVI,* indexed end-systolic volume; *ET,* left ventricular ejection time; *IMP,* index of myocardial performance; *MAM,* mitral annulus movement; *MAM %,* MAM contribution to the axial and longitudinal left ventricular shortening in systole; *PEP,* left ventricular pre-ejection time; V_{max}, maximum velocity.

REFERENCES

[1] Henein MY, Gibson DG. Normal long axis function. Heart 1999;81:111–3.

[2] Streeter DD, Spotnitz HM, Patel DP, et al. Fiber orientation in the canine left ventricle during systole and diastole. Circ Res 1969;24:339–47.

[3] Feigenbaum H. Echocardiography. In: Baunwald E, editor. Heart disease: a textbook of cardiovascular diseases. 4th ed. Philadelphia: WB Saunders; 1992, p. 84–115.

[4] Ballo PC, Quatrini I, Giacomin E, et al. Circumferential versus longitudinal systolic function in patients with hypertension: a non-linear relation. J Am Soc Echocardiogr 2007;20:298–306.

[5] Grossman W. Evaluation of systolic and diastolic function of the myocardium. In: Grossman W, editor. Cardiac catheterization and angiography. 3rd ed. Philadelphia: Lea & Febiger; 1985. p. 301–19.

[6] Borow KM, Green LH, Grossman W, Braunwald E. Left ventricular end systolic stress-shortening and strength-length relations in human. Normal values and sensitivity to inotropic state. Am J Cardiol 1982;50:1301–8.

[7] Jacobs G, Knight DH. M-mode echocardiographic measurements in non-anesthetized healthy cats: effects of body weight, heart rate, and other variables. Am J Vet Res 1985;46:1705–11.

[8] Brown DJ, Rush JE, Mac Gregor J, et al. M-mode echocardiographic ratio indices in normal dogs, cats, and horses: a novel quantitative method. J Vet Intern Med 2003;17:653–62.

[9] O'Sullivan ML, O'Grady MR, Minors SL. Assessment of diastolic function by Doppler echocardiography in normal Doberman Pinschers and Doberman Pinschers with dilated cardiomyopathy. J Vet Intern Med 2007;21:81–91.

[10] Henein MY, Gibson DG. Long axis function in disease. Heart 1999;81:229–31.

[11] De Simone G, Devereux RB, Roman MJ, et al. Assessment of left ventricular function by the midwall fractional shortening/end systolic wall stress relation in human hypertension. J Am Coll Cardiol 1994;23:1444–51.

[12] Palmieri V, Capaldo B, Russo C, et al. Left ventricular chamber and myocardial systolic function reserve in patients with type 1 diabetes mellitus: insight from traditional and Doppler tissue imaging echocardiography. J Am Soc Echocardiogr 2006;19:848–56.

[13] Aurigemma GP, Silver KH, Priest MA, Gaasch WH. Geometric changes allow normal ejection fraction despite depressed myocardial shortening in hypertensive left ventricular hypertrophy. J Am Coll Cardiol 1995;26:195–202.

[14] Gaasch WH, Zile MR, Hoshini PK, et al. Stress-shortening relations and myocardial blood flow in compensated and failing canine hearts with pressure-overload hypertrophy. Circulation 1989;79:872–83.

[15] Reichek N, Wilson J, St John Sutton M, Plappert TA, Goldberg S, Hirshfield JW. Non-invasive determination of left ventricular end-systolic stress: validation of the method and initial application. Circ 1982;65:99–108.

[16] Palmieri V, Russo C, Arezzi E, et al. Relations to longitudinal left ventricular systolic function to left ventricular mass, load, and Doppler stroke volume. Eur J Echocardiogr 2006;7:348–55.

[17] Serres F, Chetboul V, Tissier R, et al. Comparison of 3 ultrasound methods for quantifying left ventricular systolic function: correlation with disease severity and prognostic value in dogs with mitral valve disease. J Vet Intern Med 2008;22:566–77.

[18] Wyatt HL, Heng MK, Meerbaum S, et al. Cross-sectional echocardiography: II. Analysis of mathematic models for quantifying volume of the formalin-fixed left ventricle. Circulation 1980;61:1119–25.

[19] Weiss JL, Eaton LW, Kallman CH, Maughan ML. Accuracy of volume determination by two-dimensional echocardiography: defining requirements under controlled conditions in the ejecting canine left ventricle. Circulation 1983;67:889–95.

[20] Teichholz LE, Kreulen T, Herman MV, Gorlin R. Problem in echocardiographic volume determinations: echocardiographic-angiocardiographic correlations in the presence or absence of asynergy. Am J Cardiol 1976;37:7–11.

[21] Pombo JF, Troy BL, Russel RO. Left ventricular volumes and ejection fraction by echocardiography. Circulation 1971;43:480–90.

[22] Wyatt HL, Heng MK, Meerbaum S, et al. Cross-sectional echocardiography: I. Analysis of mathematic models for qualifying mass of the left ventricle in dogs. Circulation 1979;60:1104–13.

[23] Mashiro I, Nelson RR, Cohn JN. Ventricular dimensions measured non-invasively by echocardiography in the awake dog. J Appl Physiol 1976;41:953–9.

[24] Suga H, Sagawa K. Assessment of absolute volume from diameter of the intact canine left ventricular cavity. J Appl Physiol 1974;36:496–9.

[25] Brown DJ. Personal communication. 2009.

[26] Cornell CC, Kittleson MD, Della Torre P, et al. Allometric scaling of M-mode cardiac measurements in normal adult dogs. J Vet Intern Med 2004;18:311–1.

[27] Sisson DD, Daniel GB, Twardock AR. Comparison of left ventricular ejection fractions determined in healthy anesthetized dogs by echocardiography and gated equilibrium radionuclide ventriculography. Am J Vet Res 1989;50:1840–7.
[28] Borow K, Green LH, Mann T, et al. End systolic volume as a predictor of post-operative left ventricular performance in volume overload from mitral regurgitation. Am J Med 1980;68:355–63.
[29] Borgarelli M, Tarducci A, Zanatta R, Haggstrom J. Decreased systolic function and inadequate hypertrophy in large and small breed dogs with chronic mitral valve insufficiency. J Vet Intern Med 2007;21:61–7.
[30] Wandt B, Bojö L, Tolagen K, Wranne B. Echocardiography assessment of ejection fraction in left ventricular hypertrophy. Heart 1999;82:192–8.
[31] McGowan JH, Cleland JGF. Reliability of reporting left ventricular systolic function by echocardiography: a systematic review of 3 methods. Am Heart J 2003;146:388–97.
[32] Atkins CE, Curtis MB, McGuirk SM, et al. The use of M-mode echocardiography in determining cardiac output in dogs with normal, low, and high output states: comparison to thermodilution method. Vet Radiol Ultrasound 1992;33:297–304.
[33] Schober KE, Luis Fuentes V. Mitral annulus motion as determined by M-mode echocardiography in normal dogs and dogs with cardiac disease. Vet Radiol Ultrasound 2001;42:52–61.
[34] Alam R, Rosenhammer G. Atrioventricualr plane displacement and left ventricular function. J Am Soc Echocardiogr 1992;5:427–33.
[35] Tsakiris AG, Gordon GA, Padiyar R, et al. The role of displacement of the mitral annulus in left atrial filling and emptying in the intact dog. Can J Physiol Pharmacol 1978;56:447–57.
[36] Simonson JS, Schiller NB. Descent of the base of the left ventricle: an echocardiographic index of left ventricular function. J Am Soc Echocardiogr 1989;2:25–35.
[37] Pai RG, Bodenheimer MM, Pai SM, et al. Usefulness of systolic excursion of the mitral annulus as an index of left ventricular function. Am J Cardiol 1990;67:222–4.
[38] Willenheimer R, Israelsson B, Cline C, et al. Left atrioventricular plane displacement is related to both systolic and diastolic left ventricular performance in patients with chronic heart failure. Eur Heart J 1999;20:612–8.
[39] Vinereanu D, Khokhar A, Tweddel AC, et al. Estimation of global left ventricular function from the velocity of longitudinal shortening. Echocardiography 2002;19:177–85.
[40] Alam M, Wardell J, Andersson E, et al. Assessment of left centricular function using mitral annular velocities in patients with congestive heart failure with or without the presence of significant mitral regurgitation. J Am Soc Echocardiogr 2003;16:240–5.
[41] Andersen NH, Terkelsen CJ, Sloth E, Poulsen SH. Influence of preload alterations on parameters of systolic left ventricular long-axis function: a Doppler tissue study. J Am Soc Echocardiogr 2004;17:941–7.
[42] Nicolle AP, Carlos Sampedrano C, Fontaine JJ, et al. Longitudinal left ventricular myocardial dysfunction assessed by 2D colour tissue Doppler imaging in a dog with systemic hypertension and severe arteriosclerosis. J Vet Med 2005;52:83–7.
[43] Simpson KE, Devine BC, Woolley R, et al. Timing of left heart base descent in dogs with dilated cardiomyopathy and normal dogs. Vet Radiol Ultrasound 2008;49:287–94.
[44] Ahmed SS, Levinson GE, Schwartz OJ, Ettinger PO. Systolic time intervals as measures of the contractile state of the left ventricular myocardium in man. Circulation 1972;46:559–71.
[45] Burwash IG, Otto CM, Pearlman AS. Use of Doppler-derived left ventricular time intervals for non-invasive assessment of systolic function. Am J Cardiol 1993;72:1331–3.
[46] Pipers FS, Andrysco RM, Hamlin RL. A totally non-invasive method for obtaining systolic time intervals in the dog. Am J Vet Res 1978;39:1822–6.
[47] Baumwart RD, Meurs KM, Bonagura JD. Tei index of myocardial performance applied to the right ventricle in normal dogs. J Vet Intern Med 2005;19:828–32.
[48] Tei C. New non-invasive index for combined systolic and diastolic ventricular function. J Cardiol 1995;26:135–6.
[49] Dujardin KS, Tei C, Yeo TC, et al. Prognostic value of a Doppler index combining systolic and diastolic performance in idiopathic dilated cardiomyopathy. Am J Cardiol 1998;82:1072–6.
[50] Byeong-Han L, Dukes Mc-Ewan J, French AT, Corcoran BM. Evaluation of a novel Doppler index of combined systolic and diastolic myocardial performance in Newfoundland dogs with familial prevalence of dilated cardiomyopathy. Vet Radiol Ultrasound 2002;43:154–65.

8

Assessment of Diastolic Function

ÉRIC DE MADRON

Diastole Phases and Determinants, 128
Types of Diastolic Dysfunction, 129
Echocardiographic Indices of Diastolic Function, 130

Diastole Phases and Determinants

Diastole Phases

Diastole extends from the closure of the aortic valve to the end of the transmitral flow. It is divided into four phases: an isovolumic relaxation phase, a rapid filling phase due to ventricular suction, a phase during which filling is minimal (diastasis), and atrial systole [1,2]. The isovolumic relaxation phase starts when the aortic valve closes and ends when the mitral valve opens. During this phase, the left ventricular pressure drops until it becomes lower than that of the left atrium. This allows the opening of the atrioventricular valve and the filling of the ventricle. Initially, this filling occurs quickly due to ventricular suction maintaining a positive pressure gradient between the atrium and the ventricle. This gradient is influenced by atrial pressure at the beginning of diastole and the ventricular relaxation rate. This phase provides 70% to 80% of ventricle filling [1,2]. It ends when atrial and ventricular pressures equalize. Diastasis begins at this point; transmitral flow is minimal. About 5% of the ventricular filling is done during this phase. The atrial systole restores a positive pressure gradient between the atrium and ventricle, thus allowing additional filling at end-diastole (about 20% to 30% of the total ventricular filling). The diastole ends when the rapid rise of the ventricular pressure closes the atrioventricular valve (isovolumic contraction) (Figure 8-1) [1,2].

Diastolic Function Determinants

The diastolic function determinants are (1) active relaxation of the myocardium, (2) compliance of the left ventricle, (3) pump function of the left atrium and pulmonary veins, (4) heart rate, and (5) age.

Active Relaxation of the Myocardium

The active relaxation of the myocardium is a process requiring energy, hence adenosine triphosphate (ATP). During this process, calcium ions are removed from the cytoplasm against the concentration gradient. This allows actin-myosin complexes to disengage [3]. This relaxation is influenced by the status of cardiac fibers, preload and afterload levels (end-systolic volume preceding the relaxation, wall stress, peripheral vascular resistance), and the myocardial inotropic state. The rapid relaxation rate determines the speed at which the ventricular pressure drops during the isovolumic relaxation phase. This has a particular impact on the early diastolic rapid filling phase. A measure of the rapidity of this drop is the time constant *tau*. Delayed relaxation prolongs *tau* and reduces ventricular volume for a given pressure. Therefore an increase in filling pressure will be required to maintain this volume [3]. Another important factor is the degree of inotropy. During systolic contraction, the myocardium is compressed beyond its point of equilibrium and energy is stored. This energy is released during relaxation (elastic recoil), creating a suction effect. With loss of inotropy, this suction effect becomes attenuated [3].

Compliance of the Left Ventricle

Compliance is a passive function, determined by the distensibility of the ventricular cavity during its filling [3]. The pressure-volume relationship is curvilinear. It is the net result of interactions between viscoelastic properties of the myocardium, the size and architecture of the ventricle, the thickness of its walls, the interaction of the left and right ventricles, the pleural and pericardial pressures,

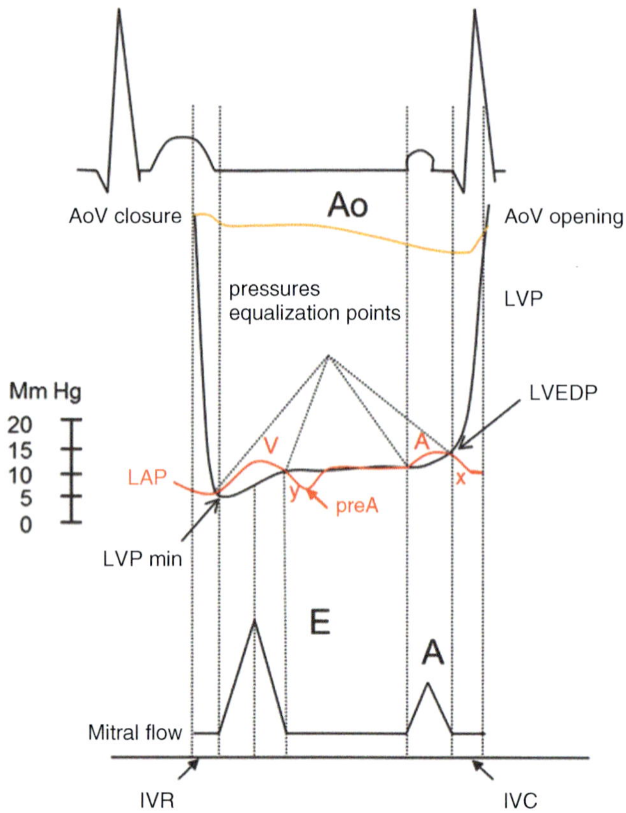

• **Fig. 8-1** Schematic representation of the correlation between aortic pressure (Ao), left ventricular pressure (LVP), left atrial pressure (LAP), and the transmitral flow in diastole. During the isovolumic relaxation phase (IVR), the LVP drops quickly to reach the level of the LAP: the mitral valve opens and the filling of the left ventricle begins (E wave). The peak of the E wave occurs when the positive atrioventricular gradient, created by ventricular suction, reaches its maximum. This corresponds to the peak of the V wave of the LAP curve. Ventricular and atrial pressures become equal again and diastolic transmitral flow stops. Atrial pressure becomes lower than ventricular pressure (y descent) reaching its minimum level: the preA wave. The atrial contraction creates another positive atrioventricular gradient, allowing the active filling of the left ventricle (A wave). The isovolumic contraction phase (IVC) and decrease in atrial pressure (x descent) then close the mitral valve. *AoV,* Aortic valve; *LVEDP,* left ventricle end-diastolic pressure; *LVP min,* left ventricular minimum pressure. (Photo credit: Éric de Madron.)

the turgidity of coronary vessels, and any component of incomplete myocardial relaxation. The characteristics of compliance will mainly affect the second half of diastole. A decrease in compliance will result in an increase in the slope of the ventricular pressure-volume curve, meaning that any increase in volume will result in a strong increase in ventricular pressure. A reduction in compliance is observed in association with fibrosis, ischemia, or infiltration of the myocardium [3].

Systolic Function of the Left Atrium

The systolic function of the left atrium is particularly important in cases of relaxation anomalies because it allows late diastolic filling to compensate for early diastolic filling deficits. This may become essential in maintaining cardiac output in case of systolic dysfunction.

Heart Rate

The heart rate has a significant influence on diastolic filling because any increase in frequency decreases the rapid filling phase as well as the duration of the isovolumic relaxation phase [4,5].

Influence of Age

In a study carried out on 92 normal dogs belonging to different age groups, Schober et al [5] showed that the left ventricle loses elasticity with age. This significantly affects the diastolic parameters of active relaxation (see below).

Types of Diastolic Dysfunction

There are three types of diastolic dysfunction. They represent a continuum and each type corresponds to a stage of progression of the cardiopathy. Diastolic dysfunctions are present in cats with hypertrophic and restrictive hyperthyroid cardiomyopathy (see Chapter 13) and in cats and dogs with hypertensive cardiomyopathy (see Chapter 15). Systolic dysfunction in dogs is also associated with diastolic dysfunction. These diastolic anomalies may even precede systolic dysfunction (see Chapter 12).

Delayed Relaxation

Anomalies in the regulation of calcium channels of the sarcolemma and a decrease in calcium recapture by the sarcoplasmic reticulum lead to an increase in intracellular calcium. This delays the disengagement of contractile elements, which leads to an increase in myocardial tension [1-3,6,7]. Therefore the left ventricle filling shifts toward late diastole, with predominance of the end-diastolic filling associated with atrial contraction. The duration of the isovolumic relaxation phase increases (Figure 8-2).

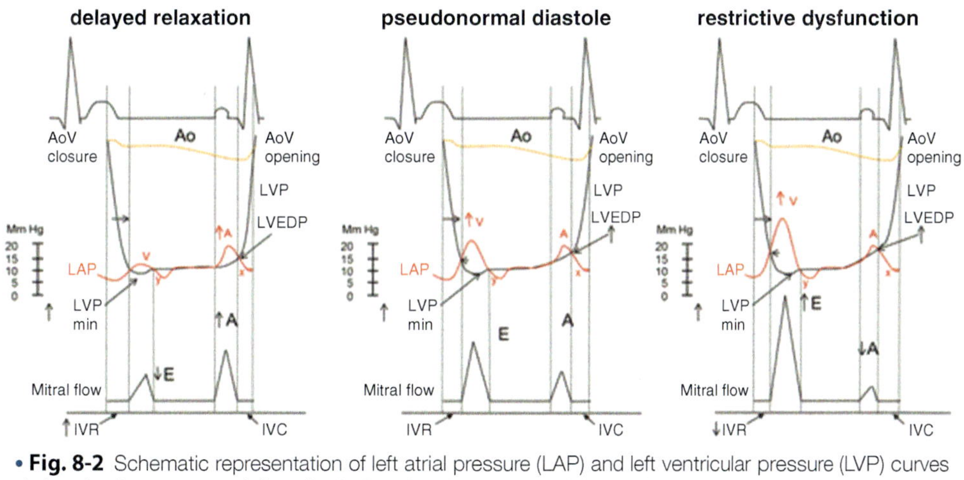

• **Fig. 8-2** Schematic representation of left atrial pressure (LAP) and left ventricular pressure (LVP) curves during the three stages of diastolic dysfunction. In the case of delayed relaxation, the rate of decrease of the LVP declines, delaying the beginning of mitral flow (the duration of the period of isovolumic relaxation [IVR] increases). Left ventricular minimum pressure (LVP min) is increased following incomplete relaxation and the early diastolic atrioventricular gradient is reduced, thus reducing the amplitude of the E wave. Increased atrial contraction compensates for the filling deficit. In the case of pseudonormal diastole, the increase of atrial pressure and the beginning of lack of compliance add to the previous phenomena. This is reflected in a shortened IVR phase (which now has a "normal" duration), an increased E wave due to the increased atrial pressure, and a reduction of A due to the reduction in compliance. The left ventricular end-diastolic pressure (LVEDP) increases. The restrictive stage of diastolic dysfunction is characterized by an even higher atrial pressure, increasing the E wave amplitude and shortening further the IVR phase. Loss of compliance is more pronounced and atrial function declines. This further reduces the end-diastolic atrioventricular gradient and therefore the A wave. *Ao,* Aortic pressure; *AoV,* aortic valve; *IVC,* isovolumic contraction. (Photo credit: Éric de Madron.)

Pseudonormal Diastole

The next stage of diastolic dysfunction is called pseudonormal diastole. It is characterized by an increase of atrial pressure, resulting in the "normalization" of early diastolic ventricular filling and of the duration of the isovolumic relaxation phase (see Chapter 9). Moreover, the increase in atrial pressure increases the length of the end-diastolic blood reflux in the pulmonary veins (see below). Compliance is also altered, leading to an increase in ventricular pressure, a reduction of the atrioventricular gradient, and therefore a reduction in the end-diastolic filling (see Figure 8-2) [1-4].

Restrictive Diastolic Dysfunction

In restrictive diastolic dysfunction, interstitial fibrosis and an increase in the left ventricular filling pressure further affect the elastic properties of the left ventricle (LV). Filling characteristics change again; early diastolic filling becomes predominant due to the increase in filling pressure whereas the end-diastolic filling becomes very attenuated due to loss of left ventricular elasticity and left atrial inotropy, leading to a reduction of the end-diastolic atrioventricular gradient (see Figure 8-2) [1-4,6,7].

Echocardiographic Indices of Diastolic Function

Echocardiography allows a noninvasive evaluation of diastolic function in humans, dogs, and cats. Many echocardiographic indices of diastolic function are derived from the aortic, mitral, and pulmonary venous blood flow spectral Doppler signals, the diastolic mitral annulus and ventricular myocardial velocities obtained using pulsed wave tissue Doppler, and the mitral flow propagation velocity obtained using color time-motion (TM) mode (Figure 8-3) [1-12].

All of these indices are variably affected by multiple factors: atrial compliance and pressure, left ventricular relaxation and elasticity, and preload and afterload conditions [1-4]. A multimodal approach is often necessary to properly identify the type of diastolic dysfunction faced. The greatest challenge is the recognition of pseudonormal diastolic dysfunction.

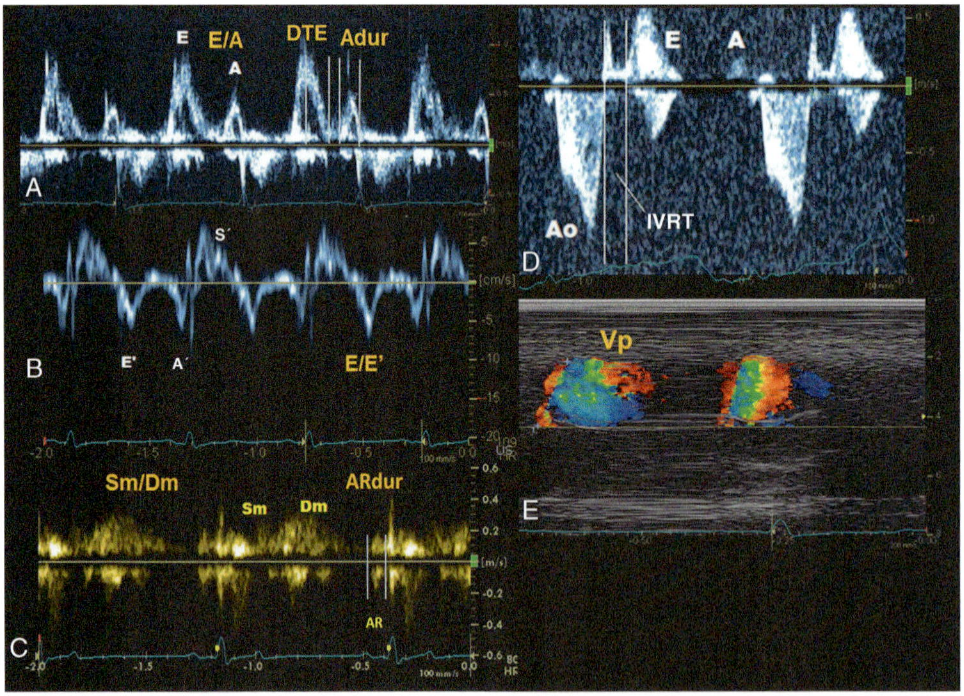

• **Fig. 8-3** Echocardiographic assessment of the diastole. A, Transmitral flow. We measure the maximal velocities of the E and A waves, the duration of the A wave (Adur), the deceleration time of the E wave (DTE), and the E/A ratio. B, Tissue Doppler of the mitral annulus. We measure the velocities of the E′ and A′ waves, as well as the E/E′ ratio. C, Pulsed wave spectral Doppler of the pulmonary venous flow. The parameters assessed are the velocities of the Sm, Dm, and AR waves; the Sm/Dm ratio; the duration of the AR wave (ARdur); and the Adur/ARdur ratio. D, Simultaneous recording of aortic flow (Ao) and mitral annulus in pulsed wave spectral Doppler mode, allowing the measurement of the isovolumic relaxation time (IVRT) of the left ventricle between the end of the aortic ejection and the beginning of the E wave. E, Color time-motion (TM) of the mitral annulus, allowing the measurement of the mitral flow propagation velocity (Vp). (Photo credit: Éric de Madron.)

Normal Diastolic Indices

Ratio of the Maximal Velocities of the Transmitral Flow E and A Waves (E/A) (Pulsed Wave Spectral Doppler)

The maximum velocity of the diastolic transmitral flow E wave is the result of the complex interaction between the atrioventricular pressure gradient, obviously influenced by atrial filling (preload), and the diastolic properties of the left ventricle, such as rate of relaxation, elastic recoil, minimum pressure, and the intraventricular pressure gradient [13-16]. The velocity of the A wave depends on the atrioventricular gradient at end-diastole, itself influenced by the compliance of the left ventricle as well as the strength of atrial contraction. The ratio of the maximum velocities of the E and A waves (E/A) is an important indicator of diastolic function. Its normal values for cats and dogs are summarized in Table 8-1. This ratio decreases with age in dogs (Table 8-2).

Deceleration Time of the E Wave

The normal values of deceleration time of the E wave (DTE) are summarized in Tables 8-1 and 8-2. In dogs, the DTE increases with age and weight and decreases with increased heart rate (see Table 8-2) [5].

TABLE 8-1 Normal Diastolic Doppler Parameters in Dogs and Cats According to Different Authors

Variable	Dogs (6-10 Years) [5] (n = 11) Median (10th-90th Percentiles)	Dogs (1-3 Years) [23] (n = 7) Average (Minimum-Maximum)	Doberman [10] (n = 10) Mean ± Standard Deviation	Cats [11] (n = 87) Mean ± Standard Deviation	Cats [22] (n = 100) Mean ± Standard Deviation	Cats [12] (n = 20) Mean ± Standard Deviation
IVRT (ms)	47 (41-65)	53 (43-62)	83 ± 14	46.2 ± 7.6	43 ± 9	55.4 ± 13.24
E_{max} (m/s)	0.69 (0.52-0.82)	0.83 (0.53-1.08)	0.768 ± 0.131	0.70 ± 0.14	0.7 ± 0.1	0.67 ± 0.13
A_{max} (m/s)	0.57 (0.45-0.70)	0.43 (0.38-0.52)	0.557 ± 0.101	0.65 ± 0.14	0.5 ± 0.1	0.59 ± 0.14
E/A	1.08 (0.98-1.70)	1.66 (1.23-2.84)	1.4 ± 0.3	1.12 ± 0.22	1.5 ± 0.3	1.19 ± 0.30
DTE (ms)	80 (49-98)	100 (75-130)	131 ± 24	ND	ND	59.90 ± 14.07
Adur (ms)	90 (68-103)	84 (62-93)	82 ± 7	52.9 ± 13.5	ND	ND
E'_{septal} (cm/s)	ND	6.8 (5.7-13.2)	ND	ND	ND	ND
E/E'_{septal}	ND	11.8 (4.0-15.1)	ND	ND	ND	ND
E'_{lat} (cm/s)	ND	9.3 (7.5-11.9)	16.5 ± 3.6	ND	5.5 ± 1.6	ND
A'_{lat} (cm/s)	ND	ND	11.3 ± 1.9	ND	2.9 ± 1.3	ND
E'/A'_{lat}	ND	ND	1.6 ± 0.7	ND	2.2 ± 1.1	ND
E/E'_{lat}	ND	8.9 (6.5-10.8)	ND	ND	ND	ND
Sm_{max} (m/s)	0.34 (0.24-0.70)	ND	0.506 ± 0.059	0.48 ± 0.14	ND	0.39 ± 0.12
Dm_{max} (m/s)	0.50 (0.36-0.75)	ND	0.494 ± 0.042	0.47 ± 0.10	ND	0.44 ± 0.09
Sm/Dm	0.79 (0.47-1.12)	ND	1.0 ± 0.1	ND	ND	0.90 ± 0.29
AR_{max} (m/s)	0.24 (0.19-0.30)	ND	0.278 ± 0.044	0.23 ± 0.06	ND	0.22 ± 0.07
ARdur (ms)	67 (57-80)	58 (56-79)	58 ± 9	53.5 ± 10.3	ND	ND
Adur/ARdur	1.33 (1.03-1.73)	1.33 (1.00-1.60)	1.5 ± 0.3	1.01 ± 0.28	ND	ND
Systolic fraction (%)	ND	ND	ND	ND	ND	62.55 ± 11.54
Vp (cm/s)	ND	63.1 (50.9-77.9)	59.7 ± 11.1	ND	ND	ND

A_{max}, Maximal velocity of A wave of the transmitral flow; *A'_{lat},* maximal velocity of the A′ wave of the lateral side of the mitral annulus; *Adur,* duration of the A wave; *AR_{max},* maximal velocity of the AR wave of the pulmonary venous blood flow; *ARdur,* duration of the AR wave of the pulmonary venous blood flow; *Dm_{max},* maximal velocity of the Dm wave of the pulmonary venous blood flow; *DTE,* deceleration time of the E wave; *E_{max},* maximal velocity of E wave of the transmitral flow; *E'_{lat},* maximal velocity of the E′ wave of the lateral side of the mitral annulus; *E'_{septal},* maximal velocity of the E′ wave of the septal side of the mitral annulus; *IVRT,* isovolumic relaxation time of the left ventricle; *ND,* not determined; *Sm_{max},* maximal velocity of the Sm wave of the pulmonary venous blood flow; *Vp,* mitral flow propagation velocity.

TABLE 8-2 Diastolic Doppler Parameter [Median (10th-90th Percentiles)] Measures in 92 Normal Dogs, Depending on Age [5]

	Age (Years)				
Variable	<2 (n = 30)	≥2 and <4 (n = 30)	≥4 and <6 (n = 13)	≥6 and <10 (n = 11)	≥10 (n = 8)
IVRT (ms)	46 (31-62)	47 (40-65)	43 (43-63)	47 (41-65)	63 (41-73)
E_{max} (m/s)	0.77 (0.63-0.93)	0.72 (0.54-0.92)	0.73 (0.52-0.91)	0.69 (0.52-0.82)	0.69 (0.52-0.81)
A_{max} (m/s)	0.48 (0.37-0.68)	0.52 (0.35-0.67)	0.49 (0.39-0.64)	0.57 (0.45-0.70)	0.65 (0.45-0.78)
E/A	1.65 (1.16-1.98)	1.35 (0.93-1.86)	1.44 (1.10-1.60)	1.08 (0.98-1.70)	1.28 (0.68-1.42)
DTE (ms)	67 (53-79)	73 (53-107)	90 (54-110)	80 (49-98)	80 (73-98)
Adur (ms)	87 (63-112)	87 (77-109)	93 (77-123)	90 (68-103)	80 (61-99)
Sm_{max} (m/s)	0.41 (0.30-0.60)	0.40 (0.31-0.53)	0.45 (0.30-0.60)	0.34 (0.24-0.70)	0.40 (0.34-0.75)
Dm_{max} (m/s)	0.57 (0.44-0.69)	0.55 (0.39-0.82)	0.51 (0.38-0.82)	0.50 (0.36-0.75)	0.57 (0.41-0.86)
Sm/Dm	0.72 (0.46-1.23)	0.68 (0.53-1.18)	0.75 (0.55-1.38)	0.79 (0.47-1.12)	0.93 (0.53-1.09)
AR_{max} (m/s)	0.21 (0.16-0.26)	0.21 (0.16-0.29)	0.21 (0.15-0.29)	0.24 (0.19-0.30)	0.26 (0.22-0.28)
ARdur (ms)	67 (53-80)	70 (53-87)	70 (53-103)	67 (57-80)	57 (48-60)
Adur/ARdur	1.19 (1.05-1.64)	1.35 (1.05-1.70)	1.47 (0.92-1.64)	1.33 (1.03-1.73)	1.42 (1.26-1.65)

A_{max}, Maximal velocity of A wave of the transmitral flow; *Adur,* duration of the A wave; *AR_{max},* maximal velocity of the AR wave of the pulmonary venous blood flow; *ARdur,* duration of the AR wave of the pulmonary venous blood flow; *Dmmax,* maximal velocity of the Dm wave of the pulmonary venous blood flow; *DTE,* deceleration time of the E wave; *E_{max},* maximal velocity of E wave of the transmitral flow; *IVRT,* isovolumic relaxation time of the left ventricle; *Sm_{max},* maximal velocity of the Sm wave of the pulmonary venous blood flow.

Isovolumic Relaxation Time

The isovolumic relaxation time (IVRT) is the interval of time between the end of aortic ejection and the beginning of ventricular filling. This is obtained from the simultaneous recording in spectral Doppler mode of the aortic and mitral flows (see Figure 8-3). To do this, the Doppler cursor is placed so as to straddle the left ventricular outflow tract and the mitral valve. The sample volume is then widened in order to record the two flows. The continuous wave spectral Doppler mode can be used in addition to the pulsed wave mode.

The normal values of the IVRT in dogs and cats are summarized in Tables 8-1 and 8-2. In dogs, the IVRT increased with age and decreases with increased heart rate [5].

Pulmonary Venous Blood Flow (Pulsed Wave Spectral Doppler)

The pulmonary venous blood flow is technically difficult to obtain but can provide important information on atrial pressure when successfully recorded. It also contributes, in association with the other modalities, to better differentiation of the different types of diastolic dysfunction [1-4,8,9]. To record pulmonary venous blood flow, the pulsed wave spectral Doppler sample volume must be placed in the medial or lateral pulmonary vein using an apical 4 chambers view.

A normal pulmonary venous blood flow is characterized by an antegrade systolic wave, sometimes biphasic (Sm); a diastolic antegrade wave (Dm); and a retrograde diastolic AR wave. The Sm wave is associated with atrial systolic filling. The Dm wave is associated with the opening of the mitral valve and the end-diastolic ventricular suction. The AR wave is associated with atrial contraction [2].

The main parameters used are the Sm/Dm ratio and the duration of the AR wave (ARdur). The normal values of these parameters are summarized in Tables 8-1 and 8-2. In dogs, the amplitude of the AR wave increases with age and heart rate [5].

Tissue Doppler of the Mitral Annulus

The velocities of the mitral annulus are measured with pulsed wave tissue Doppler. The sample volume is placed at the level of insertion of the mitral valve on the septum or the lateral wall using an apical 4 chambers view. The early diastolic E′ wave of the mitral annulus tissue Doppler is the result of the ventricular wall cardiomyocyte relaxation. This is relatively independent of the atrioventricular pressure gradient and therefore of the preload. However, this preload independence has come under some question (see Chapter 9) [2,8,17-21]. The E′ wave is significantly correlated to *tau* [8]. Other determinants of E′ are the relaxation of the left ventricle and its minimum pressure [8,18].

The A′ wave determinants are atrial function and left ventricular end-diastolic pressure [8]. Normal values of E′ and A′ waves in dogs and cats are summarized in Tables 8-1 and 8-2.

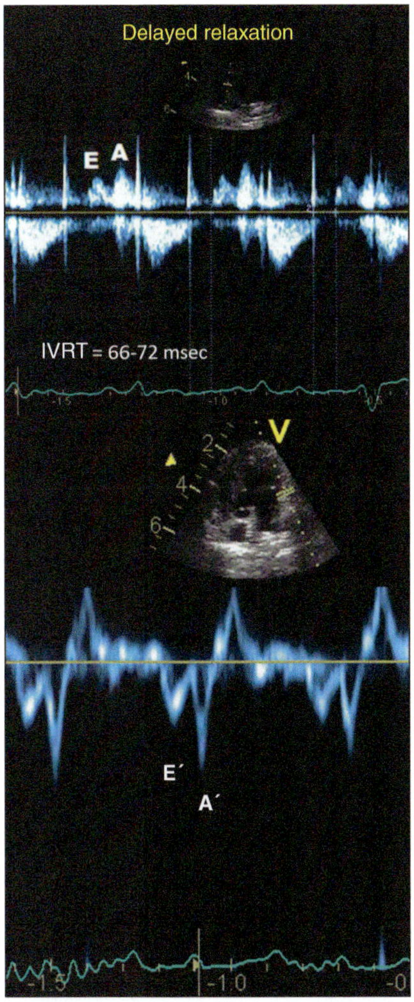

• **Fig. 8-4** Delayed ventricular relaxation in a cat with a hypertrophic cardiomyopathy. Note the lengthening of the isovolumic relaxation time (IVRT) and the inversion of the E/A (transmitral flow, *top*) and E′/A′ (tissue Doppler of the mitral annulus, *bottom*) ratios. (Photo credit: Éric de Madron.)

Color TM of the Diastolic Mitral Flow

The velocity of propagation of the mitral flow in the left ventricle (Vp) can be measured by performing a color TM of the diastolic mitral flow [1,2,4,8]. To measure this parameter, an apical 4 chambers view is used. The TM cursor is set so as to go through the center of the mitral valve and then the color Doppler mode is turned on. To get the best recording, the Nyquist limit must be reduced to 50% of the E value and the recording speed increased to 200 cm/s. The Vp will be the slope between 0 and 4 cm of the first aliasing velocity in early diastole (see Figure 8-3). Vp is an indication of ventricular relaxation that is relatively independent of preload in humans and dogs [23]. The main determinant of the Vp is the intraventricular gradient between its base and apex [1]. The mean, minimum, and maximum values of Vp in normal dogs [24] are summarized in Table 8-1.

Diastolic Dysfunctions

Delayed Relaxation

When there is delayed active relaxation, the E wave decreases, the A wave increases, and the E/A ratio decreases (Figure 8-4) [1-4,25]. These changes may become impossible to identify when the E and A waves fuse or in case of atrial fibrillation. Measurement of the IVRT allows us to overcome this limit, because IVRT can be measured in all circumstances (Figure 8-5; see also Figure 8-4). It lengthens with delayed relaxation [1-4,25]. This delay also results in a decrease of the pulmonary venous blood flow Dm wave, thus replicating the decrease of the transmitral flow E wave. The AR wave is

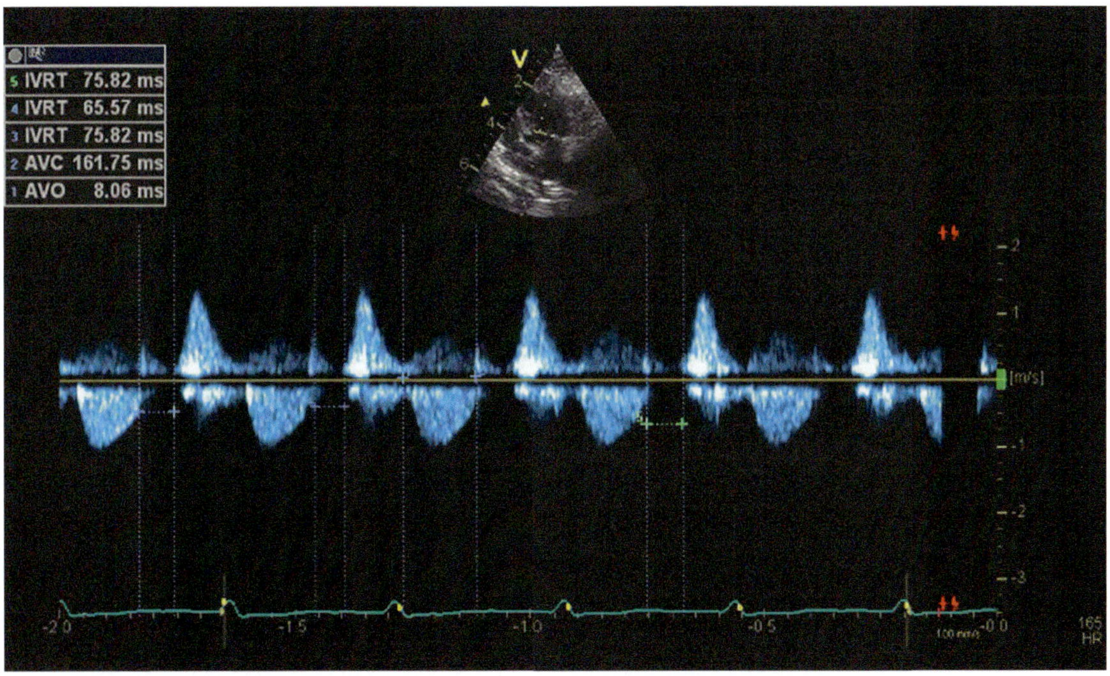

• **Fig. 8-5** Mitral and aortic flows in a cat with a hypertrophic cardiomyopathy. The isovolumic relaxation time (IVRT) is prolonged (66 to 76 ms), indicating delayed ventricular relaxation. The fusion of the E and A waves does not allow observation of the expected inversion of the E/A ratio. (Photo credit: Éric de Madron.)

not modified if the left ventricular compliance remains normal [3]. The amplitude of the mitral annulus early diastolic E′ wave decreases [1,2] while that of the A′ wave increases (see Figure 8-4).

Experimental studies performed in dogs after ligation of their circumflex coronary arteries showed that delayed relaxation results in an increase in the time interval between the beginning of the E wave and that of the E′ wave ($T_{E\text{-}E'}$) (Figure 8-6) [26]. The normal average value of $T_{E\text{-}E'}$ in dogs is 12 ms (–1 to 38) [24].

Pseudonormalization of the Diastole

The E/A ratio and IVRT normalize with pseudonormal diastolic dysfunction [1-4,8,25]. The left atrial pressure (LAP) increase, leading to pseudonormalization, results in a decrease of the Sm wave amplitude and an increase of the Dm waves amplitude. The Sm/Dm ratio decreases [1]. The decreased compliance present at this stage leads to increased resistance of the late diastolic left ventricular filling secondary to atrial contraction. The AR wave widens and its velocity increases. The ratio of the A and AR wave durations (Adur/ARdur) decreases with the LAP increase, becoming ≤1 when LAP exceeds 20 mm Hg [24,27]. The amplitude of the E′ wave remains decreased. That of the A′ wave decreases with the loss of compliance of the left ventricle (Figure 8-7). The E/E′ ratio is an index of the LAP and tends to increase with LAP (see Chapter 9) [9,27-29].

Restrictive Dysfunction

With restrictive diastolic dysfunction, the LAP is greatly increased, leading to a further increase in the amplitude of the E wave. The decrease of the compliance reduces the A wave. The E/A ratio therefore is greatly increased (>2) (Tables 8-3 and 8-4; see Figure 8-3). The marked increase in LAP reduces the IVRT, [24] which becomes shorter than normal. The decrease of the left ventricular compliance hastens the decrease of the atrioventricular pressure gradient, leading to a shorter DTE [16]. The amplitude of the pulmonary venous blood flow Sm wave is greatly decreased while that of the Dm wave increases. Theoretically, the AR wave should also increase but the decline of atrial myocardial inotropy, often present at this stage, attenuates or cancels this trend [1]. The E′ and A′ wave amplitudes are greatly reduced (Figure 8-8).

The diagnostic criteria of the different stages of diastolic dysfunction in cats and dogs are summarized in Tables 8-3 and 8-4.

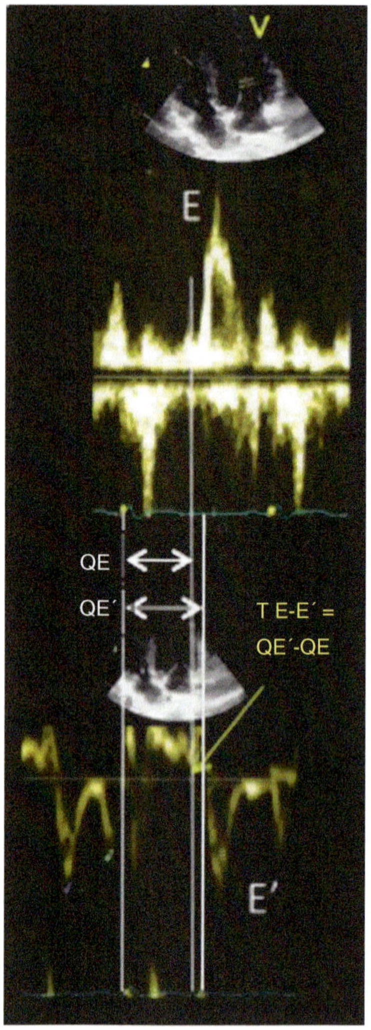

• **Fig. 8-6** Measurement of the time between the beginning of the E wave and that of the E′ wave ($T_{E\text{-}E'}$) of mitral flow by spectral Doppler and mitral annulus tissue Doppler, respectively. One measures the intervals between the beginning of the Q wave on the ECG and the beginning of the E and E′ waves. $T_{E\text{-}E'}$ is equal to QE′ – QE. (Photo credit: Éric de Madron.)

In humans, the Vp tends to decrease in advanced stages of diastolic dysfunction [1,4]. However, it can remain normal in the case of preserved ventricular ejection fraction associated with delayed relaxation [8]. The Vp is a parameter that proved to be disappointing in dogs due to its variability [24].

Figure 8-9 summarizes the changes in the mitral and pulmonary venous blood flows, mitral annulus myocardial velocities, and mitral blood flow propagation velocity with the progression of diastolic dysfunction.

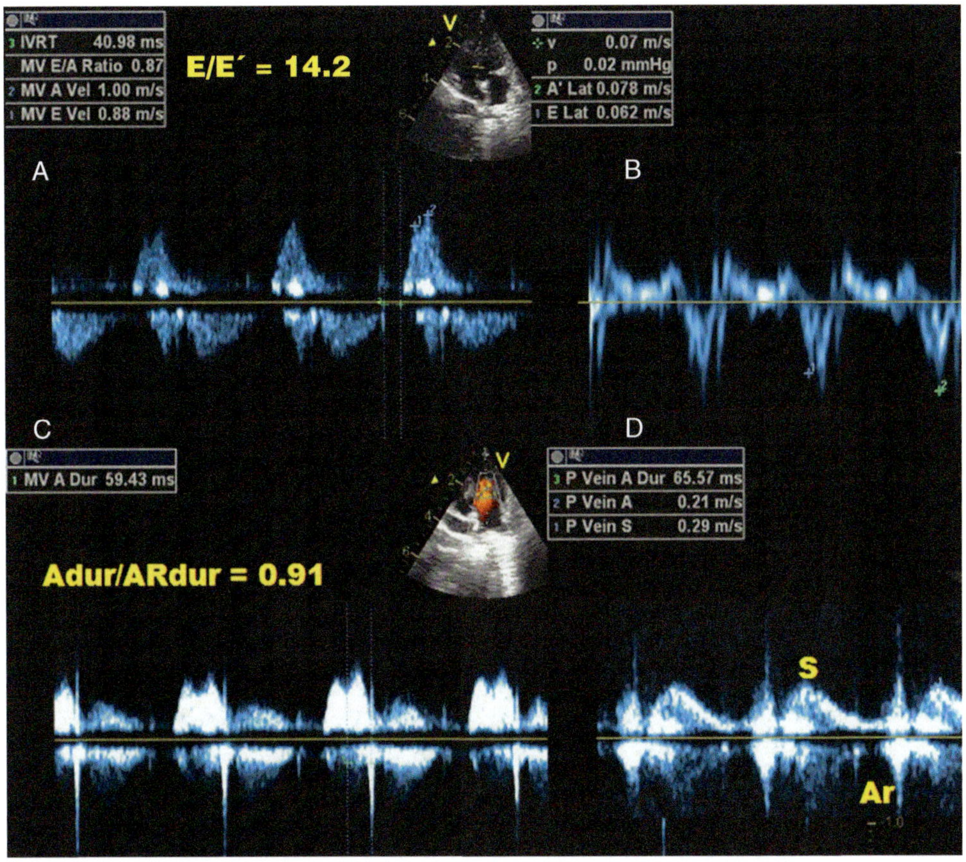

• **Fig. 8-7** Pseudonormal diastolic dysfunction in a cat with hypertrophic cardiomyopathy and congestive heart failure. The E/A ratio of the transmitral flow and the isovolumic relaxation time (IVRT) *(top left)* are normal. The E′ and A′ waves of the mitral annulus *(top right)* are of normal amplitude but the E/E′ ratio is high, compatible with a high left atrial pressure. The duration of the AR wave (ARdur) of pulmonary venous flow *(bottom right)* exceeds that of the A wave (Adur) *(bottom left)*, which also indicates a high atrial pressure. (Photo credit: Éric de Madron.)

TABLE 8-3 **Criteria for Classifying Types of Diastolic Dysfunction in Cats[12,22,25]**

Parameter	Normal Diastole	Delayed Relaxation (Stage 1a) with Normal LV Filling Pressures	Delayed Relaxation (Stage 1b) with High LV Filling Pressures	Pseudonormal Diastole (Stage 2)	Restrictive Diastole (Stage 3)
E/A	1.12 ± 0.22 [22]	<1	<1	≈1	>2
IVRT (ms)	43 ± 9 ms [22]	>60	>60	37-60	<37
Adur/ARdur	1.01 ± 0.28 [22]	≈1	≈1	≈1	< 1
AR_{max} (m/s)	0.23 ± 0.06 [22]	N	N	↑	↑↑
Sm/Dm	0.90 ± 0.29 [12]	>1	>1	≈1	<<1
E/E′	<10	<10	≥10	≥10	≥10

Adur/ARdur, Ratio of the mitral flow A wave and pulmonary venous blood flow AR wave durations; *AR_{max},* maximal velocity of the pulmonary venous blood flow AR wave; *E/A,* ratio of the maximal velocities of the transmitral flow E and A waves; *E/E′,* ratio of the mitral flow E wave and mitral annulus E′ wave velocities; *IVRT,* isovolumic relaxation time of the left ventricle; *LV,* left ventricular; *N,* normal; *Sm/Dm,* ratio of the maximal velocities of the pulmonary venous blood flow Sm and Dm waves.

TABLE 8-4 Criteria for Classifying Types of Diastolic Dysfunction in Dogs

Parameter	Normal Diastole [5] (6-10 Years)	Delayed Relaxation (Stage 1a) with Normal LV Filling Pressures	Delayed Relaxation (Stage 1b) with High LV Filling Pressures	Pseudonormal Diastole (Stage 2)	Restrictive Diastole (Stage 3)
E/A	1.08 (0.98-1.70)	<1	<1	≈1	>2
IVRT (ms)	47 (41-65)	>65	>65	41-65	<41
Adur/ARdur	1.33 (1.03-1.73)	≈1.3	≈1.3	≈1.3	<1
AR_{max} (m/s)	0.24 (0.19-0.30)	N	N	↑	↑↑
Sm/Dm	0.79 (0.47-1.12)	>0.8	>0.8	≈0.8	<<0.8
E/E′	<12	<12	≥12	≥12	≥12

Adur/ARdur, Ratio of the mitral flow A wave and pulmonary venous blood flow AR wave durations; *AR_{max}*, maximal velocity of the pulmonary venous blood flow AR wave; *E/A,* ratio of the maximal velocities of the transmitral flow E and A waves; *E/E′,* ratio of the mitral flow E wave and mitral annulus E′ wave velocities; *IVRT,* isovolumic relaxation time of the left ventricle; *LV,* left ventricular; *N,* normal; *Sm/Dm,* ratio of the maximal velocities of the pulmonary venous blood flow Sm and Dm waves.

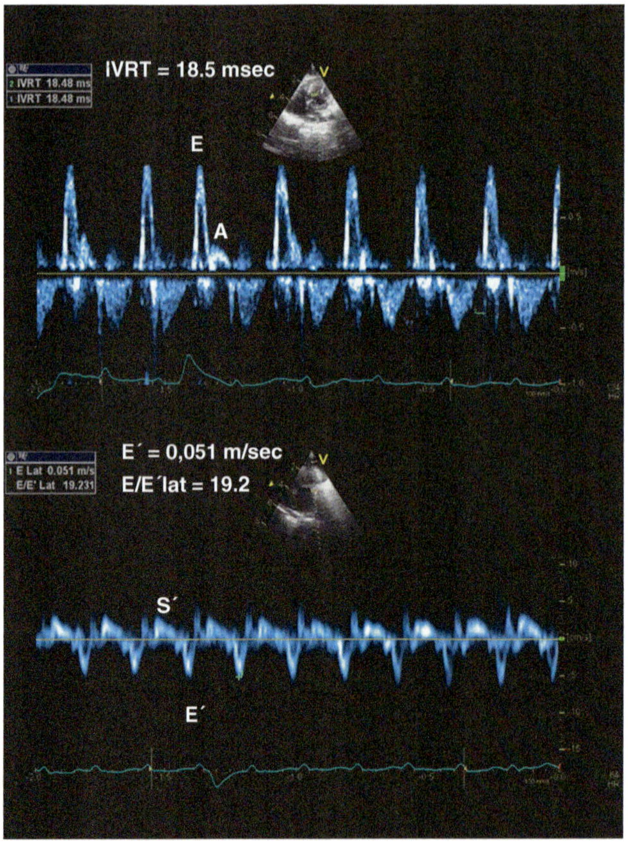

• **Fig. 8-8** Restrictive diastolic dysfunction in a cat with restrictive cardiomyopathy. The amplitude of the E wave is greatly increased whereas that of the A wave is reduced. The E/A ratio is >2. The isovolumic relaxation time (IVRT) is decreased. The E′ and A′ waves of the mitral annulus tissue Doppler are fused. The maximum velocity of this E′A′ fused wave is decreased. The E/E′ ratio is greatly increased, indicating high left atrial pressure. (Photo credit: Éric de Madron.)

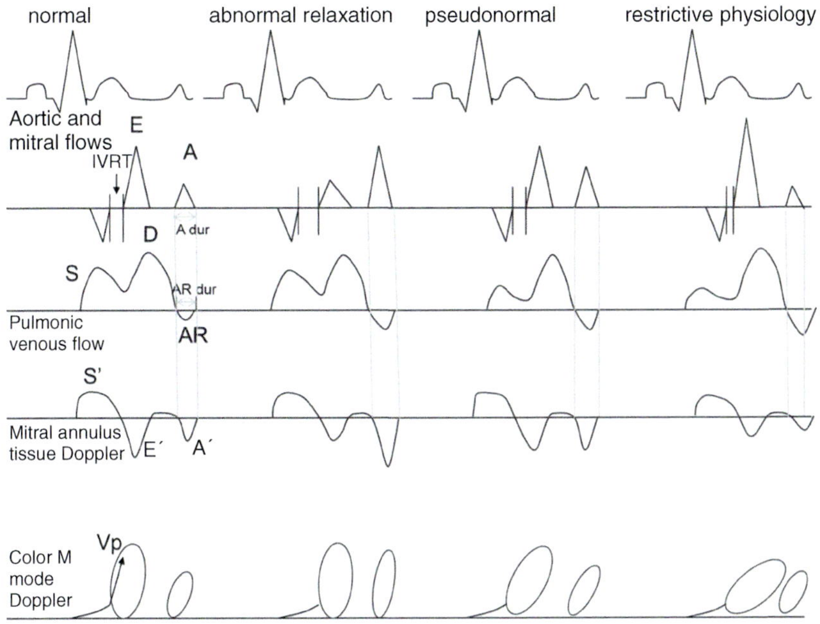

• **Fig. 8-9** The different types of diastolic dysfunction. Delayed active relaxation is characterized by lengthening of isovolumic relaxation time (IVRT) and inversion of the E/A and E′/A′ ratios. The propagation velocity (Vp) is not changed. When diastolic dysfunction becomes pseudonormal due to a rise in left atrial pressure, the E/A ratio returns to normal, IVRT also normalizes, the A′ wave decreases, and so does the Vp. When diastolic dysfunction becomes restrictive, the E/A ratio sharply rises because of the increased E wave (due to an increase in atrial pressure) and reduced A wave (because of a decrease in compliance). The IVRT decreases due to the increased left atrial pressure. The E′ and A′ waves are reduced. The duration of the AR wave (AR dur) increases and the Adur/ARdur ratio becomes <1. The Vp is greatly reduced. (Adapted with permission from Lin G, Oh JK. Echocardiographic assessment of diastolic function and diagnosis of diastolic heart failure. In: Smiseth OA, Michal T, editors. Diastolic heart failure. London: Springer; 2008, p. 149–62.)

REFERENCES

[1] Gabriel RS, Klein AL. Modern evaluation of left ventricular diastolic function using Doppler echocardiography. Curr Cardiol Rep 2009;11:231–8.

[2] Lin G, Oh JK. Echocardiographic assessment of diastolic function and diagnosis of diastolic heart failure. Diastolic heart failure. London: Springer; 2008, p. 149–62.

[3] Yamamoto K, Redfield MM, Nishimura RA. Analysis of left ventricular diastolic function. Heart 1996;75:27–35.

[4] Desai MY, Klein AL. Assessment of diastolic function by echocardiography: the practice of clinical echocardiography 2007;3:237–61.

[5] Schober KE, Luis Fuentes V. Effects of age, body weight, and heart rate on transmitral and pulmonary venous flow in clinically normal dogs. Am J Vet Res 2001;62:1447–54.

[6] Fuentes VL. Diastolic function: is it the key to successful management of many feline cardiomyopathies? J Feline Med Surgery 2003;5:51–6.

[7] Kittleson MD, Meur KM, Munro MJ, et al. Familial hypertrophic cardiomyopathy in Maine coon cats: an animal model of human disease. Circulation 1999;99:3172–80.

[8] Nagheh SF. Echocardiographic evaluation of left ventricular diastolic function. Curr Cardiovasc Imag Rep 2008;1:30–8.

[9] Schober KE, Stern JA, DaCunha DNQT, et al. Estimation of left ventricular filling pressure by Doppler echocardiography in dogs with pacing-induced heart failure. J Vet Intern Med 2008;22:578–85.

[10] O'Sullivan ML, O'Grady MR, Minors SL. Assessment of diastolic function by Doppler echocardiography in normal Doberman Pinschers and Doberman Pinschers with dilated cardiomyopathy. J Vet Intern Med 2007;21:81–91.

[11] Disatian S, Bright JM, Boon J. Association of age and heart rate with pulsed-wave Doppler measurements in healthy, non-sedated cats. J Vet Intern Med 2008;22:351–6.

[12] Santilli RA, Bussadori C. Doppler echocardiographic study of the left ventricular diastole in non-anesthetized healthy cats. Vet J 1998;156:203–15.

[13] Choong CY, Abascal VM, Thomas J, et al. Combined influence of ventricular loading and relaxation on the transmitral flow velocity profile in dogs measured by Doppler echocardiography. J Am Coll Cardiol 2000;36:1664–9.

[14] Firstenberg MS, Smedira NG, Greenberg NL, et al. Relationship between early diastolic intraventricular pressure gradients, an index of elastic recoil, and improvements in systolic and diastolic function. J Am Coll Cardiol 2000;35:201–8.
[15] Masuyama T, Yamamoto K, Uematsu M, et al. Contributors of characteristic mitral flow velocity pattern in congestive heart failure: from clinical observations back to experimental validations. J Am Soc Echocardiogr 1993;6:245–54.
[16] Ohno M, Cheng CP, Little WC. Mechanism of altered patterns of left ventricular filling during the development of congestive heart failure. Circulation 2004;89:2241–50.
[17] Nagueh SF, Sun H, Kopelen HA, et al. Hemodynamic determinants of the mitral annulus diastolic velocities by tissue Doppler. Circulation 1999;99:254–61.
[18] Jacques DC, Pinsky MR, Severyn D, Gorcsan J. Influence of alterations in loading on mitral annular velocity by tissue Doppler echocardiography and its associated ability to predict filling pressures. Chest 2004;126:1910–8.
[19] Nagueh SF, Sun H, Kopelen HA, et al. Hemodynamic determinants of the mitral annulus diastolic velocities by tissue Doppler. Circulation 1999;99:254–61.
[20] Firstenberg MS, Greenberg NL, Main ML, et al. Determinants of diastolic myocardial tissue Doppler velocities: influences of relaxation and preload. J Am Soc Echocardiogr 2005;18:1277–84.
[21] Ruan Q, Rao L, Middleton KJ, et al. Assessment of left ventricular diastolic function by early diastolic mitral annulus peak acceleration rate: experimental studies and clinical application. J Am Coll Cardiol 2001;37:278–85.
[22] Chetboul V, Carlos Sampedrano C, Tissier T, et al. Quantitative assessment of velocities of the annulus of the left atrioventricular valve and left ventricular free wall in healthy cats by use of two-dimensional color tissue Doppler imaging. Am J Vet Res 2006;67: 250–8.
[23] Garcia MJ, Smedira NG, Greenberg NL, et al. Color M-mode Doppler flow propagation velocity is a preload insensitive index of left ventricular relaxation: animal and human validation. Ultrasound Med Biol 2001;27:499–507.
[24] Schober KE, Bonagura JD, Scansen BA, et al. Estimation of left ventricular filling pressure by use of Doppler echocardiography in healthy anesthetised dogs subjected to acute volume loading. Am J Vet Res 2008;69:1034–49.
[25] Schober KE, Maerz I. Assessment of left atrial appendage flow velocity and its relation to spontaneous echocardiographic contrast in 89 cats with myocardial disease. J Vet Intern Med 2006;20:120–30.
[26] Rivas-Gotz C, Khourty DS, Manolios M, et al. Time interval between onset of mitral inflow and onset of early diastolic velocity by tissue Doppler: a novel index of left ventricular relaxation: experimental studies and clinical application. J Am Coll Cardiol 2003;42: 1463–70.
[27] Nagueh SF. Non-invasive estimation of left ventricular filling pressures. In: Smiseth OA, Michal T, editors. Diastolic heart failure. London: Springer; 2008, p. 187–202.
[28] Oyama MA, Sisson DD, Bulmer BJ, Constable PD. Echocardiographic estimation of mean left atrial pressure in a canine model of acute mitral valve insufficiency. J Vet Intern Med 2004;18:667–72.
[29] Bonagura JD, Schober KE. Can ventricular function be assessed by echocardiography in chronic canine mitral valve disease? J Small Anim Pract 2009;50: 12–24.

9

Echocardiographic Evaluation of the Left Ventricle Filling Pressure

ÉRIC DE MADRON

Left Atrial Pressure Curve, 140

Left Atrial Pressure Echocardiographic Indices, 141

Other Echocardiographic Criteria, 147

The estimation of the left ventricle filling pressure (LVFP) is particularly useful for identifying patients at risk of developing or in congestive heart failure (CHF), regardless of the underlying cardiopathy. This evaluation can help to either refine the prognosis or clarify whether left heart disease is indeed responsible for the respiratory symptoms.

Left Atrial Pressure Curve

The LVFP is equal to the diastolic atrioventricular pressure gradient, essentially determined by the left atrial pressure (LAP), in the absence of mitral valve stenosis. The LAP curve is characterized by an early diastolic peak (V wave) followed by a pressure drop after the maximal opening of the mitral valve (y descent), reaching a nadir: the pre-A wave. During diastasis, atrial and ventricular pressures are equal and slowly increase together. A second pressure peak occurs following atrial contraction (the A wave) followed by another descent (x descent) associated with the end-diastolic filling of the left ventricle (LV) (Figure 9-1) [1].

The LAP is usually measured either directly by left atrial catheterization or indirectly by recording the pulmonary capillary wedge pressure (PCWP) using pulmonary artery catheterization with a Swan-Ganz catheter. The PCWP is similar to the LAP, slightly time shifted because of the time needed for the LAP fluctuations to reach the pulmonary capillaries (see Figure 9-1) [1].

Normal LAP values in dogs are summarized in Table 9-1. The mean LAP corresponds to the area under the LAP curve during the cardiac cycle. A mean LAP or PCWP greater than 20 mm Hg, corresponding to an LVFP greater than 15 mm Hg, is associated with left-sided CHF [1].

Therefore obtaining a reliable estimation of LVFP has become a major goal of the echocardiographic exam.

TABLE 9-1 Normal Values (Median, Minimum-Maximum) of the Left Atrial Pressure (LAP) in Dogs [2]

A Wave Peak (mm Hg)	V Wave Peak (mm Hg)	Pre-A Wave (mm Hg)	Average LAP (mm Hg)
9.3 (4.8–14.5)	8.6 (4.6–15.8)	5.6 (1.9–11.9)	7.2 (2.4–14.4)

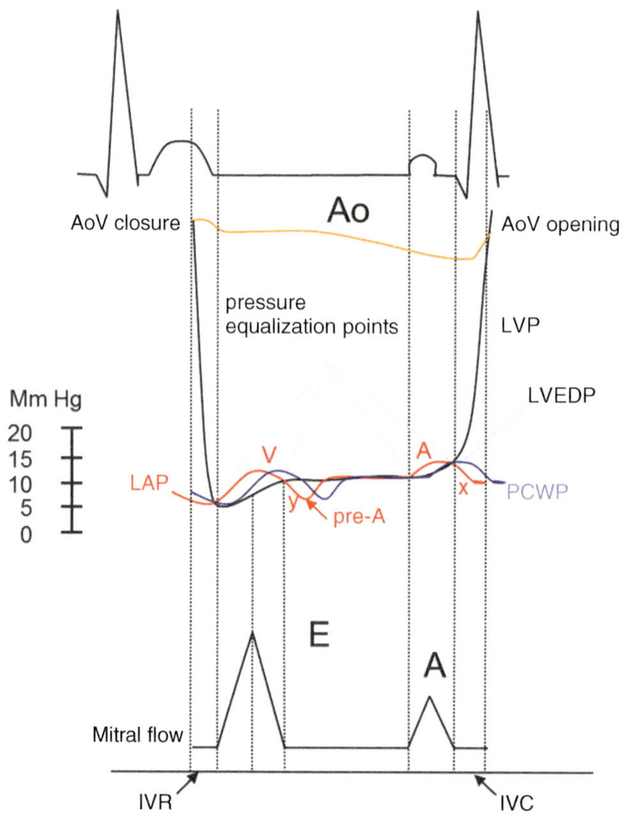

• **Fig. 9-1** Schematic representation of the relationship between the left atrial pressure (LAP), pulmonary capillary wedge pressure (PCWP), left ventricular pressure (LVP), and spectral Doppler of the transmitral flow (Mitral flow) during diastole in a normal subject. The transmitral flow E and A waves correspond to the two periods when the LAP exceeds the LVP: the V and A waves. The pre-A wave is the minimum atrial pressure immediately before the beginning of the A wave. The filling pressure of the left ventricle corresponds to the difference between LAP and LVP. It reaches its maximum in early diastole, which corresponds to the E wave peak. The peaks in the PCWP wave are slightly time shifted in relation to the LAP wave. *Ao,* Aorta diastolic pressure; *AoV,* aortic valve; *IVC,* isovolumic contraction phase; *IVR,* left ventricle isovolumic relaxation phase; *LVEDP,* left ventricle end-diastolic pressure. (Photo credit: Éric de Madron.)

Left Atrial Pressure Echocardiographic Indices

Transmitral Flow

E Wave Maximal Velocity

The maximal velocity of the diastolic transmitral E wave is the result of the complex interaction between the atrioventricular pressure gradient, obviously influenced by atrial filling (preload) [3], and the LV diastolic properties, such as relaxation rate, elastic recoil, minimum pressure, and intraventricular pressure gradient [3,4]. Transmitral flow characteristics are better explained by atrioventricular gradient changes than by absolute atrial or ventricular pressure values [5]. The latter are based on the level at which the atrial and ventricular pressures equalize, left atrial (LA) compliance, LV diastolic function, and extracardiac constraints [6]. The maximum E wave velocity tends to increase with preload but only to a certain point. A study performed in dogs with rapid pacing-induced CHF demonstrated that the LV relaxation rate slows down early in the development of CHF. This reduces the atrioventricular pressure gradient and consequently the ventricular filling rate. As CHF progresses, the increase in LAP overrides the effect of this delayed relaxation: the E wave increases [6]. Beyond a certain level of preload, the E wave amplitude will decrease because the LAP drops faster [7].

Therefore the E wave amplitude is only partially correlated to the LAP. In daily practice, in dogs with mitral regurgitation (MR), an E wave maximum velocity above 1.25 m/s (Figure 9-2) is associated with an elevated LAP and a poorer prognosis [8].

In cats, in which diastolic dysfunctions are more pronounced, a pseudonormal or restrictive ventricular filling pattern indicates an elevated LAP (see Chapter 13), as is the case in humans [5].

E Wave Deceleration Time

The decrease in LV compliance hastens the decrease of the atrioventricular pressure gradient, leading to a shorter deceleration time of the E wave (DTE) (Figure 9-3) [6].

In humans, a high-amplitude E wave associated with a shortened DTE indicates an elevated LAP and a loss of LV compliance [9]. The sensitivity and specificity of a DTE cutoff value ≤120 ms to predict a PCWP ≥20 mm Hg were 100% and 99%, respectively [9]. In another study, the DTE was the parameter that showed the best correlation with PCWP in patients with MR associated with systolic dysfunction [10].

The normal median DTE in aged dogs ranges from 80 to 100 ms [11]. Unlike in humans, the correlation between LAP and DTE revealed itself to be disappointing in normal dogs subjected to volume overload [2] as well as in dogs with spontaneous MR [12]. In another study, performed in dogs with class I, II, or III MR as defined by the International Small Animal Cardiac Health Council (ISACHC), there was no difference in the DTE between the different groups [8].

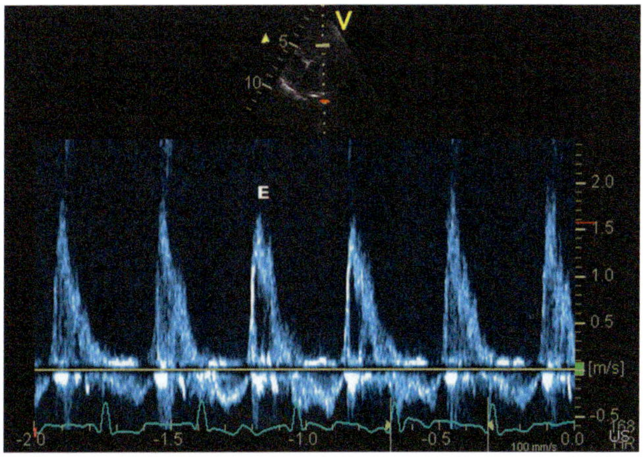

• **Fig. 9-2** Spectral Doppler of the transmitral flow in a dog with severe mitral regurgitation and pulmonary edema. The E wave amplitude reaches 1.5 m/s, compatible with elevated left atrial pressure. (Photo credit: Éric de Madron.)

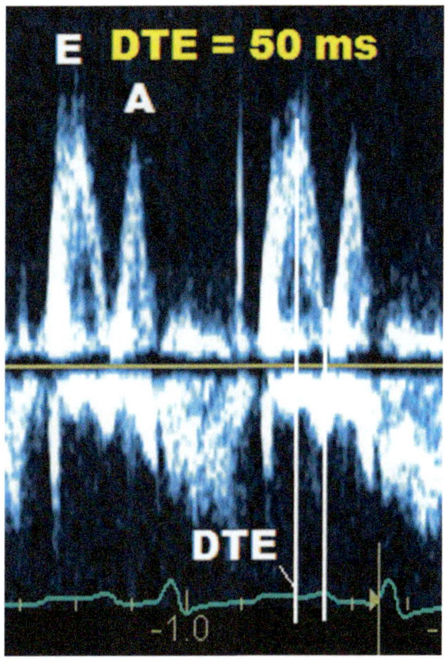

• **Fig. 9-3** Spectral Doppler of the transmitral flow in a dog with severe mitral regurgitation and pulmonary edema. In this dog, the deceleration time of the E wave (DTE) is short: 50 ms. (Photo credit: Éric de Madron.)

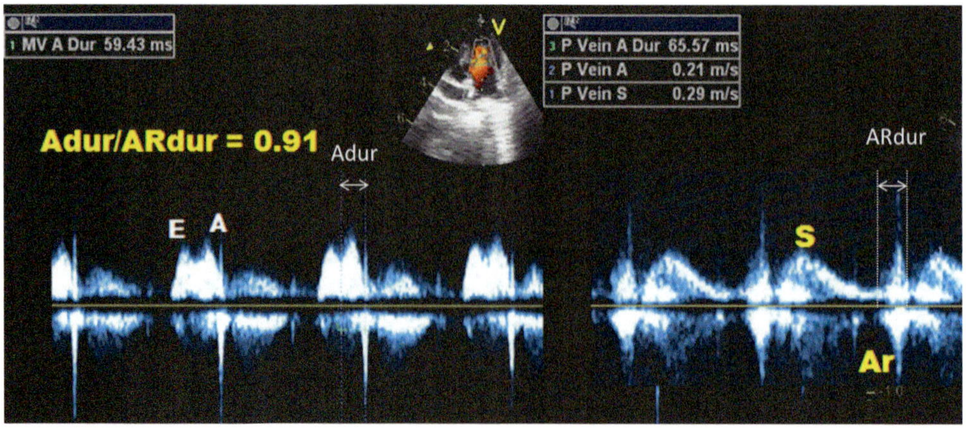

• **Fig. 9-4** Spectral Doppler of the transmitral *(right)* and pulmonary venous *(left)* flows in a cat with hypertrophic cardiomyopathy and congestive heart failure. The Adur/ARdur ratio is <1, indicating elevated left atrial pressure. (Photo credit: Éric de Madron.)

Pulmonary Venous Flow

The increase in LAP leads to increased amplitude and duration of the AR wave. The ratio of the A and AR wave durations (Adur/ARdur) decreases with the increase in LAP. It becomes <1 when the LAP is >20 mm Hg (Figure 9-4) [2].

However, the pulmonary venous flow is technically difficult to obtain in dogs and cats. Furthermore, this flow can be masked by an MR jet [13].

Ratio of the Transmitral E and Mitral Annulus E′ Wave Maximal Velocities: E/E′

The tissue Doppler early diastolic mitral annulus E′ wave is a result of the ventricular wall cardiomyocyte relaxation, which is relatively independent of the atrioventricular pressure gradient and therefore of the preload. The ratio of E and E′ wave maximal velocities (E/E′) was thus introduced to "eliminate" the influence of ventricular relaxation on the E wave and to provide a more accurate LAP index. The theoretical normal E/E′ ratio, based on a model of a pump operating at a constant volume, is 3 [14]. A validation study has demonstrated that the normal E/E′ ratio is in fact 4.2 ± 1.11 and linearly correlated with LVFP in humans [14]. Corroborating this, a good correlation between E/E′ and LVFP was demonstrated in humans with hypertrophic [15] or dilated [16] cardiomyopathy. This index can be used even in cases of sinus tachycardia with E and A wave fusion [17].

Several studies have questioned the independence of the E′ wave from preload. The influence of preload, afterload, and contractility on E′ has been demonstrated in dogs [18]. This influence seems to fade when the diastolic dysfunction worsens [18-21]. Aside from preload, the other determinants of the E′ wave are LV relaxation and minimum pressure [8,18].

Mitral Regurgitation

A study was performed in nine dogs with acute experimental MR induced by section of chordae tendineae. The authors modified the LAP with vasodilators: hydralazine and sodium nitroprusside [13]. A good correlation was obtained between E/E′ and mean LAP (Figure 9-5). However, confidence intervals were very wide, up to 20 mm Hg (Table 9-2), indicating that a significant increase in LAP was needed for the E/E′ to change. This limits the usefulness of this index for LAP calculation. However, this study also showed that an E/E′ value >9.1 indicated a 95% probability of LAP >20 mm Hg. Inversely, an E/E′ value <6 indicated a 95% probability of LAP <20 mm Hg.

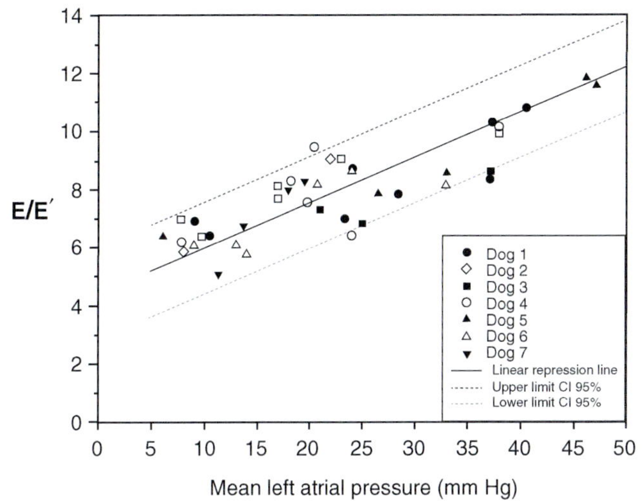

• **Fig. 9-5** Relationship between E and E′ in the left atrium average pressure in seven anesthetized dogs using isofluorane. The values for each dog were obtained after varying degrees of acute experimentally induced mitral regurgitation (chordae tendineae section) and administration of sodium nitroprusside or hydralazine to change the loading conditions. *CI,* Confidence interval. (Adapted from Oyama MA, Sisson DD, Bulmer BJ, Constable PD. Echocardiographic estimation of mean left atrial pressure in a canine model of acute mitral valve insufficiency. J Vet Intern Med 2004;18:667–72.)

TABLE 9-2 Predictive Values of Mean Left Atrial Pressure (LAP) Based on the E/E′ Ratio in Dogs with Acute Experimental Mitral Regurgitation [13]

E/E′	Predicted Mean LAP (mm Hg)	95% Confidence Intervals for Prediction (mm Hg)
5.0	3.6	–6.4-13.6
6.0	10.0	0.0-20.0
7.0	16.4	6.4-26.4
8.0	22.8	12.8-32.8
9.0	29.2	19.2-39.8
10.0	35.6	25.6-45.6
11.0	41.9	31.9-51.9
12.0	48.3	38.3-58.3

In this study, the interoperator variability of E/E′ was 8.0% ± 9.2% and that of E was 5.4% ± 3.8%. Intraoperator variability was 6.4% ± 3.6% for E/E′ and 7.9% ± 3.7% for E.

The effects of acute MR on ventricular relaxation are complex. Several studies have demonstrated that the development of acute MR leads to decreased LV elastance and delayed relaxation [22,23]. If the MR is severe, LAP increases significantly. Furthermore, the reduced afterload results in a decreased end-systolic left ventricular volume, thus increasing the elastic recoil that follows [22]. These phenomena can hide the left ventricular diastolic anomalies. The net result is an apparent "improvement" in the diastolic function, documented by the increase of E′, despite the delayed relaxation [13].

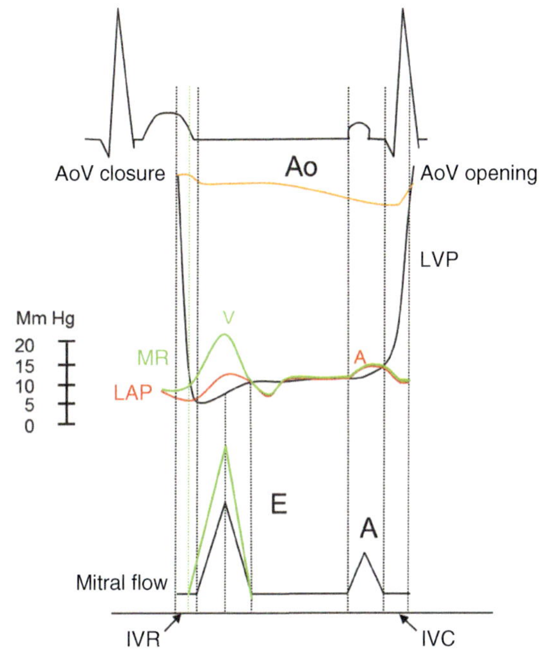

• **Fig. 9-6** Schematic representation of the relationship between left atrial pressure (LAP), left ventricular pressure (LVP), and the spectral Doppler of the transmitral flow (Mitral flow) during diastole between a normal subject *(red curve)* and a subject with mitral regurgitation (MR; *green curve*). MR is associated with a large V wave, leading to early equalization of pressures, with the mitral valve opening during the "isovolumic" relaxation (IVR) of the left ventricle, which becomes shortened. The increase of the atrioventricular gradient leads to an increase in the amplitude of the E wave. *Ao,* Aorta diastolic pressure; *AoV,* aortic valve; *IVC,* isovolumic contraction. (Photo credit: Éric de Madron.)

It is difficult to extrapolate these results obtained under experimental conditions to the evaluation of LVFP in dogs with spontaneous chronic MR. Indeed, in advanced MR, the early diastolic atrioventricular gradient is markedly increased (Figure 9-6), which can increase both the E and E′ amplitudes, in the absence of diastolic dysfunction [19]. Therefore the E/E′ ratio loses some of its effectiveness in the prediction of LVFP [18].

This can explain why the E/E′ cutoff values proposed to document elevated LVFP in spontaneous MR are more elevated than the ones proposed for cases of systolic dysfunctions, in which the atrioventricular gradient is less elevated and the diastolic dysfunction more significant. Thus Teshima et al [24] propose to use a cutoff value of 13, with 80% sensitivity and 83% specificity, to diagnose the presence of CHF in dogs with spontaneous MR. A correlation between E/E′ and the left atrium/aorta ratio has also been demonstrated. In the same fashion, Schober et al [25] propose the use of an E/E′ value >12 combined with a maximum velocity of E >1.25 m/s to predict the presence of radiographic CHF in dogs with spontaneous MR.

In humans, the DTE has been found to perform better than any other index in predicting PCWP in patients with MR [10].

Systolic Dysfunction

In human patients with ischemic cardiomyopathy, an E/E′ value <8 predicts a normal LVFP while an E/E′ value >15 indicates an elevated LVFP. Other Doppler indices must be used when E/E′ values range between 8 and 15 in order to better characterize the LVFP [16]. Another study proposes the association of an E/E′ value ≥15 and an indexed left atrial volume ≥23 mL/m^2 to identify human patients at risk of CHF [26].

The E/E′ ratio has been found to be unreliable in dogs with rapid pacing-induced systolic dysfunction leading to CHF [27]. A significant impact of preload on E′, not attenuated by significant diastolic dysfunction as well as significant LAP elevations, could explain the lack of performance of E/E′ in this study. With the same heart failure model, another study revealed that the E′ wave was delayed and no longer responded to the atrioventricular gradient [28]. Other indices using isovolumic relaxation time have been found to be more reliable, [27] however (see below).

E/E′ in Cats

The E/E′ ratio was found to be a good predictor for LVFP in human patients with hypertrophic cardiomyopathy [29]. In cats, an E/E′ value >10 has been proposed as a criterion for elevated LAP (Figure 9-7) [30].

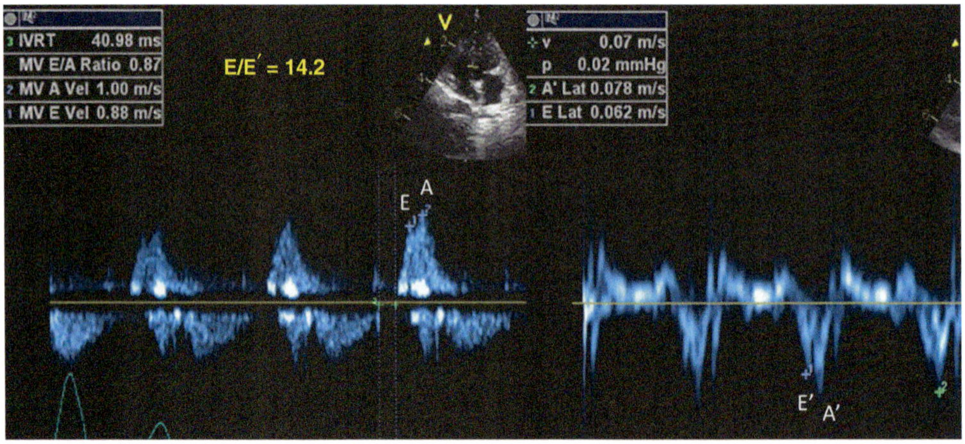

• **Fig. 9-7** Spectral Doppler of the transmitral flow *(left)* and tissue Doppler of the mitral annulus *(right)* in a cat with hypertrophic cardiomyopathy and congestive heart failure. The E/E′ ratio is 14.2, which is compatible with elevated left atrial pressure. (Photo credit: Éric de Madron.)

Ratio of the E Wave Maximal Velocity and Propagation Velocity (Vp): E/Vp

The propagation velocity of the early diastolic transmitral flow (Vp), obtained by color time-motion (TM) mode of the mitral valve (Figure 9-8), is a relatively preload-independent index of ventricular relaxation in humans and dogs [31]. However, some authors have cast doubts on this independence [32]. As with E/E′, the E/Vp capacity to predict LVFP has been evaluated. In 90 patients with various degrees of ventricular dysfunction, increasing severity of the ventricular function was associated with a progressive decrease in Vp and a significant increase in E/Vp. E/Vp was the best and sometimes the only predictor of pulmonary congestion [33]. However, Vp measurements are highly variable in humans, especially in cases of normal systolic function [34].

In dogs, the only information comes from the studies conducted by Schober et al [1,27]. In those studies, E/Vp was not correlated with LVFP and proved to be less sensitive and less specific than the other indices.

Isovolumic Relaxation Time (IVRT) and the E/IVRT Ratio

Isovolumic relaxation time (IVRT) is the time interval between the end of aortic ejection and the beginning of ventricular filling. It is obtained by simultaneously recording the aortic and mitral flows (Figure 9-9).

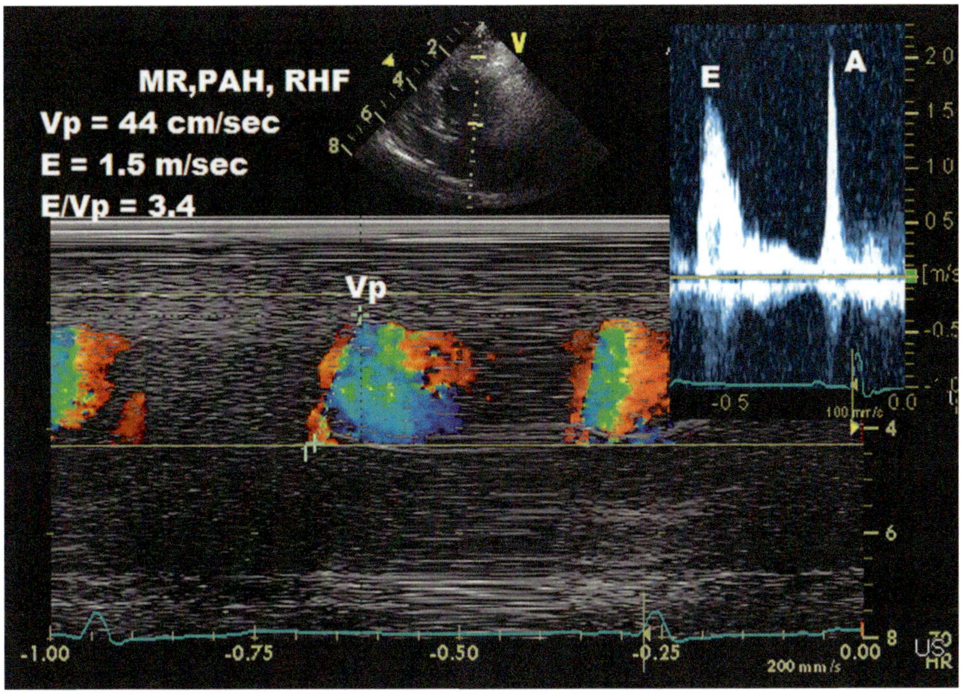

• **Fig. 9-8** Color time-motion (TM) mode and spectral Doppler of the transmitral flow in a dog with mitral regurgitation (MR), secondary pulmonary hypertension (PAH), and right-sided congestive heart failure (RHF). The E wave propagation velocity (Vp) is 44 cm/s. E wave maximum velocity is 1.5 m/s. The E/Vp ratio is therefore 3.4, significantly higher than normal values. (Photo credit: Éric de Madron.)

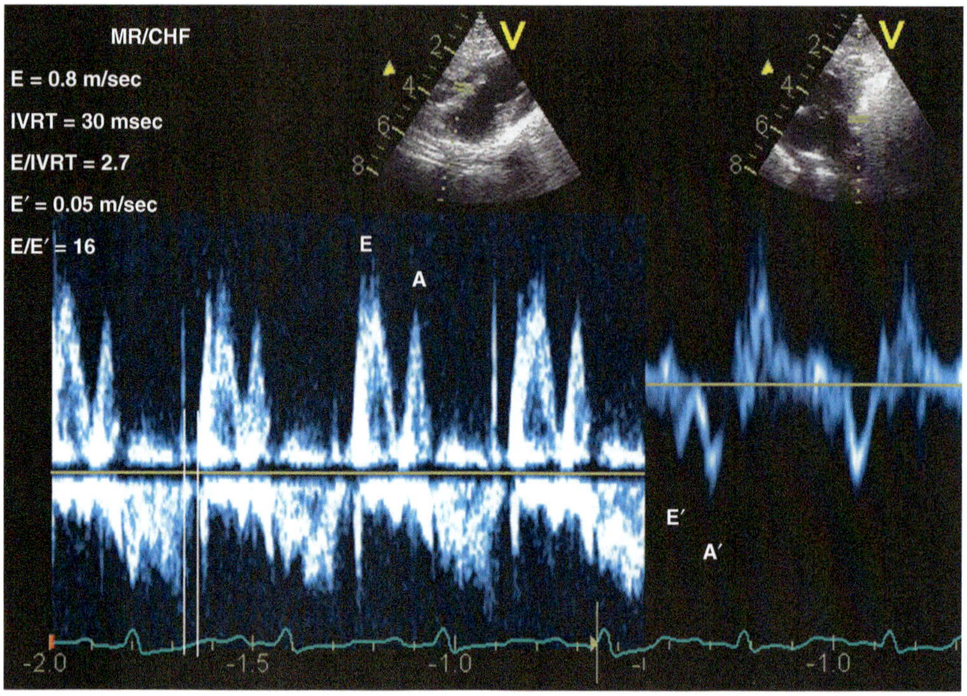

• **Fig. 9-9** Spectral Doppler of transmitral and aortic flows *(left)* and tissue Doppler of mitral annulus *(right)* in a dog with mitral regurgitation (MR) and left-sided congestive heart failure (CHF). The E/E′ ratio of 16 and E/IVRT ratio of 2.7 indicate an elevated atrial pressure. It is interesting to note that the E wave maximum velocity in this dog is not increased. *IVRT,* Isovolumic relaxation time. (Photo credit: Éric de Madron.)

The normal IVRT in the healthy aged dog varies between 41 and 73 ms [11]. Delayed relaxation lengthens IVRT whereas elevated LAP shortens it [2]. This isovolumic phase, which is not really isovolumic in the case of MR (see Figure 9-6), is subject to complex and at times contradictory influences such as the LV relaxation rate, the atrioventricular pressure gradient, and the level of LAP. In dogs, the influence of LAP becomes predominant with advanced MR. A study in human patients with primary mitral valve pathology (regurgitation or stenosis) documented a significant correlation between IVRT and PCWP, even with atrial fibrillation [35]. The best parameter was the IVRT/$T_{E\text{-}E'}$ ratio, where $T_{E\text{-}E'}$ represents the interval between the beginning of the E wave and the beginning of the E′ wave (see Chapter 8).

Schober et al [1] have demonstrated that IVRT, E/IVRT, and $T_{E\text{-}E'}$ were correlated to LAP in normal dogs submitted to volume overload. An E/IVRT value >2.2 in a normal dog in sinus rhythm predicted an average LAP ≥15 mm Hg, with 90% sensitivity and 92% specificity.

In another study, performed in dogs with rapid pacing-induced CHF in which LVFP was modified using furosemide, the best parameter predicting LAP was E/IVRT (Figure 9-10). The authors proposed the following regression equation:

$$\text{LVEDP} = 12.3 + (18.4 \times \text{E}/\text{IVRT})\ (r = 0.70;\ p < 0.01)$$

where *LVEDP* represents LV end-diastolic pressure, *E* is measured in cm/s, and *IVRT* is measured in ms [27].

It is difficult to extrapolate these conclusions to daily practice, since the dogs in the study either were normal or belonged to a model of systolic and diastolic dysfunction considerably different from the spontaneous MR we often encounter. Having said that, Bonagura and Schober [12] recommend using cutoff values of IVRT <45 ms and E/IVRT >2.5 to identify an elevated LVFP in dogs with spontaneous MR.

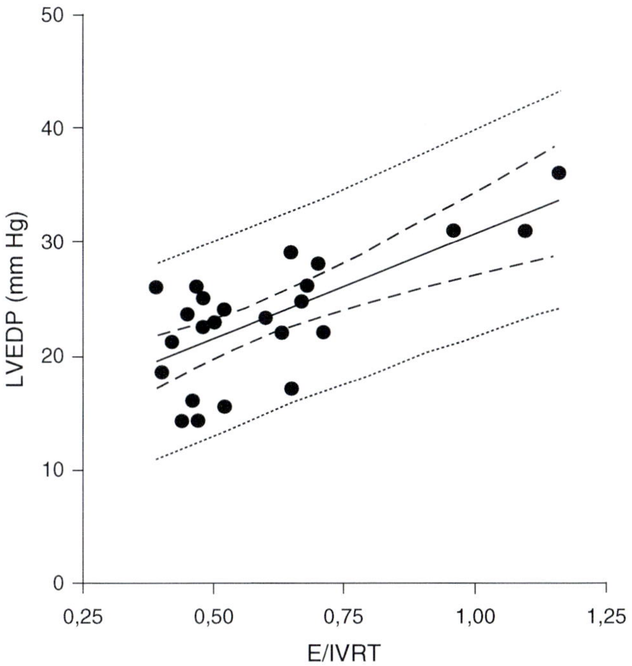

• **Fig. 9-10** Relationship between the E wave maximum velocity and the isovolumic relaxation time (IVRT) and the left ventricular end-diastolic pressure (LVEDP) in five dogs with rapid pacing-induced heart failure that were treated with furosemide. Dashed lines indicate 95% confidence interval; dotted lines indicate 95% predictive interval. (Reproduced with permission from Schober KE, Stern JA, DaCunha DNQT, et al. Estimation of left ventricular filling pressure by Doppler echocardiography in dogs with pacing-induced heart failure. J Vet Intern Med 2008;22:578–85.)

TABLE 9-3 Normal and Threshold Values for Several Doppler Indices in Dogs Indicating an Elevated Left Ventricle Filling Pressure (LVFP) [2,11,12]

Parameter	Normal Values: Average (Minimum-Maximum)	Tendency When LVFP Increases	Value Indicating Elevated LVFP
E (m/s)	0.69 (0.52-0.82)	↑	>1.2
DTE (ms)	80-100	↓	ND
E/E′	<6	↑	>12
IVRT (ms)	41-73	↓	<45
E/IVRT	1.62 (1.12-1.80)	↑	>2.5
E/Vp	1.09 (0.9-2.02)	↑	ND

DTE, Deceleration time of the E wave; *IVRT,* isovolumic relaxation time; *ND,* not determined; *Vp,* propagation velocity.

Table 9-3 displays all of the Doppler indices useful in the diagnosis of elevated LVFP in dogs.

Other Echocardiographic Criteria

A number of indirect echocardiographic criteria can also help to identify elevated LVFP.

Mitral Regurgitation

In the case of chronic MR, the regurgitant volume must be significant for CHF to appear. In fact, echocardiograms performed at the time of left-sided CHF diagnosis on 44 dogs with MR [36] revealed significant LA (LA/Ao = 1.9 ± 0.4) and LV dilations (end-diastolic volume index calculated using the Teichholz method: 143.6 ± 49.2 mL/m^2) according to the criteria used by Borgarelli et al [8]. The regurgitant fraction, calculated using the proximal isovelocity surface area (PISA) method (see Chapter 11), was also significant according to the criteria established by Gouni et al [37]: 57.5% ± 17.9%. The end-systolic volume index calculated using the Teichholz method was slightly increased: 40.4 ± 30.8 mL/m^2, although this method of calculation is questionable in dogs (see Chapters 7 and 11) (Figure 9-11).

In the case of elevated LAP, the MR jet spectral Doppler signal is shaped like a triangle, indicating a rapid decrease in the atrioventricular gradient in end-systole (Figure 9-12).

Feline Cardiomyopathy

Most cases of feline CHF are associated with at least moderate atrial dilation. However, some cats can develop severe CHF in the absence of major echocardiographic anomalies [38]. It is then essential to properly evaluate the degree of diastolic dysfunction. The pseudonormal or restrictive types of diastolic dysfunctions (see Chapter 13) are typically associated with elevated LAP, confirmed by an increase in the E/E′ ratio (Figure 9-13).

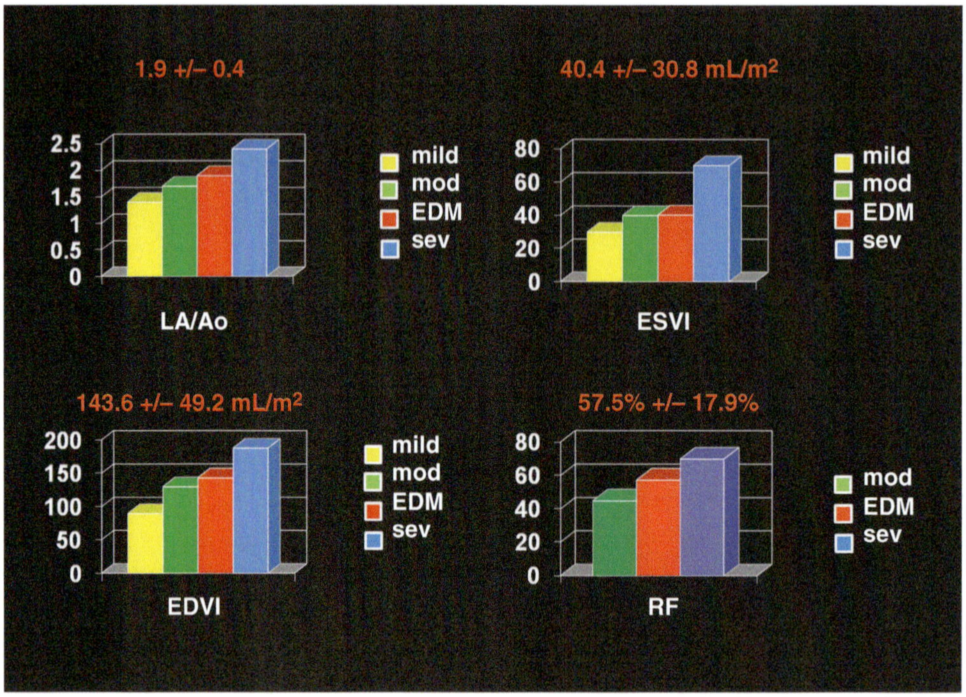

• **Fig. 9-11** Severity of mitral regurgitation (MR) at onset of congestive heart failure (pulmonary edema) in 44 dogs (*red column:* EDM). One can see that, according to several indices, the level of MR severity is at least moderate: LA/Ao (left atrium/aorta ratio), indexed end-diastolic volume calculated using the Teichholz method (EDVI) >130 mL/m², regurgitant fraction (RF) between 42% and 70%. The indexed end-systolic volume calculated using the Teichholz method (ESVI) is also slightly increased (>30 mL/m²). The yellow, green, and blue columns indicate the cutoff values used to separate the degrees of severity (mild, mod = moderate, sev = severe) according to the criteria set forth by Borgarelli et al [8] and Gouni et al [37]. (Photo credit: Éric de Madron.)

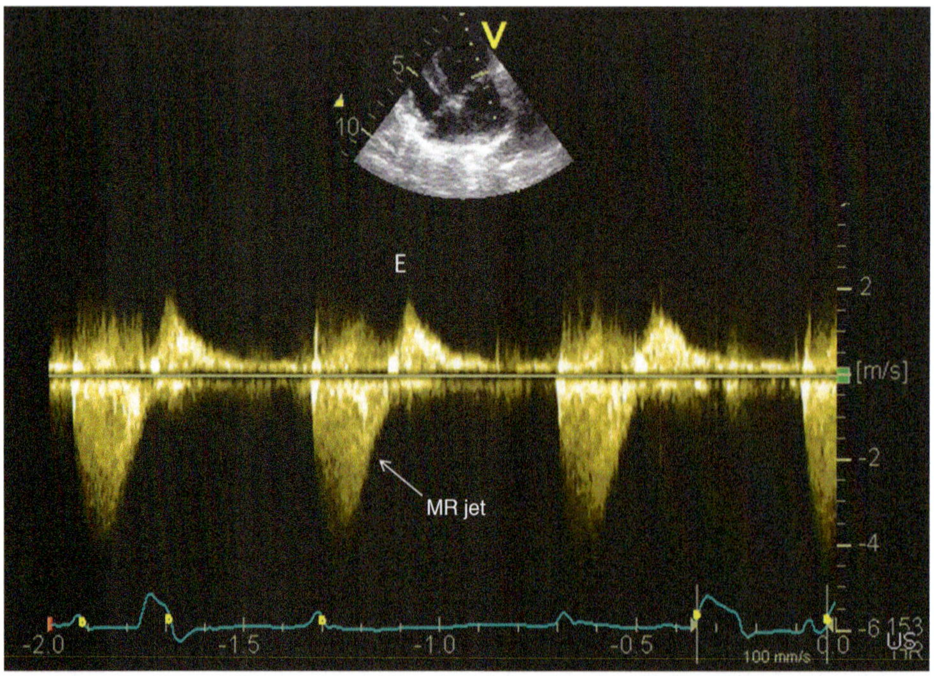

• **Fig. 9-12** Continuous wave spectral Doppler of the mitral flow in a dog with mitral regurgitation (MR) and congestive heart failure. The shape of the MR jet is triangular, indicating a rapid decrease in the atrioventricular gradient during the second part of systole, denoting increased left atrial pressure. (Photo credit: Éric de Madron.)

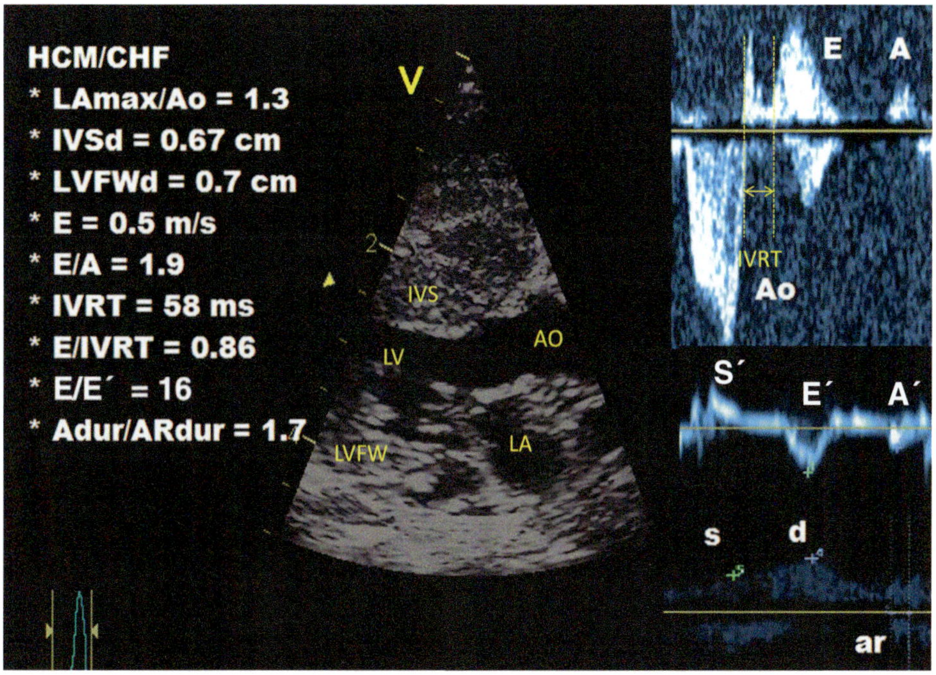

• **Fig. 9-13** Bidimensional echocardiogram *(left),* continuous wave spectral Doppler of mitral and aortic flows *(top right),* tissue Doppler of the lateral mitral annulus *(center right),* and continuous wave spectral Doppler of the pulmonary venous flow *(lower right)* in a cat with hypertrophic cardiomyopathy (HCM) and congestive heart failure (CHF). Septal (IVSd) and left ventricular free wall (LVFWd) hypertrophy is present but left atrial dilation is absent as indicated by the normal left atrium/aorta ratio (LAmax/Ao). The E/A ratio >1 and the normal isovolumic relaxation time (IVRT) indicate either normal or pseudonormal ventricular filling. The E/E′ ratio of 16, compatible with an elevated left atrial pressure, allows us to conclude that this is pseudonormal filling. E/IVRT and Adur/ARdur values remain normal, however. *LA,* Left atrium; *LV,* left ventricle. (Photo credit: Éric de Madron.)

REFERENCES

[1] Schober KE, Bonagura JD, Scansen BA, et al. Estimation of left ventricular filling pressure by use of Doppler echocardiography in healthy anesthetised dogs subjected to acute volume loading. Am J Vet Res 2008;69:1034–49.

[2] Grossman W. Cardiac catheterization. In: Braunwald E, editor. Heart disease. A Textbook of cardiovascular medicine. 4th ed. Philadelphia: WB Saunders; 1992, p. 180–203.

[3] Choong CY, Abascal VM, Thomas J, et al. Combined influence of ventricular loading and relaxation on the transmitral flow velocity profile in dogs measured by Doppler echocardiography. J Am Coll Cardiol 2000;36:1664–9.

[4] Firstenberg MS, Smedira NG, Greenberg NL, et al. Relationship between early diastolic intraventricular pressure gradients, an index of elastic recoil, and improvements in systolic and diastolic function. J Am Coll Cardiol 2000;35:201–8.

[5] Masuyama T, Yamamoto K, Uematsu M, et al. Contributors of characteristic mitral flow velocity pattern in congestive heart failure—from clinical observations back to experimental validations. J Am Soc Echocardiogr 1993;6:245–54.

[6] Ohno M, Cheng CP, Little WC. Mechanism of altered patterns of left ventricular filling during the development of congestive heart failure. Circulation 2004;89:2241–50.

[7] Yamamoto K, Masuyama T, Tanouchi J, et al. Peak early diastolic filling velocity may decrease with preload augmentation: effect of concomitant increase in the rate of left atrial pressure drop in early diastole. J Am Coll Cardiol 2003;41:1590–7.

[8] Borgarelli M, Savarino P, Crosara S, et al. Survival characteristics and prognostic variables of dogs with mitral regurgitation attributable to myxomatous valve disease. J Vet Intern Med 2008;22:120–8.

[9] Giannuzzi P, Imparato A, Temporelli PL, et al. Doppler-derived mitral deceleration time of early filling as a strong predictor of pulmonary capillary wedge pressure in postinfarction patients with left ventricular systolic dysfunction. J Am Coll Cardiol 1994;23:1630–7.

[10] Temporelli PL, Scapellato F, Corra U, et al. Chronic mitral regurgitation and Doppler estimation of left ventricular filling pressures in patients with heart failure. J Am Soc Echocardiogr 2001;14:1094–9.

[11] Schober K, Luis Fuentes V. Effect of age, body weight, and heart rate on transmitral and pulmonary venous flow in clinically normal dogs. Am J Vet Res 2001;62:1447–54.

[12] Bonagura JD, Schober KE. Can ventricular function be assessed by echocardiography in chronic canine mitral valve disease? J Small Anim Pract 2009;50:12–24.
[13] Oyama MA, Sisson DD, Bulmer BJ, Constable PD. Echocardiographic estimation of mean left atrial pressure in a canine model of acute mitral valve insufficiency. J Vet Intern Med 2004;18:667–72.
[14] Lisauskas J, Singh J, Courtois M, Kovacs SJ. The relation of the peak Doppler E-wave to peak mitral annulus velocity ratio to diastolic function. Ultrasound Med Biol 2001;27:499–507.
[15] Nagueh SF, Lakkis NM, Middleton KJ, et al. Doppler estimation of left ventricular filling pressures in patients with hypertrophic cardiomyopathy. Circulation 1999;99:254–61.
[16] Ommen SR, Nishimura RA, Appleton CP, et al. Clinical utility of Doppler echocardiography and tissue Doppler imaging in the estimation of left ventricular filling pressures: a comparative simultaneous Doppler-catheterization study. Circulation 2000;102:1788–94.
[17] Nagueh SF, Mikati I, Kopelen HA, et al. Doppler estimation of left ventricular filling pressure in sinus tachycardia: a new application of tissue Doppler imaging. Circulation 1998;98:1644–50.
[18] Jacques DC, Pinsky MR, Severyn D, Gorcsan J. Influence of alterations in loading on mitral annular velocity by tissue Doppler echocardiography and its associated ability to predict filling pressures. Chest 2004;126:1910–8.
[19] Nagueh SF, Sun H, Kopelen HA, et al. Hemodynamic determinants of the mitral annulus diastolic velocities by tissue Doppler. Circulation 1999;99:254–61.
[20] Firstenberg MS, Greenberg NL, Main ML, et al. Determinants of diastolic myocardial tissue Doppler velocities: influences of relaxation and preload. J Am Soc Echocardiogr 2005;18:1277–84.
[21] Ruan Q, Rao L, Middleton KJ, et al. Assessment of left ventricular diastolic function by early diastolic mitral annulus peak acceleration rate: experimental studies and clinical application. J Am Coll Cardiol 2001;37:278–85.
[22] Zile MR, Tomita M, Nakano K, et al. Effects of left ventricular volume overload produced by mitral regurgitation on diastolic function. Am J Physiol 1991;261:1471–80.
[23] Katayama K, Tajimi T, Guth BD, et al. Early diastolic filling dynamics during experimental mitral regurgitation in the conscious dog. Circulation 1988;78:390–400.
[24] Teshima K, Asano K, Sasaki Y, et al. Assessment of left ventricular function using pulsed tissue Doppler imaging in healthy dogs and dogs with spontaneous mitral regurgitation. Japan J Vet Science 2005;67:1207–15.
[25] Schober KE, Bonagura JD, Samii V, Zekas L. Unpublished observations. 2009.
[26] Liang HY, Cauduro S, Pellikka P, et al. Comparison of usefulness of newer echo-Doppler variables to left ventricular end diastolic pressure in predicting heart failure. J Am Coll Cardiol 2006;47:100A–1A.
[27] Schober KE, Stern JA, DaCunha DNQT, et al. Estimation of left ventricular filling pressure by Doppler echocardiography in dogs with pacing-induced heart failure. J Vet Intern Med 2008;22:578–85.
[28] Hasegawa H, Little WC, Ohno M, et al. Diastolic mitral annular velocity during the development of heart failure. J Am Coll Cardiol 2003;41:1590–7.
[29] Nagueh SF, Lakkis NM, Middleton KJ, et al. Doppler estimation of left ventricular filling pressures in patients with hypertrophic cardiomyopathy. Circulation 1998;98:1644–50.
[30] Schober KE, Maerz I. Assessment of left atrial appendage flow velocity and its relation to spontaneous echocardiographic contrast in 89 cats with myocardial disease. J Vet Intern Med 2006;20:120–30.
[31] Garcia MJ, Smedira NG, Greenberg NL, et al. Color M-mode Doppler flow propagation velocity is a preload insensitive index of left ventricular relaxation: animal and human validation. Ultrasound Med Biol 2001;27:499–507.
[32] Hsiao SH, Huang WC, Sy LC, et al. Doppler tissue imaging and color M-mode flow propagation velocity: are they really preload independent? J Am Soc Echocardiogr 2005;18:1277–84.
[33] Schwammenthal E, Popescu BA, Popescu AC, et al. Association of left ventricular filling parameters assessed by pulsed wave Doppler and color M-mode Doppler echocardiography with left ventricular pathology, pulmonary congestion, and left ventricular end diastolic pressure. Am J Cardiol 2004;94:488–99.
[34] Kidawa M, Coignard L, Drobinski G, et al. Comparative value of tissue Doppler imaging and M-mode color Doppler mitral flow propagation velocity for the evaluation of left ventricular filling pressure. Chest 2005;128:2544–50.
[35] Diwan A, McCulloch M, Lawrie GM, et al. Doppler estimation of left ventricular filling pressures in patients with mitral valve disease. Am J Cardiol 1999;83:724–7.
[36] De Madron E. Unpublished observations. 2009.
[37] Gouni V, Serres FJ, Pouchelon JL, et al. Quantification of mitral valve regurgitation in dogs with degenerative mitral valve disease by use of the proximal isovelocity surface area method. J Am Vet Med Assoc 2007;231:399–406.
[38] Bright JM, Golden AL, Daniel GB. Feline hypertrophic cardiomyopathy: variations on a theme. J Small Anim Pract 1992;33:266–74.

10

Evaluation of the Right Ventricular Global Systolic Function

ÉRIC DE MADRON

Evaluation of the Radial Systolic Function of the Right Ventricle: Shortening Fraction of the Right Ventricle, 152

Evaluation of the Longitudinal Systolic Function, 152

Indices Derived from Right Ventricular Tissue Doppler, 154

Conclusion, 155

The evaluation of the systolic function of the right ventricle (RV) is gaining attention due to its prognostic implications [1]. In humans, the techniques used to measure this function are primarily based on the measurement of the tricuspid annulus motion (or tricuspid annular plane systolic excursion; TAPSE), tissue Doppler of the ventricular wall and tricuspid annulus, and the right ventricular index of myocardial performance (RVIMP). In rare occasions, various RV shortening fractions and the RV ejection fractions, calculated using the Simpson method, have been used. In veterinary echocardiography, the methods evaluated to date include tissue Doppler, speckle tracking of the RV wall, RVIMP, and RV TAPSE.

Evaluation of the Radial Systolic Function of the Right Ventricle: Shortening Fraction of the Right Ventricle

Several RV shortening fractions have been evaluated [2]:

- The basal RV shortening fraction, obtained in the same way as the left ventricular (LV) shortening fraction, using the same time-motion (TM) view (right parasternal short axis transventricular)
- The right ventricular outflow tract shortening fraction, obtained using the right parasternal short axis transaortic TM view
- The right ventricular area shortening fraction, obtained by comparing the RV diastolic and systolic areas measured by planimetry using an apical 4-chambers view

Unfortunately, these methods are unreliable due to excessive inter- and intraobserver variability [2].

Evaluation of the Longitudinal Systolic Function

Triscupid Annulus Motion

The TAPSE is measured in a similar fashion to the mitral annulus movement (MAM), from a TM echocardiogram of the lateral rim of the tricuspid annulus obtained using an apical 4 chambers view (see Chapter 7).

Inter- and intraobserver variability of this measure are good in humans [2]. In humans, a TAPSE value below 1.5 cm predicts an RV ejection fraction below 50% with a 94% specificity, a positive predictive value of 71%, and a negative predictive value of 89% [3].

Reduced TAPSE has been noticed in patients with pulmonary hypertension following chronic obstructive pneumopathy [4].

The normal TAPSE values have been established in dogs. There is a curvilinear relationship between TAPSE and weight. The equation of correlation between TAPSE and weight (W in kg) is:

$$\text{TAPSE (cm)} = 0.17 + 0.52\,W^{1/3}$$

According to this equation, normal TAPSE values in dogs can be summarized as follows: 0 to 10 kg: 1 to 1.5 cm; 10 to 20 kg: 1.5 cm; 20 to 40 kg: 1.5 to 2 cm.

Inter- and intraobserver agreement was adequate, with a coefficient of variation <10%. Dogs with severe pulmonary hypertension (maximal velocity of the tricuspid regurgitation between 4.7 and 6.9 m/s; see Chapter 14) had TAPSE values below the reference range [5].

Tissue Doppler of the Tricuspid Annulus

The measurement of the maximal velocity of the S′ wave of the tricuspid annulus has good inter- and intraobserver coefficients of variability in humans [2]. In humans, an S′ value <10 cm predicts an RV ejection fraction <50% with a 92% specificity, a positive predictive value of 67%, and a negative predictive value of 89% [3].

One study evaluated the prognostic value of tricuspid annulus tissue Doppler parameters in patients with an LV ejection fraction <40% and congestive heart failure [1]. The authors were able to demonstrate that S′ values <10.8 cm/s, E′ early diastolic velocity values <8.9 cm/s, and a tricuspid annular acceleration during isovolumic contraction <2.52 m/s were associated with a poorer prognosis. The coexistence of S′ values <10.8 cm/s and E′ values <8.9 cm/s further worsened the prognosis [1].

Decreased maximal S′ and E′ velocities have also been documented in human patients with pulmonary thromboembolism, especially in those with higher RV systolic pressure [6].

Lower tricuspid annular S′ velocities have been documented in patients with tetralogy of Fallot several years following surgical correction, indicating persistent RV systolic dysfunction [7].

These parameters have not yet been evaluated in cats and dogs.

TABLE 10-1 Longitudinal Velocities (Mean ± Standard Deviation) Measured at the Base and Apex of the Right and Left Ventricles Using Bidimensional (2D) Color Tissue Doppler in 64 Healthy Control Dogs [8]

	Right Ventricular Free Wall		Left Ventricular Free Wall	
	Basal Segment	Apical Segment	Basal Segment	Apical Segment
Systolic S′ wave (cm/s)	12.5 ± 3.2[a,b,c,*] (7.7-18.5)	4.7 ± 1.9* (0.7-10.4*)	7.7 ± 2.5[a,b,c,*] (3.7-17.2)	2.0 ± 1.6 (0.2-6.7)
Diastolic E′ wave (cm/s)	10.3 ± 2.6[a,c,†] (5.8-17.1)	4.1 ± 1.7* (0.4-7.9)	9.1 ± 2.5[a,c] (3.2-14.7)	2.4 ± 1.5 (0.2-6.2)
Diastolic A′ wave (cm/s)	6.7 ± 1.8[a,b,*] (3.0-11.3)	1.7 ± 0.9* (0.2-3.9)	5.5 ± 1.7[a,b] (2.1-9.9)	0.6 ± 0.5 (0.1-2.5)
Diastolic E′/A′ ratio	1.6 ± 0.6 (1.0-3.4)	3.2 ± 2.6 (1.1-11.7)	1.8 ± 1.6 (0.9-4.0)	5.6 ± 5.8 (0.5-34.0)
Heart rate during examination (bpm)	93 ± 21 (48-141)		95 ± 23 (52-147)	

Note: The minimum and maximum values are shown in parentheses.
[a]The value differs significantly ($p < 0.001$) from the apical segment value from the same wall.
[b]The value differs significantly ($p < 0.001$) from the E′ wave velocity in the same segment.
[c]The value differs significantly ($p < 0.001$) from the A′ wave velocity in the same segment.
*$p < 0.001$
†$p < 0.01$. The comparisons are between the right and left myocardial velocities during the same cardiac cycle and in the same segment (basal or apical).

Right Ventricular Free Wall Velocities

Myocardial RV free wall velocities have been evaluated in dogs [8]. Normal systolic and diastolic velocities of the RV basal and apical segments have been established in a group of 6 Beagles and 64 dogs of different breeds. Inter- and intraday variability was good (3.5% to 16.1%) for the basal segment tissue Doppler variables but much higher (>15%) for those of the apical segment. The basal segment values were higher than those of the apical segment and also higher than those of the left ventricular free wall basal segment (Table 10-1). The weight and the breed had little effect on most of the variables [8].

A reduction of the systolic and diastolic tissue velocities of the base of the RV wall has been documented in dogs with pulmonary hypertension (see Chapter 14).

A reduction of the RV wall systolic velocity as well as a disappearance of the base-apex gradient was described in humans with arrhythmogenic right ventricular cardiomyopathy [9].

Systolic Time Intervals and Index of Myocardial Performance (Tei Index)

Right ventricular systolic time intervals can be obtained from the spectral Doppler signal of the pulmonic blood flow. The RVIMP, or right Tei index, is calculated from the recording of the transtricuspid and pulmonic flow spectral Doppler signals (Figure 10-1) using the same method as for the calculation of the left ventricular index of myocardial performance (LVIMP) (see Chapter 7).

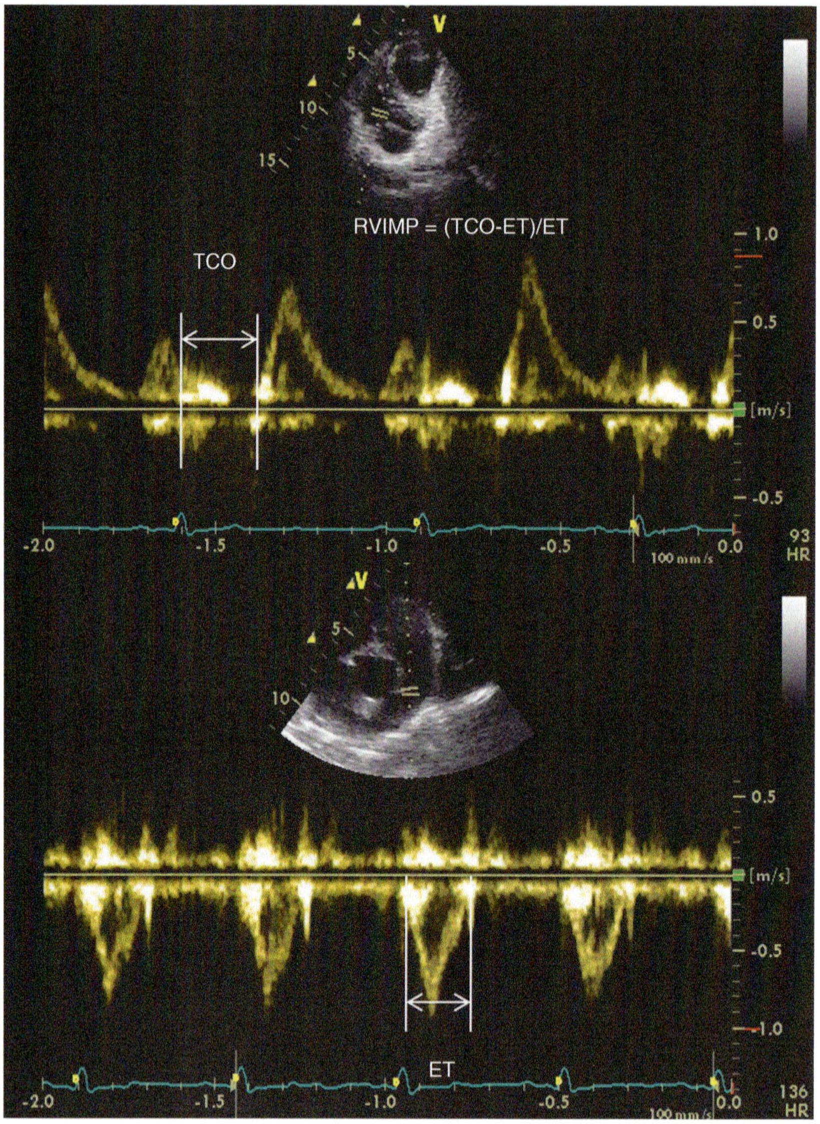

• **Fig. 10-1** Calculation of the right ventricular index of myocardial performance (RVIMP) from the spectral Doppler signals of the tricuspid and pulmonic flows. *ET,* Right ventricle ejection time; *TCO,* interval between the closing and the opening of the tricuspid valve. (Photo credit: Éric de Madron.)

In humans, the RVIMP has been shown to be useful to detect right and left systolic ventricular dysfunction. It increases with pulmonary hypertension, whether primary [10] or secondary to chronic obstructive pneumopathy [4] or to pulmonary thromboembolism [6]. In patients in congestive heart failure with a left ventricular ejection fraction <40%, a RVIMP ≥1.2 likely indicates a poor prognosis [1]. However, this index is not very specific. In humans, an RVIMP value <0.4 indicates an RV ejection fraction <50% with a 35% specificity, a positive predictive value of 29%, and a negative predictive value of 100% [3].

The normal RVIMP values and the RV systolic time intervals have both been established in dogs [11]. They are listed in Table 10-2. The authors have shown that the RVIMP was not affected by heart rate or weight. The RVIMP values were lower than the LVIMP values. RV ejection time was longer than that of the LV [11].

In another study conducted in Boxers with arrhythmogenic right ventricular cardiomyopathy, neither the IMP nor the systolic interval time intervals were able to differentiate between affected and normal boxers [12].

Indices Derived from Right Ventricular Tissue Doppler

These indices, based on strain and strain rate measurements of the right ventricle, are discussed in detail in Chapter 4. The normal RV values in dogs have been established [13] and are presented in Table 10-3.

TABLE 10-2 Systolic Time and Right Ventricular Index of Myocardial Performance [11]

Weight (kg)	3-15 (n = 15) (average ± standard deviation)	15.1-35 (n = 15) (average ± standard deviation)	35.1-55 (n = 15) (average ± standard deviation)
RVIMP	0.224 ± 0.099	0.261 ± 0.105	0.264 ± 0.077
RV PEP (ms)	46.8 ± 7.23	57.4 ± 5.15	59.8 ± 9.59
RV ET (ms)	185 ± 16	183 ± 16	194 ± 18
RV PEP/ET	0.253 ± 0.037	0.318 ± 0.050	0.309 ± 0.052

ET, Ejection time; *PEP,* pre-ejection period; *RV,* right ventricle; *RVIMP,* right ventricular index of myocardial performance.

TABLE 10-3 Longitudinal Systolic Strain Indices Calculated Using Strain Imaging and Strain Rate Imaging of the Right Ventricular Base and Apex in 30 Healthy Dogs of Various Breeds

			Correlations		
	Values	Min-Max	Age	Heart Rate (bpm)	Shortening Fraction (%)
Basal peak systolic strain (%)	–39.5 ± 5.5†‡	–50.2 - –29.5	NS	NS	NS
Basal peak systolic strain duration (ms)	223 ± 56	126-346	NS	NS	NS
Basal peak systolic strain rate (s^{-1})	–5.2 ± 0.8†‡	–7.1 - –4.0	NS	NS	NS
Apical peak systolic strain (%)	–36.3 ± 4.3*†‡	–45.7 - –28.4	NS	NS	–0.44 (p = 0.020)
Apical peak systolic strain duration (ms)	198 ± 46	67-228	NS	NS	NS
Apical peak systolic strain rate (s^{-1})	–4.7 ± 1.1*†‡	–7.1 - –2.7	NS	NS	NS

NS, Not statistically significant.
Note: These indices include the peak systolic strain (%), the peak systolic strain duration (ms), and the peak systolic strain rate (s^{-1}) expressed in mean ± standard deviation and minimum and maximum values (Min-max). The Pearson correlation coefficient is recommended when the correlation between age, heart rate, and shortening fraction is statistically significant. Unpublished data, established with a GE Vivid 5.
*p <0.01 versus corresponding value in the base.
†p <0.001 versus corresponding value in the left ventricle free wall.
‡p <0.001 versus corresponding value in the interventricular septum.

Conclusion

These new methods enable the evaluation of the right ventricular function. Some parameters, such as the various RV shortening fractions and tissue Doppler of the apical segment of the RV wall, are subject to too much variability to be useful. TAPSE and tricuspid annular velocities seem to be the most promising parameters in humans but are only starting to be evaluated in dogs. Some information is available on tissue Doppler of the RV basal wall in the dog as well as on strain and strain rate imaging. The right ventricular Tei index, or RVIMP, is easy to obtain but lacks sensitivity.

REFERENCES

[1] Meluzin J, Spiranova L, Hude P, et al. Prognostic importance of various echocardiographic right ventricular functional parameters in patients with symptomatic heart failure. J Am Soc Echocardiogr 2005;18:435–44.

[2] Pinedo M, Villacorta E, Tapia C, et al. Inter- and intra-observer variability in the echocardiographic evaluation of right ventricular function. Rev Esp Cardiol 2010;63:802–9.

[3] Miller D, Farah MG, Liner A, et al. The relation between quantitative right ventricular ejection fraction and indices of tricuspid annular motion and myocardial performance. J Am Soc Echocardiogr 2004;17:443–7.

[4] Yilmaz R, Gencer M, Ceylan E, Demirbag R. Impact of chronic obstructive pulmonary disease with pulmonary hypertension on both left ventricular systolic and diastolic performance. J Am Soc Echocardiogr 2005;18:873–81.

[5] Pariaut R, Saelinger C, Strickland KN, Beaufrère H, Reynolds CA, Vila J. Tricuspid annular plane systolic excursion (TAPSE) in dogs: reference values and impact of pulmonary hypertension. J Vet Intern Med 2012;26:1148–54.

[6] Rydman R, Larsen F, Caidhal K, Alam M. Right ventricular function in patients with pulmonary embolism: early and late findings using Doppler tissue imaging. J Am Soc Echocardiogr 2010;23:531–7.
[7] Harada K, Toyono M, Yamamoto F. Assessment of right ventricular function during exercise with quantitative Doppler tissue imaging in children late after repair of tetralogy of Fallot. J Am Soc Echocardiogr 2004;17:863–9.
[8] Chetboul V, Carlos Sampedrano C, Gouni V, et al. Quantitative assessment of regional right ventricular myocardial velocities in awake dogs by Doppler tissue imaging: repeatability, reproducibility, effect of body weight and breed, and comparison with left ventricular myocardial velocities. J Vet Intern Med 2005;19:837–44.
[9] Parthenakis FI, Patrianakos AP, Pagonidis K, et al. Arryhthmogenic right ventricular cardiomyopathy: echocardiographic and magnetic resonance imaging in a patient presenting with ventricular tachycardia. J Am Soc Echocardiogr 2007;20. 1319.
[10] Yeo TC, Dujardin KS, Tei C, et al. Value of a Doppler-derived index combining systolic and diastolic time intervals in predicting outcome in primary pulmonary hypertension. Am J Cardiol 1998;81:1157–61.
[11] Baumwart RD, Meurs KM, Bongaura JD. Tei index of myocardial performance applied to the right ventricle in normal dogs. J Vet Intern Med 2005;19:828–32.
[12] Baumwart RD, Meurs KM. An index of myocardial performance applied to the right ventricle of Boxers with arrhythmogenic right ventricular cardiomyopathy. Am J Vet Res 2008;69:1029–33.
[13] Chetboul V, Carlos Sampedrano C, Gouni V, et al. Ultrasonographic assessment of regional radial and longitudinal systolic function in healthy awake dogs. J Vet Intern Med 2006;20:885–93.

PART IV

Echocardiography of Acquired Cardiopathies

11 Assessment and Quantification of Acquired Valvular Regurgitation in Dogs, 159

12 Dilated Cardiomyopathy and Other Cardiomyopathies in Dogs, 181

13 Evaluation of Feline Cardiomyopathies, 207

14 Pulmonary Arterial Hypertension, 229

15 Dirofilariasis: Specific Bidimensional Aspects, 241

16 Cardiac Manifestations of Systemic Diseases, 245

17 Pericardial Diseases, 259

18 Cardiac Tumors, 271

11

Assessment and Quantification of Acquired Valvular Regurgitation in Dogs

ÉRIC DE MADRON

Mitral Regurgitation, 160
Tricuspid Regurgitation, 175
Aortic Regurgitation, 176
Pulmonic Regurgitation, 177

Mitral Regurgitation

Mitral regurgitation (MR) is a systolic leakage of the mitral valve, with blood flowing back from the left ventricle into the left atrium due to poor coaptation of the mitral leaflets. Only MR resulting from a primary valvular pathology is discussed in this chapter. MR secondary to either mitral annulus dilation or dynamic aspiration of the valve against the septum is discussed in its respective contexts (see Chapters 12 and 13). Mitral valve dysplasia is discussed in Chapter 19.

The main cause of MR in dogs is degenerative mitral valve disease (DMVD), formerly known as mitral endocardiosis or myxomatous degeneration. It is the most frequently encountered acquired cardiopathy in dogs [1] and affects mostly smaller animals (less than 20 kg). Cavalier King Charles Spaniels (CKCSs) are particularly predisposed to DMVD [1,2]. The prevalence of this cardiopathy ranges from 14% (breeds other than CKCS) to 40% (CKCS) [3]. Prevalence increases with age [3-5] and can affect almost 100% of CKCSs over 11 years of age [3]. Larger breed dogs such as German Shepherds can be affected by DMVD, although less frequently [6]. The characteristics of DMVD in large breeds differ in some aspects from those in small dogs (see "DMVD in large breed dogs" below).

2D and TM Echocardiographic Features of DMVD

Mitral Valve and Chordae Tendineae Anomalies

DMVD is characterized by the appearance of nodules on the free edges of the valvular leaflets, along with a thickening of the chordae tendineae. As the nodules grow, they can fuse and lead to generalized thickening of the mitral valve [7,8]. Moreover, elongation of the leaflets and stretching of the chordae tendineae are usually observed, leading to valvular leaflet prolapse in the left atrium (LA) [9]. The chordae tendineae can rupture, depriving the valve of its support and further aggravating the leakage [10]. The consequence of these abnormalities is a more or less severe MR, depending on the deformation, the degree of valvular leaflet retraction, and the condition of the chordae tendineae. Although this process affects mostly the mitral valve, the tricuspid valve and more rarely the aortic and pulmonic valves can be affected.

2D Mode

Mitral Valve Remodeling. In bidimensional (2D) mode, the mitral valve leaflets appear remodeled and thickened, with an irregular nodular aspect [11,12] (Figure 11-1).

Mitral Valve Prolapse. The presence of mitral valve prolapse (MVP) is frequently observed (97% in a cohort of CKCSs over 3 years old) [9]. It is characterized by the doming of one or two leaflets beyond the mitral valve annular plane in systole (Figure 11-2; Video 11-1). When the chordae tendineae rupture, all or part of the affected leaflet usually prolapses into the LA in systole [10]. MVP in dogs involves the anterior mitral leaflet in 48.4%, the posterior leaflet in 7.1%, and both leaflets in 44.5%. This is in contrast to humans, in whom the posterior leaflet is most frequently affected. The difference is due to the fact that, in dogs, the anterior leaflet is twice as large as the posterior leaflet [3]. The severity of the prolapse is correlated with the MR stage and the International Small Animal Cardiac Health Council (ISACHC) clinical class [13].

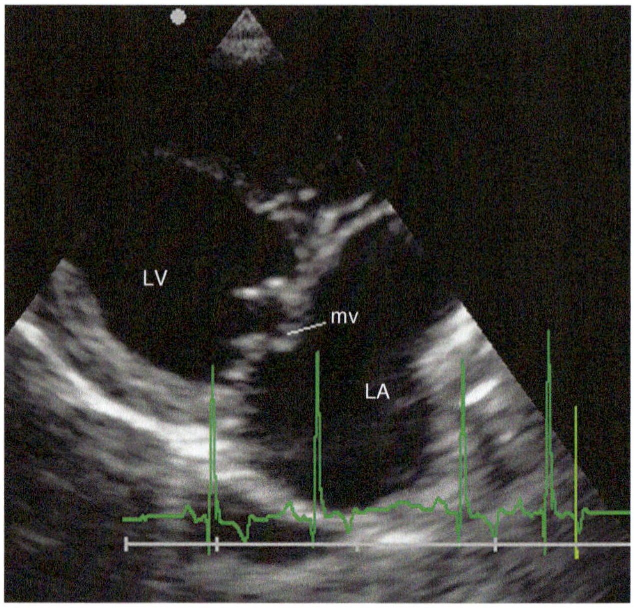

• **Fig. 11-1** Bidimensional (2D) echocardiogram (right parasternal long axis 4 chambers view) showing significant mitral valve (mv) remodeling in a dog with degenerative mitral valve disease (DMVD). The left atrium (LA) is very dilated. The left ventricle (LV) is also dilated and beginning to become spherical. (Photo credit: Éric de Madron.)

The Various Degrees of Mitral Valve Prolapse

Two reference lines are used to evaluate the degree of mitral valve prolapse (see Figure 11-2):

- Line 1, linking the ventricular aspect of the anterior and posterior mitral leaflets insertion points on the mitral annulus.
- Line 2, linking the atrial aspect of the same points.

Mild mitral valve prolapse occurs when one or both mitral leaflets bulge in systole to line 1. Moderate prolapse occurs when part of one or both leaflets bulge beyond line 1 but do not reach line 2 (see Figure 11-2). Severe prolapse occurs when the prolapsed part of the leaflets bulges beyond line 2 [13].

Chordae Tendineae Rupture. The mitral valve chordae tendineae determine the end-systolic position and tension of the mitral leaflets, and contribute to the mitral

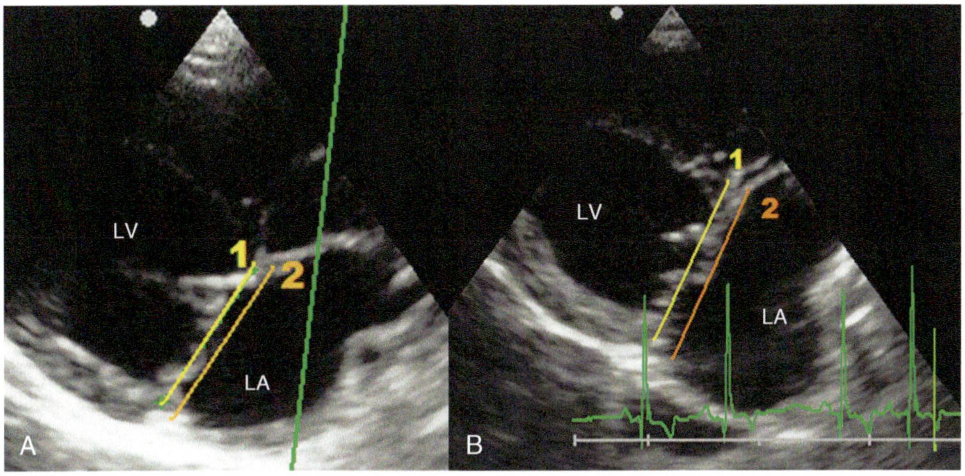

• **Fig. 11-2** Bidimensional (2D) echocardiograms (right parasternal long axis 4 chambers views) showing (A) a moderate posterior leaflet prolapse and (B) a moderate anterior leaflet prolapse of the mitral valve in two dogs with degenerative mitral valve disease (DMVD). *LA,* Left atrium; *LV,* left ventricle. (Photo credit: Éric de Madron.)

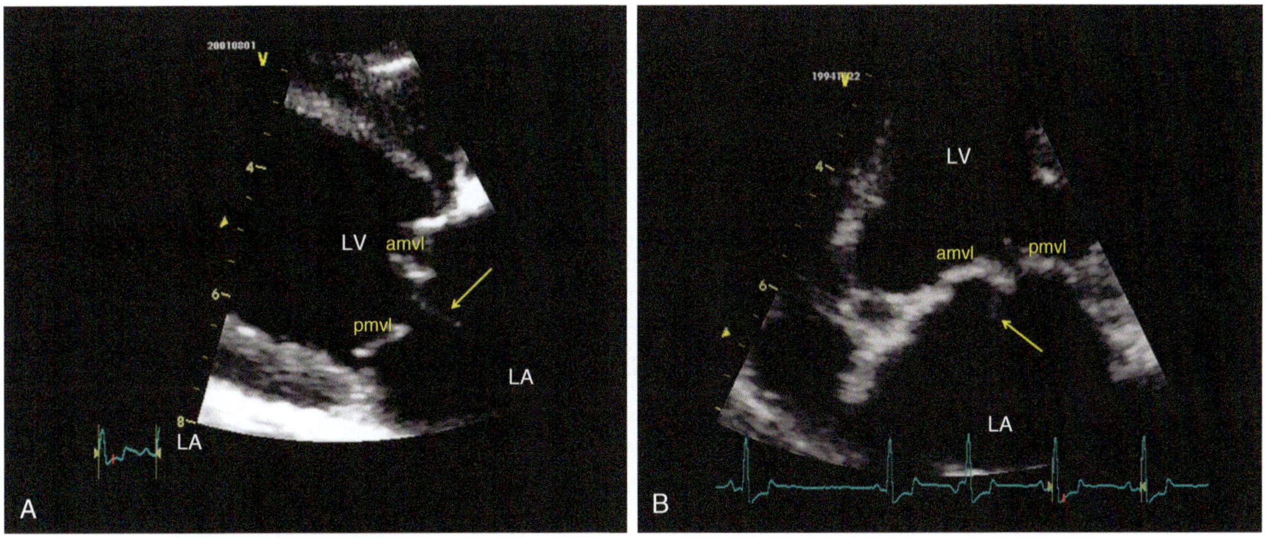

• **Fig. 11-3** Bidimensional (2D) echocardiograms obtained in dogs with degenerative mitral disease with chordae tendineae rupture (CTR). A, Both indirect signs of CTR are visible (right parasternal long axis 4 chambers view): absence of coaptation of the two leaflets in systole and prolapse of the leaflet affected by CTR (here the anterior mitral valve leaflet [amvl]) in the left atrium (LA). A portion of the ruptured chordae tendineae *(arrow)* still attached to the amvl is seen floating in the LA. B, The ruptured chordae tendineae still attached to the amvl and floating in systole in the LA is clearly visible *(arrow)* on the left apical 5 chambers view. Note the abnormal amvl curvature, bulging into the LA. *LV,* Left ventricle; *pmvl,* posterior mitral valve leaflet. (Photo credit: Valérie Chetboul.)

valve systolic closure [14]. DMVD can lead to chordae tendineae rupture, which aggravates the preexisting MR. This aggravation can be either minimal or severe, depending on the type of chordae tendineae affected (primary or secondary). Primary chordae tendineae rupture (CTR) can lead to a total loss of tension of one of the mitral valve leaflets, which then becomes flail. This often leads to abrupt aggravation of the MR, with fainting and/or acute congestive heart failure (CHF). Secondary or tertiary CTR can sometimes be detected fortuitously in still asymptomatic patients. The ruptured chordae tendineae may be seen using 2D echocardiography (Figure 11-3; Videos 11-2 and 11-3) [10,15]. In a study conducted on 706 dogs with DMVD, primary CTR was detected in 16% of the cases, with a prevalence that increased with the severity of the MR [10]. In the overwhelming majority of the cases (96.5%), the ruptured chordae tendineae were attached to the anterior leaflet of the mitral valve (see Figure 11-3). Only 3.5% of the cases suffered from posterior leaflet CTR. The MR was generally severe and symptomatic in the majority of the affected animals (75%) [10].

TM Mode

In time-motion (TM) mode, the thickening of the anterior mitral valve leaflet is also apparent. The increased transmitral flow due to the leakage increases the opening motion of the anterior mitral valve leaflet, which hits the interventricular septum in early diastole (reduced E-septum separation) (Figure 11-4) [11,12].

Left Chambers Dilation

Left Atrium

The degree of left atrial dilation depends on the severity of the leakage [16-18]. As mentioned in Chapter 2, the right parasternal long axis 5 chambers view underestimates the left atrial dimension. The right parasternal long axis 4 chambers and short axis at the heart base level views are better to fully appreciate this dilation (Figures 11-5 and 11-6). The left apical 4 chambers view allows a good appreciation of the pulmonary vein dilation as it connects to the LA (Figure 11-7; Video 11-4).

Mitral regurgitation due to CTR is a special situation. In this situation, MR could appear so suddenly that the LA has not yet had time to dilate at the time of the evaluation.

Left Ventricle

2D Mode

Dilation. The left ventricle (LV) dilates once MR becomes significant. The dilation is at first diastolic, then systolic. The increased LV internal dimensions lead to stretching of the mitral annulus and papillary muscle malalignment, which further aggravates MR [14].

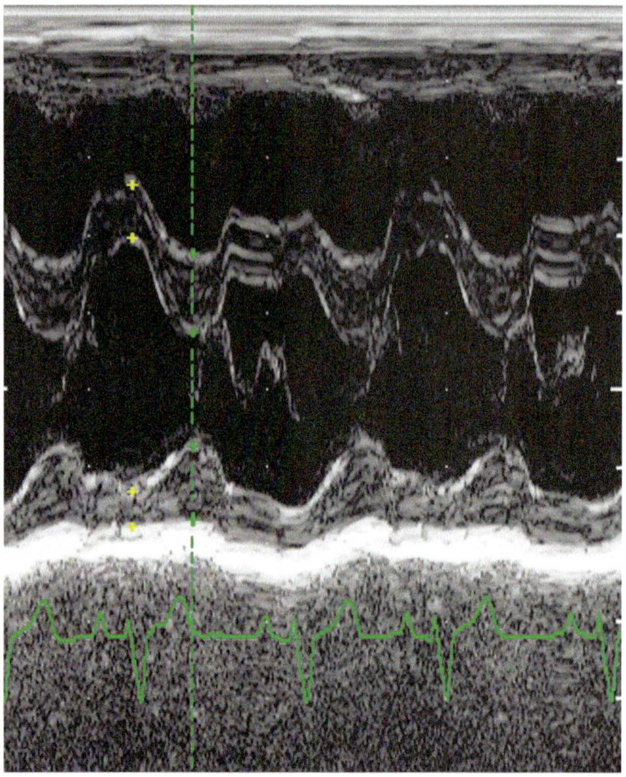

• **Fig. 11-4** Transmitral time-motion (TM) echocardiogram showing the mitral valve making contact with the interventricular septum in early diastole in a dog with degenerative mitral valve disease (DMVD). (Photo credit: Éric de Madron.)

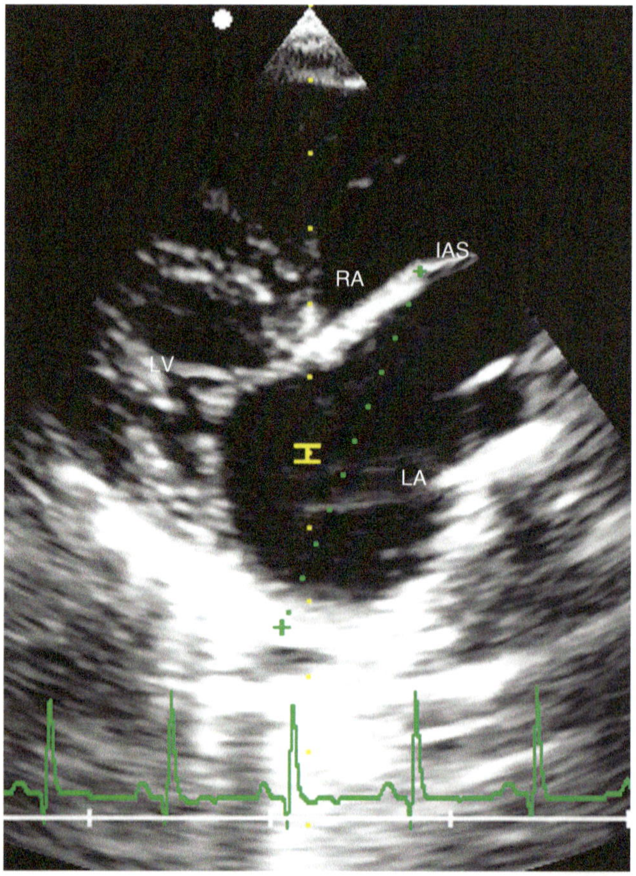

• **Fig. 11-5** Bidimensional (2D) echocardiogram (right parasternal long axis 4 chambers view) in a dog with degenerative mitral valve disease (DMVD), showing marked left atrial dilation. The interatrial septum (IAS) bulges toward the right atrium (RA). *LA,* Left atrium; *LV,* left ventricle. (Photo credit: Éric de Madron.)

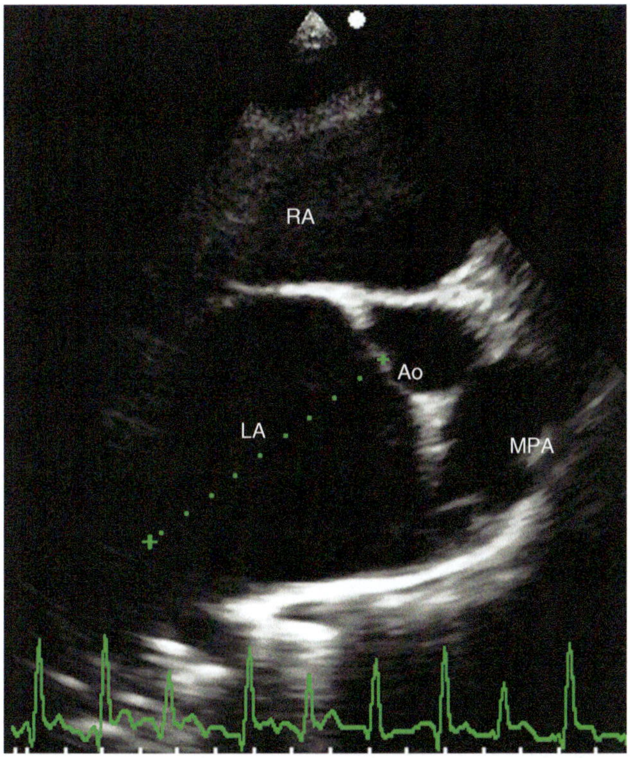

• **Fig. 11-6** Bidimensional (2D) echocardiogram (right parasternal short axis transaortic view) in a dog with degenerative mitral valve disease (DMVD), showing marked left atrial dilation. *Ao,* Aorta; *LA,* left atrium; *MPA,* main pulmonary artery; *RA,* right atrium. (Photo credit: Éric de Madron.)

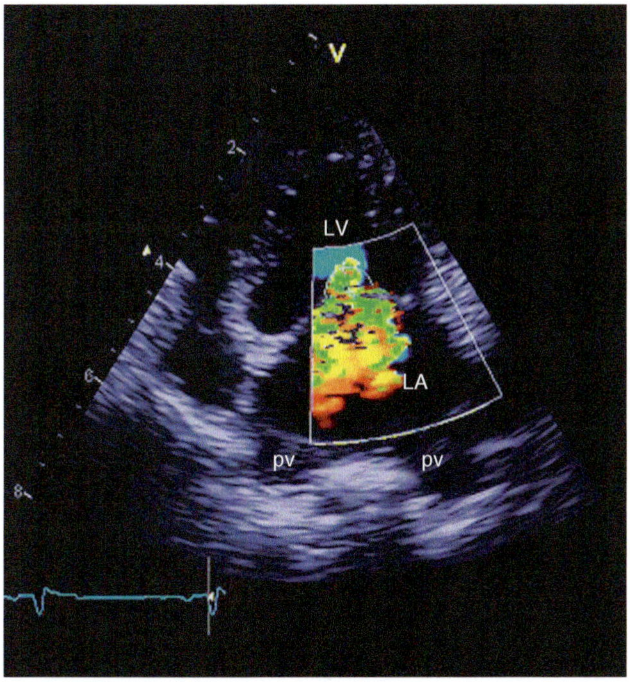

• **Fig. 11-7** Bidimensional (2D) echocardiogram (left apical 4 chambers view) in color Doppler mode in a dog with degenerative mitral valve disease (DMVD), showing marked left atrial and pulmonary vein (pv) dilation. *LA,* Left atrium; *LV,* left ventricle. (Photo credit: Éric de Madron.)

Geometric Changes. The LV becomes increasingly spherical (see Figure 11-1) as documented by the decreased sphericity index (SI = end-diastolic LV base-apex length/ internal end-diastolic LV diameter) (see Table 11-1) [19].

TM Mode

Inappropriate Eccentric Hypertrophy. The LV dilation is associated with "inappropriate" eccentric hypertrophy, as documented by the decrease in the h/r ratio, where *h* is the LV wall thickness during diastole and *r* is the LV radius in diastole [19].

Hyperdynamic Left Ventricle. The LV shortening fraction (SF) increases with MR (Figure 11-8) [16,19,20], due to increased systolic LV emptying among other causes. In fact, in the presence of MR, a large part of the ventricular stroke volume goes into the LA, a low-pressure chamber, before the intraventricular pressure raises enough to open the aortic valve and allow blood ejection into the aorta. The partial drainage of the LV during the pressure increase, along with the activation of the sympathetic system, leads to LV hyperkinesia, which is clearly visible in TM mode [11,12]. In opposition to what has been observed in normal dogs, the systolic excursion of the interventricular septum may be greater than that of the free wall (see Figure 11-8). This may result from the rightward deviation of the septum, associated or not with regional free wall dysfunction (see below) [21,22]. This hyperkinesia helps to differentiate a purely valvular (lesional) MR from a functional MR resulting from annular dilation secondary to dilated cardiomyopathy. In the latter situation, the SF of the LV is greatly decreased.

However, with severe chronic MR, the SF can decrease after this initial increase and return to a normal or subnormal value. Therefore a normal SF in a case of severe MR probably indicates the presence of systolic dysfunction [21,22]. In this situation, a hypokinetic LV free wall and hyperkinetic septum are often observed. With end-stage MR, the SF drops below normal (Figure 11-9).

End-Systolic Volume. The afterload reduction associated with primary MR makes the accurate evaluation of the left ventricular systolic function difficult. Early-onset systolic dysfunction has been shown in dogs with experimental MR induced by sectioning the chordae tendineae but this experimental model does not in any way reflect the chronic evolution of spontaneous DMVD [23,24]. The degree of systolic LV dilation seems to better reflect the actual contractility status of the LV (see Chapter 7). This is why the end-systolic volume index (ESVI) is considered to be a better systolic function parameter than SF in the case of MR, because it is less affected by afterload [25]. An ESVI can be obtained using several different methods [19,20], as discussed in Chapter 7. Planimetric methods (Simpson method and area-length formula) seem to be better suited for ventricular volume calculations in dogs [20]. The Teichholz method leads to an overestimation of ventricular volume by a factor of 2 compared to tridimensional (3D)

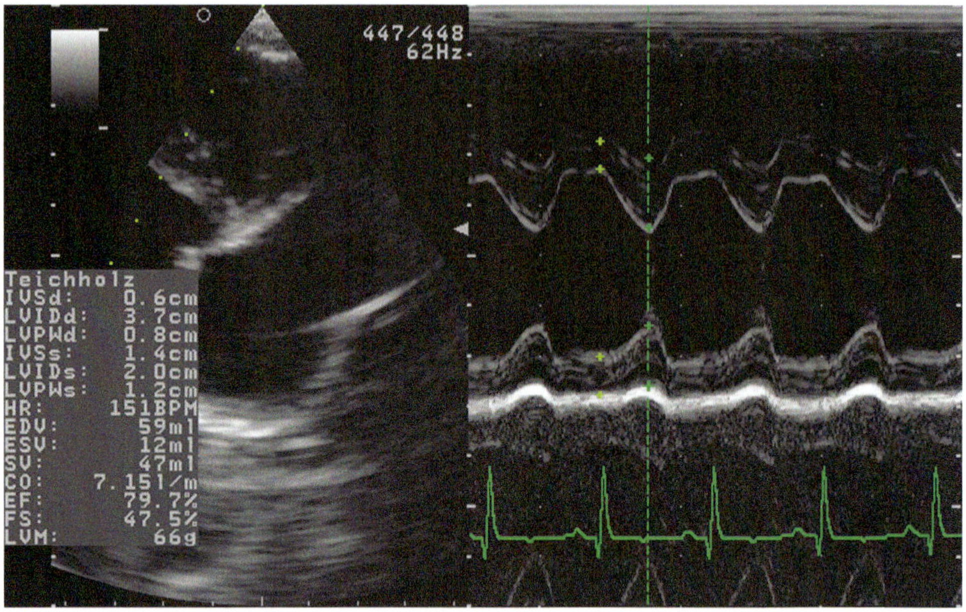

• **Fig. 11-8** Time-motion (TM) echocardiogram in a dog with degenerative mitral valve disease (DMVD) showing left ventricular hyperkinesis. The septal excursion is greater than that of the free wall of the left ventricle. (Photo credit: Éric de Madron.)

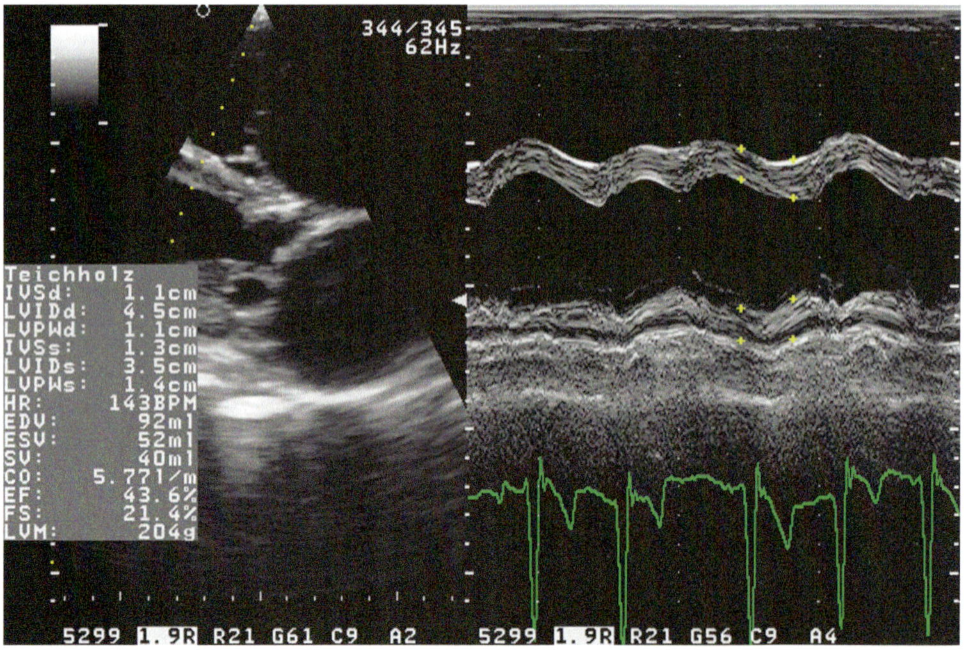

• **Fig. 11-9** Time-motion (TM) echocardiogram in a dog with chronic degenerative mitral valve disease (DMVD) showing a decreased shortening fraction (SF) of the left ventricle. (Photo credit: Éric de Madron.)

echocardiography and is therefore no longer recommended for ESVI evaluation [26].

The ESVI increases progressively with the severity of MR (see Table 11-1) [19,20] and is negatively correlated with the 5-month survival rate [20]. However, it has not been possible to identify a cutoff value above which one could state that there is systolic dysfunction, contrary to humans, in which an ESVI value >30 mL/m^2 indicates systolic dysfunction [25].

End-Diastolic Volume. In a similar fashion, the end-diastolic volume index (EDVI) can be used to evaluate the importance of the LV diastolic dilation. The EDVI increases more linearly and much faster than the ESVI with increasing MR severity (Table 11-1) [27]. Some authors have examined the changes in left atrial and left ventricular dimensions prior to and at the onset of CHF in CKCSs with DMVD. They noted that the left chamber dimensions increased rapidly during the year preceding the onset of CHF. This observation suggests

TABLE 11-1 Quantification of the Severity of Mitral Regurgitation (MR) in Dogs According to Different Criteria

Criteria	Mild MR	Moderate MR	Severe MR
Rhythm disorders	None	None	Supraventricular and ventricular premature beats, sinus tachycardia, atrial fibrillation
Mitral valve lesions	Subtle remodeling, mild prolapse	Obvious remodeling, moderate prolapse	Severe changes (chordae tendineae + valves), severe prolapse (± rupture of chordae tendineae)
Left Atrium (LA) Dimensions			
LA/Ao TM [17]	<1.7	1.7-2.4	>2.4
LAarea/AOarea 2D [17]	<4.5	4.5-8	>8
Left Ventricle (LV) Diastolic Dimensions			
EDVI (mL/m^2, Simpson method) [20]	63.6 ± 17.9	77.4 ± 25.0	101.1 ± 33.8
Sphericity index [20]	1.38 ± 0.17	1.24 ± 0.14	1.25 ± 0.17
Right Cavities Dimensions			
RV	N	N	↑
RA	N	N	↑
MPA	N	N	↑
Pericardial effusion	Absent	Rare	Often present
LV Systolic Function			
SF % [20]	42 ± 7	47.8 ± 6.9	52.7 ± 10.1
ESVI (mL/m^2, Simpson method) [20]	17.9 ± 5.2	18.9 ± 7.2	23 ± 10.1
Color Doppler of the MR Flow			
RF % (PISA) [16]	<40%	40%-70%	>70%
RJarea/LAarea [29]	<30%	30%-70%	>70%
Continuous Wave Doppler of the MR Flow			
Duration	Early systolic	Holosystolic	Pansystolic
Signal intensity	Moderate	Strong	Strong
Shape	Rectangular	Rectangular/triangular	Triangular/round
Degree of LA Pressure Elevation			
Doppler continuous waveform of MR	Rectangular	Rectangular/triangular	Triangular/round
Emax (m/s) [27]	<1	1-1.2	>1.2
IVRT (ms) [41]	>45	>45	<45
E/IVRT [41]	<2	2-2.5	>2.5
E/E′ [40]	<6	6-9.1	>9.1
Systolic pulmonary arterial pressure in mm Hg (estimated from the maximum velocity of the TR flow spectral Doppler signal) [20]	39.1 ± 17	56 ± 31.1	74.5 ± 27.4

2D, Bidimensional mode; *Ao*, aorta; *AOarea*, aortic cross-sectional area; *EDVI*, end-diastolic volume index; *E/E′*, ratio of the transmitral flow E wave and the pulsed wave tissue Doppler E′ wave of the mitral annulus; *Emax*, maximum E wave amplitude of the diastolic transmitral flow; *ESVI*, end-systolic volume index; *IVRT*, left ventricle isovolumic relaxation time; *LAarea*, left atrial area; *MPA*, main pulmonary artery; *N*, normal; *PISA*, proximal isovelocity surface area; *RA*, right atrium; *RF*, regurgitant fraction; *RJarea/LAarea*, ratio of the left atrial and regurgitant jet areas; *RV*, right ventricle; *SF*, shortening fraction; *TM*, time-motion mode; *TR*, tricuspid regurgitation.

that the rate of dilation of the left chambers could be used as a criterion of imminent decompensation [28].

The PREDICT (prediction of first onset of congestive heart failure in dogs with degenerative mitral valve disease) study identified several indicators of imminent onset of CHF such as: a LVIDd /Ao ratio >3 and a serum level of the N terminal of the pro-brain natriuretic peptide (NT-proBNP) >1500 pmol/l. These two indicators were associated with an odd ratio of 6. Dogs in the CHF group of this study had higher heart rate, radiographic vertebral heart score, systolic and diastolic left ventricular diameters, left atrial dilation, higher tricuspid regurgitation velocity and NT pro-BNP levels [29].

Another study has shown that key parameters associated with a rapid deterioration of the clinical status were: the LVIDd/Ao and LVIDd/LVFWd and LA/Ao ratios, the mitral E wave amplitude and E/A ratio [30]. Dogs in which the LA/Ao ratio increased by more than 2% per month were more at risk of cardiac death. The time to document a 10% increase of the E/A ratio was 4 months in dogs that died due to their heart disease [30].

Right Chambers Dilation

It is important to understand that DMVD is not strictly limited to valvular lesions. As seen above, the remodeling process also involve the LA and LV [19,20,23,24]. In addition, a vascular complication—pulmonary arterial hypertension (PAH)—arises in 14% of cases [31]. The prevalence and degree of PAH increase with the severity of MR (see Table 11-1; Table 11-2; see "Prevalence of pulmonary arterial hypertension" below) [31].

The right chambers can dilate once PAH becomes significant (Figure 11-10; Video 11-5).

Dilation of the main pulmonary artery and annulus can be observed. With severe PAH, systolic and diastolic flattening of the interventricular septum, leading to paradoxical septal motion, can be observed on the right parasternal short axis transventricular view [32]. If right-sided CHF is present, echocardiography can reveal pleural effusion, hepatic congestion, and the presence of ascites.

Pericardial Effusion

Pericardial effusion can be seen in advanced cases, due to increase in the pericardial veins pressure (Figure 11-11; Video 11-6). More rarely, erosion of the left atrial wall by the regurgitant jet can lead to atrial rupture accompanied by intrapericardial hemorrhage, which could lead to cardiac tamponade. In this case, an intrapericardial thrombus is often visible (Figure 11-12) [33].

Interatrial Septum Rupture

Interatrial septum rupture is a fairly rare complication of severe MR in dogs. This rupture usually occurs in the thinnest parts of the interatrial septum, near the oval

TABLE 11-2 Prevalence of Pulmonary Arterial Hypertension and Pulmonary Arterial Pressure Values (Systolic and Diastolic) According to ISACHC Clinical Status and the Degree of Mitral Regurgitation in 617 Dogs with Degenerative Mitral Valve Disease [29]

Variable	Percentage of Dogs with PAH	PAPs (mm Hg)	PAPd (mm Hg)
ISACHC Ia	3	46 ± 17.8	16
ISACHC Ib	16.9	56.5 ± 20	21.2 ± 6.0
ISACHC II	26.7	52.4 ± 19.9	20.8 ± 4.9
ISACHC III	72.2	65 ± 22.6	22.7 ± 6.9
RJarea/LAarea <30%	0	NE	NE
RJarea/LAarea 30%-70%	2.3	41.5 ± 5	NE
RJarea/LAarea >70%	19.9	56.3 ± 21.5	21.4 ± 5.8

ISACHC, International Small Animal Cardiac Health Council; *LAarea,* left atrial area; *NE,* not evaluated; *PAH,* pulmonary arterial hypertension (maximal tricuspid regurgitation velocity >2.5 m/s or maximal end-diastolic velocity of pulmonic regurgitation >2 m/s); *PAPd,* end-diastolic pulmonary arterial pressure, evaluated using spectral Doppler; *PAPs,* systolic pulmonary arterial pressure, evaluated using spectral Doppler; *RJarea,* regurgitant jet area.

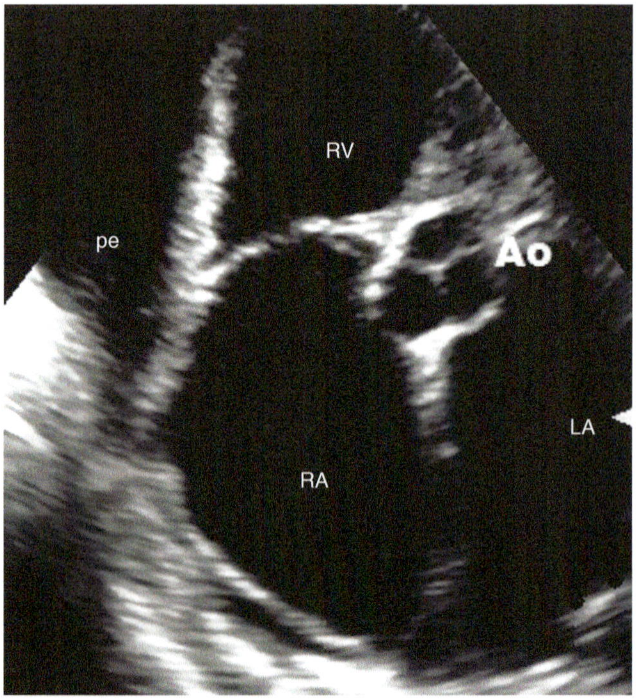

• **Fig. 11-10** Bidimensional (2D) echocardiogram (left apical 5 chambers view) showing marked right atrial (RA) and right ventricular (RV) dilation in a dog with tricuspid regurgitation secondary to pulmonary arterial hypertension (PAH) secondary to degenerative mitral valve disease (DMVD). Pericardial effusion (pe) is visible along the right ventricle wall. The left atrium (LA) is also markedly dilated. *Ao,* Aorta. (Photo credit: Éric de Madron.)

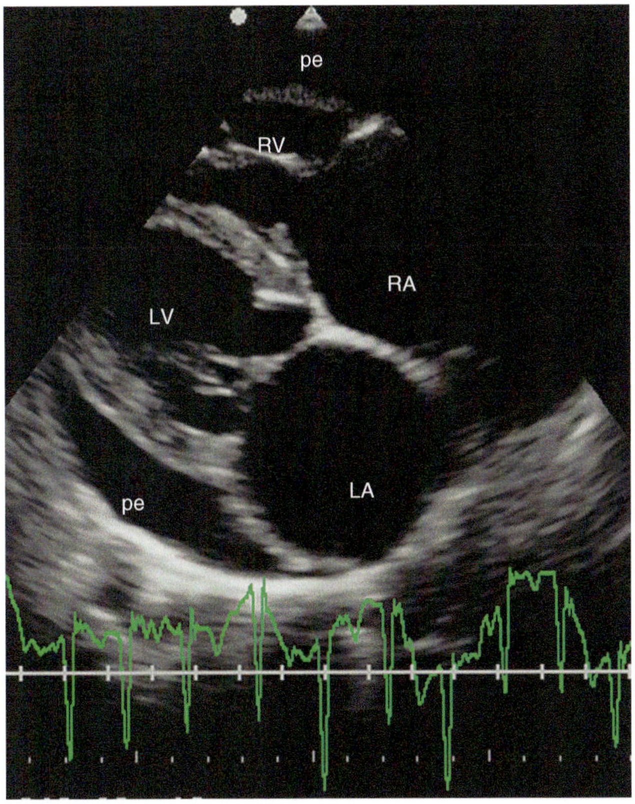

• **Fig. 11-11** Bidimensional (2D) echocardiogram (right parasternal long-axis 4 chambers view) showing significant pericardial effusion (pe) in a dog with advanced degenerative mitral valve disease (DMVD). Both the right atrium (RA) and the left atrium (LA) are dilated. *LV,* Left ventricle; *RV,* right ventricle. (Photo credit: Éric de Madron.)

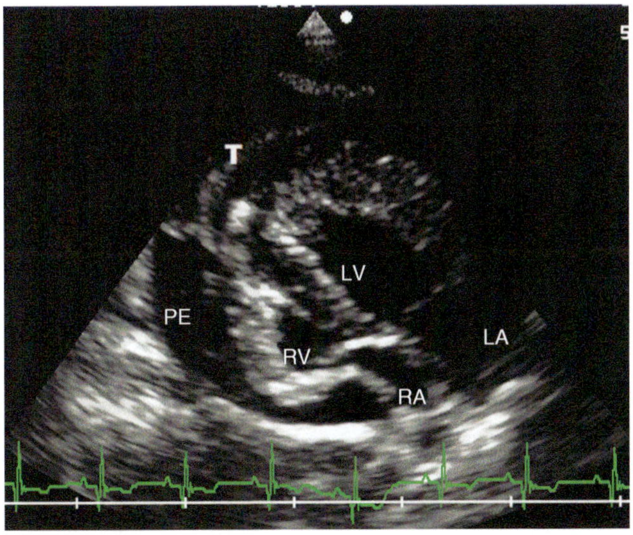

• **Fig. 11-12** Bidimensional (2D) echocardiogram (left apical 4 chambers view) in a dog with degenerative mitral valve disease (DMVD) and left atrial wall tear. A pericardial effusion (PE) is visible along with right atrial wall collapse and an intrapericardial thrombus (T) at the level of the cardiac apex. *LA,* Left atrium; *LV,* left ventricle; *RA,* right atrium; *RV,* right ventricle. (Photo credit: Éric de Madron.)

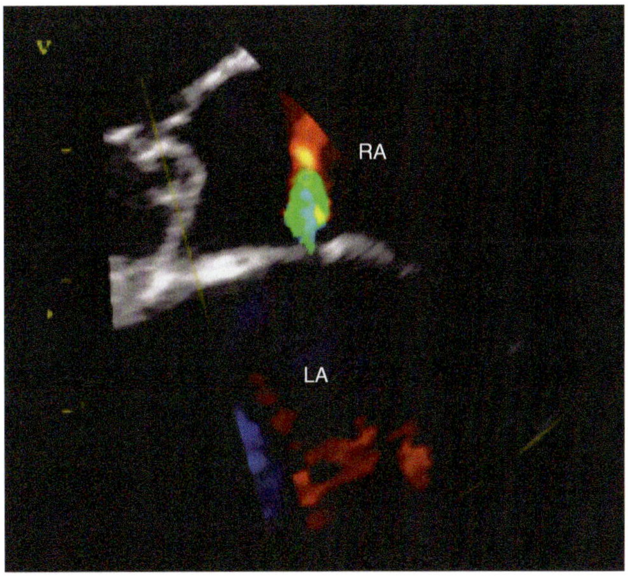

• **Fig. 11-13** Small acquired atrial septal defect (1.8 mm) in a dog with degenerative mitral valve disease (right parasternal long axis 4 chambers view). The turbulent left-to-right shunt flow is observed in the right atrium (RA) by color Doppler. Maximum velocity as evaluated by continuous wave spectral Doppler was 2.5 m/s, indicating a 24 mm Hg gradient between the left atrium (LA) and RA. Note that the interatrial septum is deviated to the right due to the elevated left atrial pressure. (Photo credit: Valérie Chetboul.)

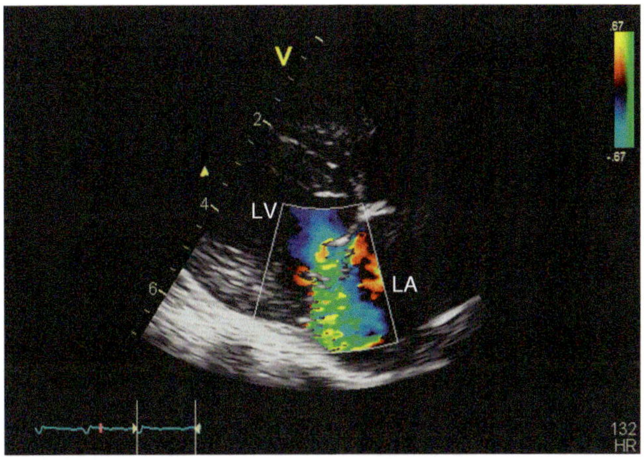

• **Fig. 11-14** Bidimensional (2D) echocardiogram in color Doppler mode (right parasternal long axis 4 chambers view) in a dog with degenerative mitral valve disease (DMVD). The color Doppler shows the mitral regurgitation jet, here directed posteriorly toward the left atrial free wall. *LA,* Left atrium; *LV,* left ventricle. (Photo credit: Éric de Madron.)

foramen (Figure 11-13) [34]. The subsequent atrial septal defect, usually associated with a left-to-right shunt, can actually be beneficial since it allows left atrial pressure reduction. However, a larger interatrial shunt can lead to right-sided CHF.

Color and Spectral Doppler Characteristics of DMVD

Color Doppler

The MR can be detected directly in color Doppler mode. A turbulent jet with a mosaic aspect is observed in systole in the LA. This jet can be either eccentric and directed toward the interatrial septum or the LA lateral wall, which may lead to left atrial wall tear (Figure 11-14; Video 11-7), or central (Figure 11-15; Video 11-8) [16,17,35,36].

On the left apical 4 chambers view (see Figure 11-15), the MR jet is made up of three components. First, in the LV, one can observe a hemisphere directly upstream of the mitral valve: the convergence zone or proximal isovelocity surface area (PISA) zone (see below). Next, the jet forms a sort of narrow "vein" when going through the valve: the *vena contracta*. Finally, the flow disperses itself into the LA.

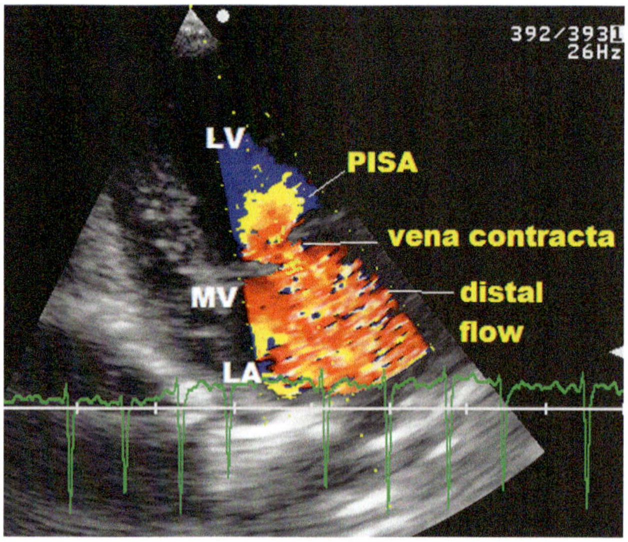

• **Fig. 11-15** Color Doppler of a mitral regurgitation jet. Note the somewhat hemispheric turbulent flow convergence zone (PISA) immediately upstream of the mitral valve in the left ventricle (LV), the vena contracta through the mitral valve (MV), and the distal area (distal flow) where the regurgitant flow disperses into the left atrium (LA). (Photo credit: Éric de Madron.)

Spectral Doppler

Regurgitant Flow

The continuous wave spectral Doppler shows a high-velocity turbulent flow (Figure 11-16) [37-39].

Indeed, the maximum velocity of this flow is correlated to the LV-LA systolic pressure gradient by the Bernoulli equation (see Chapter 2). This LV-LA gradient depends on systolic systemic arterial pressure [40]. The shape of the continuous wave spectral Doppler envelope of the MR jet can reveal the status of myocardial contractility as well as LA pressure. A rectangular envelope denotes adequate LV contractility and normal LA pressure. A rounded envelope reveals a decline in LV inotropy. A triangular envelope, as shown in Figure 11-16, reveals elevated atrial pressures [37-39].

Diastolic Transmitral Flow

The transmitral flow pulsed wave spectral Doppler is characterized by an increase of the E wave due to increased transmitral volume (Figure 11-17) [27,35].

Aortic Flow

The aortic flow pulsed wave Doppler reveals a shortened ejection time due to decreased forward aortic stroke volume [35].

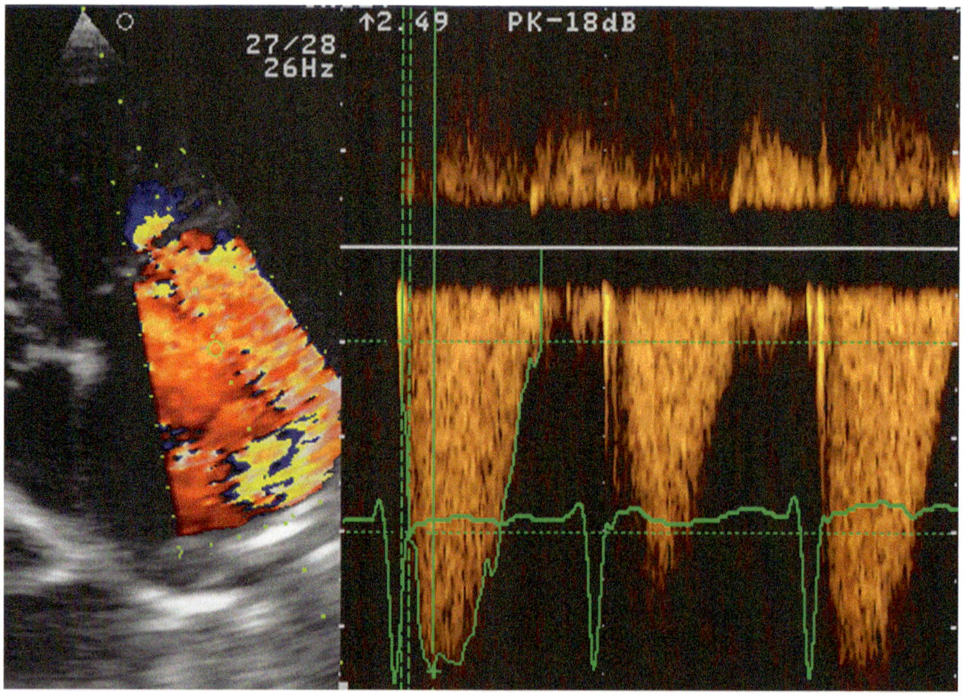

• **Fig. 11-16** Continuous wave Doppler of a mitral regurgitation jet in a dog. The Doppler cursor is well positioned in the regurgitant flow, observed in color Doppler mode on the left apical 4-chambers view *(left panel)*. The turbulent flow, recorded in continuous wave Doppler mode, is systolic and moves away from the transducer; it is therefore displayed as negative *(right panel)*. The triangular shape of this jet indicates left atrial pressure elevation. (Photo credit: Éric de Madron.)

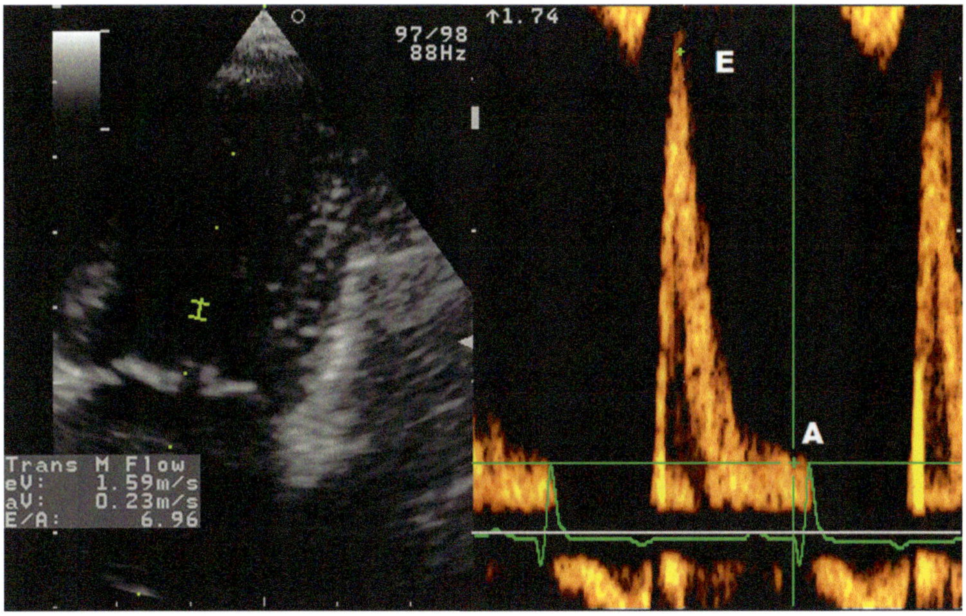

• **Fig. 11-17** Pulsed wave Doppler of the transmitral diastolic flow in a dog with degenerative mitral valve disease (DMVD). The E wave has a markedly elevated velocity (1.59 m/s) compared to the A wave (0.23 m/s). This denotes very severe mitral regurgitation with elevated left atrial pressure. (Photo credit: Éric de Madron.)

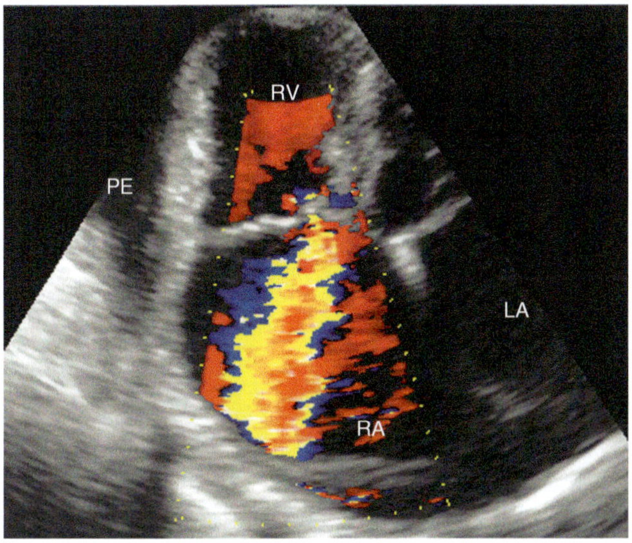

• **Fig. 11-18** Bidimensional (2D) echocardiogram (left apical 4 chambers view) in color Doppler mode displaying a large tricuspid regurgitation jet due to pulmonary arterial hypertension (PAH) secondary to degenerative mitral valve disease (DMVD). *LA,* Left atrium; *PE,* pericardial effusion; *RA,* right atrium; *RV,* right ventricle. (Photo credit: Éric de Madron.)

Tricuspid Flow

With PAH (pulmonary artery systolic pressure >30 mm Hg), tricuspid regurgitation (TR), which is often present and considered physiologic in normal dogs, worsens (Figure 11-18). Its maximum velocity will then rise above 2.5 m/s (Figure 11-19) [31] (see Chapter 14). One must distinguish passive from active PAH. Passive PAH reflects elevated left atrial pressure and is not associated with precapillary pulmonary vasoconstriction. It is usually seen in cases of cardiogenic pulmonary edema. The TR velocity can reach values up to 3.5 m/s. With active PAH, there is precapillary vasoconstriction leading to TR velocity values >3,5 m/s. Active PAH is typically associated with signs of right-sided forward (syncopes, exercise intolerance) and backward (ascites, pleural effusion) hear failure. The lungs become "protected" from pulmonary edema.

Pulmonic Flow

With PAH, the pulmonic ejection flow can become asymmetric (see Chapter 14).

Interrogation of the pulmonic regurgitation (PR) flow can also help to confirm the presence of PAH when the end-diastolic PR V_{max} exceeds 2 m/s (Figure 11-20) [31].

Tissue Doppler Characteristics of DMVD

Mitral Annulus Pulsed Wave Tissue Doppler

The effects of MR on the early diastolic movement of the mitral annulus (E′ wave analyzed in pulsed wave tissue Doppler imaging [TDI] mode) are complex. Several studies have shown that the development of acute MR leads not only to decreased LV elastance but also to delayed relaxation [41,42]. In theory, this should result in a decreased E′ wave. However, the amplitude of the E′ is also influenced by the preload increase [43]. Moreover, the reduction of the afterload due to the ventricular drainage in the LA leads to a decreased LV end-systolic volume, resulting in increased subsequent elastic recoil. The diastolic function

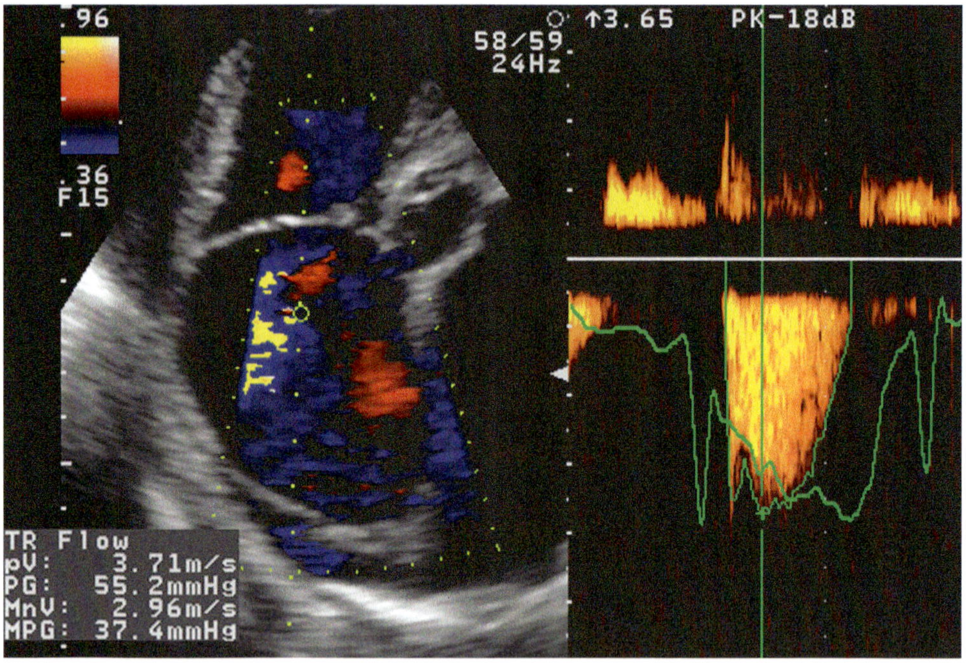

• **Fig. 11-19** Continuous wave spectral Doppler of a tricuspid regurgitation jet in a dog with pulmonary arterial hypertension (PAH) secondary to chronic degenerative mitral valve disease (DMVD). The maximum velocity, reaching 3.71 m/s, is elevated, indicating a 55 mm Hg gradient between the right ventricle and right atrium. (Photo credit: Éric de Madron.)

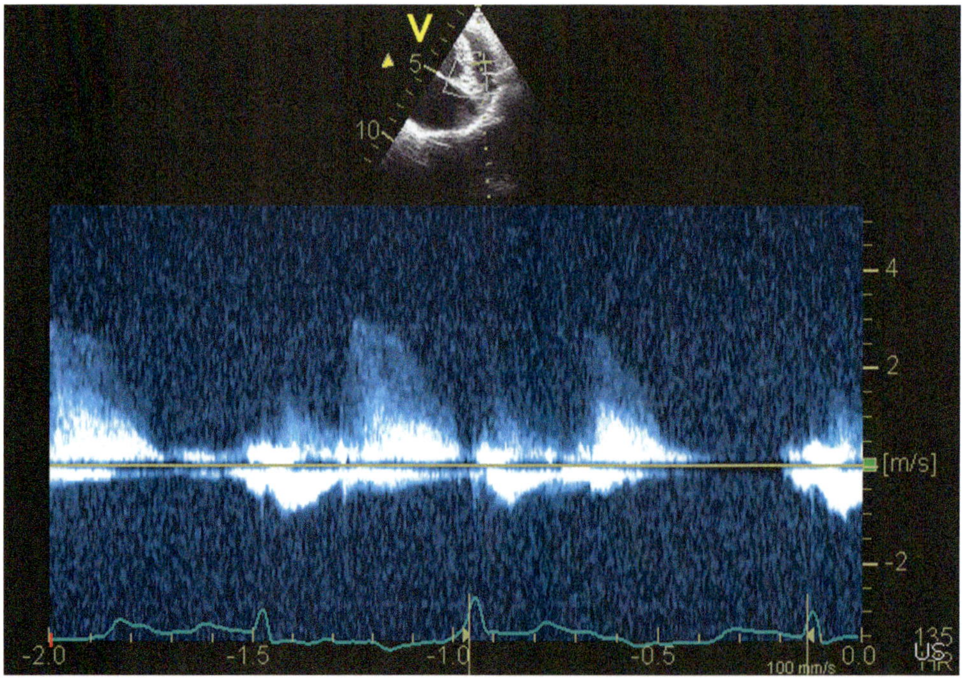

• **Fig. 11-20** Continuous wave Doppler of a pulmonic regurgitation jet in a dog with pulmonary arterial hypertension (PAH) secondary to chronic degenerative mitral valve disease (DMVD). Early diastolic velocities are elevated, reaching 3 m/s, indicating a 36 mm Hg pressure gradient between the main pulmonary artery and the right ventricle. They then drop rapidly to slightly more than 1 m/s in end-diastole. A rapid drop of the pulmonic regurgitation flow velocities during diastole indicates an elevated diastolic right ventricular pressure. (Photo credit: Éric de Madron.)

apparently becomes "improved" despite delayed relaxation [41,44]. The net result is an increase in the E′ wave, as long as the diastolic dysfunction remains minimal.

Right Ventricular Tissue Doppler

Few data regarding TDI alterations associated with DMVD are currently available. A study compared TDI and strain and strain rate parameters in 61 dogs with DMVD (with or without CHF) to those obtained in 10 normal dogs. The two groups were not comparable in age, however, and the intraday coefficient of variation (CV) of several important measurements was >15% [45]. No radial systolic function impairment was found in dogs with DMVD. To the contrary, an increase in LV longitudinal basal and apical systolic free wall velocities was observed in animals in CHF when compared to control animals and those not in CHF. A similar increase, in all likelihood mostly due to the elevated heart rate associated with CHF, was found for several longitudinal and radial diastolic parameters. Finally, the difference between the time-to-peak intervals of the longitudinal velocities of the LV free wall and interventricular septum were significantly greater in dogs with DMVD than in control animals, possibly indicating intraventricular dyssynchrony. However, the intraday variability of this parameter was very large (CV of 43.8%) [45], meaning that confirmation of this finding will require more prospective studies.

Tissue Doppler in Cases of Pulmonary Arterial Hypertension

This is discussed in Chapter 14.

Speckle Tracking in DMVD

Speckle tracking mode allows the evaluation of the radial and longitudinal systolic strain and strain rate of the LV wall, allowing the assessment of regional synchronism. Regional dysfunctions associated with MR, particularly involving the LV free wall, can thus be highlighted (Figure 11-21) [46].

Left Ventricular Tei Index

The LV Tei index (see Chapter 7) increases with the progression of the clinical signs in dogs with MR due to the shortened ejection time. This suggests systolic dysfunction in severe MR [47].

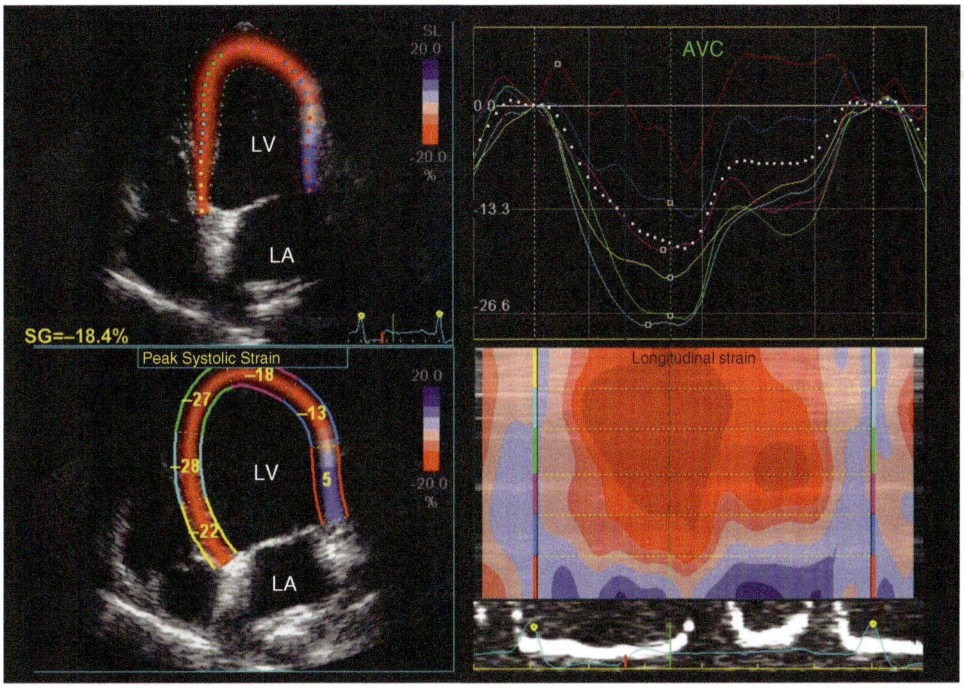

• **Fig. 11-21** Left ventricular (LV) longitudinal strain anomaly analyzed by speckle tracking from the left apical 4 chambers view in a dog with degenerative mitral valve disease (DMVD). The walls of the LV have been divided into six equidistant segments. The longitudinal strain color code is superimposed on the bidimensional (2D) image *(top left)* and displayed as a function of time *(bottom right)*. *(Bottom left)*, The peak longitudinal systolic strain value for each of the six segments analyzed is superimposed on the 2D color image. Five of the six segments shorten during systole (negative strain, reaching its maximum prior to or at the end of systole). However, the strain values are heterogeneous (ranging from −28% to −13%). Furthermore, the longitudinal strain in a segment (at the base of the LV free wall, *red curve*) is abnormal (it is positive instead of negative with a value of +5%). This dyskinesia is also visible on the 2D views *(top and bottom left)* and in color time-motion (TM) mode *(bottom right)*, where the positive strain is displayed in blue (instead of red). The color TM mode also shows the heterogeneity of the strain of the other five segments. *AVC*, Aortic valve closure; *LA*, left atrium. (Photo credit: Valérie Chetboul.)

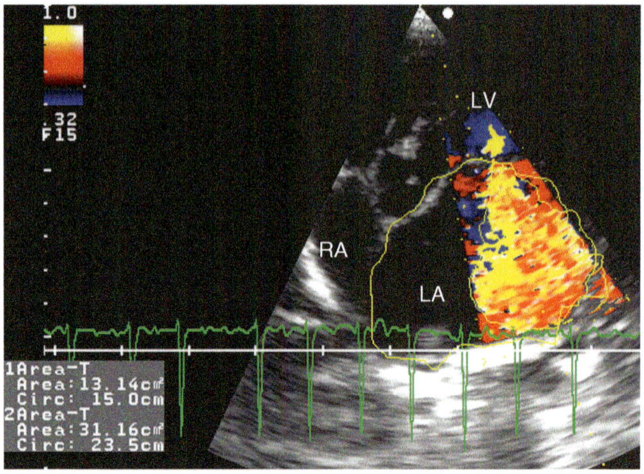

• **Fig. 11-22** Bidimensional (2D) echocardiogram (left apical 5 chambers view) in color Doppler mode in a dog with degenerative mitral valve disease (DMVD). The regurgitant jet area (RJarea) can be measured and compared to the left atrium area (LAarea). In this case, the RJarea/LAarea ratio is 42.2%, indicating moderate mitral regurgitation. *LA*, Left atrium; *LV*, left ventricle; *RA*, right atrium. (Photo credit: Éric de Madron.)

Mitral Leakage Quantification

Color Doppler Methods

Evaluation of the Distal Regurgitant Jet Area

This semiquantitative method involves tracking the contour of the regurgitant flow visualized on the left apical 4 chambers view in color Doppler mode to obtain its area (regurgitant jet area [RJarea]) and to compare it to the LA area (LAarea), measured on the same view. One then obtains the ratio of the regurgitant jet and left atrial areas (RJarea/LAarea) (Figure 11-22).

The repeatability and reproducibility of this technique are good with a trained operator (interday and intraday variability <10%) [16]. An RJarea/LAarea ratio <30% indicates mild MR, a ratio of 30% to 70% indicates moderate MR, and a ratio >70% indicates severe MR (see Table 11-1) [16,31]. However, the RJarea/LAarea has limitations: it is influenced by the systolic arterial pressure, left atrial pressure, and jet direction (eccentric versus central) as well as the transducer frequency and gain level [16,17].

PISA Method

Principles. The PISA (acronym for *proximal isovelocity surface area*) method is based on the fluid dynamic principle stipulating that when a flow approaches a circular orifice, it forms concentric semi-circles of decreasing surfaces and increasing velocities [48]. When applied to the situation of MR, the circular orifice is the regurgitant orifice at the level of coaptation of the mitral valve leaflets and the concentric semi-circles are isovelocity areas (PISA zones, also known as convergence zones) forming upstream of the valve (see Figure 11-15; Video 11-9). According to the law of conservation of mass, the flow rate in each of these PISA zones is equal to the regurgitant flow rate. These PISA zones are relatively hemispheric in shape. The flow rate in these zones is equal to the surface of the hemisphere $2\pi r^2$, where r is the radius of the isovelocity zone, multiplied by the Nyquist limit of the velocity.

This flow rate is equal to the regurgitant flow rate (RFR), still according to the law of conservation of mass. Once the flow is calculated, the regurgitant orifice area (ROA) can be obtained by dividing the RFR by the maximum velocity (V_{max}) of the regurgitant flow obtained by continuous wave spectral Doppler:

$$\text{ROA}\left(\text{in cm}^2\right) = \text{RFR}\,(\text{in mL/s})\,/V_{\text{max}}\,(\text{in cm/s})$$

This gives us the instantaneous maximal ROA. The regurgitant volume (RV) is then calculated by multiplying the ROA by the area under the curve (velocity-time integral [VTI]) of the continuous wave spectral Doppler signal of the regurgitant flow:

$$\text{RV}\,(\text{in mL}) = \text{ROA}\left(\text{in cm}^2\right) \times \text{VTI}\ (\text{in cm})$$

Finally, the regurgitant fraction (RF) can be calculated using the following formula:

$$\text{RF}\,(\%) = \text{RV}\,(\text{in mL})\,/\text{RV}\,(\text{in mL}) + \text{AOSV}\,(\text{in mL})$$

where *AOSV* is the aortic stroke volume (calculated using the average of three aortic flow VTIs multiplied by the aortic area) [16,17,48].

To calculate the RV using the PISA method, a color Doppler of the MR flow on the left apical 4 chambers view must be obtained. The flow convergence zone radius is measured above the mitral valve. For this zone to be as hemispheric as possible, the base line is lowered (in the direction of the flow) until the Nyquist limit is around 18 to 39 cm/s (Figure 11-23, *A*). An overly low Nyquist limit will lead to an overestimation of the convergence area and a limit that is too high will lead to an underestimation. It is recommended that the PISA radius be measured over three consecutive cardiac cycles [17].

The second measurement requires a tracing of the contour of the continuous wave Doppler envelope of the regurgitant jet. From this, the maximum velocity (V_{max} in cm/s) and the VTI (in cm) of the envelope will be derived (Figure 11-23, *B*).

The third measurement will be of the aortic flow VTI in order to calculate the AOSV (Figure 11-23, *C*).

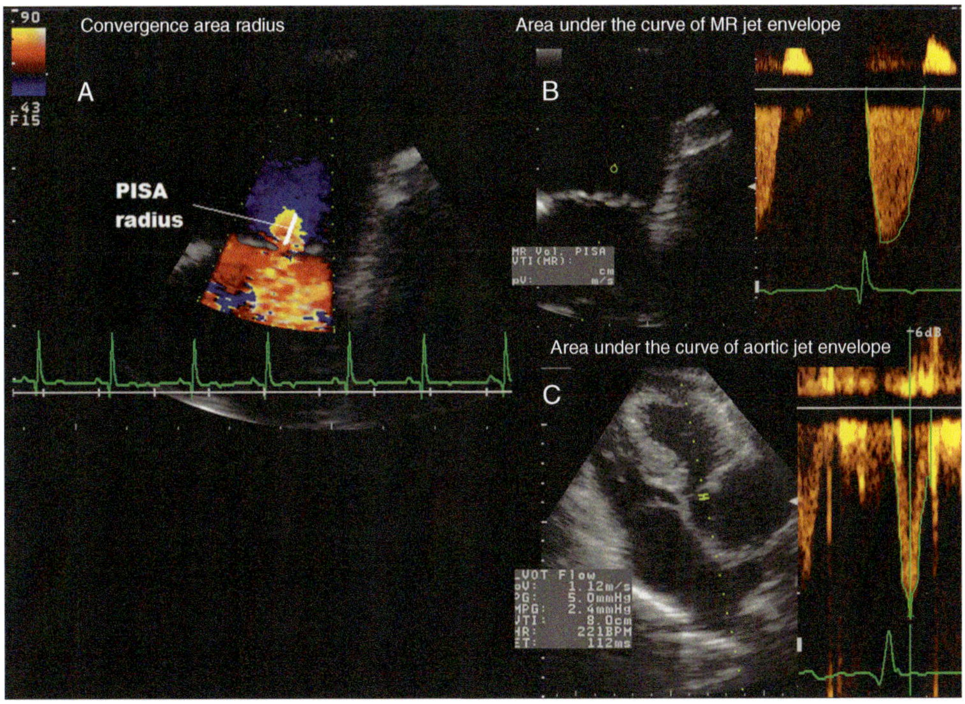

• **Fig. 11-23** Mitral regurgitation (MR) quantification using the proximal isovelocity surface area (PISA) method. A, Measurement of the convergence area radius using color Doppler of the MR jet after lowering the Nyquist limit to 18 to 39 cm/s. B, Measurement of the area under the curve (velocity-time integral) of the spectral envelope of the MR jet. C, Measurement of the area under the curve (velocity-time integral) of the spectral envelope of the systolic transaortic flow. (Photo credit: Éric de Madron.)

Factors Affecting PISA

Geometric Factors. The PISA method is more accurate for central jets. If the jet is eccentric or oblique, the RFR can be overestimated. On some echocardiographic machines, it is possible to correct this by measuring the angle between the mitral leaflet and the end of the PISA region [48]. However, it can sometimes be difficult to discern the exact location of the orifice and the shape of the convergence zone. Any error at this phase will be squared, noticeably affecting the RFR. The PISA method must be used only if the jet is holosystolic. In addition, the presence of multiple regurgitant jets, sometimes observed in dogs with severe MR, precludes the use of this method [49,50].

Technical Factors. The contour of the convergence zone changes with the stage of the regurgitation. Smaller zones are flattened, which leads to an underestimation of the RFR, and larger zones are elliptical, which leads to an overestimation of the RFR [48].

It is important to measure the radius in the center of the convergence zone, where the flow is parallel to the radius, rather than on the sides, where the regurgitant flow is perpendicular to the radius (causing a loss of echoes) [48].

Finally, the shape of the regurgitant orifice influences the results obtained. Indeed, the PISA method assumes a circular orifice. If the orifice is rectangular, the RFR will be underestimated [48].

Results in Dogs. Calculation of the RF in dogs using the PISA method has been evaluated by several authors [16, 17]. The repeatability and reproducibility of this technique are good with a trained operator (intraday and interday CV for RF of 8% and 11%, respectively) [16].

Volumetric Methods Using Pulsed Wave Spectral Doppler

The RV also may be determined by calculating the difference between the total stroke volume (SV_{total}) of the LV (see above) and the AOSV:

$$\text{RV (in mL)} = SV_{total} - \text{AOSV}$$

The SV_{total} can be estimated using either a planimetric method (see Chapter 7, "Planimetric methods") or the pulsed wave Doppler signal of the diastolic mitral flow (SV_{total} = area under the mitral flow curve × area of the mitral annulus) [48].

Staging of the Mitral Regurgitation

The goals of the Doppler echocardiographic examination are not only to diagnose MR but also to stage it in order to establish a prognosis and the best treatment. Usually MR can be classified as minimal, moderate, or severe.

Several direct and indirect criteria can be used for this purpose (see Table 11-1).

Degree of Left Atrial Dilation

The degree of LA dilation is correlated with the severity of the MR. The LA/Ao or LAarea/AOarea ratios have been used to quantify the severity of the MR [16,17]. A significant correlation has been shown between the LA/Ao ratio and the RF (see below) as well as the systolic pulmonary arterial pressure (PAPs) [16]. An LA/Ao ratio >1.7 has been shown to be associated with a poorer prognosis [27].

Left Ventricular Remodeling and Kinetics

The LV becomes increasingly spherical and hyperkinetic as the MR progresses (see Table 11-1). The ESVI (calculated using a planimetric method) increases significantly with the MR ISACHC classification. This increase has a negative impact on the prognosis at 5 months in cases of DMVD [20].

Shape of the Spectral Doppler Signal of the Regurgitant Flow

A rectangular envelope denotes still normal left atrial pressure. A triangular envelope, however, indicates elevation of left atrial pressure. A rounded envelope reveals declining LV inotropy (Figure 11-24) [51].

Regurgitant Fraction

A wide range of MR severity was demonstrated by Gouni et al [16] in dogs with asymptomatic DMVD. Close to one third of these dogs had an RF >30%. Another study conducted by the same group showed that dogs with asymptomatic DMVD and an RF >30% had greater plasma concentration of NT-proBNP and were more likely to decompensate in the following year than were dogs with an RF <30% [52]. Therefore RF is an important criterion to stratify the risk of developing CHF and the prognosis in dogs with DMVD, as established in human medicine [53,54].

The RF has also been shown to be more elevated in dogs with ISACHC class III MR (72.8 ± 9.5%) than those with ISACHC class II MR (57.9 ± 20.1%) or ISACHC class I MR (40.7 ± 19.2%) [9]. Similar results were reported by Kittleson et al [17] in a small number of animals (see Table 11-1). The RF is also correlated with the intensity of the murmur, the ISACHC class, the RJarea/LAarea ratio, the LA/Ao ratio, and PAPs [16].

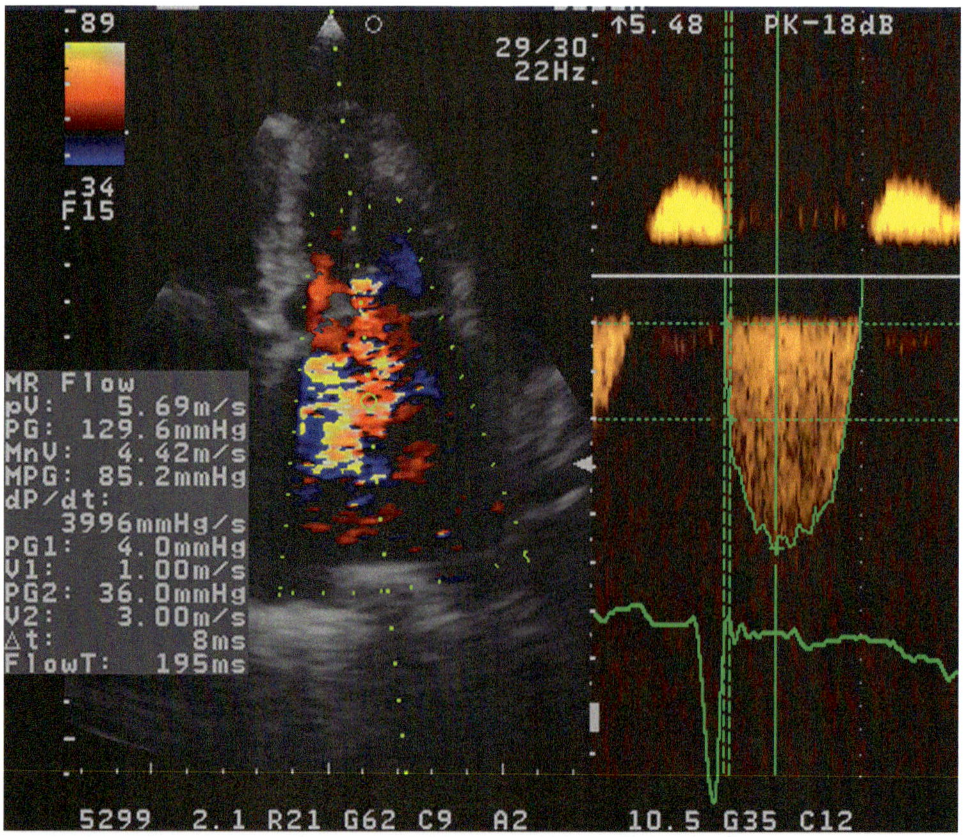

• Fig. 11-24 Continuous wave Doppler of a mitral regurgitation jet showing a rounded envelope, which is a marker of declining left ventricular inotropy. (Photo credit: Éric de Madron.)

Based on recommendations in humans [53] and the data in dogs with DMVD [16,17], the following classification can be proposed:

- RF <30%: very moderate MR
- RF between 30% and 50%: moderate MR
- RF between 50% and 70%: severe MR
- RF >70%: very severe MR

Evaluation of the Left Atrial Pressure

The progression of MR affects several Doppler parameters, mostly because of the increase in left atrial pressure (LAP). Indeed, this increase in LAP results in a shortening of the LV isovolumic relaxation time (IVRT) and an increase in the transmitral flow E wave maximum velocity and E/E′ and E/IVRT ratios. This is discussed in more detail in Chapter 9.

The proposed threshold values for identification of elevated LAP (>20 mm Hg) in dogs with DMVD are E >1.25 m/s, E/E′ >12, IVRT <45 ms, and E/IVRT >2.5 [22,55].

Prevalence of Pulmonary Arterial Hypertension

The more the MR worsens, the greater the prevalence of PAH, rising from 3% (ISACHC class Ia) to 17% (ISACHC class Ib) to 27% (ISACHC class II) to 72% (ISACHC class III) (see Table 11-2) [31].

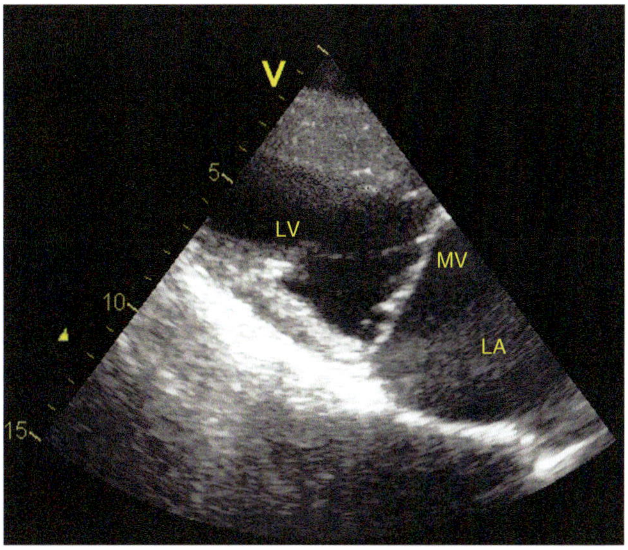

• **Fig. 11-25** Bidimensional (2D) echocardiogram (right parasternal long axis 4 chambers view) in a German Shepherd with primary mitral regurgitation. The mitral valve (MV) is relatively thin and prolapses slightly. The left atrium (LA) is markedly dilated. The left ventricle (LV) is normal in size and its contractility is preserved (in time-motion [TM] mode, image not provided here). (Photo credit: Éric de Madron.)

DMVD in Large Breed Dogs

DMVD does affect medium to large breeds (Brittany Spaniel, Irish Setter, German Shepherd, etc.), although less frequently [6]. Several characteristics differentiate this cardiopathy from DMVD in small dogs. First, the mitral valve is not as remodeled as it is in small dogs. It is usually thinner, elongated, and often prolapsed (Figure 11-25). Second, the LV systolic dysfunction seems to be more pronounced in larger breeds than in small dogs, with a marked increase of the ESVI [19,55]. Atrial fibrillation is often observed [55]. PAH may also be present.

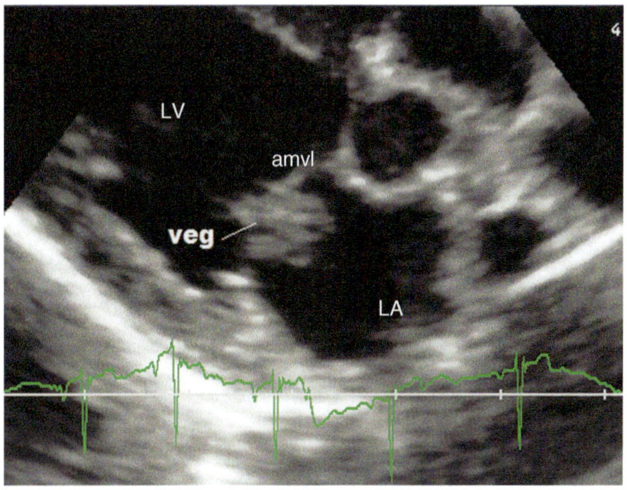

• **Fig. 11-26** Bidimensional (2D) echocardiogram (right parasternal long axis 5 chambers view) in a dog with bacterial endocarditis of the mitral valve. A vegetation (veg) is present on the anterior leaflet of the valve (amvl). *LA,* Left atrium; *LV,* left ventricle. (Photo credit: Éric de Madron.)

Mitral Valve Bacterial Endocarditis

Valvular bacterial endocarditis is characterized by the formation of a platelet, fibrin, and bacterial agglomerate adhering to the surface of one of the cardiac valves, thus creating a masslike lesion called vegetation. The aortic valve is the most commonly affected valve. The mitral valve also can be affected, either in association with the aortic valve (see below) or alone [4,57].

Changes due to endocarditis can range from discrete thickening of one of more leaflets or cusps to a burgeoning and calcified mass (Figure 11-26).

Mitral valve vegetation can be difficult to differentiate from DMVD lesions. The clinical context is essential to establish the proper diagnosis. Bacterial endocarditis is usually (but not always) accompanied by fever, neutrophilia, and at times polyarthritis [57].

Tricuspid Regurgitation

Trivial or mild physiologic tricuspid regurgitation (TR) is often present in normal dogs [36]. The TR jet is eccentric (most frequently lateral) and occupies less than 5% of the right atrial area. Pathologic TR is much less frequent than MR. Causes of acquired pathologic TR include degenerative tricuspid valve disease and TR associated with PAH (see above) [31].

Echocardiographic Characteristics

2D and TM Echocardiography

With degenerative tricuspid valve disease, thickening of the tricuspid valve can be harder to detect than the mitral valve remodeling associated with DMVD because the leaflets are smaller. The consequences of TR need to be sought out, such as dilation of the right chambers (atrium then ventricle), best detected on an apical 4 chambers view (see Figure 11-10). If the TR is severe, the interventricular septal motion becomes paradoxical, mostly in diastole due to the right ventricular volume overload [32]. In cases of severe TR, caudal vena cava and hepatic vein dilation, hepatomegaly, ascites, or pleural effusion may be observed [18].

Color Doppler

The color Doppler mode reveals the TR flow on the right parasternal long axis 4 and 5 chambers views. This jet may be seen even better on the left apical 4 chambers view (see Figure 11-18).

Spectral Doppler

Spectral Doppler interrogation of the TR flow reveals a turbulent flow in the right atrium [36-38]. The measurement of the maximum velocity of the TR flow is used to calculate the pressure gradient between the right ventricle and right atrium and to estimate the right ventricular systolic pressure and the PAPs (see Figure 11-19; see above).

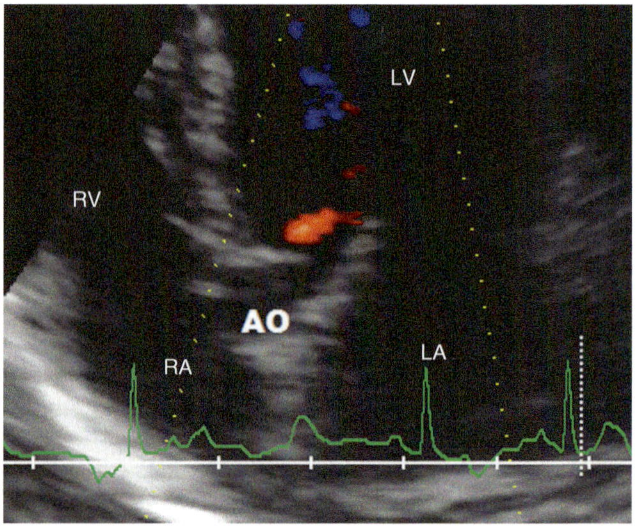

• **Fig. 11-27** Bidimensional (2D) echocardiogram (left apical 5 chambers view) in color Doppler mode in a dog with aortic regurgitation *(red flame)*. *AO,* Aorta; *LA,* left atrium; *LV,* left ventricle; *RA,* right atrium; *RV,* right ventricle. (Photo credit: Éric de Madron.)

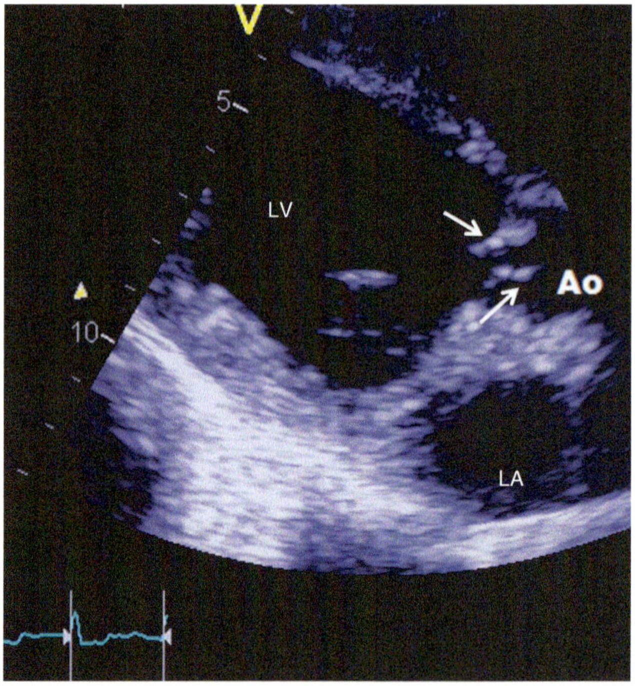

• **Fig. 11-28** Bidimensional (2D) echocardiogram (right parasternal long axis 5-chambers view) in a dog with aortic valve bacterial endocarditis. The vegetation appears in the form of a hyperechoic thickening of the aortic cusps, which are markedly deformed *(arrows)*. *Ao,* Aorta; *LA,* left atrium; *LV,* left ventricle. (Photo credit: Éric de Madron.)

Aortic Regurgitation

A trivial or mild aortic regurgitation (AR), without physiologic consequences, can sometimes be seen in older dogs. This AR is due to mild degeneration of the aortic cusps (Figure 11-27).

Significant acquired AR is rare in small animals. Usually, pathologic AR results from bacterial valvular endocarditis (see below) [56-59].

Echocardiographic Characteristics

2D and TM Echocardiography

Dilation of the Left Ventricle and Anomalies of Mitral Valve Movement

If the AR is significant, the main anomalies include LV dilation with increased SF, diastolic vibration of the median part of the anterior mitral valve leaflet, and possibly premature mitral valve closure in the case of massive AR [18,60].

Aortic Regurgitation Due to Bacterial Endocarditis: Visualization of the Vegetation

When aortic bacterial endocarditis is present, one or several aortic valve cusps appear thickened and hyperechoic (Figure 11-28). Sometimes the vegetation can take the aspect of a mass [18,56-59].

Color Doppler

Color Doppler reveals a turbulent diastolic flow traveling from the aortic valve toward the LV on either a right parasternal long axis view centered on the LV outflow tract or on a left apical 5 chambers view (Figure 11-29).

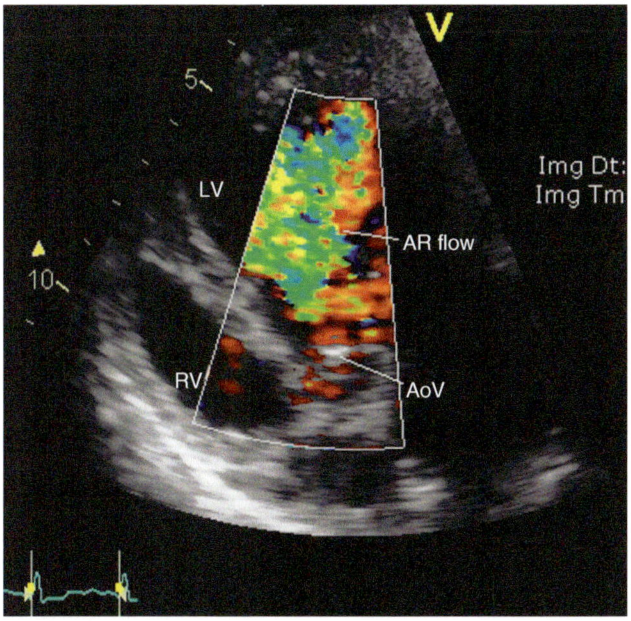

• **Fig. 11-29** Bidimensional (2D) echocardiogram (left apical 5 chambers view) in color Doppler mode in the same dog as in Figure 11-28 showing the turbulent aortic regurgitant jet (AR flow). Its colorimetric area is quite extensive and reaches the apex of the left ventricle (LV) (compare to Figure 11-27). *AoV,* Aortic valve; *RV,* right ventricle. (Photo credit: Éric de Madron.)

The greater the regurgitation, the further the regurgitant jet extends into the LV [37,38,48].

Spectral Doppler

The spectral Doppler interrogation of the AR flow confirms the turbulent nature of the diastolic flow (Figure 11-30).

In the case of acute AR, as is usual in the case of endocarditis, the regurgitant flow velocity sharply decreases during diastole, indicating elevated intraventricular pressure [37,38].

In the case of chronic regurgitation, the ventricle has the time to distend and the AR flow is typically plateau-shaped.

Pulmonic Regurgitation

Trivial or mild pulmonic regurgitation (PR) is often present in normal dogs [36]. Pathologic PR results from either valvular malformation (pulmonic valve dysplasia) or another disease disturbing pulmonary arterial hemodynamics, such as a patent ductus arteriosus or pulmonary arterial hypertension [18].

2D and TM Echocardiography

Only PR secondary to pulmonic valve dysplasia is associated with visible valvular changes, including thickening of valve leaflets and poststenotic dilation of the

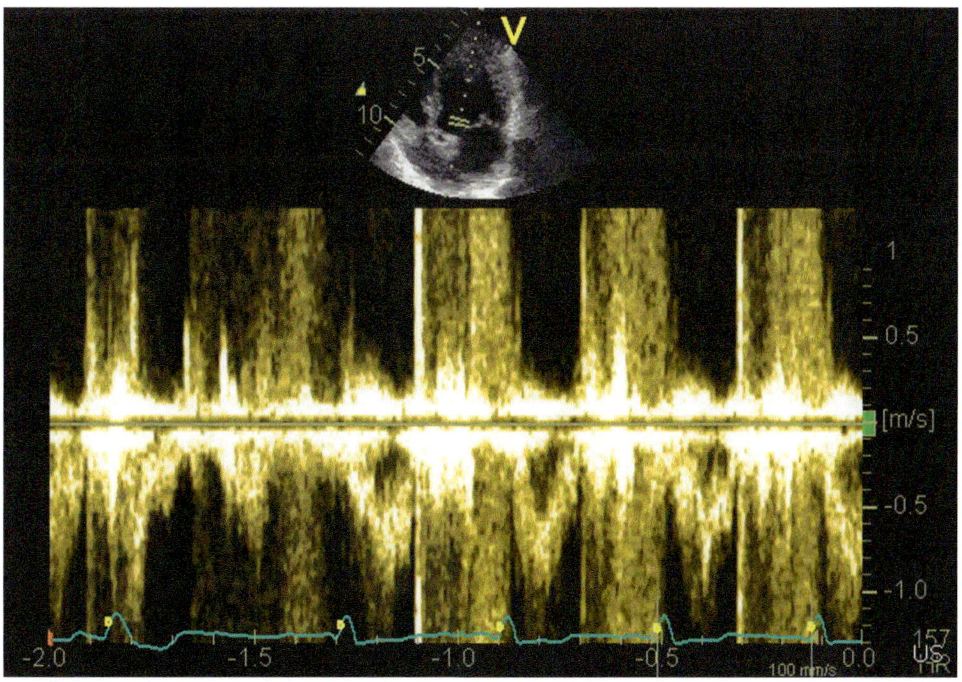

• **Fig. 11-30** Pulsed wave Doppler of an aortic regurgitant flow in a dog with aortic valve bacterial endocarditis (apical 5 chambers view). The diastolic aortic regurgitant flow is turbulent. Its high velocity creates an aliasing phenomenon. (Photo credit: Éric de Madron.)

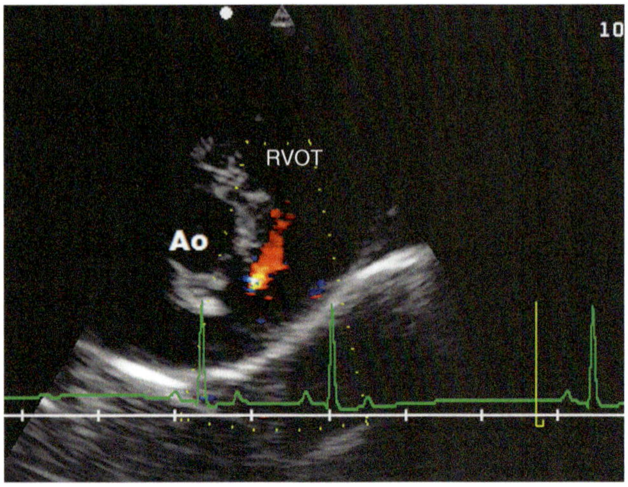

• **Fig. 11-31** Bidimensional (2D) echocardiogram (right parasternal short axis transaortic view) in color Doppler mode in a dog with mild pulmonic regurgitation *(red flame)*. This pulmonic regurgitation can be considered physiologic due to its weak colorimetric extension into the right ventricular outflow tract (RVOT) and low velocity (absence of aliasing, maximum scale: 66 cm/s). *Ao,* Aorta. (Photo credit: Éric de Madron.)

main pulmonary artery (see Chapter 19) [18]. In other cases of PR, the valve appears normal. In the case of PR secondary to PAH, dilation of the main pulmonary artery, pulmonic valve annulus, and right ventricular outflow tract may be present.

Color Doppler

The PR flow can be identified with color Doppler on the right parasternal short axis transaortic view. It appears as a red flame (in the absence of PAH, the velocities are low, therefore there is no aliasing) traveling from the pulmonic valve toward the right ventricular outflow tract in diastole (Figure 11-31; Video 11-10).

Spectral Doppler

A positive diastolic flow traveling from the main pulmonary artery toward the right ventricle outflow tract is recorded. If the pulmonary arterial pressure is normal, the maximum end-diastolic velocity of this flow is generally <1 m/s (and does not exceed 2 m/s) [37,38]. In the case of PAH, this velocity increases (see above; see Figure 11-20).

REFERENCES

[1] Sisson D, Kvart C, Darke PGC. Acquired valvular heart diseases of dogs and cats. In: Fox PR, Sisson D, Moise S, editors. Textbook of canine and feline cardiology: principles and clinical practice. 2nd ed. Philadelphia: WB Saunders; 1999, p. 536–65.

[2] Kvart C, Häggstrom J. Acquired valvular heart disease. In: Ettinger SJ, Feldman EC, editors. Textbook of veterinary internal medicine; 2005;6:1022–39.

[3] Chetboul V, Tissier R, Villaret F, et al. Epidemiological, clinical, echo-Doppler characteristics of mitral valve endocardiosis in Cavalier King Charles in France: a retrospective study of 451 cases (1995 to 2003). Can Vet J 2004;45:1012–5.

[4] Beardow AW, Buchanan JW. Chronic mitral valve disease in Cavalier King Charles Spaniels: 95 cases (1987-1991). J Am Vet Med Assoc 1993;203:1023–9.

[5] Serfass P, Chetboul V, Carlos Sampedrano C, et al. Retrospective study of 942 small sized-dogs: prevalence of left apical systolic heart murmur and left-sided heart failure, critical effects of breed, and sex. J Vet Cardiol 2006;8:1–8.

[6] D'Agnolo G, Tarducci A, Santilli RA, et al. Comparison of primary mitral valve disease in German Shepherd dogs and in small breeds. Am J Vet Res 2001;62:1447–54.

[7] Kogure K. Pathology of chronic mitral valve disease in the dog. Jpn J Vet Sci 1980;42:323–35.

[8] Whitney JC. Observations on the effects of age on the severity of heart valve lesions in the dog. J Small Anim Pract 1974;15:511–22.

[9] Pedersen HD, Lorentzen KA, Kristensem BO. Echocardiographic mitral valve prolapse on cavalier King Charles Spaniels: epidemiology and prognostic significance for regurgitation. Vet Record 1999;144:315–20.

[10] Serres F, Chetboul V, Tissier R, et al. Chordae tendineae rupture in dogs with degenerative mitral valve disease: prevalence, survival, and prognostic factors (114 cases, 2001-2006). J Vet Intern Med 2007;21:258–64.

[11] Dennis MO, Nealeigh RC, Pyle RL, et al. Echocardiographic assessment of normal and abnormal valvular function in Beagle dogs. Am J Vet Res 1978;39:1591–8.

[12] Pipers FS, Bonagura JD, Hamlin RL, Kittleson M. Echocardiographic abnormalities of the mitral valve associated with left-side heart diseases in the dog. J Am Vet Med Assoc 1981;179:580–6.

[13] Terzo E, di Marcello M, McAllister H, et al. Echocardiographic assessment of 537 dogs with mitral valve prolapse and leaflet involvement. Vet Radiol Ultrasound 2009;50:416–22.

[14] O'Gara P, Sugeng L, Lang R, et al. The role of imaging in chronic degenerative mitral regurgitation. JACC Cardiovasc Imaging 2008;1:221–37.

[15] Jacobs GJ, Calvert CA, Mahaffey MB, Hall DG. Echocardiographic detection of flail left atrioventricular valve cusp from ruptured chordae tendinae in 4 dogs. J Vet Intern Med 1995;9:341–6.

[16] Gouni V, Serres FJ, Pouchelon JL, et al. Quantification of mitral valve regurgitation in dogs with degenerative mitral valve disease by use of the proximal isovelocity surface area method. J Am Vet Med Assoc 2007;231:399–406.
[17] Kittleson MD, Brown WA. Regurgitant fraction measured by using the proximal isovelocity surface area method in dogs with chronic myxomatous mitral valve disease. J Vet Intern Med 2003;17:84–8.
[18] Moise NS. Echocardiography. In: Fox PR, editor. Canine and feline cardiology. New York: Churchill Livingstone; 1988, p. 113–56.
[19] Borgarelli M, Tarducci A, Zanatta R, Haggstrom J. Decreased systolic function and inadequate hypertrophy in large and small breed dogs with chronic mitral valve insufficiency. J Vet Intern Med 2007;21: 61–7.
[20] Serres F, Chetboul V, Tissier R, et al. Comparison of 3 ultrasound methods for quantifying left ventricular systolic function: correlation with disease severity and prognostic value in dogs with mitral valve disease. J Vet Intern Med 2008;22:566–77.
[21] Boon JA. Acquired heart disease: mitral insufficiency. In: Boon JA, editor. Manual of veterinary echocardiography. Baltimore: Williams & Wilkins; 1998. p. 261–86.
[22] Bonagura JD, Schober KE. Can ventricular function be assessed by echocardiography in chronic canine mitral valve disease? J Small Anim Pract 2009;50: 12–24.
[23] Dell'italia LJ, Balcells E, Meng QC, et al. Volume-overload cardiac hypertrophy is unaffected by ACE inhibitor treatment in dogs. Am J Physiol 1997;273: H961–70.
[24] Pat B, Killingsworth C, Denney T, et al. Dissociation between cardiomyocyte function and remodeling with beta-adrenergic receptor blockade in isolated canine mitral regurgitation. Am J Physiol Heart Circ Physiol 2008;295:H2321–7.
[25] Borow KM, Green LH, Mann T, et al. End systolic volume as a predictor of postoperative left ventricular performance volume overload from valvular regurgitation. Am J Med 1980;68:655–63.
[26] Tidholm A, Westling AB, Höglund K, et al. Comparisons of 3-, 2-dimensional, and M-mode echocardiographical methods for estimation of left chamber volumes in dogs with and without acquired heart disease. J Vet Intern Med 2010;24:1414–20.
[27] Borgarelli M, Savarino P, Corsara S, et al. Survival characteristics and prognostic variables of dogs with mitral regurgitation attributable to myxomatous valve disease. J Vet Int Med 2008;22:120–8.
[28] Lord P, Hansson K, Kvart C, Häggström J. Rate of change of heart size before congestive heart failure in dogs with mitral regurgitation. J Small Anim Pract 2010;51:210–8.
[29] Reynolds CA1, Brown DC, Rush JE, Fox PR, Nguyenba TP, Lehmkuhl LB, Gordon SG, Kellihan HB, Stepien RL, Lefbom BK, Meier CK, Oyama MA. Prediction of first onset of congestive heart failure in dogs with degenerative mitral valve disease: the PREDICT cohort study. J Vet Cardiol 2012;14:193–202.
[30] Hezzell MJ, Boswood A, Moonarmart W, Elliott J. Selected echocardiographic variables change more rapidly in dogs that die from myxomatous mitral valve disease. J Vet Cardiol 2012;14:269–79.
[31] Serres FJ, Chetboul V, Tissier, et al. Doppler echocardiography-derived evidence of pulmonary arterial hypertension in dogs with degenerative mitral valve disease: 86 cases (2001–2005). J Am Vet Med Assoc 2006;229:1772–8.
[32] De Madron E, Bonagura JD, O'Grady MR. Normal and paradoxical septal motion in the dog: an echocardiographic study. Am J Vet Res 1985;46:1832–41.
[33] Sadanaga KK, MacDonald MJ, Buchanan JW. Echocardiography and surgery in a dog with left atrial rupture and hemopericardium. J Vet Intern Med 1990;4:216–21.
[34] Peddle GD, Buchanan JW. Acquired atrial septal defects secondary to rupture of the atrial septum in dogs with degenerative mitral valve disease. J Vet Cardiol 2010;12:129–34.
[35] Kisslo J, Adams DB, Belkin RN. Doppler color flow imaging. New York: Churchill Livingstone; 1988. p. 87–112.
[36] Miller RW, Bonagura JD. Doppler color flow imaging. In: Report from the VIIth Annual Veterinary Medical Forum; San Diego 1989, p. 823–29.
[37] Hatle L, Angelsen B. Doppler ultrasound in cardiology. Philadelphia: Lea & Febiger; 1985, p. 97–292.
[38] Goldberg SJ, Allen HD, Marx GR, Finn CJ. Doppler echocardiography. Philadelphia: Lea & Febiger; 1985, p. 55–137.
[39] de Madron E. Rôle de l'échocardiographie Doppler en mode continu et pulsé dans le diagnostic et l'évaluation de la sévérité des cardiopathies des petits animaux (1re et 2e parties). Prat Med Chir Anim Comp 1991;26:23–42.
[40] Tou SP, Adin DB, Estrada AH. Echocardiographic estimation of systemic systolic blood pressure in dogs with mild mitral regurgitation. J Vet Intern Med 2006;20:1127–31.
[41] Zile MR, Tomita M, Nakano K, et al. Effects of left ventricular volume overload produced by mitral regurgitation on diastolic function. Am J Physiol 1991;261:H1471–80.

[42] Katayama K, Tajimi T, Guth BD, et al. Early diastolic filling dynamics during experimental mitral regurgitation in the conscious dog. Circulation 1988;78:390–400.
[43] Nagueh SF, Sun H, Kopelen HA, et al. Hemodynamic determinants of the mitral annulus diastolic velocities by tissue Doppler. Circulation 1999;99:254–61.
[44] Oyama MA, Sisson DD, Bulmer BJ, Constable PD. Echocardiographic estimation of mean left atrial pressure in a canine model of acute mitral valve insufficiency. J Vet Intern Med 2004;18:667–72.
[45] Tidholm A, Ljungwall I, Hoglund K, et al. Tissue Doppler and strain imaging in dogs with myxomatous mitral valve disease in different stages of congestive heart failure. J Vet Intern Med 2009;23:1197–207.
[46] Chetboul V, Tissier R. Echocardiographic and Doppler assessment of canine degenerative mitral valve disease. J Vet Cardiol 2012;14:127–48.
[47] Teshima K, Asano K, Iwanaga K, et al. Evaluation of left ventricular Tei index (index of myocardial performance) in healthy dogs and dogs with mitral regurgitation. J Vet Med Sci 2007;69:117–23.
[48] Hung J. Quantification of valvular regurgitation. In: Otto CM, editor. The practice of clinical echocardiography. Philadelphia: Saunders Elsevier; 2007;14: 405–29.
[49] Utsunomiya T, Ogawa T, Doshi R, et al. Doppler color flow "proximal isovelocity surface area" method for estimating volume flow rate: effects of orifice shape and machine factors. J Am Coll Cardiol 1991;17:1103–11.
[50] Simpson IA, Shiota T, Gharib M, Sahn DJ. Current status of flow convergence for clinical applications: is it a leaning tower of "PISA"? J Am Coll Cardiol 1996;27:504–9.
[51] Asano K, Masui Y, Masuda K, Fujinaga T. Noninvasive estimation of cardiac systolic function using continuous-wave Doppler echocardiography in dogs with experimental mitral regurgitation. Aust Vet J 2002;80:25–8.
[52] Serres F, Pouchelon JL, Poujol L, et al. Plasma N-terminal pro-B-type natriuretic peptide concentration helps to predict survival in dogs with symptomatic degenerative mitral valve disease regardless of and in combination with the initial clinical status at admission. J Vet Cardiol 2009;11:103–21.
[53] Zoghbi WA, Enriquez-Sarano M, Foster E, et al. American Society of Echocardiography. Recommendations for evaluation of the severity of native valvular regurgitation with two-dimensional and Doppler echocardiography. J Am Soc Echocardiogr 2003;16:777–802.
[54] Enriquez-Sarano M, Avierinos JF, Messika-Zeitoon D, et al. Quantitative determinants of the outcome of asymptomatic mitral regurgitation. N Engl J Med 2005;352:875–83.
[55] Teshima K, Asano K, Sasaki Y, et al. Assessment of left ventricular function using pulsed tissue Doppler imaging in healthy dogs and dogs with spontaneous mitral regurgitation. Jpn J Vet Science 2005;67:1207–15.
[56] Lombard CW, Buergelt CD. Vegetative bacterial endocarditis in dogs: echocardiographic diagnosis and clinical signs. J Small Anim Pract 1983;24:325–39.
[57] Miller MW, Sisson D. Infective endocarditis. In: Fox PR, Sisson D, Moise S, editors. Textbook of canine and feline cardiology: principles and clinical practice. 2nd ed. Philadelphia: WB Saunders; 1999, p. 567–80.
[58] Bonagura JD, Pipers FS. Echocardiographic features of aortic valve endocarditis in a dog, a cow and a horse. J Am Vet Med Assoc 1983;182:595–9.
[59] Ettinger SJ. Valvular diseases. In: Ettinger SJ, editor. Textbook of veterinary internal medicine: diseases of the dog and cat. 3rd ed Philadelphia: WB Saunders; 1989, p. 1031–50.
[60] Feigenbaum H. Acquired valvular heart diseases. In: Feigenbaum H, editor. Echocardiography. 3rd ed. Philadelphia: Lea & Febiger; 1981, p. 276–84.

12

Dilated Cardiomyopathy and Other Cardiomyopathies in Dogs

VALÉRIE CHETBOUL

Primary Dilated Cardiomyopathy, 182
Other Cardiomyopathies, 194

Cardiomyopathies are highly heterogeneous cardiopathies that, in the past 20 years, have been the topic of nosographic discussions directly linked to increased knowledge (mostly in genetics) [1,2]. At this time, cardiomyopathies are defined as cardiac muscle disorders that could lead to mechanical and/or electrical malfunctions of the heart [1,2]. It is common practice to distinguish between intrinsic and extrinsic cardiomyopathies [1]. Unlike intrinsic cardiomyopathies, extrinsic cardiomyopathies (still referred to as "specific"), as indicated by their name, are the result of "extramyocardial" disorders, whether cardiovascular in origin (ischemia, valvulopathies, cardiac rhythm disorders, arterial hypertension) or systemic (including immune-mediated, nutritional, infectious, toxic, endocrine, or neuromuscular diseases).

The most common cardiomyopathy in dogs is an intrinsic cardiomyopathy known as primary dilated cardiomyopathy (PDCM) [3-9]. PDCM is a degenerative myocardial disease that is not secondary to any other disorder (as opposed to other dilated cardiomyopathies secondary to taurine or L-carnitine deficiencies, for example). It is the second most frequently encountered acquired cardiomyopathy in dogs after degenerative mitral valve disease. This is why most of this chapter is devoted to PDCM. Some specific cardiomyopathies will be covered in the second part of the chapter.

Primary Dilated Cardiomyopathy

In its classical form, PDCM is characterized by inotropic impairment leading to the dilation of one of the two ventricles (usually the left) or both ventricles simultaneously. Arrhythmias may precede the systolic dysfunction (ventricular arrhythmias in the Doberman Pinscher and atrial fibrillation in the Irish Wolfhound) [10,11].

PDCM mainly affects male dogs, usually young large breed adults (with the exception of the Cocker Spaniel and the Portuguese Water Dog) [3,7,12]. The prevalence of this disease, which is variable according to literature, is quite high in certain breeds. It affects 25% of Irish Wolfhounds and 47% to 58% of Doberman Pinschers [4,7,11,13-15].

PDCM has been shown to be hereditary in several breeds [16]. An autosomal dominant transmission with incomplete penetrance has thus been reported in the Doberman Pinscher, the Irish Wolfhound, and the Newfoundland [17-19]. In contrast, an autosomal recessive transmission has been described for the juvenile PDCM form in the Portuguese Water Dog. Transmission linked to the X chromosome has been shown in the Great Dane [20,21].

Changes in Bidimensional and TM Echocardiography

Description

Bidimensional (2D) and time-motion (TM) echocardiographic anomalies associated with classical forms of PDCM are dependent on the stage of the disease [3,4,7,22-27].

1. Early PDCM is characterized by moderate decrease in inotropy, documented by the reduction of the shortening fraction (SF) and the systolic left ventricular dilation. The left ventricular diastolic diameter remains normal, similar to the other cardiac cavities (Figure 12-1).

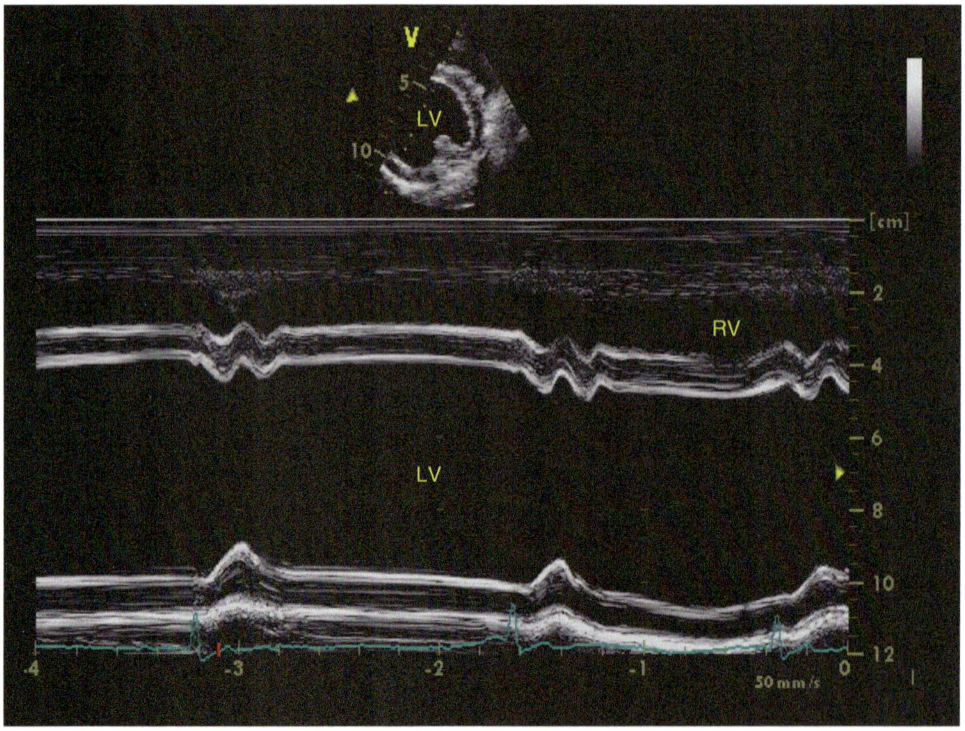

• **Fig. 12-1** Transventricular time-motion (TM) echocardiogram in an exercise-intolerant Weinberger with early dilated cardiomyopathy without congestive heart failure. The cardiomyopathy is characterized in this instance by a slightly decreased shortening fraction (22%) as well as a reduced systolic wall thickness (10% thickening). In addition (not visible on this TM echocardiogram), the left ventricle was rounded (sphericity index = 1) and the ejection fraction, calculated using the Simpson method, was <40% (39%). *LV,* Left ventricle; *RV,* right ventricle. (Photo credit: Valérie Chetboul.)

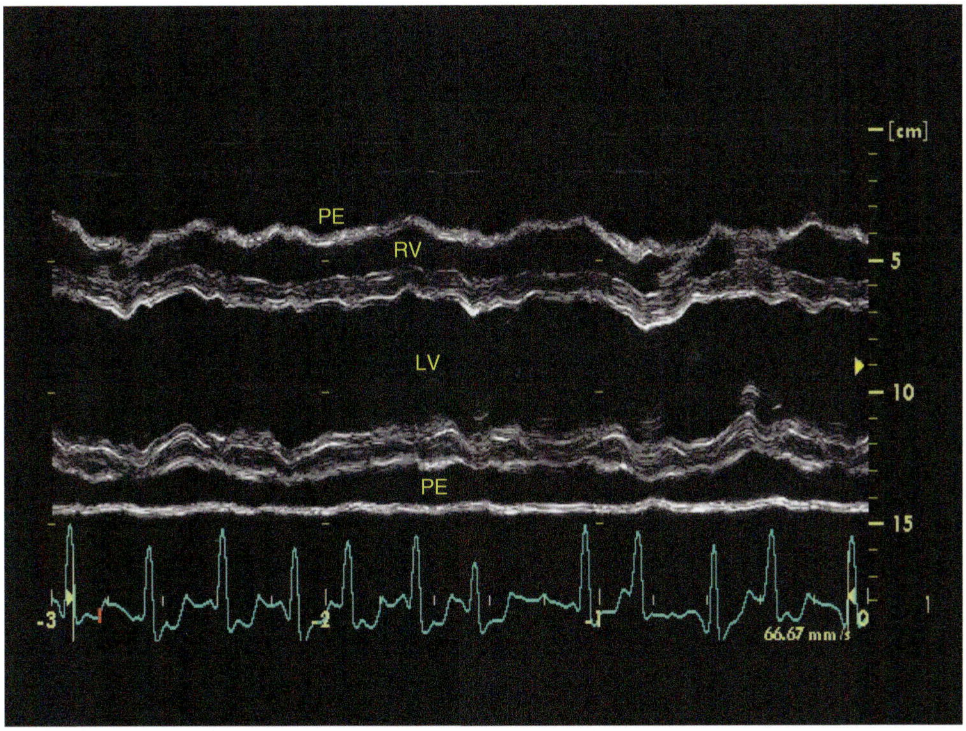

• **Fig. 12-2** Transventricular time-motion (TM) echocardiogram of a Bordeaux Mastiff with advanced dilated cardiomyopathy and congestive heart failure. In this instance, cardiomyopathy is characterized by a markedly decreased shortening fraction (12%), left ventricular systolic dilation, decreased systolic wall thickness, pericardial effusion (PE), and atrial fibrillation, documented by the concomitant electrocardiographic trace. *LV,* Left ventricle; *RV,* right ventricle. (Photo credit: Valérie Chetboul.)

2. As the disease progresses, the systolic dysfunction becomes more pronounced (the SF can even drop below 10%) and the left ventricular dilation becomes systolic and diastolic (Figure 12-2). Dalmatians and Doberman Pinschers are known for their tendency to develop marked chambers dilations.
3. Although systolic dysfunctions are generally diffuse and homogeneous, some myocardial zones can be more affected than others, hence the importance of evaluating the left ventricular inotropism not just in a single dimension (i.e., the SF in TM mode) but in two dimensions, keeping in mind the global left ventricular geometry. Indeed, the left ventricular morphology changes as PDCM progresses and a single short axis view can only imperfectly reflect this tridimensional change. Planimetric methods (such as the Simpson method) (Figure 12-3), using the endocardial contour of the long axis of the left ventricular chamber, take into account the global left ventricular morphology. This is why the American and European echocardiography societies are recommending the Simpson method for evaluation of the left ventricular volumes [26]. This formula allows one to calculate these volumes in end-systole and end-diastole and from these to calculate the ejection fraction (EF) (expressed in % and defined as the difference of the two volumes divided by the end-diastolic volume). An EF <40% is classically considered a sign of reduced inotropy in dogs.
4. End-diastolic and end-systolic ventricular volumes calculated using the Simpson method can also be indexed to the body area (end-diastolic volume index [EDVI] and end-systolic volume index [ESVI]). These two indices, calculated using this method, have been proven to be more sensitive than TM mode–derived parameters in detecting early forms of PDCM in the Doberman Pinscher. An EVSI >55 mL/m^2 allows the diagnosis of PDCM with 94.4%

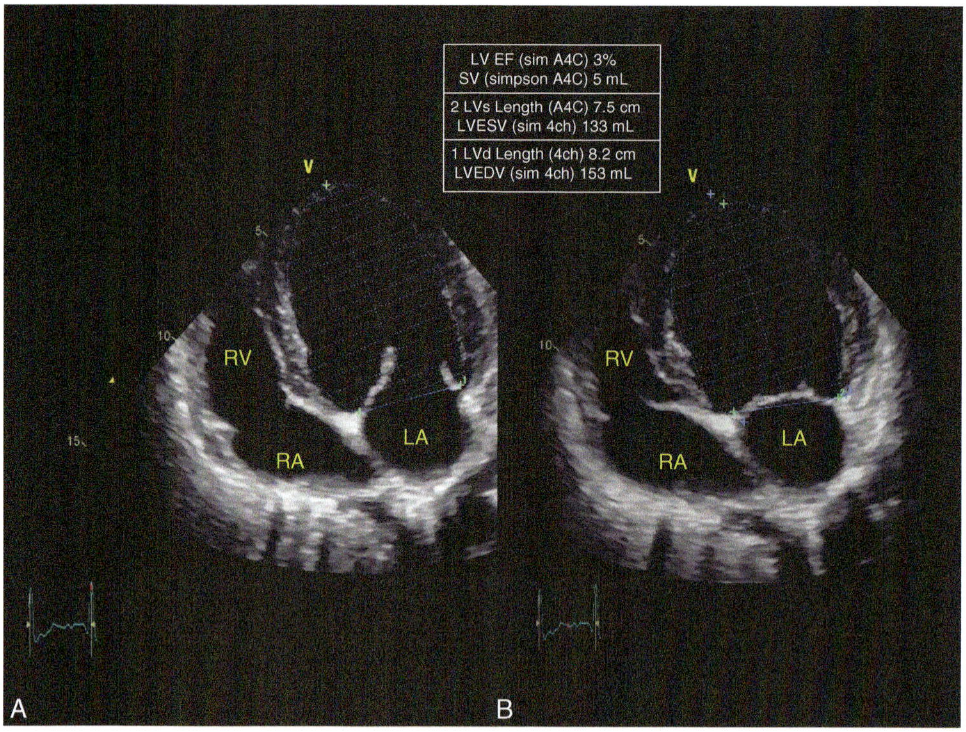

• **Fig. 12-3** Calculation of the left ventricular volumes in (A) end-diastole and (B) end-systole using the Simpson monoplane method, from a left apical 4 chambers view in a Doberman Pinscher with dilated cardiomyopathy. The Simpson monoplane method consists of determining the left ventricular volume by tracing the endocardial contour of the aforementioned cavity on a single 4 chambers view. The ventricular area thus delimited is cut into a series of "slices" or "disks" of equal thickness, perpendicular to the long axis of the left ventricle. The sum of these volumes is equal to the total left ventricular volume. The ejection fraction (defined as the difference of the ventricular diastolic and systolic volumes divided by the diastolic volume) is then calculated. In this particular case, it has collapsed (3%). *LA,* Left atrium; *RA,* right atrium; *RV,* right ventricle. (Photo credit: Valérie Chetboul.)

sensitivity and 97% specificity, while an EVDI >95 mL/m^2 allows this diagnosis with 96.9% sensitivity and 94.4% specificity [23]. In contrast, TM left ventricular diameters have a lower sensitivity in the detection of PDCM in this breed (maximum sensitivity of 71.6% for an end-diastolic left ventricular diameter >49 mm) [23].

5. The thickness of the myocardial walls decreases with the progression of the disease (initially in systole—see Figures 12-1 and 12-2—then in diastole).
6. Alongside these chamber dilations and decreased inotropy, the left ventricular cavity becomes more spherical (Video 12-1). This ventricular morphologic change is made more obvious by the concomitant hypotrophy, or even atrophy, of the papillary muscles (Figure 12-4 and Video 12-2). This can be documented by the sphericity index (SI) calculation. The SI is defined as the ratio between the end-diastolic base-apex left ventricle (LV) length divided by the end-diastolic diameter of the same cavity measured in TM mode. The base-apex length is measured on a right parasternal long axis or left apical 4 chambers view. It is best to select the view that will allow an optimal view of the apex [4,22]. The SI, usually ≥1.65, decreases gradually with the progression of PDCM.

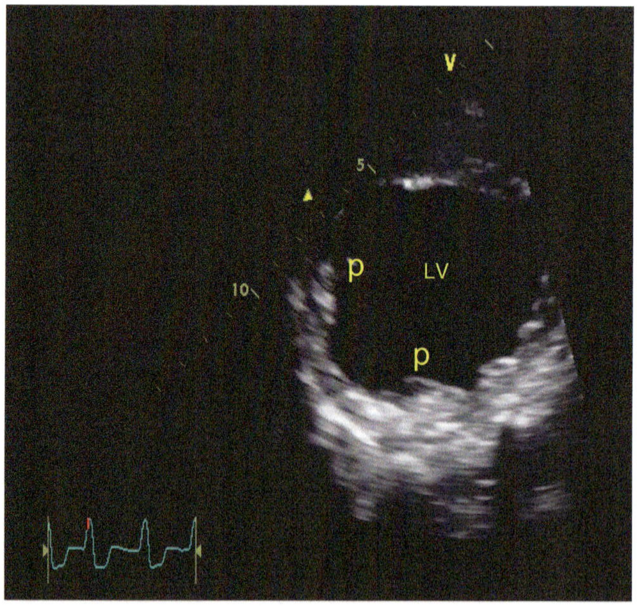

• **Fig. 12-4** Bidimensional (2D) echocardiogram (right parasternal short axis transventricular view) in a Newfoundland with advanced dilated cardiomyopathy. Note the atrophy of the two left papillary muscles (p) and the abnormal rounded shape of the dilated left ventricular cavity (LV). (Photo credit: Valérie Chetboul.)

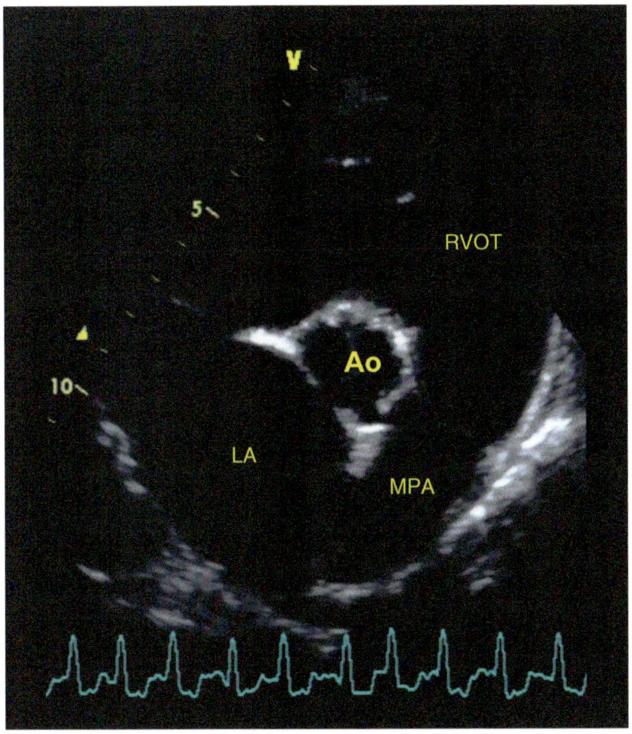

• **Fig. 12-5** Left atrial dilation in a Boxer with dilated cardiomyopathy, atrial fibrillation, and congestive heart failure. This right parasternal short axis transaortic view shows marked left atrial dilation (LA/Ao ratio = 2.1). Note also the dilation of the right ventricular outflow tract (RVOT) due to the combination of right-sided cardiac dysfunction and pulmonary arterial hypertension. *Ao,* Aorta; *LA,* left atrium; *MPA,* main pulmonary artery. (Photo credit: Valérie Chetboul.)

7. Next, left atrial dilation appears (Figure 12-5) due to various causes: LV end-systolic pressure increase (preventing optimal left atrial drainage) and presence of systolic mitral regurgitation (Figure 12-6). Mitral regurgitation results from both mitral leaflets and LV remodeling. The latter leads to mitral annulus stretching and altered tension of the chordae tendineae because of the shrinkage of the papillary muscles. All of these factors play a role in decreasing the systolic leakproofness of the mitral apparatus.
8. More advanced cases of PDCM are characterized by right atrial and ventricular dilation. These right cardiac changes have two causes: pulmonary arterial hypertension (secondary to left myocardial changes discussed above) and the presence of right myocardial lesions. In the most severe cases, the four cardiac cavities are simultaneously dilated at the time of diagnosis.
9. Signs of congestive heart failure (CHF) (see Figure 12-2) are present in the final stages of classical PDCM: pleural effusion, pericardial effusion, caudal vena cava dilation, venous hepatic congestion, and ascites.
10. Complications due to thrombosis associated with canine PDCM are very rare. They are generally seen only in association with acute tachyarrhythmias and marked cavity dilation (Figure 12-7).

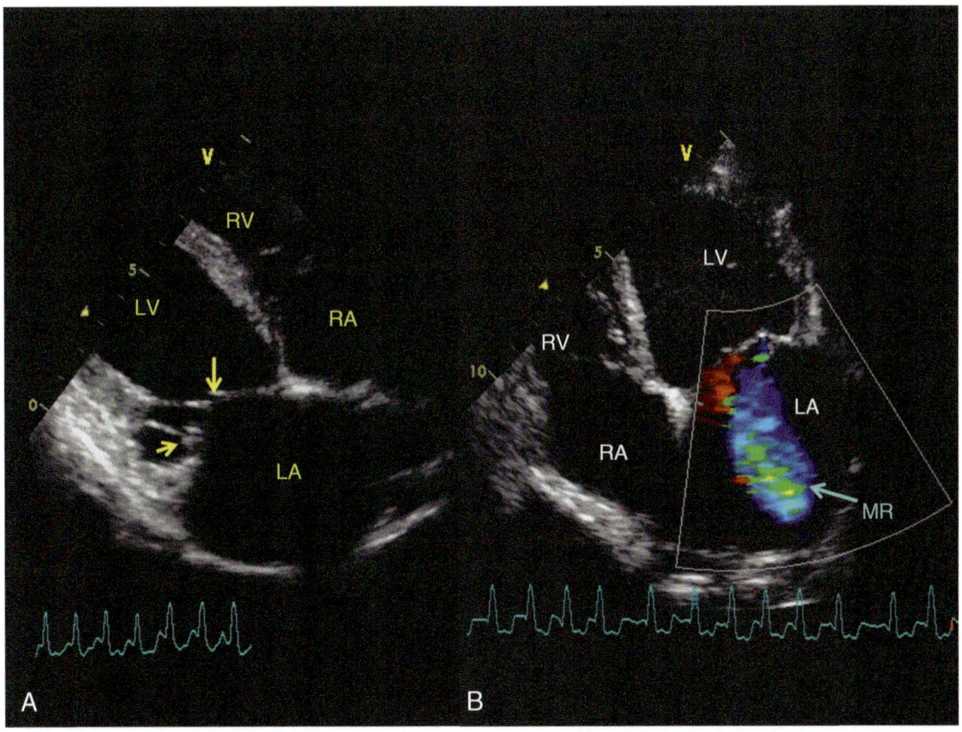

• **Fig. 12-6** Bidimensional (2D) echocardiograms in a Boxer with dilated cardiomyopathy (the same animal as in Figure 12-5): (A) right parasternal long axis 4 chambers view and (B) left apical 4 chambers view in color Doppler mode. Note the thickening of the mitral leaflets *(arrows)* and left chordae tendineae in part A. These mitral lesions associated with left ventricular dilation explain the systolic mitral regurgitation (MR) seen in color Doppler mode in part B and hence the left apical systolic murmur detected by cardiac auscultation. *LA,* Left atrium; *LV,* left ventricle; *RA,* right atrium; *RV,* right ventricle. (Photo credit: Valérie Chetboul.)

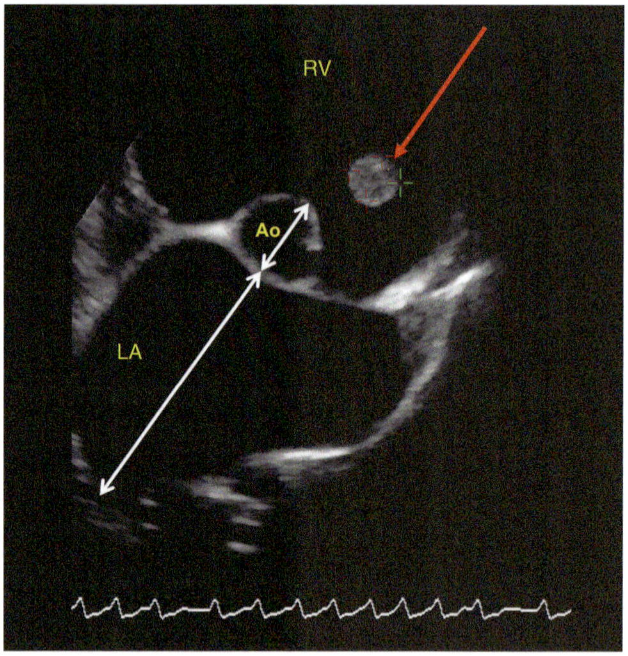

• **Fig. 12-7** Documentation of a thrombus *(red arrow)* at the entrance of the right ventricular outflow tract in a dog with dilated cardiomyopathy. This right parasternal short axis transaortic view also shows marked left atrial dilation (LA/Ao ratio = 3.3). *Ao,* Aorta; *LA,* left atrium; *RV,* right ventricle. (Photo credit: Valérie Chetboul.)

11. The other indirect signs of myocardial function impairment in TM mode are:
    A. Transmitral TM view:
        a. Increased E-septal separation between the mitral E point and the interventricular septum (Figure 12-8). Contrary to former assumptions, this anomaly (due to a reduction in the movement of the mitral leaflets because of decreased left atrial drainage) is not an early sign of systolic dysfunction but rather a late sign.
        b. Doming (known as "B" notch) of the anterior mitral valve leaflet at the end of its diastolic motion (associated with delayed closing of the mitral leaflets due to the elevated left ventricular end-diastolic filling pressure). This doming is only observed with marked left chambers dilation, often accompanied by CHF.
        c. Absence of the mitral A point during atria fibrillation (see Figure 12-8).
    B. Transaortic TM view:
        a. Decreased amplitude of the aortic cusps opening and sometimes even absence of opening with some ventricular contractions (Figure 12-9).
        b. Increase in the pre-ejection period (PEP) and pre-ejection/ejection time ratio (PEP/ET >0.4). However, the PEP/ET ratio is a fairly

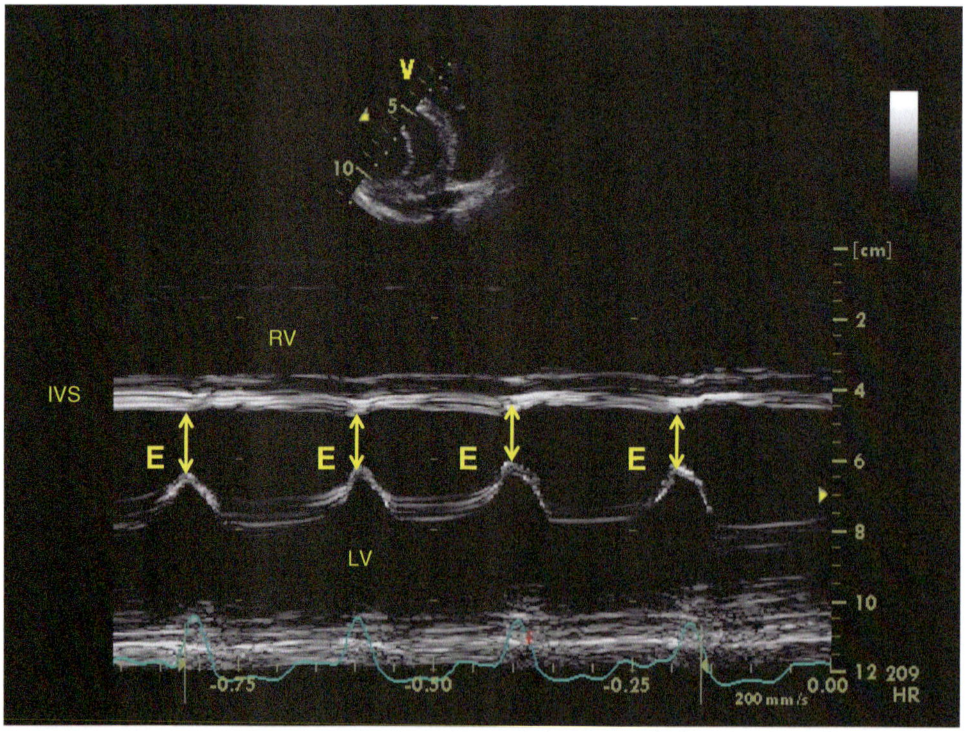

• **Fig. 12-8** Transmitral time-motion (TM) echocardiogram in a Boxer with dilated cardiomyopathy. The distance *(double arrows)* between the mitral E point and the interventricular septum (IVS) is increased (14 mm). Note the absence of the mitral A point due to the presence of atrial fibrillation. *LV,* Left ventricle; *RV,* right ventricle. (Photo credit: Valérie Chetboul.)

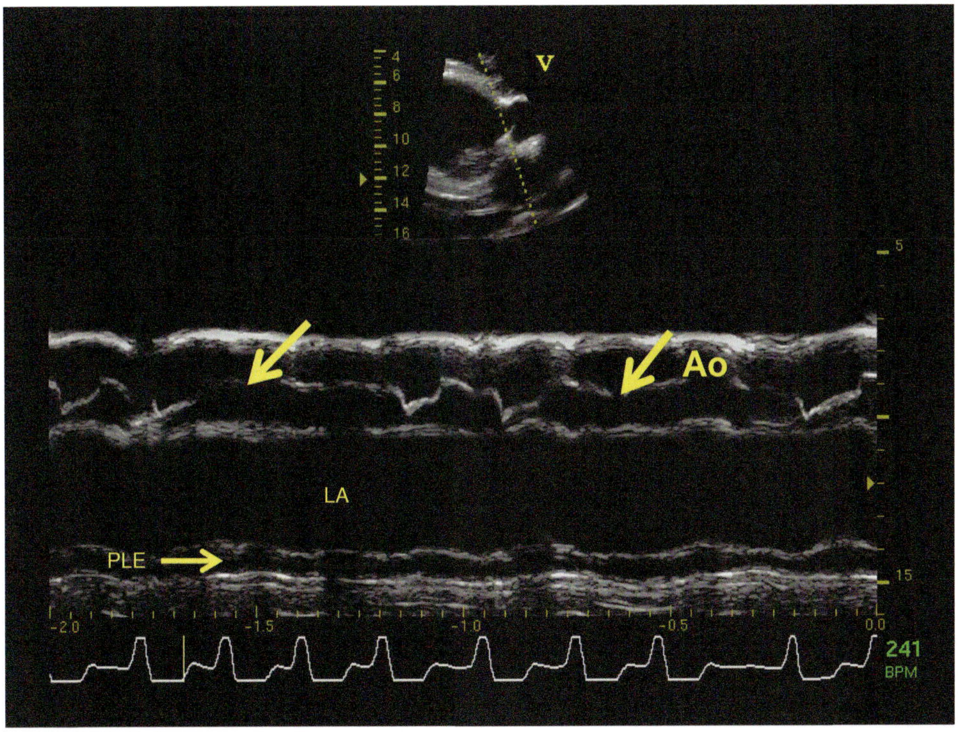

• **Fig. 12-9** Transaortic time-motion (TM) echocardiogram in a dog with dilated cardiomyopathy and atrial fibrillation. Note that some ventricular depolarizations are not followed by aortic valve opening *(arrows)*. *Ao,* Aorta; *LA,* left atrium; *PLE,* pleural effusion. (Photo credit: Valérie Chetboul.)

insensitive indicator of myocardial dysfunction. It can remain normal even in the more advanced forms of PDCM. It is therefore a minor diagnostic criterion of PDCM.

The European Society of Veterinary Cardiology (ESVC) has proposed a scoring system to establish the echocardiographic diagnosis of PDCM, as is already the case in humans [4]. This system defines major and minor diagnostic criteria:

- *Major criteria:* left ventricular systolic or diastolic dilation, increased left ventricular sphericity (decreased SI), decreased SF or EF (Simpson method).
- *Minor criteria:* ventricular arrhythmias in some breeds (such as Boxers and Doberman Pinschers), atrial fibrillation, increased E-septal separation, PEP/ET >0.4, equivocal SF values, left atrial or biatrial dilation.

By assigning 3 points to each major criterion present and 1 point to each minor criterion present, a score of 6 or more favors PDCM. Even though this scoring system has not yet been validated in dogs with PDCM, it has been shown to be positively correlated with the heart rate and negatively correlated with several systolic function indices (subendocardial and subepicardial radial systolic myocardial velocities, basal longitudinal systolic myocardial velocities, and radial systolic strain) [22].

Special Cases

Compared to humans, the difficulty in diagnosing canine PDCM (especially the asymptomatic or "occult" forms) comes largely from the breed- and weight-related variations in cavity dimensions and systolic function indices.

In the Doberman Pinscher, left ventricular diameters ≥49 mm in diastole and ≥42 mm in systole are usually considered compatible with PDCM (assuming exclusion of other causes of dilation) [23,25]. These criteria differ slightly between authors (e.g., >50 mm and >40 mm for Calvert et al [27]) and also can vary according to body weight. An E-septal separation >9 mm and a SF ≤25% are also indicative of possible PDCM [27]. A SF between 26% and 29% can be considered equivocal [27].

In the Irish Wolfhound, left ventricular diameters >61.2 mm in diastole and >41 mm in systole, a SF <25%, an EVSI >41 mL/m^2, and an E-septal separation >10 mm are indicative of PDCM [7,28].

Differential Diagnosis

Decreased systolic function with left chambers dilation can also be a complication of other cardiopathies, which must be excluded prior to confirming PDCM [4]. These include:

- Some congenital cardiopathies: patent ductus arteriosus, mitral valve dysplasia.

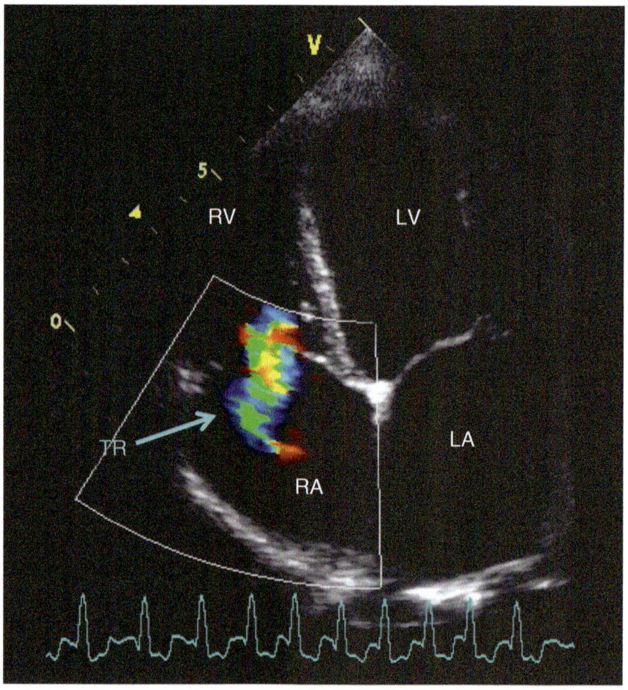

• **Fig. 12-10** Systolic pulmonary arterial hypertension in a Boxer with dilated cardiomyopathy with generalized congestive heart failure (pulmonary edema and ascites). This left apical 4 chambers view shows a turbulent jet of tricuspid regurgitation (TR) with an important colorimetric area (491 mm²). *LA,* Left atrium; *LV,* left ventricle; *RA,* right atrium; *RV,* right ventricle. (Photo credit: Valérie Chetboul.)

- Some acquired cardiopathies: degenerative mitral valve disease (which can affect large breed dogs [29] like PDCM), aortic regurgitation secondary to endocarditis.
- Sustained tachyarrhythmia leading to cardiomyopathies referred to as "tachy-induced."

A decrease in the systolic function can also have an extracardiac origin: taurine and L-carnitine deficiencies, hypothyroidism, or medications (especially anthracyclines).

Finally, a decreased SF can be observed in athletic animals and can accompany bradycardia.

Changes in Conventional Doppler Mode

Anomalies associated with PDCM observed in conventional Doppler mode include, either in isolation or combined [4,24,30]:

- Presence of mitral regurgitation (see "Description" above; see Figure 12-6).
- Presence of high-velocity tricuspid regurgitation when systolic pulmonary arterial hypertension is present (Figures 12-10 and 12-11) and the presence of a high-velocity diastolic pulmonic regurgitation in cases of diastolic pulmonary arterial hypertension.

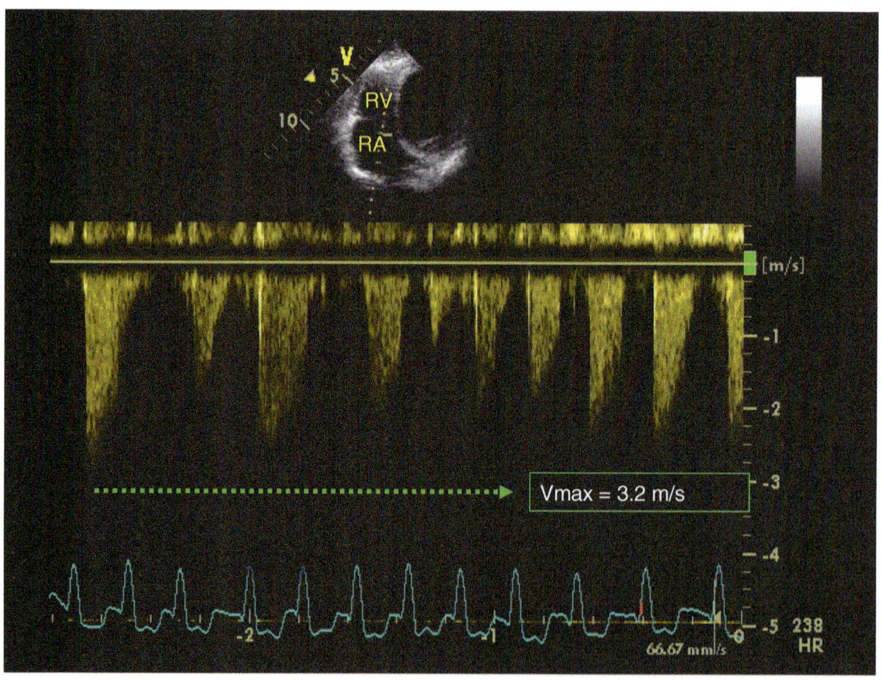

• **Fig. 12-11** Systolic pulmonary arterial hypertension in a Boxer with dilated cardiomyopathy (same dog as in Figure 12-10). The maximal velocity of the tricuspid regurgitation is measured on the continuous wave Doppler signal of the regurgitant jet, obtained from a left apical 4 chambers view. Note that, in this dog, the spectral envelopes (negative because the regurgitant jet moves away from the transducer) can vary from one cycle to the next due to atrial fibrillation. The maximal regurgitant jet velocity (Vmax) is 3.2 m/s. According to the Bernoulli equation, the maximum right ventricular–right atrial systolic pressure gradient that governs this regurgitation is $4 \times 3.2^2 = 41$ mm Hg. The right atrial pressure can be estimated at 15 mm Hg due to the presence of ascites (right-sided heart failure). The right ventricular systolic pressure (generally equivalent to the systolic pulmonary arterial pressure) is therefore elevated, estimated at 41 + 15 = 56 mm Hg. *RA,* Right atrium; *RV,* right ventricle. (Photo credit: Valérie Chetboul.)

- A restrictive mitral profile (Figure 12-12) characterized by a large E wave (due to left atrial pressure increase), a small A wave, and a decrease in the deceleration time of the E wave. A short deceleration time of the E wave (<80 ms) was shown to have a better negative prognostic value than other echocardiographic indices or even the stage of heart failure and presence of atrial fibrillation [30].
- Absence of the mitral A wave during atrial fibrillation (see Figure 12-12).
- Decrease in the maximal velocity of the transaortic flow, whose envelope becomes symmetric (Figure 12-13).

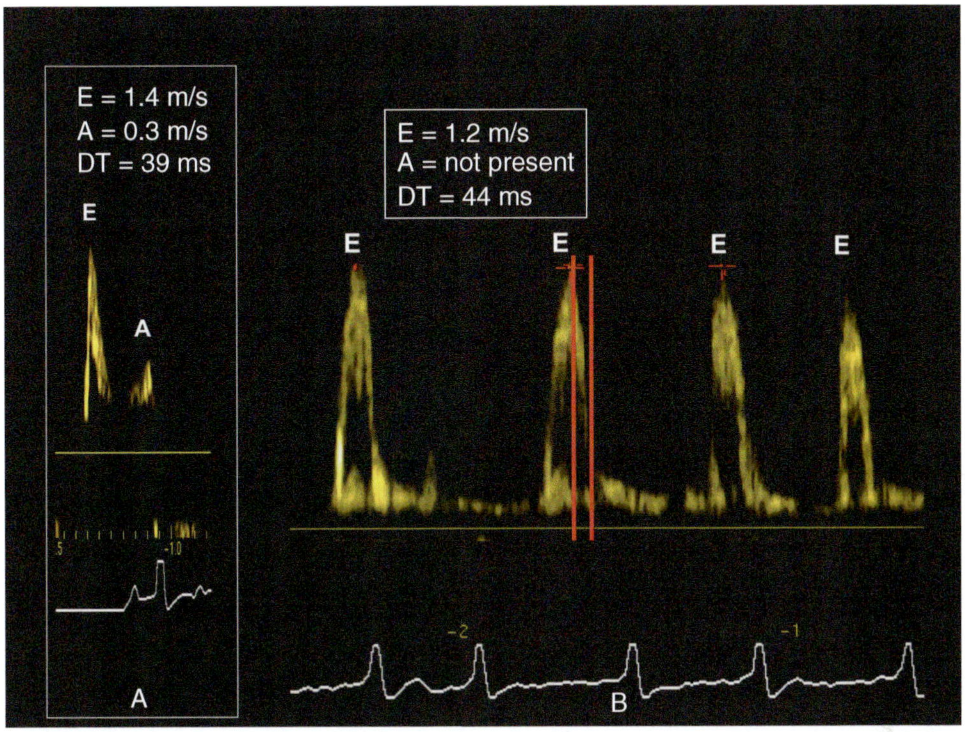

• **Fig. 12-12** Examples of mitral Doppler anomalies in two dogs with dilated cardiomyopathy (pulsed wave Doppler mode). A, The E and A mitral waves are present but the deceleration time (DT) is short (39 ms). B, The A wave is absent because of atrial fibrillation and the deceleration time is shortened (44 ms). (Photo credit: Valérie Chetboul.)

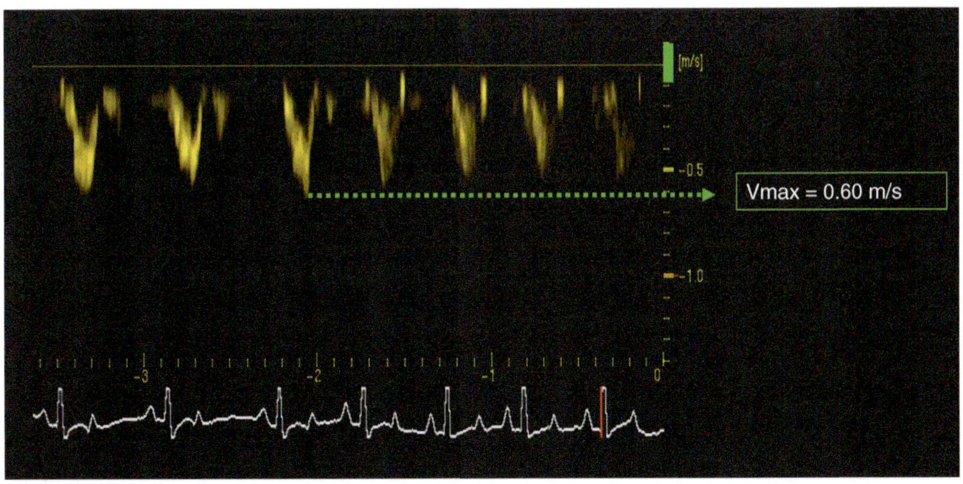

• **Fig. 12-13** Examples of transaortic flow anomalies in a dog with dilated cardiomyopathy (pulsed wave Doppler mode). The transaortic flow maximal velocity (Vmax = 0.6 m/s) is reduced (minimum reference value [31] = 0.9 m/s). Note also the disappearance of the normal bladelike aspect (the spectral envelope shape resembles that of a transpulmonic flow). (Photo credit: Valérie Chetboul.)

Changes in Tissue Doppler and Related Techniques

As validated in the awake dog in 2D color mode, myocardial tissue Doppler (or tissue Doppler imaging [TDI]; see details in Chapter 4) has allowed our team to demonstrate for the first time that canine PDCM is associated with not only radial but also longitudinal myocardial dysfunction of the left ventricular free wall [22,32,33].

Radial dysfunction is primarily systolic and is characterized by a decreased endoepicardial systolic gradient and reduced subepicardial and subendocardial radial systolic velocities (Figures 12-14 and 12-15) [22]. This systolic dysfunction may be present before the appearance of 2D and TM echocardiographic changes, thus contributing to the early diagnosis of PDCM [34]. In addition, but more rarely, postsystolic contractions may be observed, most likely due to ischemic phenomena (see Figure 12-15).

The left longitudinal dysfunction is characterized by decreased basal systolic velocities, leading to a decreased base-apex systolic gradient [22]. However, this longitudinal systolic impairment is less important than the radial impairment and not as well correlated as the latter to the heart failure stage, the ESVC score, or even the SI and SF [22]. To the contrary, the left longitudinal diastolic function is more frequently impaired than the radial one (Figure 12-16). Likewise, the left longitudinal motion is more frequently associated with postsystolic contractions [22].

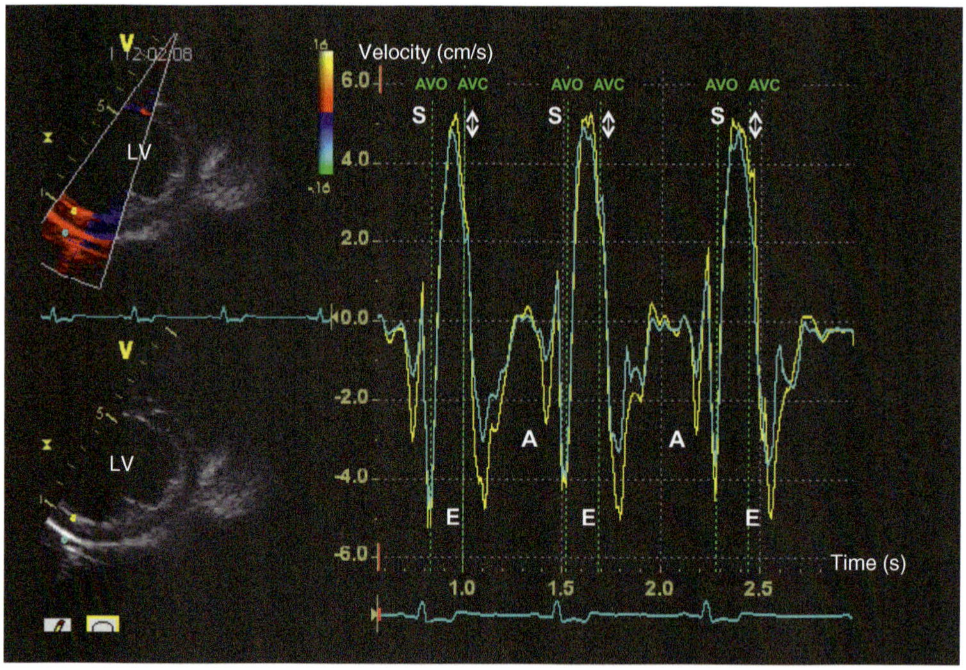

• **Fig. 12-14** Impairment of the left radial systolic and diastolic function analyzed by color bidimensional (2D) tissue Doppler imaging (TDI) in a dog with dilated cardiomyopathy. *Top left,* The color-coded velocities are superimposed in real time on a right parasternal short axis transventricular cross-section. The left ventricular free wall myocardial velocities are analyzed simultaneously in two circular segments, each measuring 2 mm in diameter: a subendocardial segment *(yellow)* and a subepicardial segment *(green)*. In both segments, each wave includes a positive systolic wave reaching its maximum at S and two negative E and A waves, concomitant with early diastole and end-diastole, respectively. The tracings obtained show that the subendocardium moves more rapidly *(yellow curve)* than the subepicardium *(green curve)* during both systole and diastole, thus defining an intramyocardial speed gradient throughout the cardiac cycle. Meanwhile, the systolic gradient is greatly reduced *(white double arrows)*, confirming a radial systolic dysfunction. *AVC,* Aortic valve closing; *AVO,* aortic valve opening; *LV,* left ventricle. (Photo credit: Valérie Chetboul.)

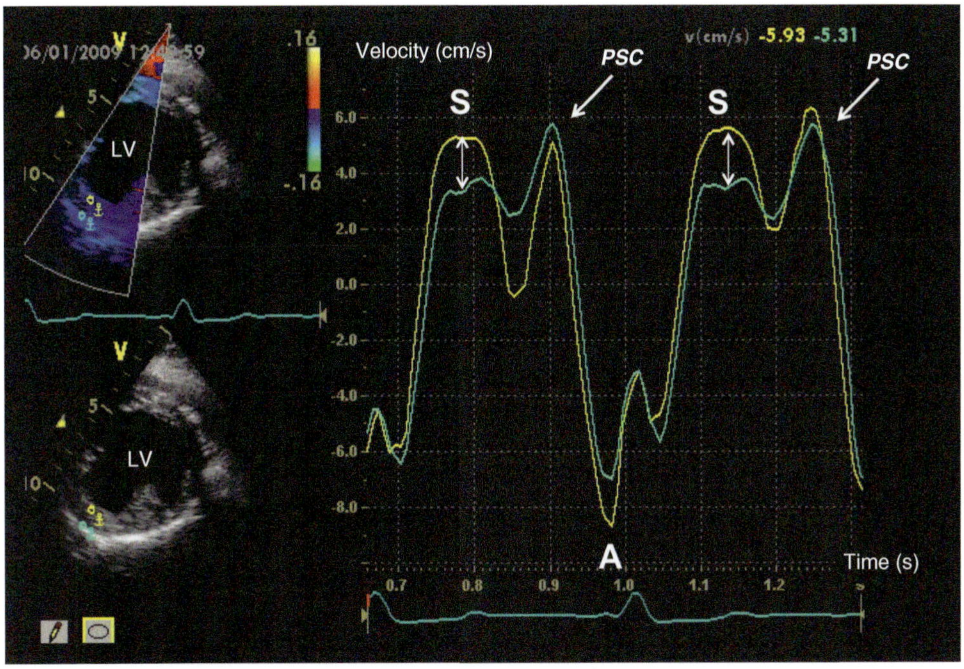

• **Fig. 12-15** Impairment of the left radial systolic and diastolic functions analyzed by color bidimensional (2D) tissue Doppler imaging (TDI) in a dog with dilated cardiomyopathy (same dog as in Figure 12-14). Functional myocardial anomalies include a decreased systolic gradient *(white double arrows)*, the presence of postsystolic contraction (PSC) leading to the disappearance of the early diastolic E wave, and the presence of a single high-amplitude end-diastolic A wave. *LV,* Left ventricle; *S,* systolic peak wave. (Photo credit: Valérie Chetboul.)

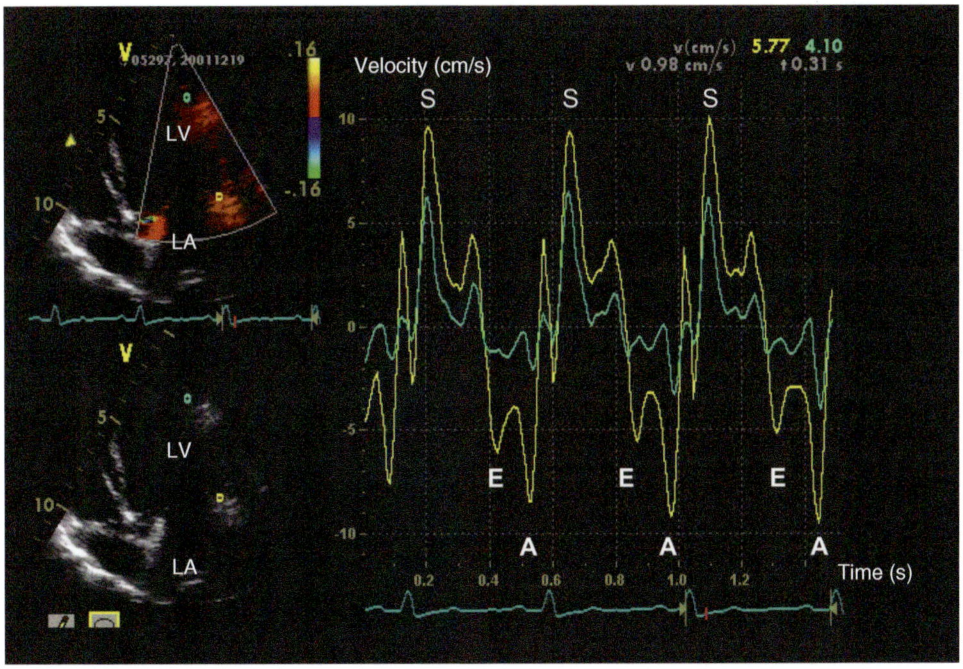

• **Fig. 12-16** Impairment of the left longitudinal diastolic function analyzed using color bidimensional (2D) tissue Doppler imaging (TDI) in a dog with dilated cardiomyopathy (same animal as in Figure 12-14). *Top left,* The color-coded velocities are superimposed in real time on a left apical 4 chambers cross-section. The TDI analysis was performed on two circular segments, each measuring 2 mm in diameter, of the left ventricular free wall, one at the base *(yellow curve)* and one at the apex *(green curve)*. In both segments, each wave includes a positive systolic wave reaching its maximum at S and two negative waves, E and A, concomitant with early diastole and end-diastole, respectively. At the base, as at the apex, the impaired diastolic function is characterized by an E/A ratio <1. *LA,* Left atrium; *LV,* left ventricle. (Photo credit: Valérie Chetboul.)

Another TDI change associated with PDCM is decreased right longitudinal systolic velocities (linked to right myocardial degeneration and/or pulmonary arterial hypertension). This right-sided dysfunction is found even in the absence of conventional echocardiographic right heart changes (namely chamber dilation). Intra- and interventricular asynchrony may also be present (Figure 12-17).

The left longitudinal and radial myocardial dysfunction can also be documented using strain imaging, a technique derived from TDI that allows quantification of the regional myocardial strain, expressed as a percentage (see details in Chapter 4) [32]. The changes observed in strain imaging include decreased left radial and longitudinal systolic strain values and the presence of postsystolic contractions (Figures 12-18 and 12-19) [22]. A negative correlation has been demonstrated between the radial systolic strain and the stage of heart failure, as well as the ESVC score. A positive correlation was observed with the SI as well as the SF. However, none of these correlations were found for longitudinal systolic strain.

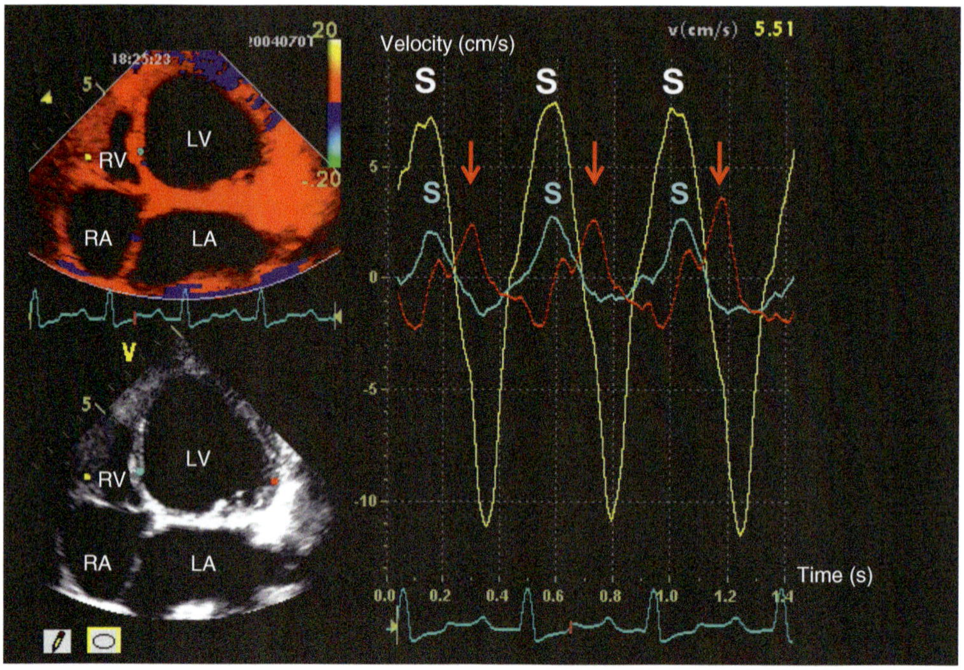

• **Fig. 12-17** Example of interventricular asynchrony analyzed using color bidimensional (2D) tissue Doppler imaging (TDI) in a dog with dilated cardiomyopathy. Longitudinal velocity profiles obtained in three basal segments of the left ventricular free wall *(red)*, the interventricular septum *(green)*, and the right ventricular myocardial wall *(yellow)* display delayed peak systolic velocity of the left wall *(arrows)* with respect to the other two segments. The maximum velocity is in fact recorded after the end of the T wave (on the electrocardiogram trace); it is a postsystolic contraction. *Top left,* The color-coded velocities are superimposed on the left apical 4 chambers cross-section. *LA,* Left atrium; *LV,* left ventricle; *RA,* right atrium; *RV,* right ventricle; *S,* maximum systolic myocardial velocity. (Photo credit: Valérie Chetboul.)

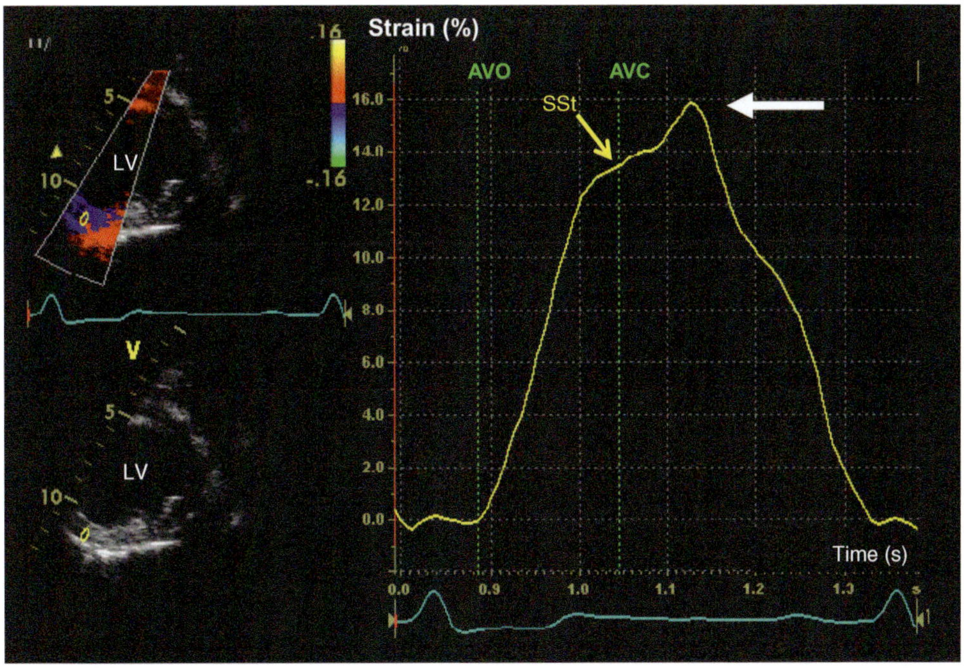

• **Fig. 12-18** Example of impaired left ventricular free wall radial segment strain analyzed using strain imaging in a dog with dilated cardiomyopathy. The systolic radial strain (or strain) is positive, as normally expected. However, its maximal value (SSt) between the opening (AVO) and closure (AVC) of the aortic valve is greatly decreased (13.5%; normal range = 45% to 87% [35]). In addition, a postsystolic contraction *(white arrow)* is present and it has a greater amplitude than SSt. Size of the region of interest (ROI): 5 mm/3 mm. *LV,* Left ventricle. (Photo credit: Valérie Chetboul.)

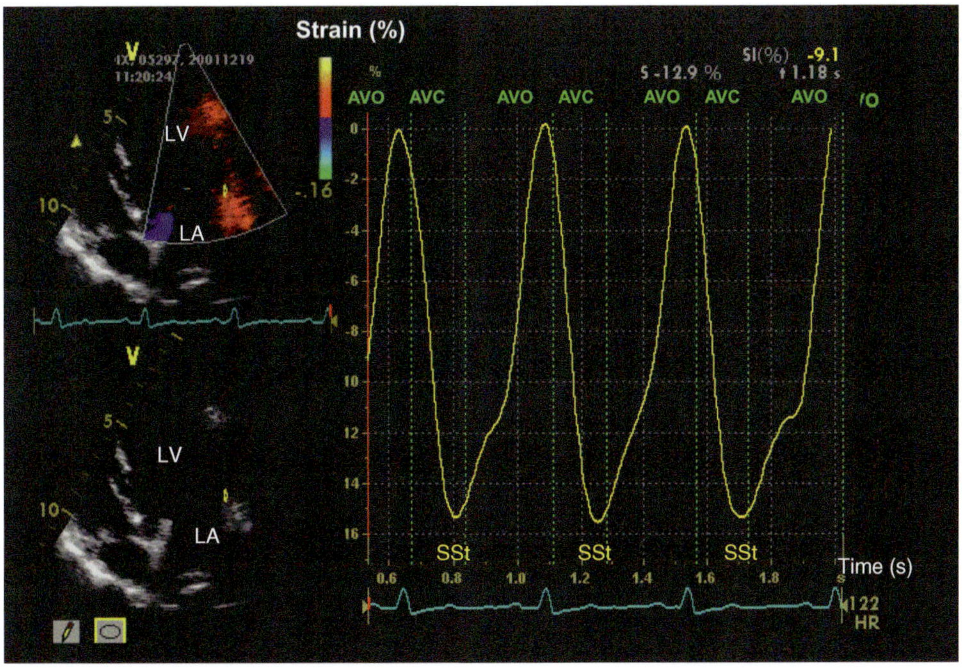

• **Fig. 12-19** Example of impaired longitudinal myocardial function analyzed at the left ventricular free wall base using strain imaging in a dog with dilated cardiomyopathy. The longitudinal systolic strain is negative and maximal at the end of systole, as normally expected. However, its absolute maximal value (SSt) is decreased (15.8%; normal range = 19% to 35% [35]). Size of the region of interest (ROI): 5 mm/3 mm. *AVC,* Aortic valve closure; *AVO,* aortic valve opening; *LA,* left atrium; *LV,* left ventricle. (Photo credit: Valérie Chetboul.)

Changes in Speckle Tracking Imaging

Contrary to TDI and derived modalities, speckle tracking imaging, based on a grayscale imaging modality, allows a "non-Doppler" evaluation of myocardial motion, this evaluation being angle independent (see details in Chapter 4) [36]. Therefore the analysis by speckle tracking imaging of the radial myocardial dysfunction associated with PDCM is complete. It is performed simultaneously on all segments making up the left myocardium (Figures 12-20 and 12-21) and, unlike TDI, is not limited to a portion of the left ventricular wall. This radial dysfunction includes, in isolation or in combination, the same abnormalities described by TDI and strain imaging: decreased systolic radial strain and presence of postsystolic radial contractions with or without early systolic stretching (see Figure 12-20 and Video 12-3). To these, we can add radial segmental asynchronism undetectable by Doppler techniques (see Figure 12-21).

PDCM is also characterized by global longitudinal myocardial dysfunction with segmental dyskinesia and asynchronism, readily detectable by speckle tracking imaging (Figure 12-22, Video 12-4). Finally, speckle tracking imaging has demonstrated that PDCM was associated with reduced left myocardial basal and apical torsion motions, leading to a reduction of the torsion of the entire left ventricle [37].

Other Cardiomyopathies

Hypertensive canine cardiomyopathy and other cardiomyopathies secondary to endocrine or metabolic disorders are discussed in Chapter 16. The only cardiomyopathies discussed here are cardiomyopathies associated with neuromuscular diseases, arrhythmogenic right ventricular cardiomyopathy, and uremic and hypertrophic cardiomyopathies.

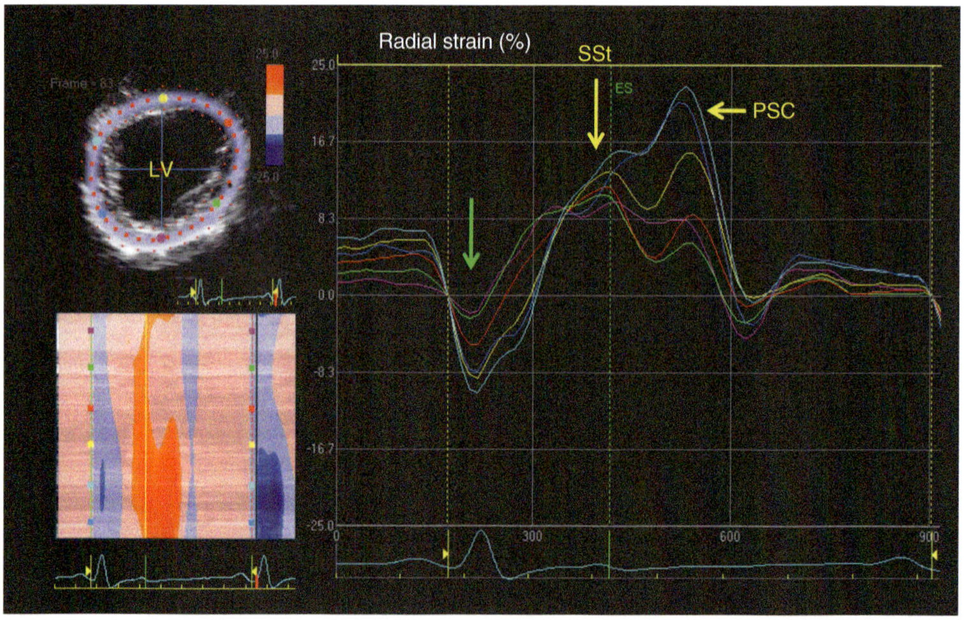

• **Fig. 12-20** Example of impaired left ventricular free wall radial segmental strain analyzed using speckle tracking imaging in a dog with dilated cardiomyopathy. Six traces of radial strain (%) as a function of time are recorded in six left myocardial ventricular wall and septum segments. Note that the strain of the six segments is abnormal: it begins with an early systolic shortening *(green arrow)*, followed by a weak positive strain (SSt), and ends, after the end of systole (ES), with a postsystolic contraction (PSC) of much greater amplitude than SSt in some segments. The color-coded strain is superimposed in real time on the bidimensional (2D) image *(top left)* and displayed as a function of time *(lower right)*. *LV,* Left ventricle. (Photo credit: Valérie Chetboul.)

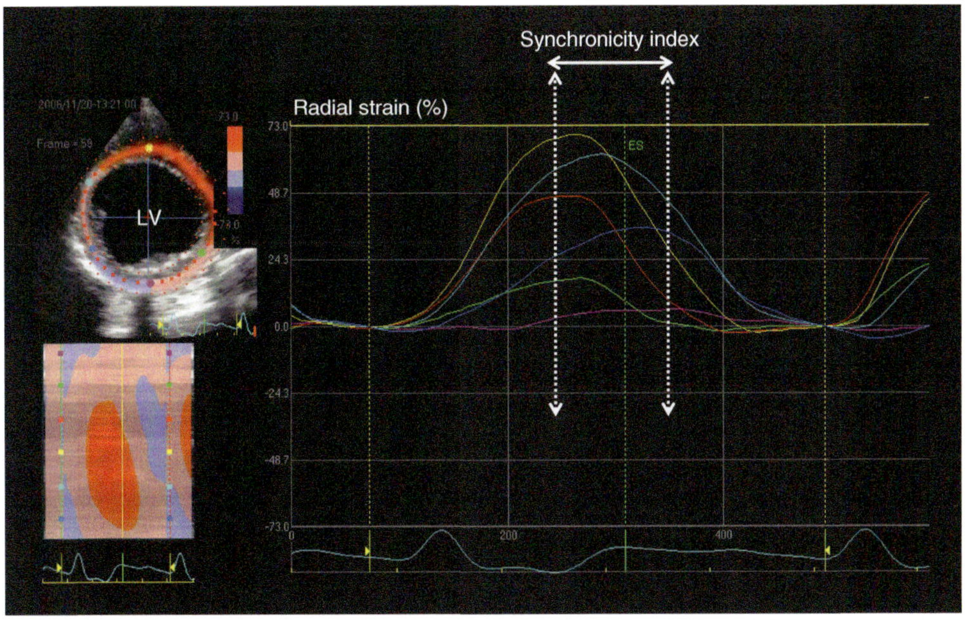

• **Fig. 12-21** Another example of impaired left ventricular free wall radial segment analyzed using speckle tracking imaging in a dog with dilated cardiomyopathy. Six traces of radial strain (%) as a function of time are recorded in six myocardial segments of the left ventricular free wall and the septum. Note that the strain of the six segments is abnormal: it is, as normally expected, positive but the strain peaks are not synchronous. Some appear prior to and others appear after the end of systole (ES). The synchronism index (interval between the first and last peak systolic strains) is increased (104 ms; normal range [33] = 0 to 45 ms). The color-coded strain is superimposed in real time on the bidimensional (2D) image *(top left)* and displayed as a function of time *(lower right)*. This last image confirms at a glance dyssynchrony between the six segments. *LV,* Left ventricle. (Photo credit: Valérie Chetboul.)

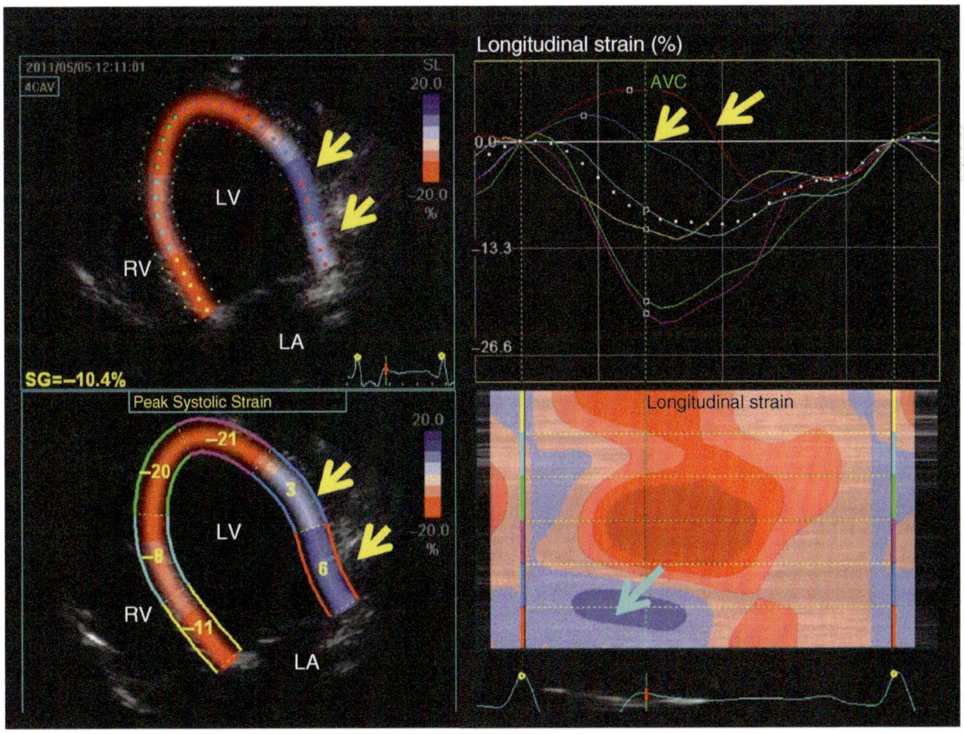

• **Fig. 12-22** Example of impaired left longitudinal segmental strain analyzed using speckle tracking imaging in a dog with dilated cardiomyopathy (left apical 4 chambers view). *Top left,* The color-coded longitudinal strain is superimposed on the bidimensional (2D) image with *(lower left)* the longitudinal peak systolic strain value displayed for each of the six segments analyzed (in this case, –21% to 6%). The absolute value of the peak global longitudinal strain (SG) is abnormally low (10.4%). In addition, left ventricular free wall dyskinesia is present, confirmed by the different segment colors (abnormally blue color of the left ventricular free wall segments showing positive instead of negative strain). This dyskinesia is seen again on the display of strain as a function of time *(blue arrow on lower right)*. Finally, the six curves of longitudinal strain as a function of time *(top right)* confirm the heterogeneity of the strain of the different segments, two of which *(yellow arrows)* have an opposite behavior to the other four (positive strain instead of negative). *AVC,* Aortic valve closure; *LA,* left atrium; *LV,* left ventricle; *RV,* right ventricle. (Photo credit: Valérie Chetboul.)

Cardiomyopathies and Neuromuscular Diseases

As in humans, a number of canine neuromuscular diseases are associated with musculoskeletal lesions and cardiomyopathies. The latter can be either dilated (Figures 12-23 to 12-29) or hypertrophic (Figures 12-30 and 12-31). The most studied is the cardiomyopathy associated with Golden Retriever muscular dystrophy (GRMD), a hereditary disease related to Duchenne disease in humans, linked to the X chromosome, and resulting from a spontaneous mutation of the dystrophin coding gene [38]. GRMD cardiomyopathy is characterized by necrotic myocardial lesions, replaced by fibrous, fatty, and mineralized zones. Initially, lesions are located mainly in the median and basal regions of the left ventricular free wall and interventricular septum, as well as in the papillary muscles. On 2D and TM echocardiograms, these appear as hyperechoic plaques without chamber dilation, or inotropic impairment (see Figure 12-23) [38]. At this stage, radial systolic function impairment, frequently associated with diastolic longitudinal dysfunction, is already detected by TDI (see Figures 12-24 and 12-25) [39,40]. Speckle tracking imaging enables identification of the signs of systolic dysfunction of PDCM: systolic strain reduction (longitudinal and radial), frequent presence of postsystolic contractions, dyskinesia, and segmental asynchrony (see Figures 12-26 and 12-27). As the disease progresses, the lesions involve the entire myocardium and the systolic dysfunction becomes evident in 2D and TM modes, either of a single (see Figure 12-28) or of both left walls (see Figure 12-29). For several months the left atrium remains normal in size (see Figure 12-28), then dilates, signaling the first step toward CHF.

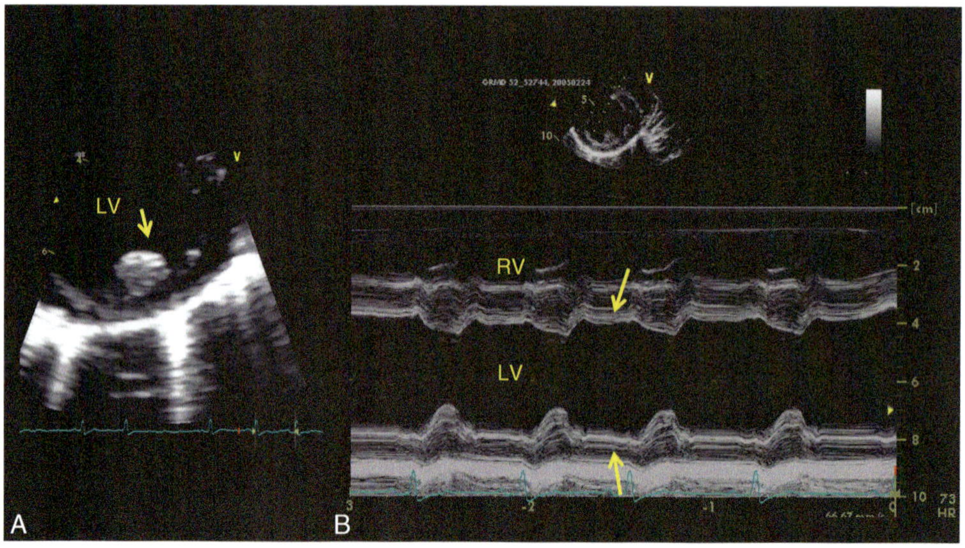

• **Fig. 12-23** Examples of early cardiomyopathy associated with hereditary myopathy (Golden Retriever muscular dystrophy [GRMD]). In this 4-month-old Golden Retriever puppy with GRMD, conventional echocardiography changes include the presence of hyperechoic areas of fibrosis and mineralization *(arrows)* in the left papillary muscles (A, right parasternal short axis transventricular view) and in the interventricular septum and left ventricular free wall (B, transventricular time-motion [TM] view). At this point, inotropy still "appears" normal (SF = 39% in panel B). *LV,* Left ventricle; *RV,* right ventricle. (Photo credit: Valérie Chetboul.)

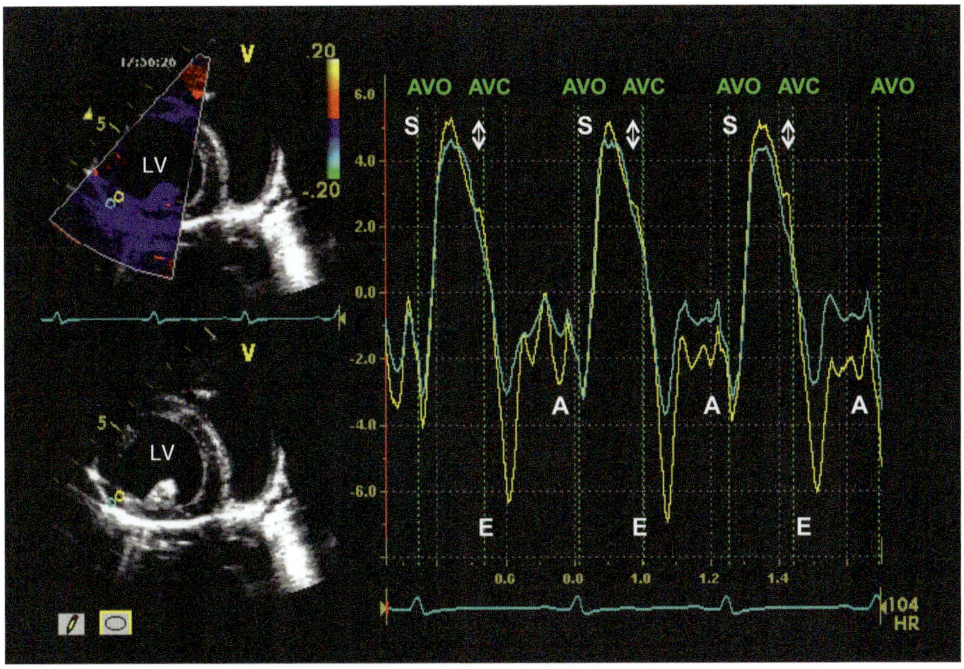

• **Fig. 12-24** Early impairment of the left ventricular free wall radial systolic function in a 4-month-old Golden Retriever puppy with Golden Retriever muscular dystrophy (GRMD) analyzed using color bidimensional (2D) tissue Doppler imaging (TDI). This systolic dysfunction, undetectable by conventional echography, is characterized by a significant decrease in the endoepicardial radial systolic gradient *(white double arrows)*. *Top left,* The color-coded velocities are superimposed in real time on the right parasternal short axis transventricular cross-section. The left ventricular free wall myocardial velocities are analyzed simultaneously in two circular segments of 2-mm diameter: a subendocardial segment *(yellow)* and a subepicardial segment *(green)*. *A,* Peak end-diastolic velocity; *AVC,* aortic valve closure; *AVO,* aortic valve opening; *E,* peak early diastolic velocity; *LV,* left ventricle; *S,* peak systolic velocity. (Photo credit: Valérie Chetboul.)

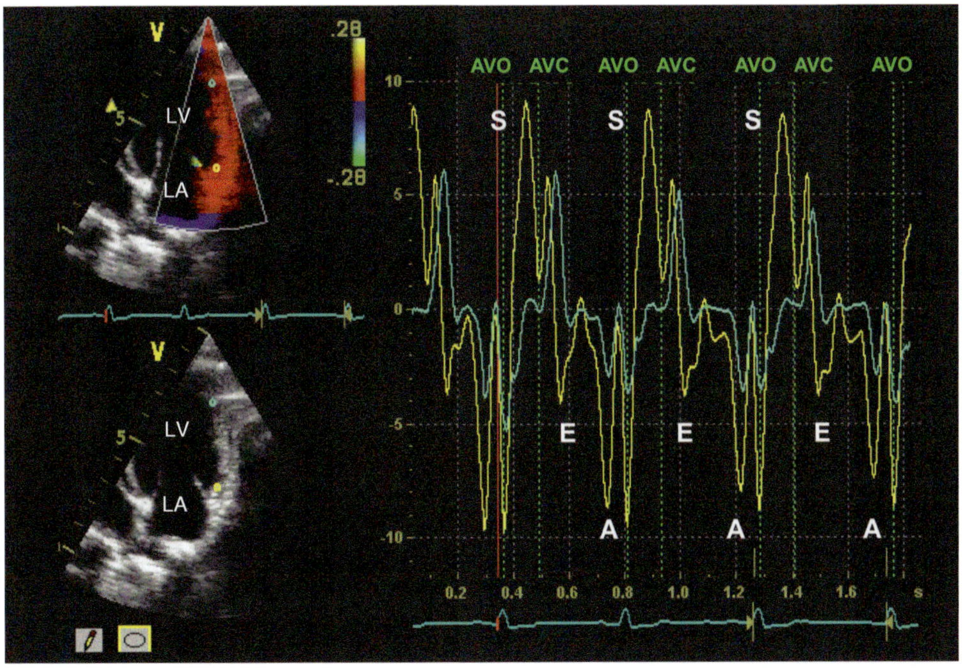

• **Fig. 12-25** Early impairment of the left ventricular free wall longitudinal diastolic function in a Golden Retriever puppy with Golden Retriever muscular dystrophy (GRMD) analyzed using color bidimensional (2D) tissue Doppler imaging (TDI). This diastolic dysfunction, not detectable by conventional Doppler (mitral E/A ratio >1), is characterized by inversion of the early diastolic and end-diastolic waves (E/A ratio <1). *Top left,* The color-coded velocities are superimposed in real time on the left apical 4 chambers cross-section. The left ventricular wall myocardial velocities are analyzed simultaneously at the base and apex (2-mm-diameter circular segments, *yellow* and *green* respectively). *A,* Peak end-diastolic velocity; *AVC,* aortic valve closure; *AVO,* aortic valve opening; *E,* peak early diastolic velocity; *LA,* left atrium; *LV,* left ventricle; *S,* peak systolic velocity. (Photo credit: Valérie Chetboul.)

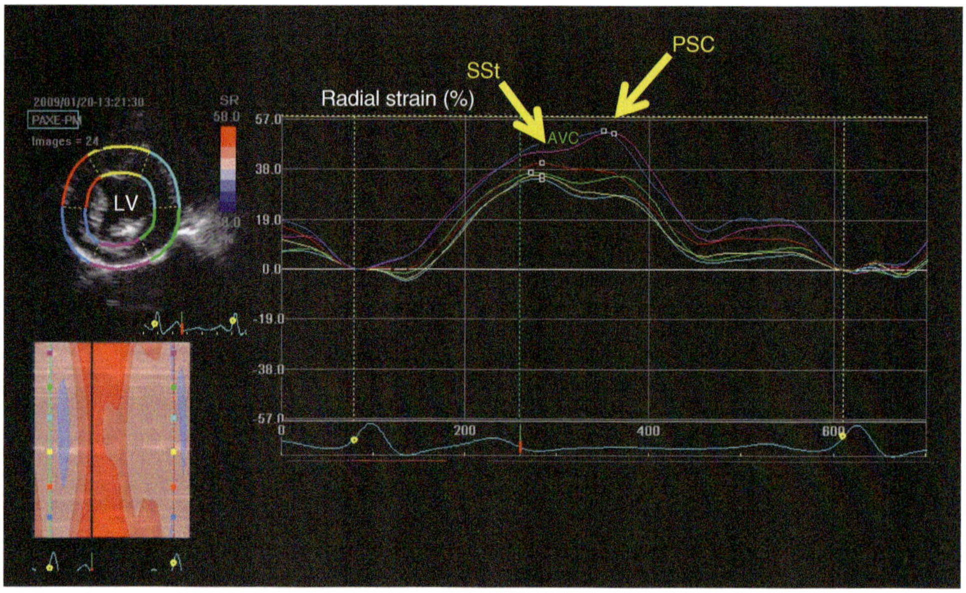

• **Fig. 12-26** Example of impaired left ventricular free wall radial segmental strain analyzed using speckle tracking imaging in a 4-month-old Golden Retriever puppy with Golden Retriever muscular dystrophy (GRMD). Six traces of radial strain (%) as a function of time are recorded in six left ventricular wall and septum myocardial segments. The radial systolic strain is, as normally expected, positive over the six analyzed segments. However, its maximum value (SSt) is reached after the aortic valve closure (AVC). In addition, a postsystolic contraction (PSC), with a greater amplitude than SSt, is present in two of the six segments. The color-coded strain is superimposed in real time on the bidimensional (2D) image *(top left)* and displayed as a function of time *(lower left)*. *LV,* Left ventricle. (Photo credit: Valérie Chetboul.)

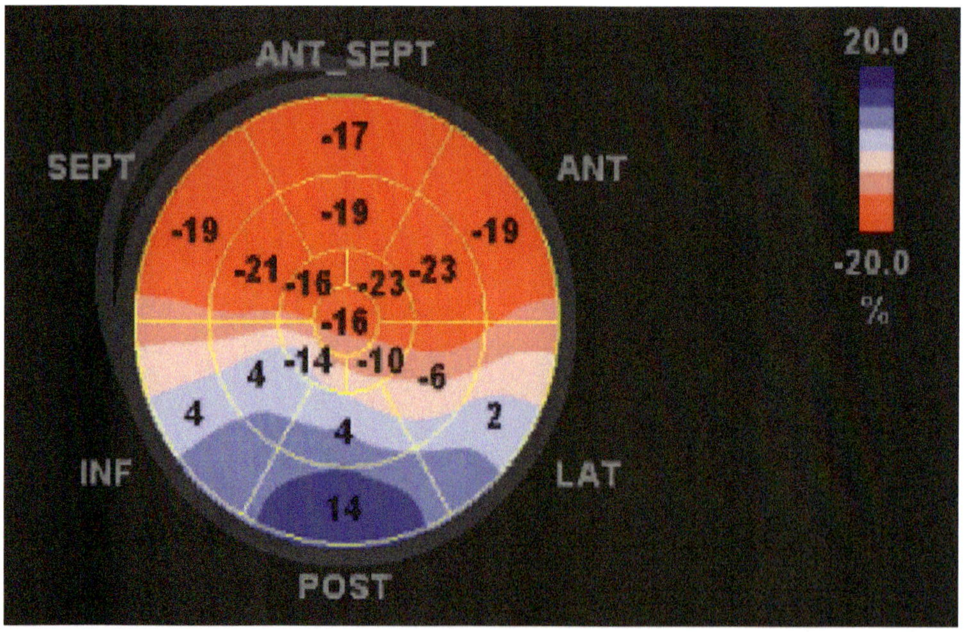

• **Fig. 12-27** Example of asynchrony detected using AFI *(automated function imaging)* using bull's eye mapping in a 4-month-old Golden Retriever puppy with Golden Retriever muscular dystrophy (GRMD). The peak longitudinal strains of the different myocardial segments (total of 18) are displayed on the same schematic drawing (left ventricle as seen from the apex), with color coding of the values. In this puppy, conventional echocardiography could not reveal any abnormality. However, several myocardial segments of the interventricular septum and of the left ventricular free wall are here coded in *blue,* already revealing the presence of segmental dyskinesia. Their longitudinal strain is positive (not negative, as in other normal segments coded in *red*). Note, in addition, the abnormal heterogeneity of the longitudinal peak systolic strain values. (Photo credit: Valérie Chetboul.)

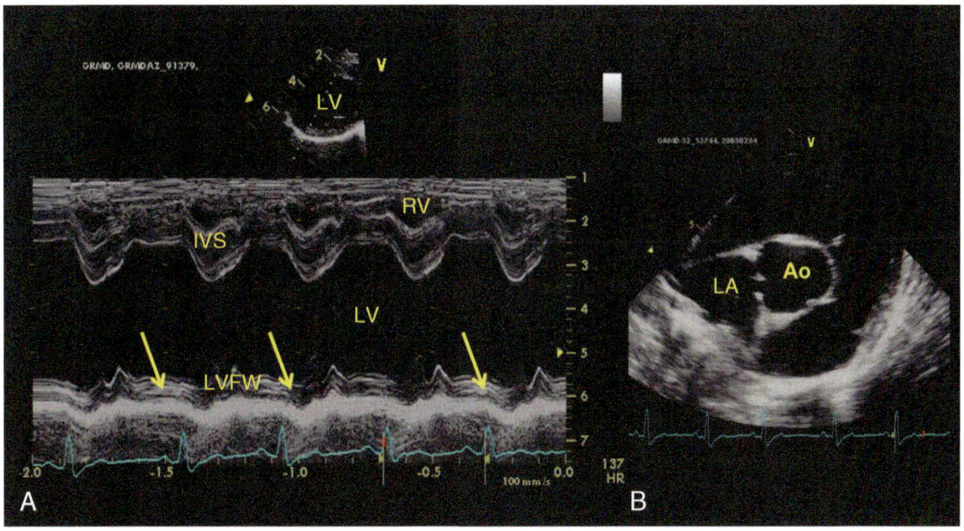

• **Fig. 12-28** Example of cardiomyopathy associated with hereditary myopathy (Golden Retriever muscular dystrophy [GRMD]). A, The transventricular time-motion (TM) echocardiogram of this 6-month-old Golden Retriever puppy with myopathy shows left ventricular free wall (LVFW) hypokinesia (compared to the still strong motion of the interventricular septum [IVS]). Note the presence of hyperechoic plaques *(arrows)* in the left myocardial wall. B, This free wall hypokinesia is not yet accompanied by left atrial dilation (right parasternal short axis transaortic view). *Ao,* Aorta; *LA,* left atrium; *LV,* left ventricle; *RV,* right ventricle. (Photo credit: Valérie Chetboul.)

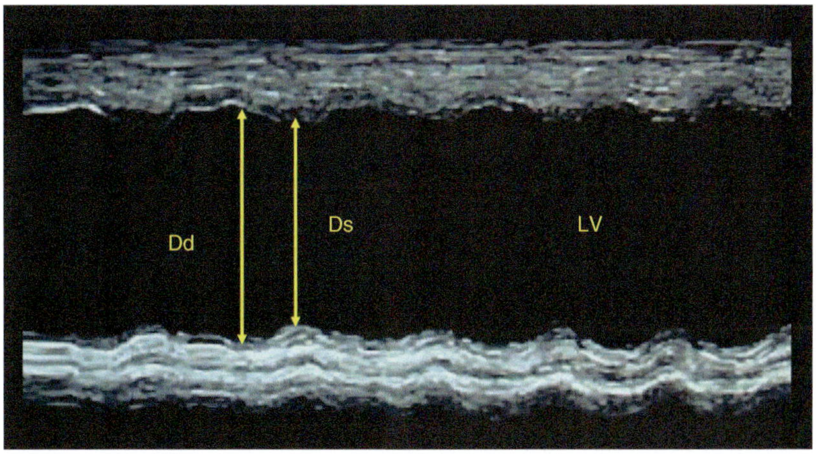

• **Fig. 12-29** Example of advanced dilated cardiomyopathy associated with hereditary myopathy (Golden Retriever muscular dystrophy [GRMD]). In this adult dog with GRMD, the transventricular time-motion (TM) echocardiogram shows marked left ventricular free wall and interventricular septum hypokinesia (SF = 8%). Note the small difference between the diastolic (Dd) and systolic (Ds) diameters of the left ventricle (LV). (Photo credit: Valérie Chetboul.)

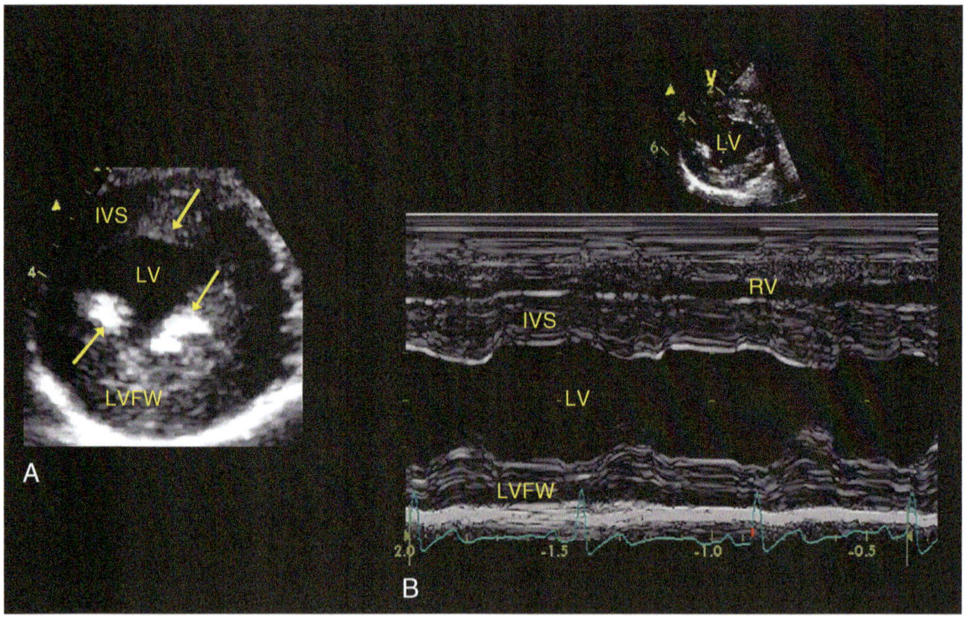

• **Fig. 12-30** Example of cardiomyopathy associated with lipid myopathy in a 1-year-old Fox Terrier mix. A, Conventional echocardiographic changes include the presence of hyperechoic areas *(arrows)* in the left papillary muscles, the latter being hypertrophied. B, No other kinetic or morphologic anomaly of the ventricle (LV) is visible on the transventricular time-motion (TM) echocardiogram, except for the myocardial wall thickness, which is in the upper limits of the normal range. *IVS,* Interventricular septum; *LVFW,* left ventricular free wall; *RV,* right ventricle. (Photo credit: Valérie Chetboul.)

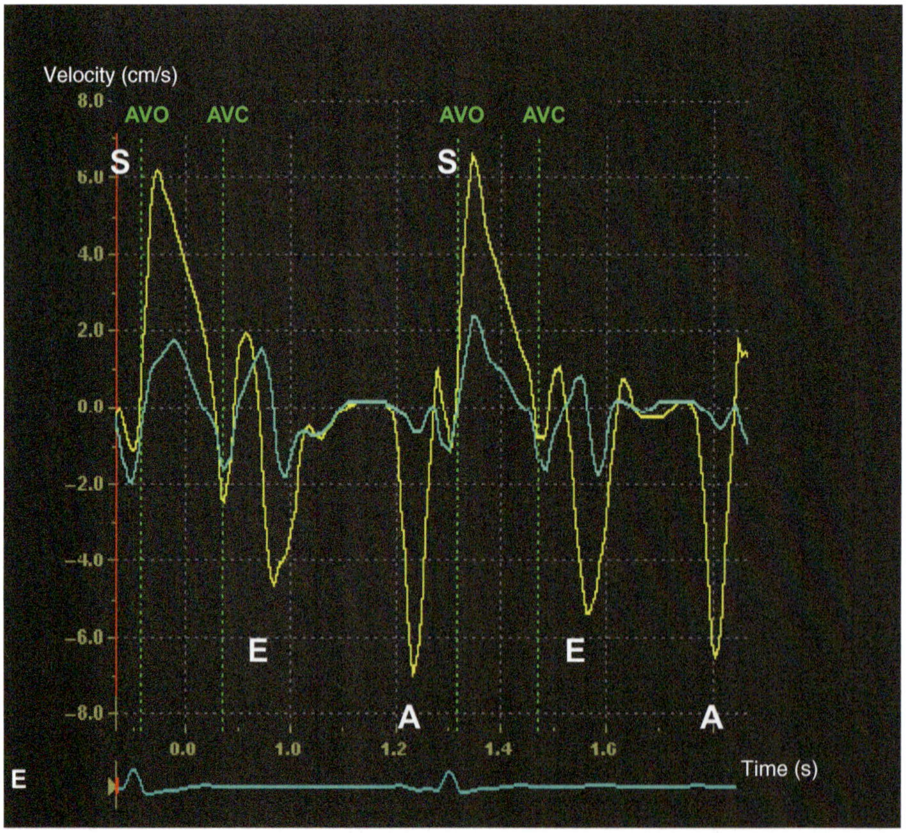

• **Fig. 12-31** Impaired left ventricular free wall longitudinal diastolic function analyzed by color bidimensional (2D) tissue Doppler imaging (TDI) in a 1-year-old Fox Terrier mix with lipid myopathy (same animal as in Figure 12-30). This diastolic dysfunction, not detectable using conventional Doppler (mitral E/A ratio >1), is characterized by inversion of the early diastolic and end-diastolic waves (E/A ratio <1) at the base but not at the apex (*yellow* and *green* curves, respectively). *A,* Peak end-diastolic velocity; *AVC,* aortic valve closure; *AVO,* aortic valve opening; *E,* peak early diastolic velocity; *S,* peak systolic velocity. (Photo credit: Valérie Chetboul.)

Arrhythmogenic Right Ventricular Cardiomyopathy

This cardiomyopathy, described mainly in the Boxer, is a familial cardiopathy with an autosomal dominant mode of transmission, incomplete penetrance, and variable expression. It is linked to a mutation of the striatin-coding gene located on chromosome 17 [16, 41-47]. Arrhythmogenic right ventricular cardiomyopathy is characterized by fatty or fibrofatty infiltration of the right myocardium, which can also involve the left myocardium to a lesser degree as the disease progresses. Arrhythmias are the dominant clinical expression of the disease (mainly ventricular premature beats and right ventricular tachycardias), potentially leading to syncopes or even sudden death. These arrhythmic forms, similar to those in humans, are not associated with myocardial dysfunction according to conventional echography or pulsed wave Doppler (right Tei index and PEP/ET) [47]. However, right ventricular dysfunction has been documented by magnetic resonance imaging (MRI) in some affected Boxers [46]. Therefore the diagnosis of these arrhythmic forms does not rely on conventional echo-Doppler examinations but rather on electrocardiography or, even better, Holter examination. In the other cases (Figures 12-32 and 12-33), a dilation of the right chambers (ventricle or ventricle and atrium), sometimes marked (even aneurysmal), can be observed in association or not with signs of right-sided CHF (caudal vena cava dilation, venous hepatic congestion, ascites, pleural effusion). The echocardiographer must exclude other causes of right cardiac dilation (pulmonary arterial hypertension and tricuspid valve dysplasia) before establishing the diagnosis for this cardiomyopathy.

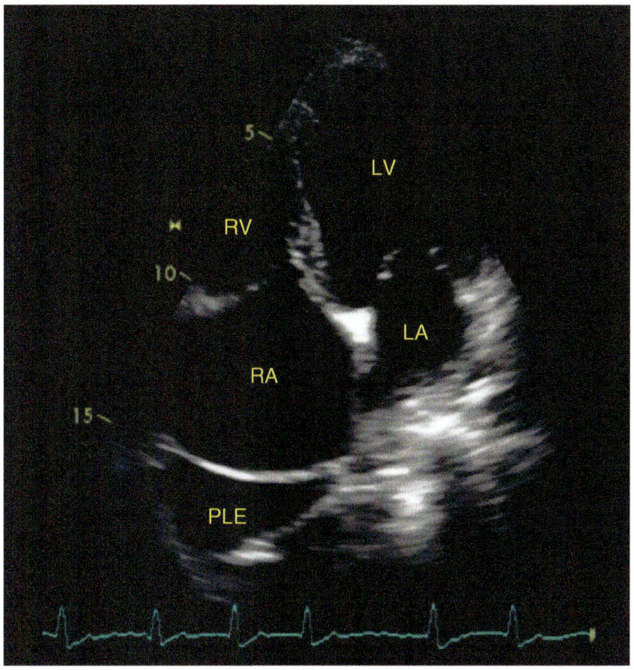

• **Fig. 12-32** Left apical 4 chambers view in a dog with arrhythmogenic right ventricular cardiomyopathy (with atrial fibrillation). Note the marked dilation of the right chambers and the presence of pleural effusion (PLE). *LA,* Left atrium; *LV,* left ventricle; *RA,* right atrium; *RV,* right ventricle. (Photo credit: Valérie Chetboul.)

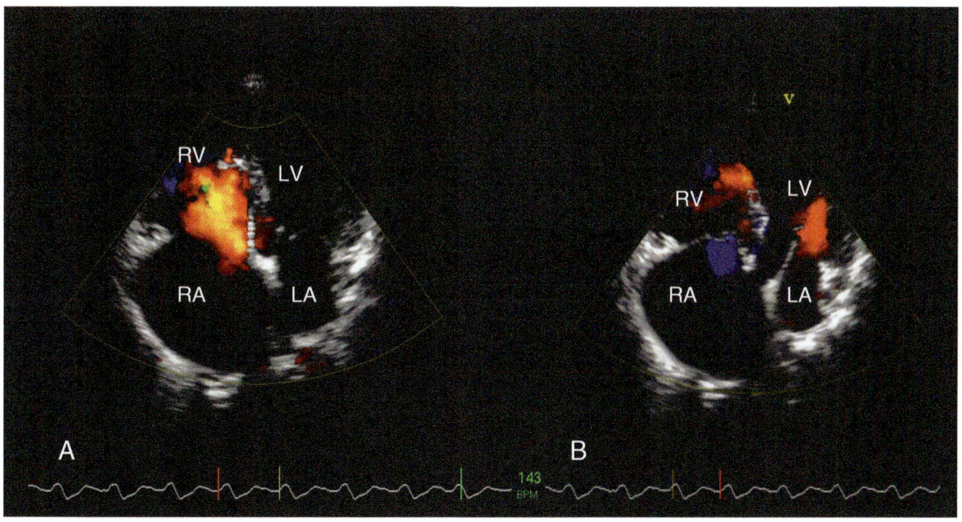

• **Fig. 12-33** Left apical 4 chambers view in a Boxer displaying arrhythmogenic right ventricular cardiomyopathy (with atrial fibrillation and bundle branch block). The marked dilation of the right chambers is apparent in these two photos. In addition, marked interventricular asynchrony is also present: (A) when the tricuspid valve is open, as evidenced by the transtricuspid flow color-coded in *red,* the mitral valve is closed. Inversely (B), when the mitral valve is open, as evidenced by the transmitral flow color-coded in *red*, the tricuspid valve is closed (note the presence of a discrete tricuspid regurgitation in *blue*). *LA,* Left atrium; *LV,* left ventricle; *RA,* right atrium; *RV,* right ventricle. (Photo credit: Valérie Chetboul.)

Uremic Cardiomyopathy

Very few data are available in dogs regarding the echocardiographic description of uremic cardiomyopathy, which is associated with chronic renal failure. As in humans [48, 49], uremic cardiomyopathy is most often characterized by myocardial hypertrophy associated or not with chamber dilation (Figure 12-34). The myocardium appears remodeled, hyperechoic, and heterogenous due to interstitial fibrosis and mineralization. Diastolic dysfunction, sometimes associated with systolic impairment, is often seen in TDI mode. These left ventricular changes are multifactorial and may be due to anemia, sodium and water retention (accounting for volume overload), systemic arterial hypertension, changes in the metabolism of phosphorus and calcium, uremia, endocrine disorders involving the renin-angiotensin-aldosterone system, and parathormone (accounting for hypertrophy and wall remodeling).

Canine Hypertrophic Cardiomyopathy

Primary hypertrophic cardiomyopathy is a rare cardiopathy in dogs, which is why so few descriptions have been published [7,50-53]. 2D and TM echocardiographic changes most often include symmetric concentric hypertrophy of the left ventricle associated with a hyperechoic myocardial change, more marked in the subendocardial and papillary muscle regions (Figure 12-35) with or without secondary left atrial dilation. The mitral leaflets are most affected by changes. As in cats, subaortic obstructive forms with left ventricular outflow tract obstruction and systolic anterior motion of the mitral valve have been described. Differential diagnosis mainly includes hypertensive cardiomyopathy (see Chapter 16), drug-induced cardiomyopathies [54] (Figure 12-36), inflammatory cardiomyopathies (myocarditis), and infiltrative cardiomyopathies (amyloidosis, tumoral).

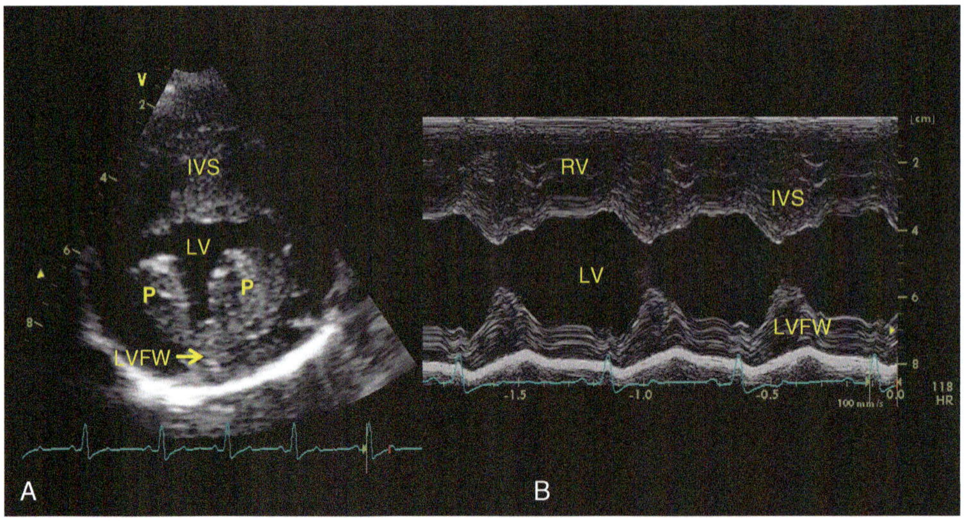

• **Fig. 12-34** Uremic cardiomyopathy in a German Shepherd with nonhypertensive chronic glomerulonephritis for 1 year. A, Conventional echocardiographic changes include a mildly heterogeneous myocardium (hyperechoic speckling distributed in a diffuse fashion, more visible at the end of the papillary muscles). B, In addition, concentric left ventricular hypertrophy is documented by the transventricular time-motion (TM) echocardiogram. *IVS,* Interventricular septum; *LV,* left ventricle; *LVFW,* left ventricular free wall; *P,* papillary muscles; *RV,* right ventricle. (Photo credit: Valérie Chetboul.)

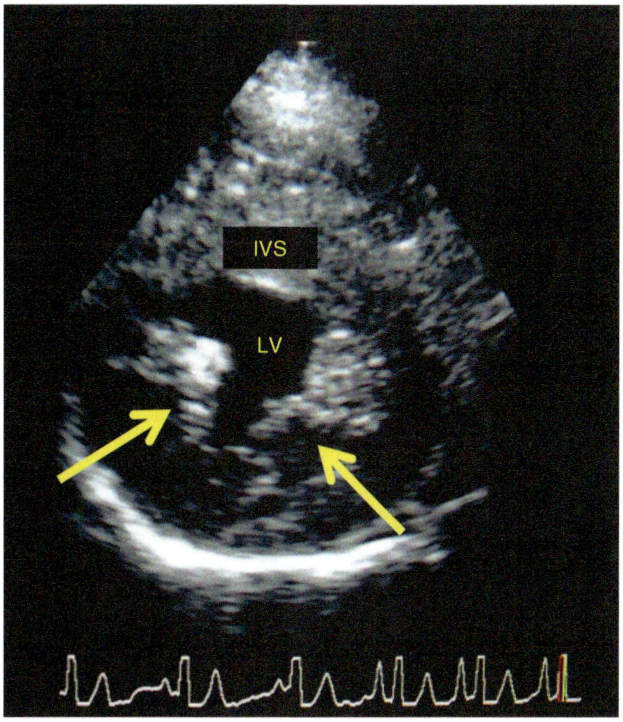

• **Fig. 12-35** Primary hypertrophic cardiomyopathy in a 5-year-old Jack Russell Terrier (right parasternal short axis transventricular view). The symmetric concentric hypertrophy is significant. In addition, hyperechoic plaques, distributed throughout the myocardium, are visible, especially near the endocardium and in the left papillary muscles *(arrows)*. *IVS,* Interventricular septum; *LV,* left ventricle. (Photo credit: Valérie Chetboul.)

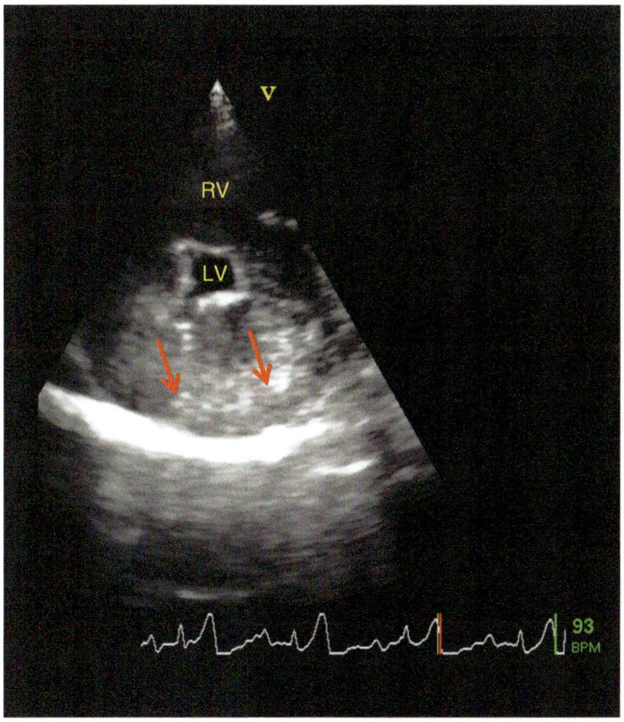

• **Fig. 12-36** Example of hypertrophic cardiomyopathy in a German Shepherd receiving Pimobendan (off-label prescription) over a period of 10 months at a dose of 0.66 mg/kg twice a day (*Cardiovascular Toxicology* [51]). The symmetric concentric hypertrophy is marked. In addition, hyperechoic plaques *(arrows)* are present in the myocardium. This end-systolic frame demonstrates that the left ventricular postsystolic residue is very low. Note the presence of a large T wave associated with myocardial hypertrophy on the concomitant electrocardiographic trace (sign of myocardial hypoxia). *LV,* Left ventricle; *RV,* right ventricle. (Photo credit: Valérie Chetboul.)

REFERENCES

[1] Richardson P, McKenna W, Bristow M, et al. Report of the 1995 World Health Organization/International Society and Federation of Cardiology Task Force on the Definition and Classification of Cardiomyopathies. Circulation 1996;93:841–2.

[2] Thiene G, Corrado D, Basso C. Revisiting definition and classification of cardiomyopathies in the era of molecular medicine. Eur Heart J 2008;29:144–6.

[3] Kittleson MD, Kienle RD. Primary myocardial disease leading to chronic myocardial failure (dilated cardiomyopathy and related diseases). In: Kittelson MD, editor. Small animal cardiovascular medicine. 2nd ed. St. Louis: Mosby; 1998, p. 319–46.

[4] Dukes-McEwan J, Borgarelli M, Tidholm A, et al. Proposed guidelines for the diagnosis of canine idiopathic dilated cardiomyopathy (The ESVC Taskforce for Canine Dilated Cardiomyopathy). J Vet Cardiol 2003;2:7–19.

[5] Tidholm A, Jonsson L. A retrospective study of canine dilated cardiomyopathy (189 cases). J Am Anim Hosp Assoc 1997;33:544–50.

[6] Martin MW, Stafford Johnson MJ, Celona B. Canine dilated cardiomyopathy: a retrospective study of signalment, presentation and clinical findings in 369 cases. J Small Anim Pract 2009;50:23–9.

[7] Oyama MA. Canine cardiomyopathy. In: Tilley LP, Smith FWK, Oyama MA, Sleeper MM, editors. Manual of canine and feline cardiology 2008;4:139–50.

[8] Monnet E, Orton EC, Salman M, Boon J. Idiopathic dilated cardiomyopathy in dogs: survival and prognostic indicators. J Vet Intern Med 1995;9:12–7.
[9] Tidholm A, Häggström J, Borgarelli M, Tarducci A. Canine idiopathic dilated cardiomyopathy. Part I: Aetiology, clinical characteristics, epidemiology and pathology. Aust Vet J 162: 92–107.
[10] Calvert CA, Hall G, Jacobs G, Pickus C. Clinical and pathologic findings in Doberman Pinschers with occult cardiomyopathy that died suddenly or developed congestive heart failure: 54 cases (1984–1991). J Am Vet Med Assoc 1997;210:505–11.
[11] Vollmar AC. The prevalence of cardiomyopathy in the Irish Wolfhound: a clinical study of 500 dogs. J Am Anim Hosp Assoc 2000;36:125–32.
[12] Sleeper MM, Henthorn PS, Vijayasarathy C, et al. Dilated cardiomyopathy in juvenile Portuguese Water Dogs. J Vet Intern Med 2002;16:52–62.
[13] Tidholm A, Jonsson L. Dilated cardiomyopathy in the Newfoundland: a study of 37 cases (1983–1994). J Am Anim Hosp Assoc 1996;32:465–70.
[14] Calvert CA, Jacobs GJ, Smith DD, et al. Association between results of ambulatory electrocardiography and development of cardiomyopathy during long-term follow-up of Doberman Pinschers. J Am Vet Med Assoc 2000;216:34–9.
[15] Wess G, Schulze A, Butz V, et al. Prevalence of dilated cardiomyopathy in Doberman Pinschers in various age groups. J Vet Intern Med 2010;24:533–8.
[16] Meurs KM. Genetics of cardiac disease in the small animal patient. Vet Clin North Am Small Anim Pract 2010;40:701–15.
[17] Meurs KM, Fox PR, Norgard M, et al. A prospective genetic evaluation of familial dilated cardiomyopathy in the Doberman Pinscher. J Vet Intern Med 2007;21:1016–20.
[18] Philipp U, Broschk C, Vollmar A, Distl O. Evaluation of tafazzin as candidate for dilated cardiomyopathy in Irish Wolfhounds. J Hered 2007;98:506–9.
[19] Dukes-McEwan J, Jackson IJ. The promises and problems of linkage analysis by using the current canine genome map. Mamm Genome 2002;13:667–72.
[20] Werner P, Raducha MG, Prociuk U, et al. A novel locus for dilated cardiomyopathy maps to canine chromosome 8. Genomics 2008;91:517–21.
[21] Meurs KM, Miller MW, Wright NA. Clinical features of dilated cardiomyopathy in Great Danes and results of a pedigree analysis: 17 cases (1990–2000). J Am Vet Med Assoc 2001;218:729–32.
[22] Chetboul V, Gouni V, Carlos Sampedrano C, et al. Assessment of regional systolic and diastolic myocardial function using tissue Doppler and strain imaging in dogs with dilated cardiomyopathy. J Vet Intern Med 2007;21:719–30.
[23] Wess G, Mäurer J, Simak J, Hartmann K. Use of Simpson's method of disc to detect early echocardiographic changes in Doberman Pinschers with dilated cardiomyopathy. J Vet Intern Med 2010;24:1069–76.
[24] Boon JA. Acquired heart disease. In: Boon JA, editor. Manual of veterinary echocardiography. Baltimore: The Williams & Wilkins Co; 1998, p. 261–382.
[25] O'Grady MR, O'Sullivan ML, Minors SL, Horne R. Efficacy of benazepril hydrochloride to delay the progression of occult dilated cardiomyopathy in Doberman Pinschers. J Vet Intern Med 2009;23:977–83.
[26] Lang RM, Bierig M, Devereux RB, et al. American Society of Echocardiography's Nomenclature and Standards Committee; Task Force on Chamber Quantification; American College of Cardiology Echocardiography Committee; American Heart Association; European Association of Echocardiography; European Society of Cardiology. Eur J Echocardiogr 2006;7:79–108.
[27] Calvert CA, Jacobs GJ, Smith DD, et al. Association between results of ambulatory electrocardiography and development of cardiomyopathy during long-term follow-up of Doberman Pinschers. J Am Vet Med Assoc 2000;216:34–9.
[28] Vollmar AC. Echocardiographic measurements in the Irish Wolfhound: reference values for the breed. J Am Anim Hosp Assoc 1999;35:271–7.
[29] Borgarelli M, Zini E, D'Agnolo G, et al. Comparison of primary mitral valve disease in German Shepherd dogs and in small breeds. J Vet Cardiol 2004;6:27–34.
[30] Borgarelli M, Santilli RA, Chiavegato D, et al. Prognostic indicators for dogs with dilated cardiomyopathy. J Vet Intern Med 2006;20:104–10.
[31] Chetboul V, Gouni V, Carlos Sampedrano C, et al. Use of quantitative two-dimensional color tissue Doppler imaging for assessment of left ventricular radial and longitudinal myocardial velocities in dogs. Am J Vet Res 2005;66:953–61.
[32] Chetboul V. Tissue Doppler imaging: a promising technique for quantifying regional myocardial function. J Vet Cardiol 2002;4:7–12.
[33] Chetboul V, Gouni V, Carlos Sampedrano C, et al. Assessment of repeatability, reproducibility, and effect of anesthesia on determination of radial and longitudinal left ventricular velocities via tissue Doppler imaging in dogs. Am J Vet Res 2004;65:909–15.

[34] Chetboul V, Carlos Sampedrano C, Testault I, Pouchelon JL. Use of tissue Doppler imaging to confirm the diagnosis of dilated cardiomyopathy in a dog with equivocal echocardiographic findings. J Am Vet Med Assoc 2004;225:1877–80.
[35] Chetboul V, Carlos Sampedrano C, Gouni V, et al. Ultrasonographic assessment of regional radial and longitudinal systolic function in healthy awake dogs. J Vet Intern Med 2006;20:885–93.
[36] Chetboul V, Serres F, Gouni V, et al. Radial strain and strain rate by two-dimensional speckle tracking echocardiography and the tissue velocity based technique in the dog. J Vet Cardiol 2007;9:69–81.
[37] Chetboul V, Serres F, Gouni V, et al. Non-invasive assessment of systolic left ventricular torsion by 2-dimensional speckle tracking imaging in the awake dog: repeatability, reproducibility, and comparison with tissue Doppler imaging variables. J Vet Intern Med 2008;22:342–50.
[38] Moise NS, Valentine BA, Brown CA, et al. Duchenne's cardiomyopathy in a canine model: electrocardiographic and echocardiographic studies. J Am Coll Cardiol 1991;17:812–20.
[39] Chetboul V, Escriou C, Tessier D, et al. Tissue Doppler imaging detects early asymptomatic myocardial abnormalities in a dog model of Duchenne's cardiomyopathy. Eur Heart J 2004;25:1934–9.
[40] Chetboul V, Carlos C, Blot S, et al. Tissue Doppler assessment of diastolic and systolic alterations of radial and longitudinal left ventricular motions in Golden Retrievers during the preclinical phase of cardiomyopathy associated with muscular dystrophy. Am J Vet Res 2004;65:1335–41.
[41] Fernández del Palacio MJ, Bernal LJ, Bayón A, et al. Arrhythmogenic right ventricular dysplasia/cardiomyopathy in a Siberian Husky. J Small Anim Pract 2001;42:137–42.
[42] Basso C, Fox PR, Meurs KM, et al. Arrhythmogenic right ventricular cardiomyopathy causing sudden cardiac death in Boxer dogs: a new animal model of human disease. Circulation 2004;109:1180–5.
[43] Meurs KM. Boxer dog cardiomyopathy: an update. Vet Clin North Am Small Anim Pract 2004;34:1235–44.
[44] Meurs KM, Mauceli E, Lahmers S, et al. Genome-wide association identifies a deletion in the 3′ untranslated region of striatin in a canine model of arrhythmogenic right ventricular cardiomyopathy. Hum Genet 2010;128:315–24.
[45] Oxford EM, Danko CG, Kornreich BG, et al. Ultrastructural changes in cardiac myocytes from Boxer dogs with arrhythmogenic right ventricular cardiomyopathy. J Vet Cardiol 2011;13:101–13.
[46] Baumwart RD, Meurs KM, Raman SV. Magnetic resonance imaging of right ventricular morphology and function in boxer dogs with arrhythmogenic right ventricular cardiomyopathy. J Vet Intern Med 2009;23:271–4.
[47] Baumwart RD, Meurs KM. An index of myocardial performance applied to the right ventricle of Boxers with arrhythmogenic right ventricular cardiomyopathy. Am J Vet Res 2008;69:1029–33.
[48] London GM, Fabiani F, Marchais SJ, et al. Uremic cardiomyopathy: an inadequate left ventricular hypertrophy. Kidney Int 1987;31:973–80.
[49] El-Husseini AA, Sheashaa HA, Hassan NA, et al. Echocardiographic changes and risk factors for left ventricular hypertrophy in children and adolescents after renal transplantation. Pediatr Transplant 2004;8:249–54.
[50] Washizu M, Takemura N, Machida N, et al. Hypertrophic cardiomyopathy in an aged dog. J Vet Med Sci 2003;65:753–6.
[51] Marks CA. Hypertrophic cardiomyopathy in a dog. J Am Vet Med Assoc 1993;203:1020–2.
[52] Pang D, Rondenay Y, Hélie P, et al. Sudden cardiac death associated with occult hypertrophic cardiomyopathy in a dog under anesthesia. Can Vet J 2005;46:1122–5.
[53] Sisson D, O'Grady MR, Calvert CA. Myocardial diseases of dogs. In: Fox PR, Sisson D, Moise NS, editors. Textbook of canine and feline cardiology. 2nd ed. Philadelphia: WB Saunders; 1999, p. 601–6.
[54] Tissier R, Chetboul V, Moraillon R, et al. Increased mitral valve regurgitation and myocardial hypertrophy in two dogs with long-term pimobendan therapy. Cardiovasc Toxicol 2005;5:43–51.

13

Evaluation of Feline Cardiomyopathies

ÉRIC DE MADRON

Hypertrophic Cardiomyopathies, 208
Restrictive Cardiomyopathies, 218
Dilated Cardiomyopathies, 222
Atypical Cardiomyopathies, 224
Thrombotic Risk Assessment, 225

Cardiomyopathies are myocardial diseases. These cardiopathies are the most frequently encountered type of acquired heart disease in cats. There are three main types of cardiomyopathies: hypertrophic cardiomyopathy (HCM), restrictive cardiomyopathy (RCM), and dilated cardiomyopathy (DCM). This classification is based on morphologic and hemodynamic criteria (systolic and diastolic function anomalies) [1]. In a retrospective study of 106 cats, HCM was the most frequent cardiomyopathy (57.5%), RCM the second most frequent (20.7%), and DCM the third most frequent (10.4%).

A few atypical cardiomyopathies affected the rest of the cohort [2]. These included undetermined cardiomyopathies (UCMs), those associated with excessive moderator bands, right ventricular cardiomyopathy, and noncompaction of the left ventricle.

Hypertrophic Cardiomyopathies

Myocardial changes due to HCM may appear at any age, even though most of the animals affected are young adults. Certain breeds (particularly Persian, British Shorthair, Ragdoll, and Maine Coon) are predisposed to HCM [1, 3]. HCM in cats, as in humans, has a familial pattern and is suspected of having a genetic origin. A genetic mutation of the *MyBPC3* (myosin binding protein C3) gene has been identified in the Maine Coon and the Ragdoll [4].

HCM is characterized by myocardial hypertrophy affecting mostly the left ventricle (LV) and sometimes the right ventricle (RV) [5]. This hypertrophy can take very diverse aspects [6]. It leads to diastolic anomalies resulting in congestive heart failure (CHF). These diastolic anomalies worsen with the progression of the disease. Similarly, myocardial remodeling may develop with time. Finally, cats with HCM can develop intracardial thrombi [1] and evaluating this risk is an important goal of the echocardiographic examination.

2D and TM Echocardiographic Characteristics

Left Ventricular Hypertrophy

2D Mode

Variability of Hypertrophy. LV hypertrophy can take on many aspects, which makes the HCM group highly heterogeneous [2]. Indeed, this hypertrophy can be either symmetric or asymmetric, focal or generalized, affecting to diverse degrees the interventricular septum (Figure 13-1, *A*), the left ventricular free wall (Figure 13-1, *B*), or the papillary muscles (Figure 13-1, *C*). It can also affect the base or the apex of the ventricle (Figure 13-1, *D*). Some cats have limited hypertrophy in the basal region of the septum (Figure 13-1, *E*). This hypertrophy can also be generalized, affecting in a symmetric fashion both left ventricular walls (see Figure 13-1). It can also be lateral or medial (Figure 13-2). These various facets of HCM are also shown in Videos 13-1 to 13-8.

A study performed on 15 cats with HCM confirmed this phenotypic heterogeneity [6]. The hypertrophy was segmental in 11 cats, diffuse in 3, and minimal with systolic anterior movement (SAM) of the mitral valve in 1 cat. The free wall was affected in 53% of the cases, the basal septum in 60%, the anteromedial segment in 27%, and the anterolateral segment in 7%. The hypertrophy involved two different regions in 27% of the cases and more than two regions in 7% [6].

Therefore the bidimensional (2D) examination of the LV must be thorough and comprehensive, with evaluation of its long and short axes, basal and apical regions, and the papillary muscles. In the cat, a left ventricular

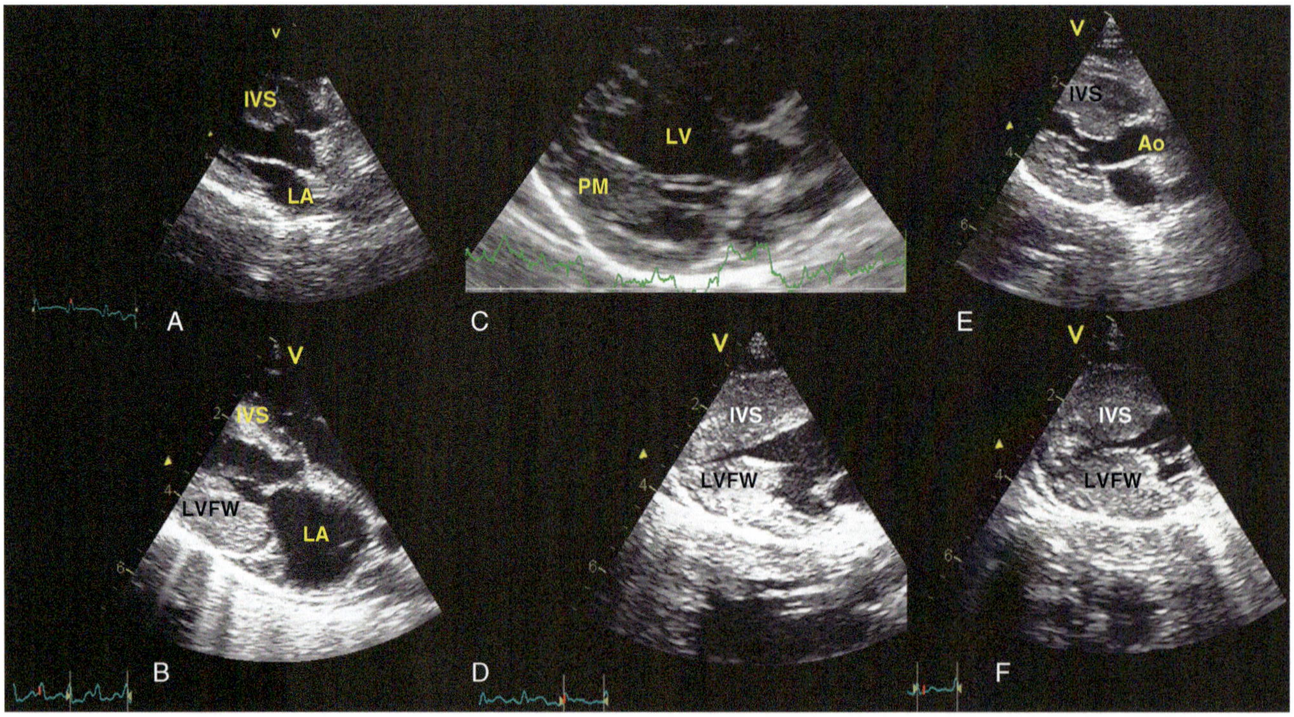

• **Fig. 13-1** Echocardiograms (right parasternal long axis views) of several cats with hypertrophic cardiomyopathy (HCM) illustrating the different types of hypertrophy. **A**, Asymmetric hypertrophy affecting the septum. **B**, Left ventricular free wall hypertrophy. **C**, Hypertrophy mainly affecting one of the papillary muscles. **D**, Apical hypertrophy. **E**, Basal septum hypertrophy. **F**, Hypertrophy affecting the entire left ventricular myocardium. The myocardial heterogeneity denotes the presence of fibrosis. *Ao*, Aorta; *IVS*, interventricular septum; *LA*, left atrium; *LV*, left ventricle; *LVFW*, left ventricular free wall; *PM*, papillary muscle. (Photo credit: Éric de Madron.)

wall segment end-diastolic thickness ≥6 mm is a widely accepted criterion of hypertrophy [6-8].

This hypertrophy can be accompanied by a heterogeneous myocardial echogenicity, corresponding to local fibrosis (see Figure 13-1, *B and D* and Video 13-9).

In the particular case of HCM associated with feline hypertrophic muscular dystrophy (resulting from the mutation of the dystrophin coding gene), the myocardium appears thick and diffusely hypoechoic, usually with multiple hyperechoic foci indicating areas of mineralization [9].

The left ventricular chamber is normal or reduced in diameter and contracts normally [7,8]. In rare cases, an aneurysmal dilation of the left ventricular apex can be observed [5].

A study performed on 18 cats with HCM reported concomitant right ventricular free wall hypertrophy in 11% of the cases [5].

Myocardial Remodeling. In humans, advanced HCM (5% to 10% of patients) is characterized by reduced wall thickness, left ventricular chamber dilation, shortening fraction (SF) reduction, and progression toward CHF. A study documented a similar progression in four cats with HCM followed over a period of 8 years [10]. Progressive dilation of the LV and left atrium (LA) as well as a reduction of the SF were observed. Subendocardial and myocardial fibrosis, as well as multifocal infarcts, was present in three of these cats, indicating that ischemic phenomena were involved in the remodeling process [11]. Echocardiographically, the presence of thin and hypocontractile myocardial areas adjacent to still hypertrophied segments characterizes remodeling (Figure 13-3 and Video 13-10).

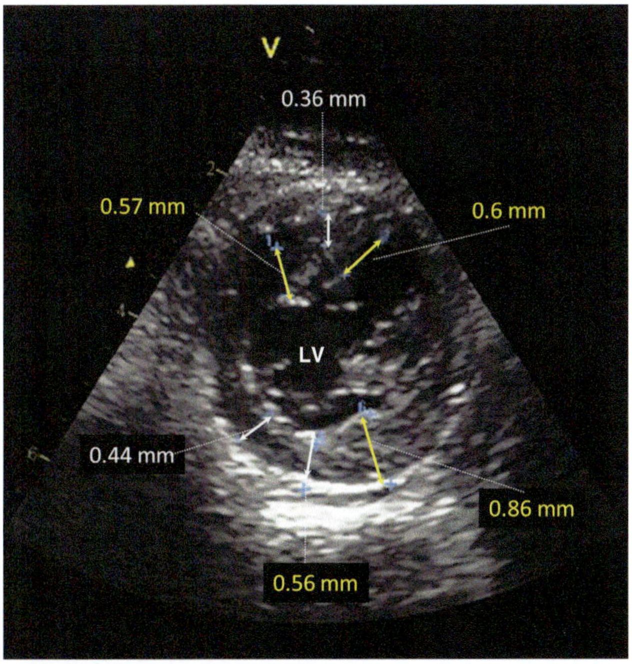

• Fig. 13-2 Echocardiogram (right parasternal short axis view) of a cat with hypertrophic cardiomyopathy (HCM). The selected image was taken in end-diastole. The hypertrophy here is highly heterogeneous and affects only certain segments of the left ventricular walls: the lateral (cranial) segments of the interventricular septum and of the free wall. *LV,* Left ventricle. (Photo credit: Éric de Madron.)

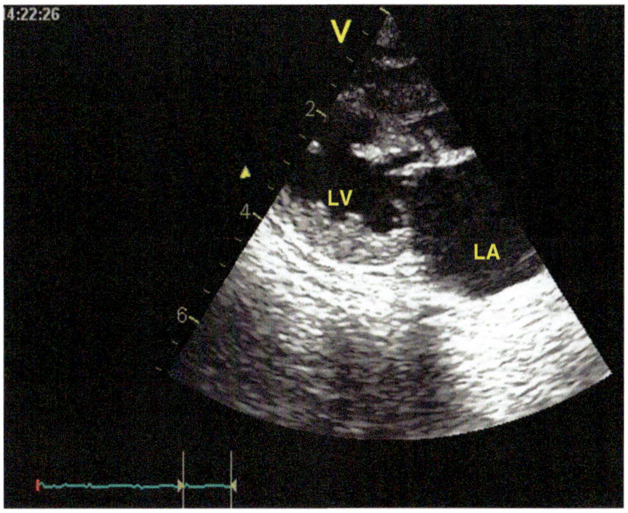

• Fig. 13-3 Echocardiogram (right parasternal long axis view) of a cat with hypertrophic cardiomyopathy (HCM) and heterogenous left myocardial changes. Note the variations in thickness of the free wall and septum, with some areas being hypertrophied while others are thinner. *LA,* Left atrium; *LV,* left ventricle. (Photo credit: Éric de Madron.)

Systolic Anterior Movement of the Mitral Valve. In 33% to 42% of the cases of HCM in cats [1,2], SAM of the mitral valve is observed, the anterior leaflet making contact with the septum in end-systole (Figure 13-4).

This abnormal movement causes a dynamic obstruction of the left ventricular outflow tract (DOLVOT), which can lead to significant pressure gradients between the left ventricle and the aorta (see below). This SAM is the result of hemodynamic factors (aspiration during systole of the anterior mitral valve leaflet against the septum due to a Venturi effect created by eddy currents) [12-14] as well as mechanical (mitral valve leaflet elongation and anterior displacement of the papillary muscles, leading to loss of leaflet support) [1] and geometric factors (angle between the interventricular septum and the aortic axis) (see below).

Pericardial and Pleural Effusion. In cats, a small pericardial effusion is observed in 7% of the cases [2], especially when the hypertrophy is marked. Pleural effusion can also be observed when CHF is present (Figure 13-5).

Intraventricular Thrombus. A thrombus, appearing as a hyperechoic mass floating in the LV (sometimes even obstructing the outflow tract), can be observed. However, intracavitary thrombi are mainly located in the LA (see below) [15].

TM Mode

The time-motion (TM) mode allows one to objectively document and quantify ventricular hypertrophy, as long as it affects the median part of the LV (Figure 13-6).

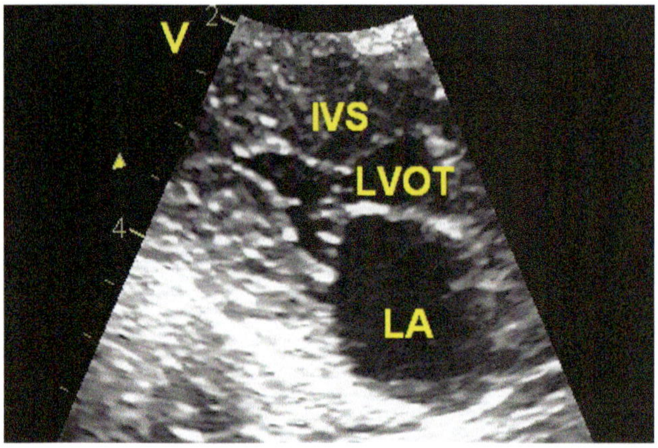

• **Fig. 13-4** Echocardiogram (right parasternal long axis 5 chambers view) of a cat with hypertrophic cardiomyopathy (HCM) and systolic anterior movement (SAM) of the mitral valve. The anterior leaflet of the mitral valve is in contact with the septum (IVS) in end-systole, partially obstructing the left ventricular outflow tract (LVOT). *LA,* Left atrium. (Photo credit: Éric de Madron.)

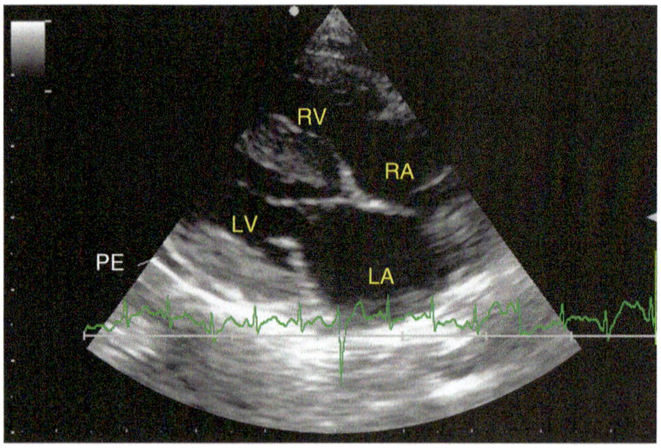

• **Fig. 13-5** Echocardiogram (right parasternal long axis 4 chambers view) of a cat with hypertrophic cardiomyopathy (HCM). A small posterior pericardial effusion (PE) is present. *LA,* Left atrium; *LV,* left ventricle; *RA,* right atrium; *RV,* right ventricle. (Photo credit: Éric de Madron.)

As stated earlier, a septal or left ventricular free wall end-diastolic thickness ≥6 mm is a criterion of myocardial hypertrophy [7,8].

However, to optimally interpret wall thickness, it is strongly recommended to take into account the body weight of the cat by comparing the measured thicknesses to the normal theoretical allometric values and aortic ratios (see Chapter 2).

With HCM, the LV end-diastolic internal diameter is either normal or reduced and the SF is either normal or increased [7,8]. The mitral valve SAM, if present, is easily detected in TM mode (Figure 13-7).

Dilation of the Atria

Dilation

Left atrial dilation is present in HCM with significant diastolic dysfunction (see below). As in dogs, this dilation can be evaluated by measuring the three left atrial diameters—LA TM, LA 2D, and LAmax—using the right parasternal long axis 4 and 5 chambers and short axis transaortic views.

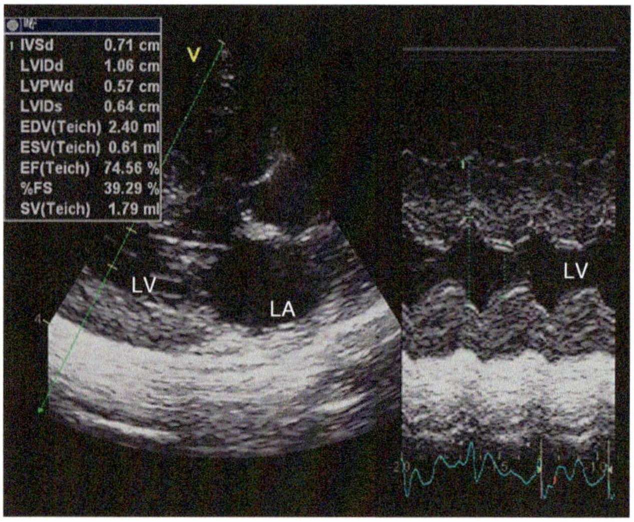

• **Fig. 13-6** Echocardiogram in time-motion (TM) mode of the left ventricle in a cat with asymmetric hypertrophic cardiomyopathy (HCM). The septal end-diastolic thickness is increased (0.71 cm). The free wall thickness is in the upper range of normal (0.57 cm). The internal left ventricular end-systolic and end-diastolic diameters and the shortening fraction (39%) are normal. *LA,* Left atrium; *LV,* left ventricle. (Photo credit: Éric de Madron.)

Spontaneous Echocardiographic Contrast/Thrombi

The presence of spontaneous echoes in the LA, a marker of thrombotic risk, should be sought systematically. This blood "hyperechogenicity," observed in 11.5% of HCM cases, is a result of ultrasonic reflection on red blood cell aggregates whirling in the LA (Figure 13-8 and Video 13-11) [2]. These hyperechoic spirals (also called "smoke") also must be looked for in the left atrial appendage. To accomplish this, an oblique right parasternal short axis view should be used.

More rarely, an intraatrial thrombus can be observed, especially when marked left atrial dilation is present [1,16].

Color and Spectral Doppler Characteristics

Color Doppler

Dynamic Obstruction

Mitral valve SAM leads to DOLVOT, with an increase of the systolic pressure gradient between the LV and the aorta. HCM is then said to be obstructive. This obstruction is dynamic, meaning that its degree is variable (depending on the systolic phase, contractility, and loading conditions). It may not necessarily be present at rest. In that case, it can be provoked by pharmacologic interventions that increase contractility (isoproterenol) or reduce ventricular filling (sodium nitroprusside) [12,13]. This obstruction can also be exacerbated by increased heart rate. It can accompany subaortic septal hypertrophy. A study performed in human

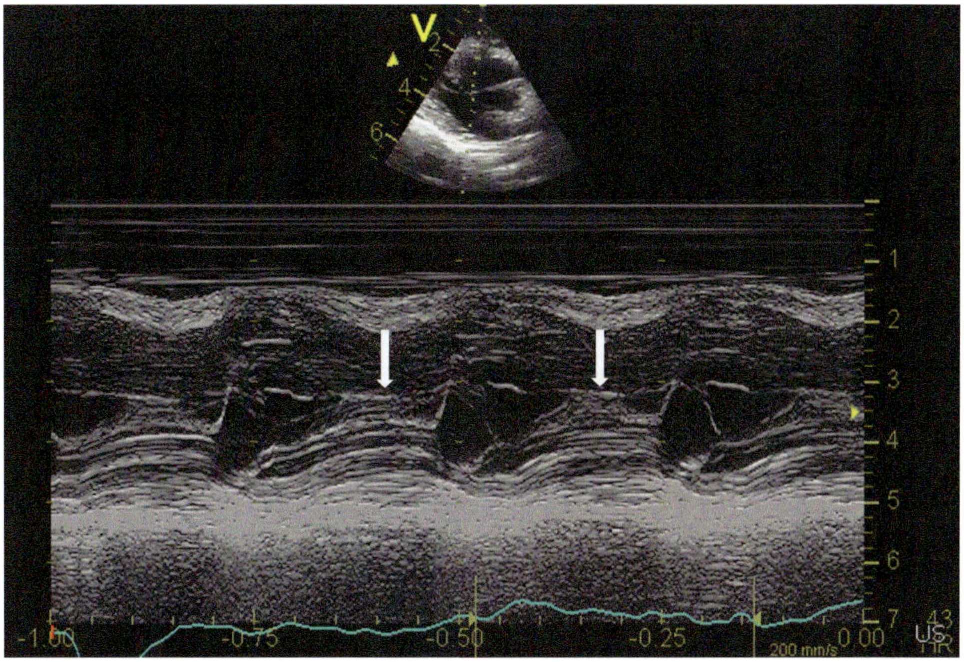

• **Fig. 13-7** Echocardiogram in time-motion (TM) mode of a mitral valve of a cat with asymmetric hypertrophic cardiomyopathy (HCM). Note the systolic anterior movement *(arrows)* of the mitral valve. (Photo credit: Éric de Madron.)

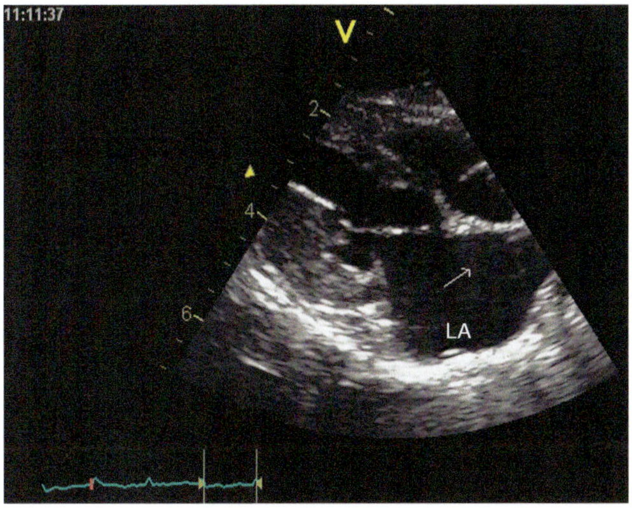

• **Fig. 13-8** Echocardiogram (right parasternal long axis 4 chambers view) of a cat with hypertrophic cardiomyopathy (HCM). The left atrium (LA) is markedly dilated. Note the spontaneous echo contrast *(arrow)* due to intracavitary blood stasis. (Photo credit: Éric de Madron.)

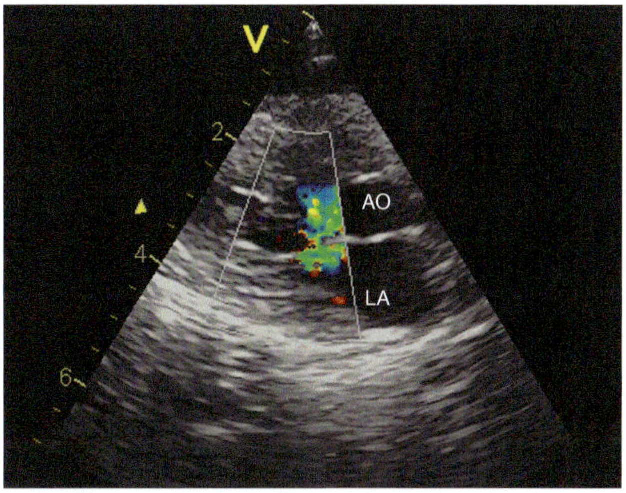

• **Fig. 13-9** Echocardiogram (right parasternal long axis 5 chambers view) in color Doppler mode of a cat with hypertrophic cardiomyopathy (HCM) and systolic anterior movement (SAM) of the mitral valve. A turbulence is visible in the left ventricular outflow tract. As well, a small mitral regurgitation is visible. *Ao,* Aorta; *LA,* left atrium. (Photo credit: Éric de Madron.)

patients with either HCM or hypertensive cardiopathy has revealed that DOLVOT was not correlated with basal septum thickness but rather with the angle formed by the interventricular septum and the aortic root axis. The greater the angle, the greater the chances of DOLVOT [17].

In cases of dynamic obstruction associated with HCM, color Doppler reveals a systolic turbulent mosaic in the LV outflow tract (Figure 13-9 and Video 13-12).

In the case of marked concentric left ventricular hypertrophy, dynamic stenosis can also occur at the level of the papillary muscles, causing left intraventricular obstruction in end-systole.

A dynamic obstruction of the right ventricular outflow tract (DORVOT) can also be observed (Figure 13-10 and Video 13-13) but is not specific to HCM and also may be found in normal cats [18].

Mitral Regurgitation

Aspiration of the mitral valve against the septum in systole can cause mitral regurgitation, visible in color

Doppler mode (Figure 13-11 and Video 13-14). This regurgitation is usually eccentric and mild.

Spectral Doppler

Dynamic Obstruction of the Left Ventricular Outflow Tract

Spectral Doppler documents the presence of a high-velocity turbulent transaortic flow. Typically, the high-velocity transaortic flow associated with obstructive HCM is asymmetric, reaching its maximum velocity at the end of systole (Figure 13-12). This peak velocity can vary from one systole to the other depending on the heart rate.

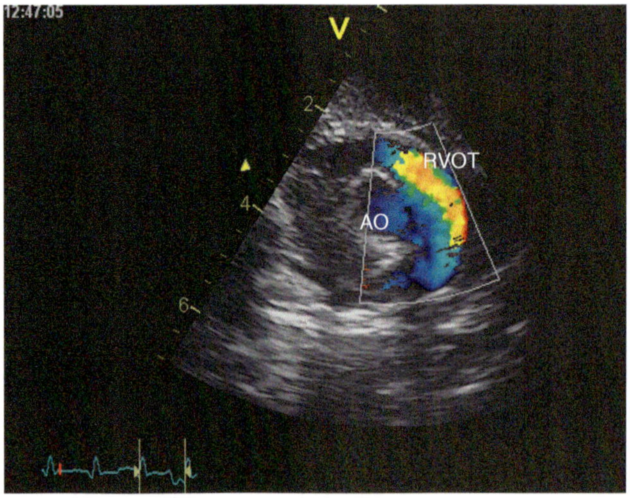

• **Fig. 13-10** Echocardiogram (right parasternal short axis transaortic view) in color Doppler mode of a cat with hypertrophic cardiomyopathy (HCM) and dynamic obstruction of the right ventricular outflow tract (RVOT). *Ao,* Aorta. (Photo credit: Éric de Madron.)

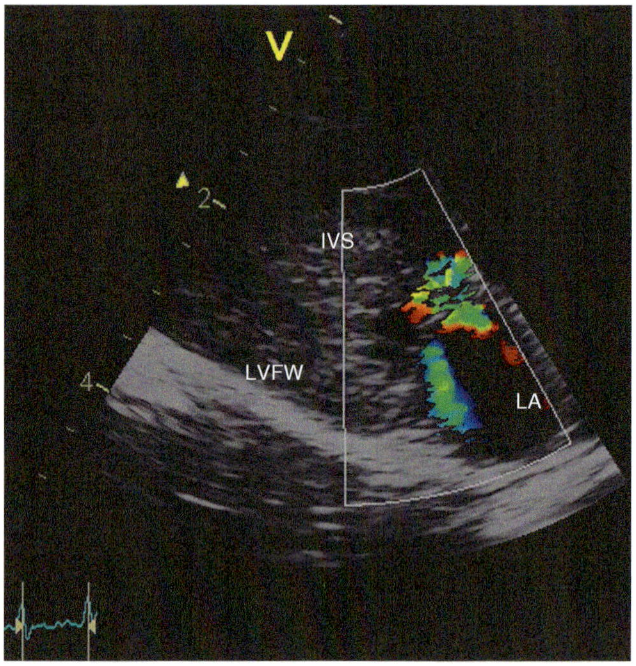

• **Fig. 13-11** Echocardiogram (right parasternal long axis view) in color Doppler mode of a cat with hypertrophic cardiomyopathy (HCM) and systolic anterior movement (SAM) of the mitral valve. An eccentric mitral regurgitation flow is readily visible in the left atrium (LA). *IVS,* Interventricular septum; *LVFW,* left ventricular free wall. (Photo credit: Éric de Madron.)

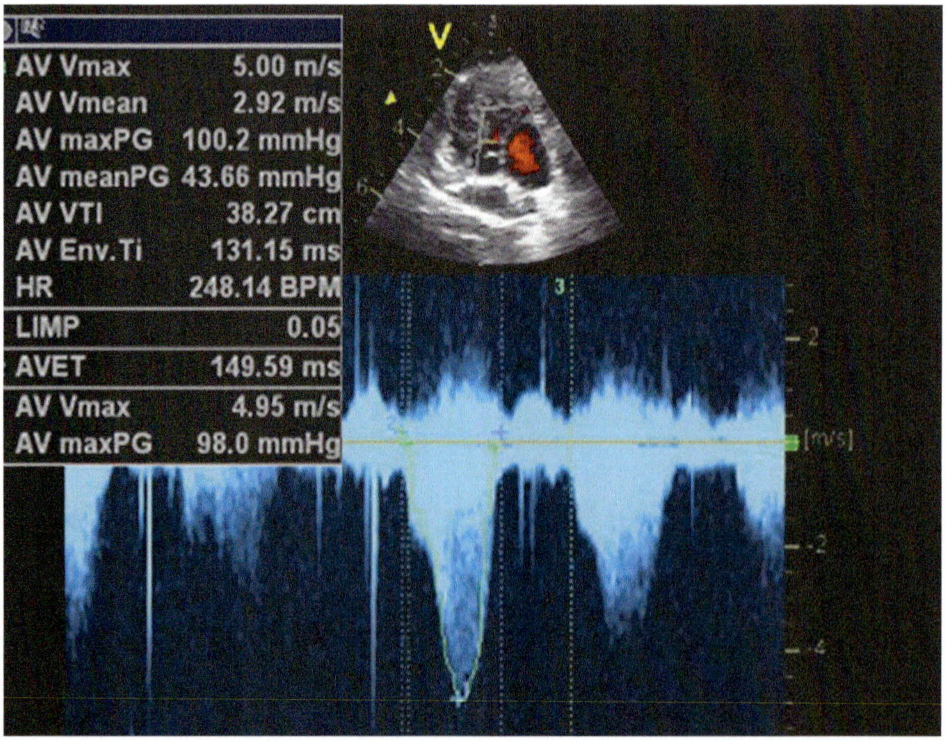

• **Fig. 13-12** Continuous wave Doppler mode echocardiogram of a cat with hypertrophic cardiomyopathy (HCM) and dynamic obstruction of the left ventricular outflow tract (DOLVOT). The aortic systolic flow has a beveled shape with a peak velocity reached late in systole. The maximum pressure gradient is variable but high. In this case, it reaches 100 mm Hg. (Photo credit: Éric de Madron.)

In humans with obstructive HCM, the ejection time (measured on the aortic systolic ejection flow) is increased and systolic velocities decrease rapidly once the peak velocity is reached [19]. The peak velocities can also vary from one systole to the next, depending on the heart rate.

In obstructive HCM, the LV-aorta pressure gradient can range from 20 mm Hg to more than 120 mm Hg. This increase in the left intraventricular pressure can then lead to subendocardial ischemia and increased myocardial oxygen consumption, and can even stimulate myocardial hypertrophy [1]. In humans, the presence of a DOLVOT can lead to sudden death [20,21]. The risk is particularly high in patients with a significant gradient at rest [22]. This correlation has not been confirmed in cats [23].

Evaluation of the Diastolic Function

Diastolic anomalies associated with HCM are multifactorial in origin, resulting from the combination of cardiomyocytes disorganization, fibrosis lesions, and myocardial ischemia [24]. The disruption of cardiomyocytes is frequently observed in severe HCM in the Maine Coon cat and is identified to a varying degree (30% to 62%) in other breeds [1,25,26]. It is interesting to note that diastolic dysfunction is not limited to the hypertrophied myocardial segments (see below).

The type of diastolic dysfunction (see Chapter 8) depends on the stage of the disease (Table 13-1) [27]. Thus an initially normal diastolic function will evolve into delayed relaxation with normal filling pressure (Figure 13-13) and then into abnormal relaxation with elevated filling pressure. The increased atrial pressure along with a loss of LV elasticity leads to the next phase, called the pseudonormal phase (Figure 13-14). Finally, myocardial remodeling and fibrosis lead to the restrictive stage (Figure 13-15) [16].

TABLE 13-1 Classification Criteria for Diastolic Dysfunction Types in Cats [16, 39, 40]

Parameter	Normal Diastole	Delayed Relaxation with Normal LV Filling Pressure (Stage 1a)	Delayed Relaxation with Elevated LV Filling Pressure (Stage 1b)	Pseudonormal Diastole (Stage 2)	Restrictive Diastole (Stage 3)
E/A	1.12 ± 0.22 [38]	<1	<1	≈1	>2
IVRT (ms)	43 ± 9 [38]	>60	>60	37-60	<37
Adur/ARdur	1.01 ± 0.28 [38]	≈1	≈1	≈1	<1
ARmax (ms)	0.23 ± 0.06 [38]	N	N	↑	↑↑
S/D	0.90 ± 0.29 [39]	>1	>1	≈1	<<1
E/E′	<10	<10	≥10	≥10	≥10

Adur/ARdur, Ratio of the duration of the transmitral flow A wave and the duration of the pulmonary venous flow AR wave; *ARmax,* maximum velocity of the pulmonary venous flow AR wave; *E/A,* ratio of the transmitral flow E and A waves; *E/E′,* ratio of the transmitral flow E wave and pulsed wave tissue Doppler of the mitral annulus E′ wave; *IVRT,* left ventricle isovolumic relaxation time; *LV,* left ventricular; *S/D,* ratio of the pulmonary venous flow S and D wave velocities.

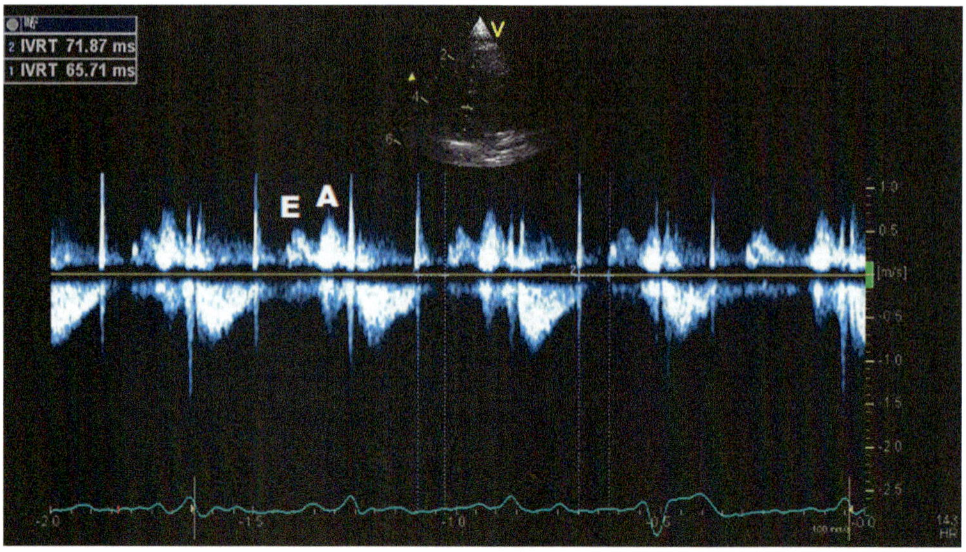

• **Fig. 13-13** Pulsed wave spectral Doppler of the transmitral and aortic flows documenting delayed relaxation in a cat with hypertrophic cardiomyopathy (HCM). The E/A ratio is inverted and the isovolumic relaxation time (IVRT) is prolonged, with values ranging from 66 to 72 ms. (Photo credit: Éric de Madron.)

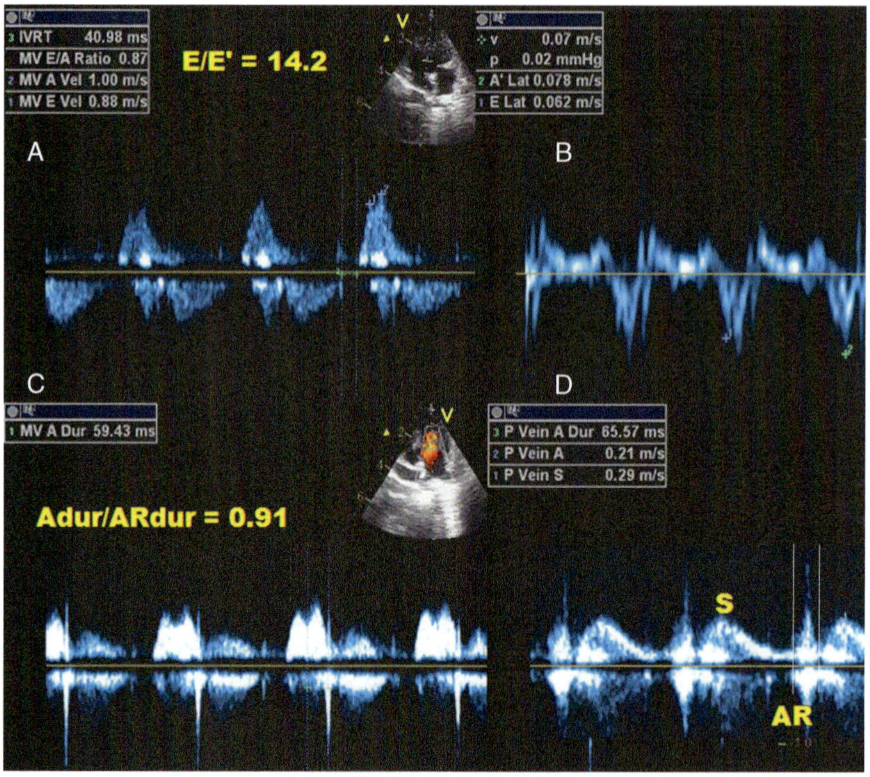

• **Fig. 13-14** Pulsed wave spectral Doppler of the transmitral (A, C) and aortic (A) flows, pulsed wave tissue Doppler of the mitral annulus (B), and pulsed wave spectral Doppler of the pulmonary venous flow (D) in a cat presenting with hypertrophic cardiomyopathy (HCM) and pseudonormal diastolic function. The E/A ratio remains close to 1 and the isovolumic relaxation time (IVRT) is normal. In contrast, the E/E′ ratio is high, indicating elevated left atrial pressure. The Adur/ARdur ratio is <1, indicating early restrictive physiology. (Photo credit: Éric de Madron.)

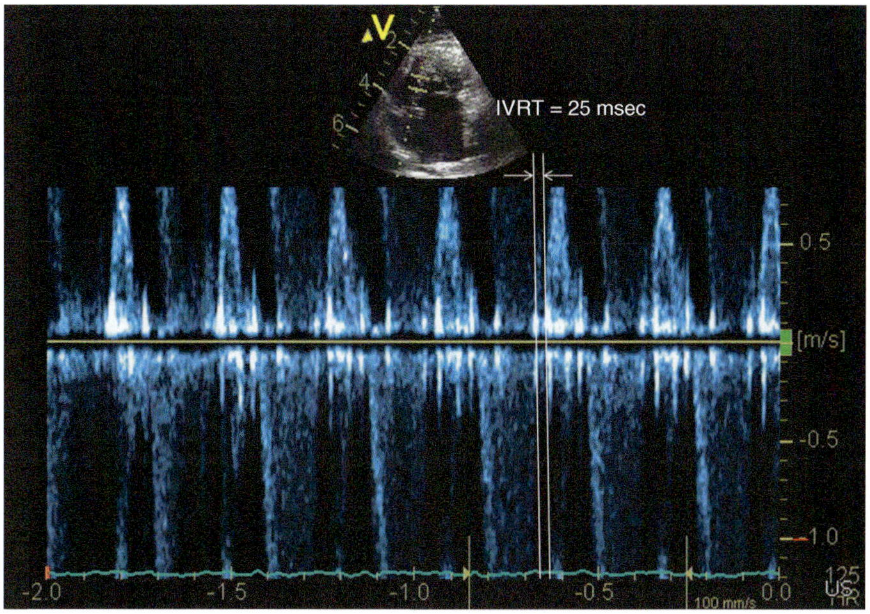

• **Fig. 13-15** Pulsed wave Doppler of the transmitral and aortic flows in a cat with hypertrophic cardiomyopathy (HCM) and restrictive diastolic dysfunction. The isovolumic relaxation time (IVRT) is shortened. The turbulent aortic flow with aliasing indicates concomitant left ventricular outflow tract obstruction. (Photo credit: Éric de Madron.)

Measurement of the isovolumic relaxation time (IVRT) is crucial to assess the degree of diastolic dysfunction associated with HCM, because the E and A as well as the E′ and A′ waves are often fused in cats, due to their elevated heart rate. However, the IVRT value by itself may sometimes be misleading. Indeed, diastolic dysfunction could be present (and confirmed by tissue Doppler; see below) with a still normal IVRT.

Tissue Doppler

Pulsed Wave Tissue Doppler of the Mitral Annulus

The amplitude of the lateral mitral annulus E′ or of the fused E′ and A′ ($E'A'_{sum}$) waves, measured using a left apical 4 chambers view, decreases in HCM due to ventricular relaxation impairment (Figure 13-16) [28].

These tissue Doppler anomalies of the annulus can be present early on, even prior to the appearance of hypertrophy. This has been documented in Maine Coon cats with an abnormal genotype (*MyBPC3* mutation) when no myocardial hypertrophy had yet been detected using conventional echocardiographic examination [28].

The maximum velocity of the mitral annulus S′ wave is also reduced in HCM, illustrating a systolic dysfunction not detectable by TM mode [29].

An E/E′ ratio ≥10 is compatible with elevated left atrial pressure (see Chapter 9) [16].

Tissue Doppler of the Left Myocardium and Septum

Tissue Doppler left myocardial and septal abnormalities associated with HCM are predominantly diastolic and more pronounced for the longitudinal motion than for the radial motion. They include [29-33]:

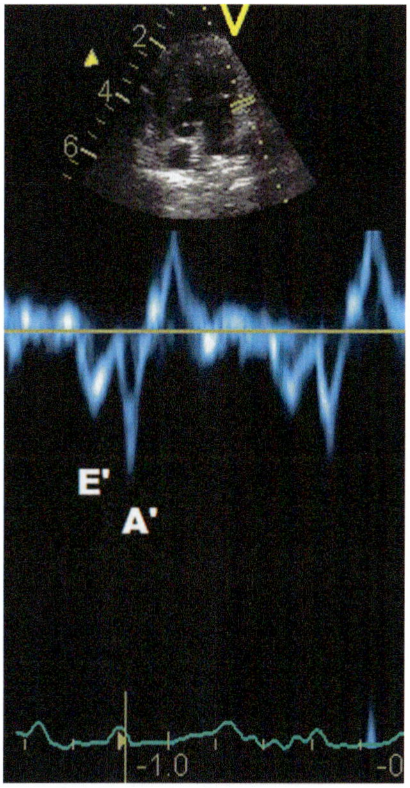

• **Fig. 13-16** Mitral annulus pulsed wave tissue Doppler demonstrating delayed relaxation in a cat with hypertrophic cardiomyopathy (HCM). The E′/A′ ratio is inverted. (Photo credit: Éric de Madron.)

- Decreased early diastolic velocities (E_{DTI})
- End-diastolic velocity increase (A_{DTI}) with decrease in E_{DTI}/A_{DTI} ratio (Figures 13-17 to 13-19)

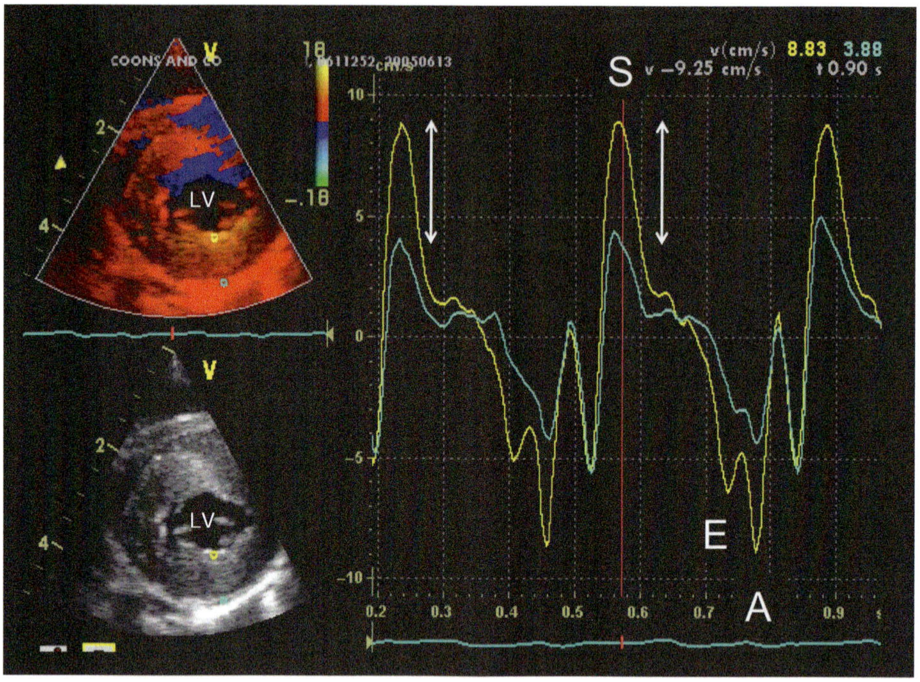

• **Fig. 13-17** Impaired left radial myocardial function analyzed by color bidimensional (2D) tissue Doppler imaging (TDI) in a Maine Coon cat with hypertrophic cardiomyopathy (HCM). Myocardial velocities are analyzed simultaneously in two circular segments of 1-mm diameter: a subendocardial segment *(yellow)* and a subepicardial segment *(green)* of the left ventricular free wall. The myocardial function impairment is systolic and diastolic, and characterized by an increased systolic S wave, an increased endoepicardial systolic gradient *(white double arrows)*, and early diastolic and end-diastolic wave inversion (E and A, respectively), with an E/A ratio <1. *LV,* Left ventricle. (Photo credit: Valérie Chetboul.)

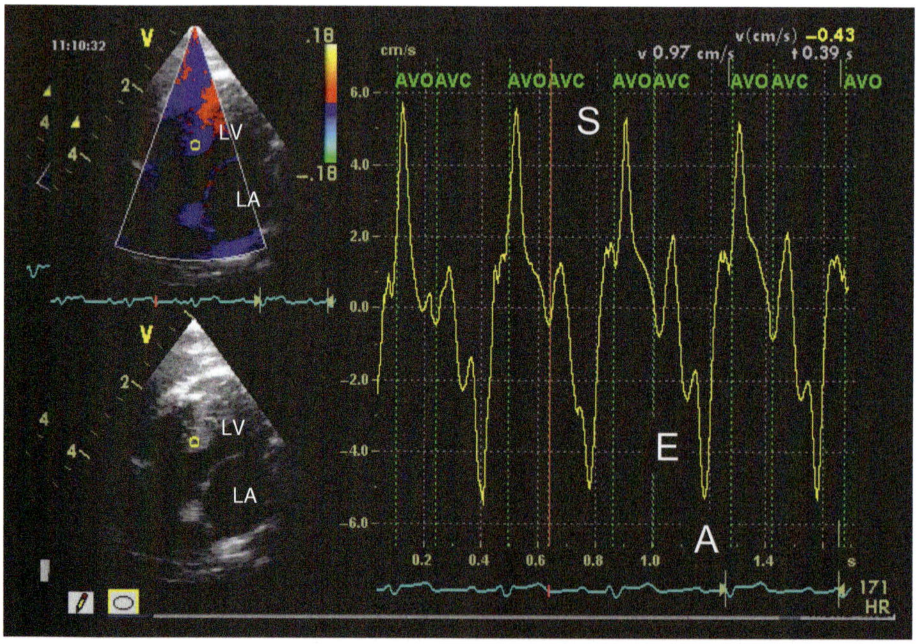

• **Fig. 13-18** Impaired septal longitudinal myocardial function analyzed by color bidimensional (2D) tissue Doppler imaging (TDI) in a Maine Coon cat with hypertrophic cardiomyopathy (HCM). Myocardial velocities are analyzed in a circular segment of 2-mm diameter located at the base of the interventricular septum. The myocardial function impairment is diastolic and characterized by early diastolic and end-diastolic wave inversion (E and A, respectively), with an E/A ratio <1. *AVC,* Aortic valve closure; *AVO,* aortic valve opening; *LA,* left atrium; *LV,* left ventricle. (Photo credit: Valérie Chetboul.)

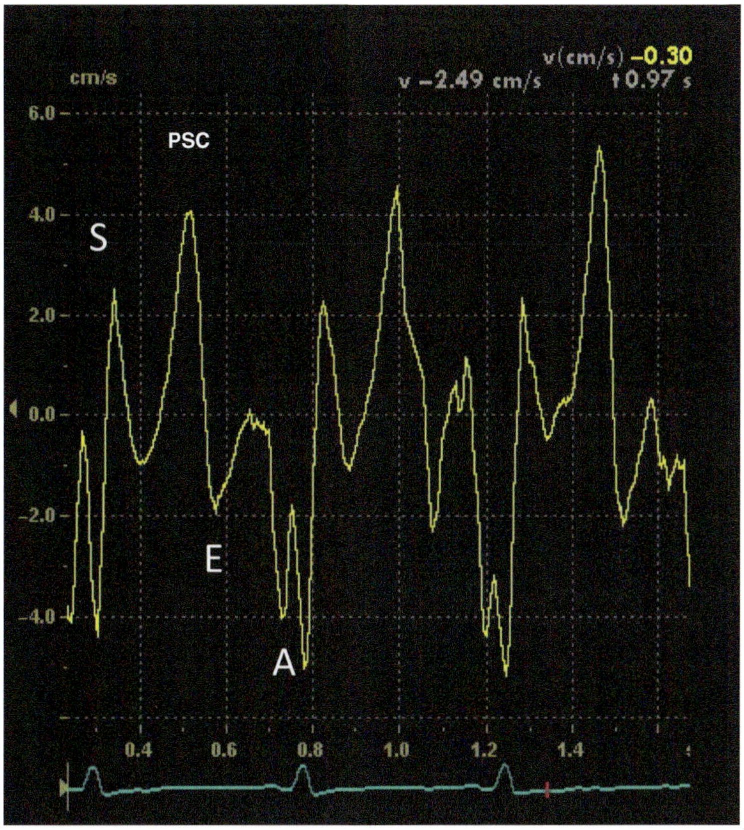

• **Fig. 13-19** Impaired left longitudinal myocardial function analyzed by color bidimensional (2D) tissue Doppler imaging (TDI) in a Maine Coon cat with hypertrophic cardiomyopathy (HCM). Myocardial velocities are analyzed in a circular segment of 2-mm diameter located at the base of the ventricular free wall. The myocardial function impairment is systolic and diastolic, and characterized by the presence of a postsystolic contraction (PSC) of greater amplitude than the systolic S wave as well as early diastolic and end-diastolic wave inversion (E and A, respectively), with an E/A ratio <1. (Photo credit: Valérie Chetboul.)

- Reduced early diastolic endoepicardial and left ventricular free wall base-apex gradients
- Increased end-diastolic endoepicardial and left ventricular free wall base-apex gradients
- Increased radial and especially longitudinal IVRT

In Maine Coon cats, heterozygous for the *MyBPC3* mutation but free of LV hypertrophy, a significant decrease in E_{DTI}/A_{DTI} was demonstrated in the longitudinal movement of the basal interventricular septum (in comparison to wild homozygous animals).

The magnitude of the changes of direction of the myocardial motion during the isovolumic contraction and relaxation phases is also decreased in cats with HCM [30].

In normal cats, septal systolic and diastolic velocities are higher than free wall velocities. This physiologic difference disappears in cats with HCM [29].

Systolic dysfunction is also present in HCM, often initially characterized by radial hyperkinesia (with increased systolic velocities and gradients), followed by a decrease in longitudinal ventricular systolic velocities (radial systolic velocities being, at this stage, often normal or reduced) [29,31]. An S′ wave corresponding to a postsystolic contraction is noted in almost 25% of feline HCM cases, particularly for the left and/or right septal longitudinal movement [29]. This myocardial systolic dysfunction is usually undetectable by conventional echocardiographic examination (normal SF).

The systolic and diastolic myocardial alterations described above can be observed in regions of the myocardium that are still not affected by hypertrophy. This observation, made during both spontaneous "classical" and dystrophic HCM, confirms the high sensitivity of tissue Doppler imaging (TDI) in the diagnosis of regional myocardial dysfunction as well as its importance in early HCM screening [31,32].

Speckle Tracking

Speckle tracking mode enables the documentation of the same dysfunctions detected by TDI. A decrease in the

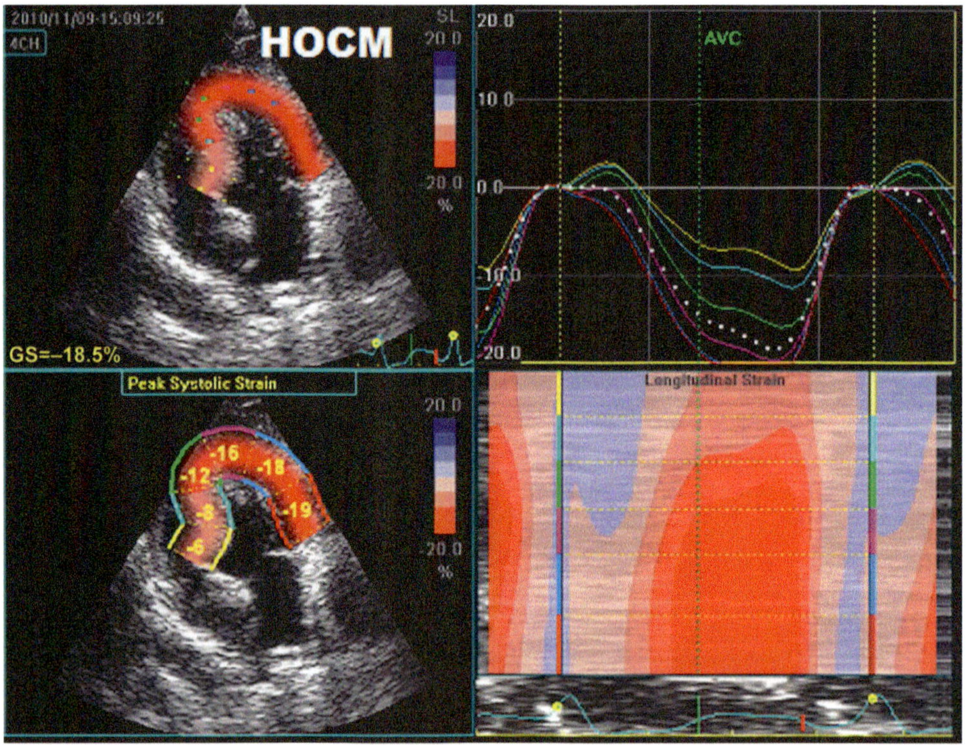

• **Fig. 13-20** Speckle tracking of the left ventricle (longitudinal movement) in a cat with hypertrophic obstructive cardiomyopathy (HOCM) characterized by hypertrophy of the base of the septum. The maximum longitudinal systolic strain of the basal segment of the septum is slightly lower *(pink)* than that of other segments of the left ventricle *(red)*, indicating mild hypokinesia of the hypertrophied area. *AVC,* Aortic valve closure; *GS,* global strain. (Photo credit: Éric de Madron.)

peak systolic strain, a sign of myocardial hypokinesia, is often noted within the hypertrophied area (Figure 13-20) and even in apparently normal segments, according to 2D and TM echocardiography (Figure 13-21). The longitudinal systolic strain is most frequently affected; the radial strain generally remains normal (see Figure 13-21). These local dysfunctions can lead to dyskinesia, the affected segment stretching in systole and contracting in diastole (Figure 13-22).

Restrictive Cardiomyopathies

Restrictive cardiomyopathy (RCM) represents 7% to 24% of feline cardiomyopathies and comes in two forms: myocardial and so-called endomyocardial [1-3]. The myocardial form in cats is idiopathic and noninfiltrative (no amyloid deposits, unlike in humans) [1]. Fibrosis of the endocardium is discrete and multifocal. In the endomyocardial form, fibrosis of the endocardium is predominant and often located at the apex of the LV. The ventricular chamber is distorted, sometimes with obliteration of its apical area as well as intraventricular stenosis. The mitral apparatus can be fused and distorted. The etiology of this form includes hypereosinophilic syndrome [1,34], endomyocarditis, and endomyocardial fibrosis of the LV [1,3].

Echocardiographic Characteristics

2D and TM Echocardiography

In both forms of RCM, the thickness of the LV walls is typically normal or in the upper limits of the normal range. The LV chamber is normal to slightly dilated (Figures 13-23 and 13-24) with a normal or slightly reduced left ventricular SF (Figure 13-25 and Videos 13-15 and 13-16) [1]. Regional dyskinesia (Video 13-17) is sometimes observed (see "Speckle tracking" below). In the endomyocardial form, focal hyperechogenicity of the endocardium associated with endomyocardial plaques can be observed [2,7].

In the case of endomyocarditis or endocardial fibroelastosis [1,3,34], the endocardium often appears

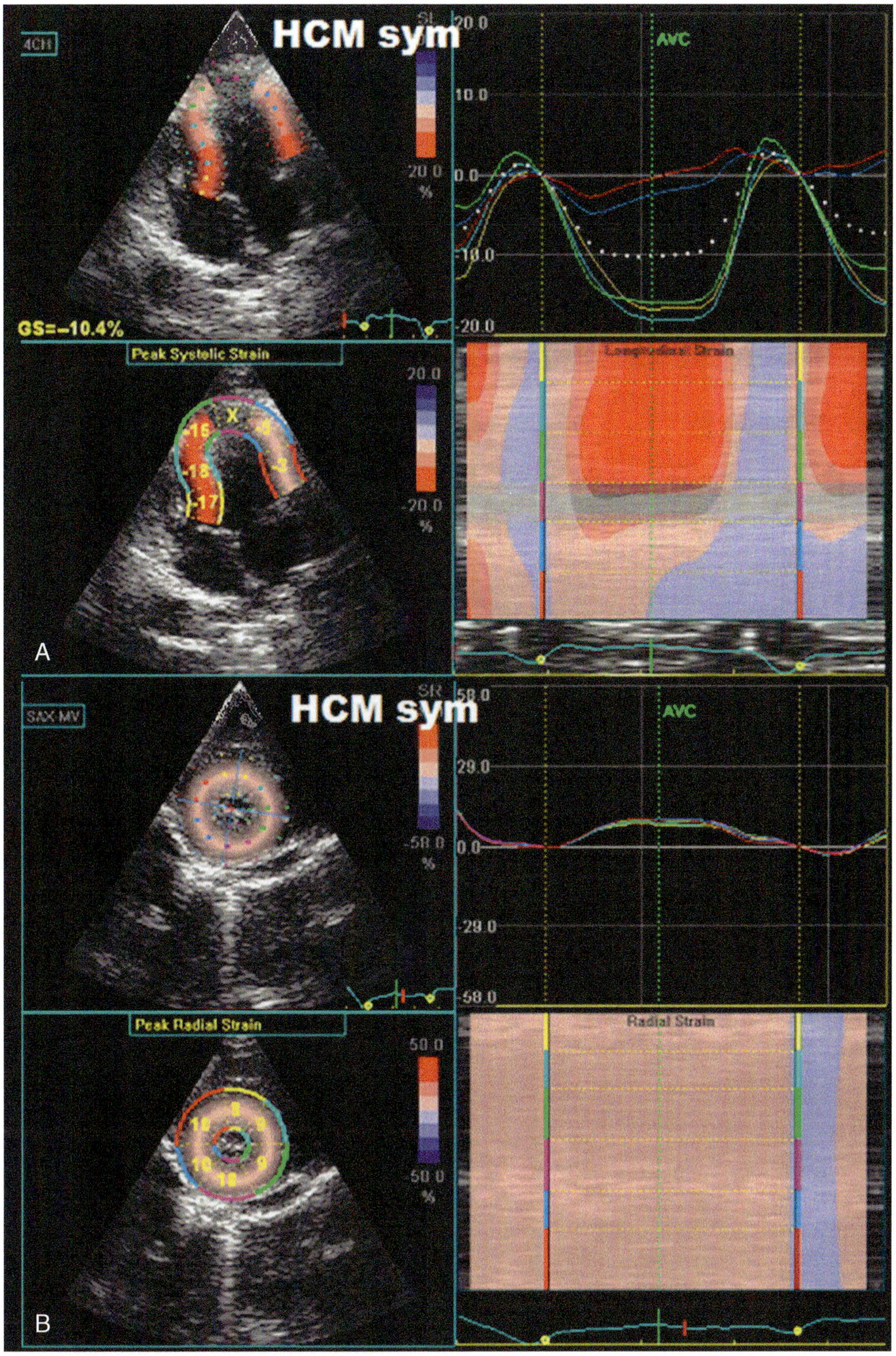

• **Fig. 13-21** Speckle tracking of the left ventricular radial (A) and longitudinal (B) movement in a cat with slightly obstructive symmetric hypertrophic cardiomyopathy (HCM sym). A, The peak longitudinal systolic strain of the left ventricular free wall basal and lateral segments is weaker *(colored pale pink and numbered −3 and −5)* than that of other segments of the left ventricle *(colored red and numbered −16, −18, and −17)*, indicating relative regional hypokinesia of the left ventricular free wall. B, However, the maximum radial systolic strain is uniform though generally decreased *(light pink)* in all left ventricular segments. *AVC,* Aortic valve closure; *GS,* global strain. (Photo credit: Éric de Madron.)

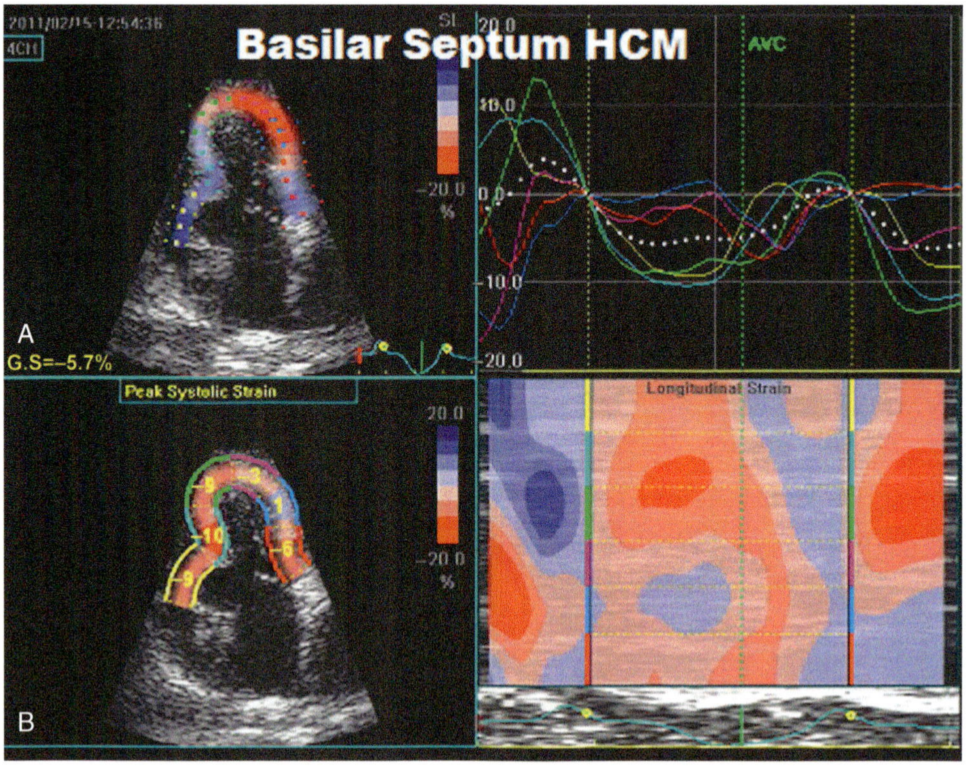

• **Fig. 13-22** Speckle tracking of the left ventricle (longitudinal movement) in a cat with hypertrophic cardiomyopathy (HCM) characterized by significant hypertrophy of the base of the septum. The apicolateral left ventricular free wall segment behaves in a paradoxic manner (dyskinesia), contracting in diastole (A, *red zone*) and stretching in systole (B, *blue zone numbered 1*). The peak systolic strain of all left ventricular segments *(pale pink)* is globally decreased. All septal segments contract normally *(light red and dark red)*. *AVC,* Aortic valve closure; *GS,* global strain. (Photo credit: Éric de Madron.)

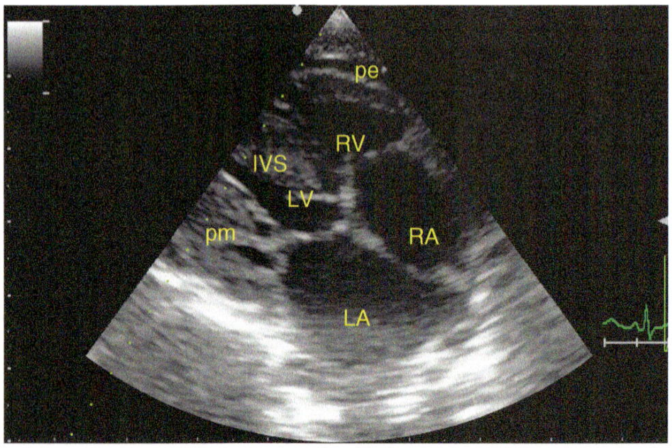

• **Fig. 13-23** Bidimensional (2D) echocardiogram (right parasternal long axis 4 chambers view) in a cat with restrictive cardiomyopathy (RCM). The appearance of the left ventricle (LV) is relatively normal. The right ventricle (RV) is slightly dilated. The two atria are markedly dilated. A small anterior pericardial effusion (pe) is present. *IVS,* Interventricular septum; *LA,* left atrium; *PM,* papillary muscle; *RA,* right atrium. (Photo credit: Éric de Madron.)

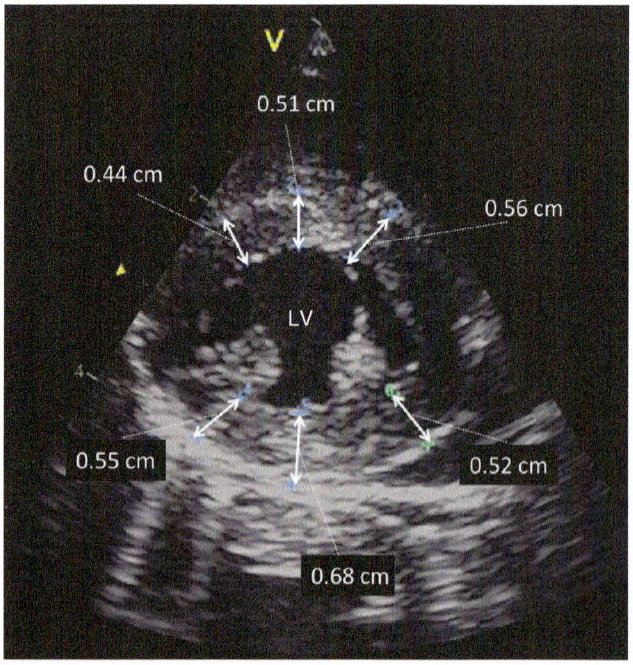

• **Fig. 13-24** Bidimensional (2D) echocardiogram (right parasternal short axis transventricular view) in a cat with restrictive cardiomyopathy (RCM). The appearance of the left ventricle (LV) is fairly normal for most of the examined segments. The end-diastolic wall thickness is at the upper limit of normal. In some areas, myocardial heterogeneity can be observed. Hyperechoic plaques can also be seen (fibrosis). (Photo credit: Éric de Madron.)

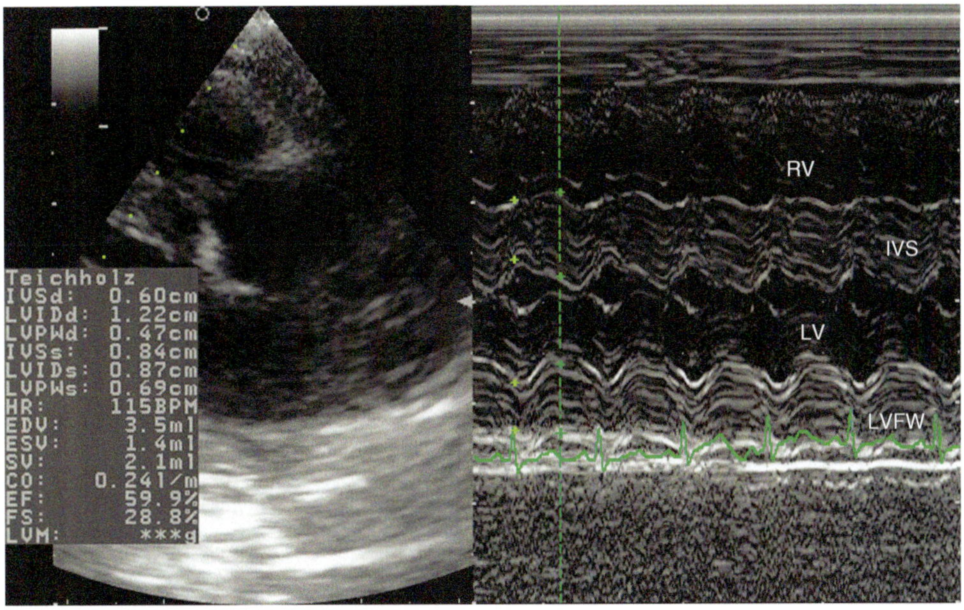

• **Fig. 13-25** Time-motion (TM) echocardiogram (right parasternal transventricular view) in a cat with restrictive cardiomyopathy (RCM). The contractility of the left ventricle (LV) is relatively normal. The left ventricular free wall (LVFW) is slightly thicker than normal. The serrated appearance of the myocardium of the LVFW and the septum (IVS) is consistent with myocardial fibrosis. *RV,* Right ventricle. (Photo credit: Éric de Madron.)

hyperechoic and diffusely thickened. Intraventricular bands distorting the ventricular cavity can sometimes be observed.

Marked dilation of the atria is usually present (Figure 13-26 and Video 13-18). Spontaneous echo contrast (SEC) is present in the LA in 22.7% of cats with RCM (see Video 13-11) [2].

A small pericardial effusion can be observed in 9.1% of cases (see Figure 13-23) [2].

Color Doppler

RCM is typically not associated with dynamic left and right ventricular outflow tract obstructions. However, a systolic turbulence may be noted in cases of intraventricular stenosis. It is sometimes possible to observe a mitral regurgitation jet.

Spectral Doppler

Spectral Doppler allows the documentation of a predominantly restrictive diastolic dysfunction. Indeed, the myocardial fibrosis, a salient feature of RCM, leads to increased ventricular myocardial stiffness, adding to the ventricular relaxation disorders already present. This loss of compliance will greatly reduce end-diastolic filling. Weakening atrial contractility compounds this. At the same time, the left atrial pressures are elevated, exaggerating the early diastolic filling (see Chapter 8) [27].

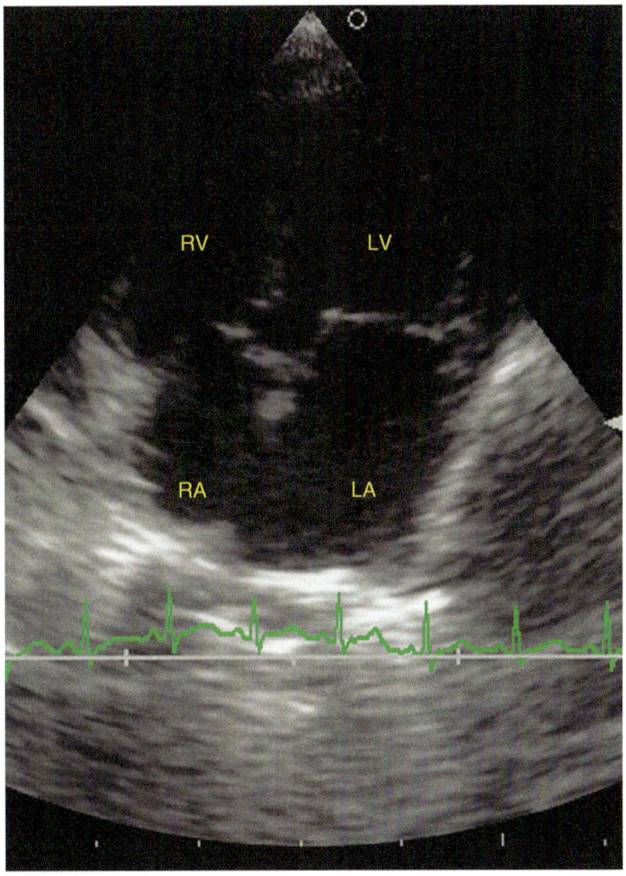

• **Fig. 13-26** Bidimensional (2D) echocardiogram (left apical 5 chambers view) in a cat with restrictive cardiomyopathy (RCM). Note the biatrial dilation. *LA,* Left atrium; *LV,* left ventricle; *RA,* right atrium; *RV,* right ventricle. (Photo credit: Éric de Madron.)

Therefore the transmitral flow is characterized by an increased E wave, a reduced A wave, and an increased E/A ratio. The IVRT is decreased (Figure 13-27). The E′ and A′ waves are decreased. The RA wave amplitude is greatly increased and the Adur/ARdur ratio becomes <1 (see Chapter 8) [16].

Speckle Tracking

Myocardial fibrosis can affect regional left ventricular segmental kinesis. Speckle tracking mode allows the visualization of these dyskinetic areas, behaving in an opposite fashion to that of the normal segments (longitudinal systolic stretching and diastolic shortening) (Figure 13-28).

Dilated Cardiomyopathies

Dilated cardiomyopathy (DCM) has become rare in the feline species since taurine supplementation in processed cat foods [35]. The prevalence of DCM is currently 10.4% [1,2]. Females are most affected. The average age of affected cats is 9 years [1,2]. Siamese and Abyssinians seem to be predisposed [1,36].

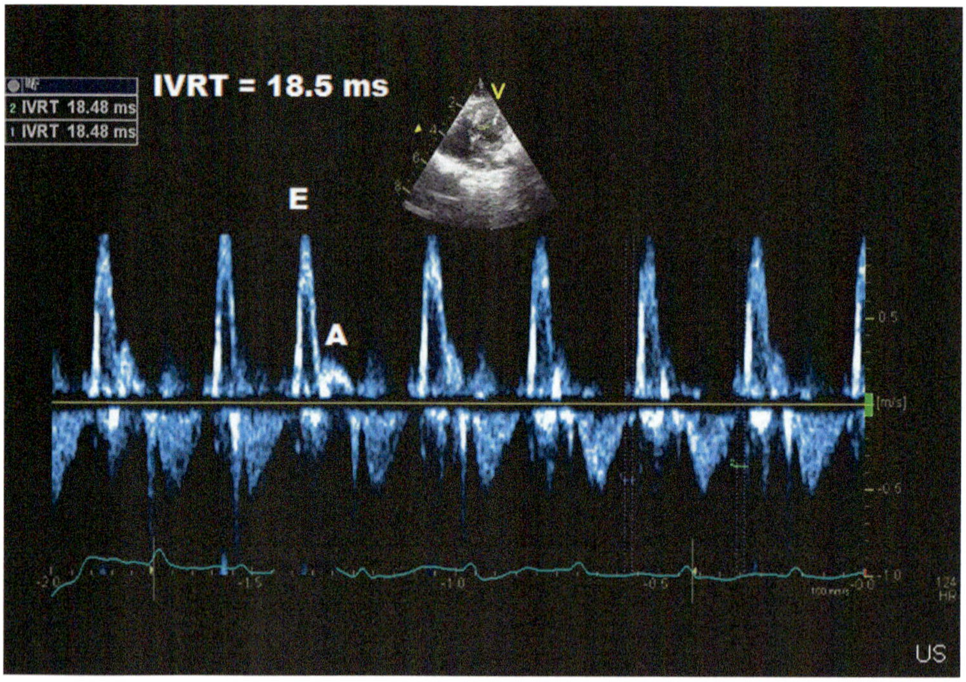

• **Fig. 13-27** Pulsed wave spectral Doppler of the transmitral flow in a cat with restrictive cardiomyopathy (RCM) and severe restrictive diastolic dysfunction. The maximum E wave velocity is increased (reaching 1 m/s), indicating high atrial pressure; the E/A ratio is >2; and the isovolumic relaxation time (IVRT) is greatly shortened (18.5 ms). (Photo credit: Éric de Madron.)

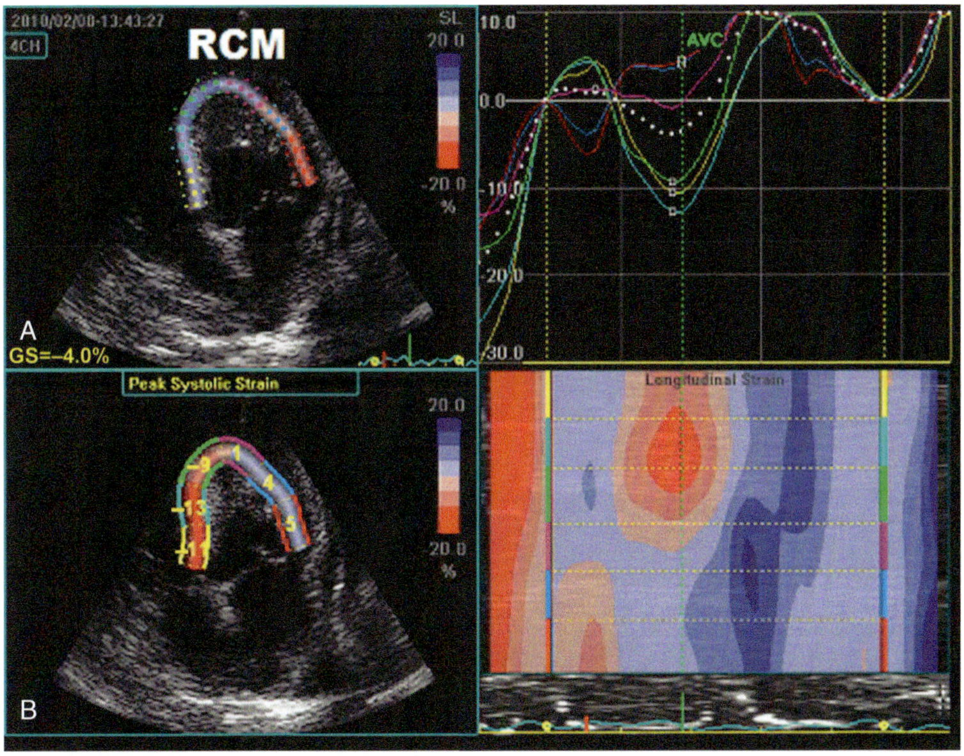

• **Fig. 13-28** Speckle tracking of the left ventricle (longitudinal movement) in a cat with restrictive cardiomyopathy (RCM). A, In diastole, all segments are stretching *(blue)*, except for the basal part of the free wall. B, Note the inversion of the peak longitudinal systolic strain in most of the left ventricular free wall, stretching rather than contracting in systole *(blue)*. This indicates significant dyskinesia of these segments. The septum contracts normally *(red)*. *AVC,* Aortic valve closure; *GS,* global strain. (Photo credit: Éric de Madron.)

Echocardiographic Characteristics

2D and TM Echocardiography

In its typical form, DCM is characterized by decreased inotropy with dilation of the four cardiac cavities. The LV becomes spherical and contractility indices are markedly decreased. The left ventricular walls are thinner than normal (Figures 13-29 and 13-30; Video 13-19) [7].

The mitral valve opens only slightly in diastole due to low flow, resulting in increased E-septum distance [7]. Delayed mitral valve closure is sometimes observed due to the increased atrial and left ventricular end-diastolic pressures [7].

Pericardial effusion and intraatrial SECs are present in 18.2% of cases [2].

Color Doppler

Color Doppler allows the detection of any functional mitral or tricuspid regurgitation secondary to annular dilation. Degenerative atrioventricular lesions can also lead to these systolic regurgitations.

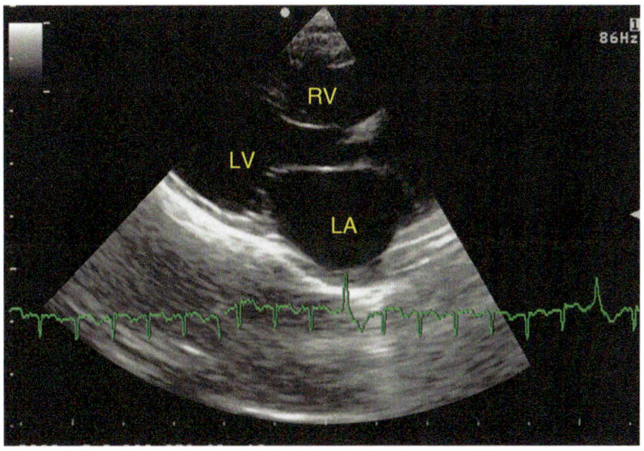

• **Fig. 13-29** Bidimensional (2D) echocardiogram (right parasternal long axis 4 chambers view) in a cat with dilated cardiomyopathy (DCM). The four cavities are dilated. The left ventricular walls are thin. *LA,* Left atrium; *LV,* left ventricle; *RV,* right ventricle. (Photo credit: Éric de Madron.)

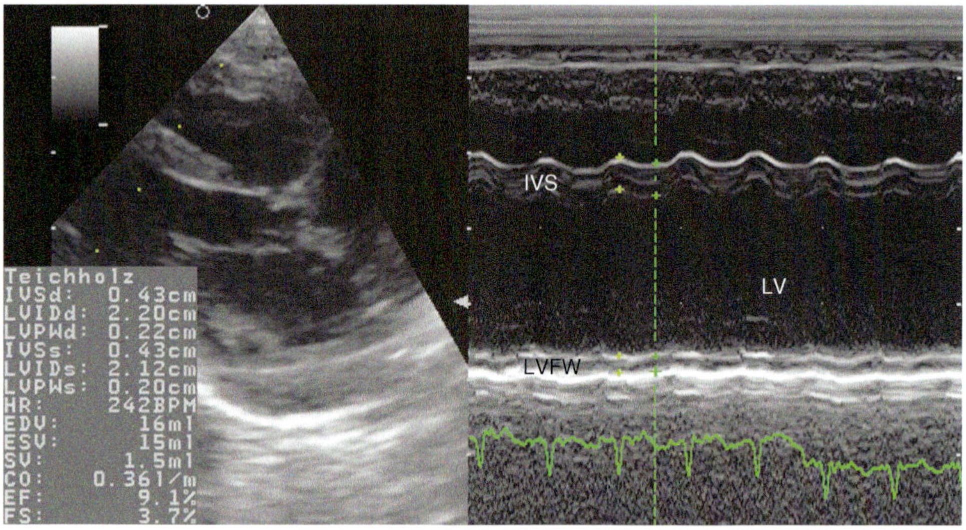

• **Fig. 13-30** Time-motion (TM) echocardiogram (transventricular view) in a cat with dilated cardiomyopathy (DCM). The end-systolic and end-diastolic left ventricular internal diameters are increased. The left ventricular walls are thin and hypokinetic. The shortening fraction has collapsed (SF = 3.7%). *IVS,* Interventricular septum; *LV,* left ventricle; *LVFW,* left ventricular free wall. (Photo credit: Éric de Madron.)

Spectral Doppler

Spectral Doppler reveals low-velocity aortic and pulmonary ejection flows.

Diastolic dysfunction accompanies and sometimes precedes systolic dysfunction. It can range from delayed relaxation to restrictive dysfunction (see above) [27].

Atypical Cardiomyopathies

"Undetermined" Cardiomyopathies

Some cats have echocardiographic anomalies that do not correspond to any of the above categories. Typically there is a combination of focal hypertrophy of the LV with regional hypokinesia, marked atrial dilatation, and mitral regurgitation [2] (Video 13-20). These are called undetermined cardiomyopathies (UCMs). The prevalence of UCM is 10.4% [2]. It is possible that a majority of these UCMs are in fact advanced HCM with significant LV remodeling. The echocardiographer should endeavor to outline the morphologic and predominant hemodynamic abnormalities in order to best describe this type of cardiomyopathy.

Excessive Moderator Bands

Moderator bands or "pseudotendons" are intraventricular fibrous bands. Echocardiographically, they appear as hyperechoic bands connecting the left ventricular free wall or one of the papillary muscles to the septum. Discrete and isolated bands do not affect LV hemodynamics and are often found in normal cats [1]. However, thick or excessive moderator bands (Figure 13-31) can affect diastolic filling and cause restrictive diastolic dysfunction, resulting in dilation of the LA. These bands can also disturb ventricular ejection (Figure 13-32). Moderate ventricular hypertrophy can also be observed [1].

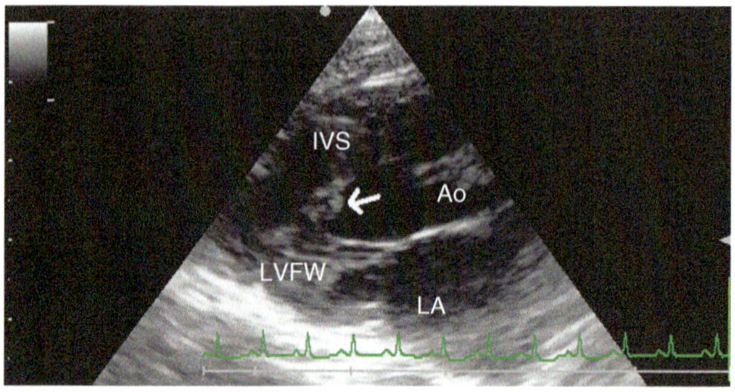

• **Fig. 13-31** Bidimensional (2D) echocardiogram (right parasternal long axis 5 chambers view) in a cat with a large moderator band in the left ventricle. This one appears as a strip of heterogeneous tissue connecting the septum to one of the papillary muscles *(arrow)*, thus restraining dilation of the middle of the left ventricular chamber. *Ao,* Aorta; *LA,* left atrium; *LVFW,* left ventricular free wall; *IVS,* interventricular septum. (Photo credit: Éric de Madron.)

Right Ventricular Cardiomyopathies

Right ventricular cardiomyopathies represent 2% to 4% of all feline cardiomyopathies [1]. They are related to the arrhythmogenic right ventricular cardiomyopathy described in the Boxer, with fibrofatty infiltration of the myocardium [1]. The echocardiographic examination reveals segmental or diffuse dilation of the RV, sometimes with localized aneurysms; significant right atrial dilation; abnormal morphology of the trabeculae; paradoxic movement of the interventricular septum; and an often significant tricuspid valve regurgitation [1,6,36]. In some cases,

LA dilatation and systolic dysfunction of the LV can also be observed [1,6]. Arrhythmias may also be present [37].

Noncompaction of the Left Ventricle

Noncompaction of the LV is a rare disorder characterized by hypertrabeculation of the endomyocardium. The subsequent crypts communicate with the ventricular chamber. The crypts represent an interruption of the normal development and compaction of the ventricle. They are present in the fetus and allow nutrients to access the myocardium in the absence of coronary arteries. In the affected individual, this leads to a spongy myocardium with multiple small channels indenting the endocardium. These channels do not connect to coronary vascularization [38].

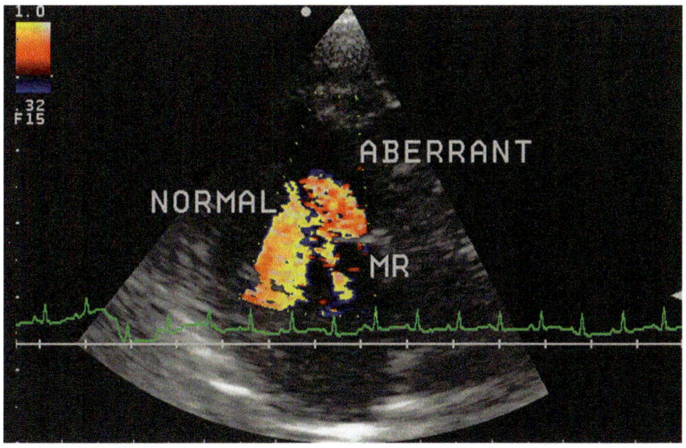

• **Fig. 13-32** Echocardiogram in color Doppler mode (left apical 5 chambers view) in a cat with a large moderator band in the left ventricle. The intraventricular flow splits into two parts at the level of the moderating band: one part heads as normal toward the left ventricular outflow tract (NORMAL) and the other part heads toward the mitral valve (ABERRANT). Mitral regurgitation (MR) is also present. (Photo credit: Éric de Madron.)

Thrombotic Risk Assessment

Arterial thrombosis is a serious complication of feline cardiomyopathies leading to significant morbidity and mortality. This complication is observed in 36% to 48% of HCM, 29% of RCM, 25% of DCM, and 14% of cardiomyopathies associated with excessive moderator bands [1,23].

The thrombus usually forms in the LA. One of the early signs is the presence of SEC swirling in the LA [16]. Contributing factors are intraatrial blood stasis resulting from atrial dilation, impaired left atrial contractility, endothelial lesions prompting platelet adhesion, and release of procoagulant factors [16].

Thromboembolic risk identification is important, as it will affect the decision making regarding the prescription of anticoagulants.

Atrial Dilation

Cats with intraatrial SEC tend to have a more dilated LA ($LAmax_{syst}$ >2.4 cm) than those without (Table 13-2).

Atrial Function

In HCM cases, the atrial function declines and this can lead to blood stasis setting the stage for thrombus formation. In the study by Schober and Maerz [16], two parameters have been used to evaluate this function (see Table 13-2): the LA shortening fraction (LASF%) and the LA fractional area change (LAFAC%).

LASF% calculation uses the LA septolateral systolic and diastolic diameters ($LAmax_{syst}$ and $LAmax_{diast}$), obtained using the right parasternal long axis 4 chambers view:

$$LASF\,\% = (LAmax_{syst} - LAmax_{diast})/LAmax_{syst} \times 100$$

TABLE 13-2 Significantly Different Parameters in Cats with (SEC+) and without (SEC–) Spontaneous Intraatrial Echo Contrast [16]

Variable	SEC+	SEC–
LAmax (mm)	2.4 (1.34-3.1)	1.9 (1.36-3.25)
LASF%	10 (0-37)	20 (1-45)
LAFAC%	9 (0-42)	30 (0-61)
Peak wave 1 (m/s)	0.16 (0.09-0.25)	0.30 (0.07-1.35)
Peak wave 2 (m/s)	0.15 (0.06-0.30)	0.32 (0.19-0.85)
LAA V_{max} (m/s)	0.15 (0.07-0.23)	0.33 (0.08-1.35)

LAA V_{max}, Maximum velocity of left intraatrial appendage flow; *LAFAC%*, left atrial fractional area change; *LAmax*, septolateral systolic atrial diameter; *LASF%*, left atrium shortening fraction; *Peak wave 1*, maximum velocity of wave 1 of the left intraatrial appendage flow; *Peak wave 2*, maximum velocity of wave 2 of the left intraatrial appendage flow.

The systolic and diastolic areas of the LA ($LAarea_{syst}$ and $LAarea_{diast}$) are measured using the same view and the LAFAC% is calculated using the following equation:

$$LAFAC\% = (LAarea_{syst} - LAarea_{diast})/LAarea_{syst} \times 100$$

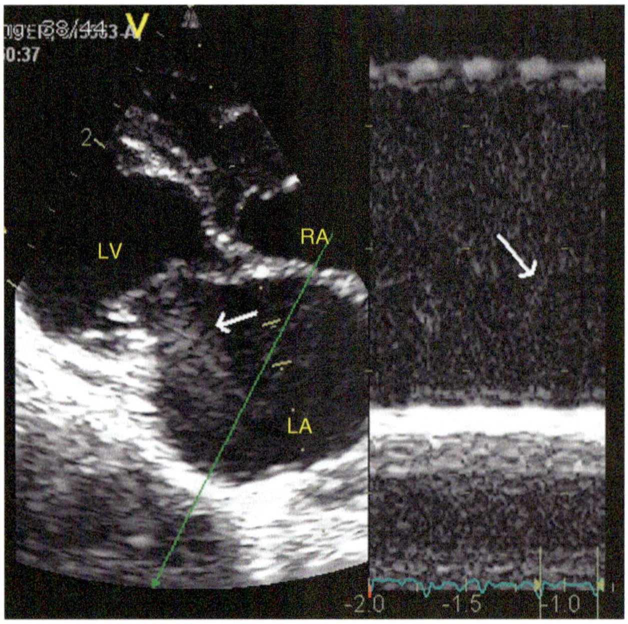

• **Fig. 13-33** Bidimensional (2D) (right parasternal long axis 4 chambers view) *(left image)* and time-motion (TM) *(right image)* echocardiograms of the left atrium in a cat with advanced restrictive cardiomyopathy (RCM). The left atrium (LA) is markedly dilated and hypocontractile. Spontaneous echographic contrast is visible *(arrows)*. This indicates an elevated risk of thrombosis. *LV,* Left ventricle; *RA,* right atrium. (Photo credit: Éric de Madron.)

The atrial function in cats with intraatrial SEC is significantly lower than that in cats without SEC (see Table 13-2; Figure 13-33 and Video 13-21) [16].

Intraatrial Velocities

The measurement of blood velocities in the left atrial appendage allows the documentation of blood stasis and the identification of cats at risk for thrombosis. These velocities are measured by positioning the sample volume in the left atrial appendage and using an oblique right parasternal short axis view (Figure 13-34). The flow thus obtained is characterized by two waves: wave 1, negative and end-diastolic, corresponding to the end-diastolic emptying of the LA, and wave 2, positive and early systolic corresponding to atrial filling.

The maximum velocities of the left atrial appendage waves in cats with SEC tend to be much lower than in cats without SEC. A maximum value of these velocities <0.20 m/s predicts the presence of SEC and indicates a greater risk of thrombus formation (Figure 13-35) [16].

Global Context

In the study by Schober and Maerz [16], HCM was present in 24.5% of SEC cases, RCM in 25%, DCM in 33.3%, and UCM in 20%. The majority of cats (63.2%) with SEC displayed advanced diastolic dysfunction of a restrictive type. None of these cats had normal diastolic function. The majority of the animals (68.4%) were also in CHF.

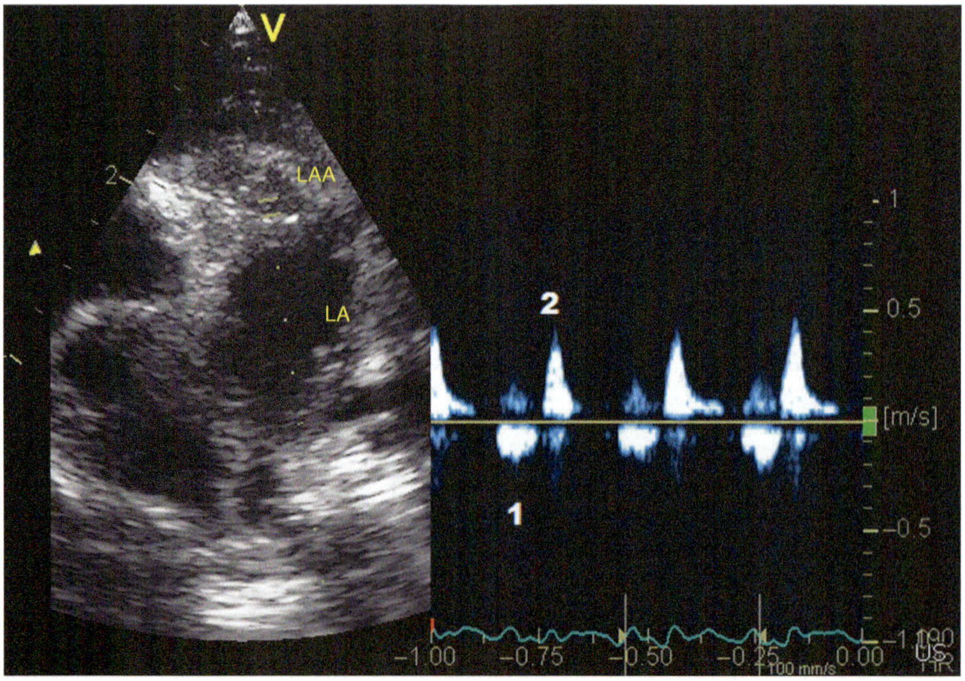

• **Fig. 13-34** Example of a spectral Doppler recording of normal blood flow in the left atrial appendage (LAA) of a cat, characterized by wave 1, negative and end-diastolic corresponding to the end-diastolic emptying of the left atrium (LA), and wave 2, corresponding to atrial filling. (Photo credit: Éric de Madron.)

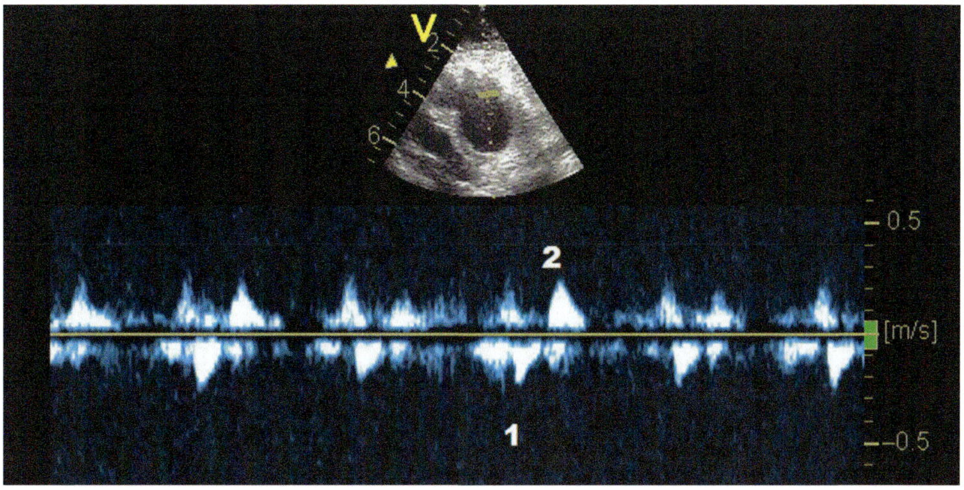

• **Fig. 13-35** Spectral Doppler of blood flow in the left atrial appendage illustrating reduced waves 1 and 2 maximum velocities (≤0.2 m/s), indicating a high risk of thrombosis. (Photo credit: Éric de Madron.)

REFERENCES

[1] Fox PR. Feline cardiomyopathies. In: Fox PR, Moise NS, Sisson D, editors. Textbook of canine and feline cardiology: principles and clinical practice. 1999;2: 621–78.

[2] Ferasin L, Sturgess CP, Cannon MJ, et al. Feline idiopathic cardiomyopathy: a retrospective study of 106 cats (1994–2001). J Feline Med Surg 2003;5:151–9.

[3] Tilley LP, Liu SK, Gilberston SR, et al. Primary myocardial disease in the cat. Am J Pathol 1977;87:493–522.

[4] Meurs KM, Sanchez X, David RM, et al. A cardiac myosin binding protein C mutation in the Maine coon cat with familial hypertrophic cardiomyopathy. Hum Mol Gen 2005;14:3587–93.

[5] Bright JM, Golden AL, Daniel GB. Feline hypertrophic cardiomyopathy: variations on a theme. J Small Anim Pract 1992;33:266–74.

[6] Paige CF, Abbott JA, Elvinger F, Pyle RL. Prevalence of cardiomyopathy in apparently healthy cats. J Am Vet Med Assoc 2009;234:1398–403.

[7] Bonagura JD. Feline echocardiography. J Feline Med Surg 2000;2:147–51.

[8] Fox PR, Liu SK, Maron BJ. Echocardiographic assessment of spontaneously occurring feline hypertrophic cardiomyopathy: an animal model of human disease. Circulation 1995;92:2645–51.

[9] Gaschen L, Lang J, Lin S, et al. Cardiomyopathy in dystrophin-deficient hypertrophic feline muscular dystrophy. J Vet Intern Med 1999;13:346–56.

[10] Baty CJ, Malarkey DE, Atkins CE, et al. Natural history of hypertrophic cardiomyopathy and aortic thromboembolism in a family of domestic shorthair cats. J Vet Intern Med 2001;15:595–9.

[11] Cesta MF, Baty CJ, Keene BW, et al. Pathology of end stage remodeling in a family of cats with hypertrophic cardiomyopathy. Vet Pathol 2005;42:458–67.

[12] Murgo JP, Alter BR, Dorethy JF, et al. Dynamics of left ventricular ejection in obstructive and non-obstructive hypertrophic cardiomyopathy. J Clin Invest 1980;66:1369–82.

[13] Gardin JM, Dabestani A, Glasgow GA, et al. Echocardiographic and Doppler flow observations in obstructed and non-obstructed hypertrophic cardiomyopathy. Am J Cardiol 1985;56:614–21.

[14] Woo A, Wigle ED, Rakowski H. Echocardiography in the evaluation and management of patients with hypertrophic cardiomyopathy. In: Otto CM, editor. The practice of clinical echocardiography. 3rd ed. Philadelphia: WB Saunders; 2007, p. 653–78.

[15] Venco L. Ultrasound diagnosis: left ventricular thrombus in a cat with hypertrophic cardiomyopathy. Vet Radiol Ultrasound 1997;38:467–8.

[16] Schober KE, Maerz I. Assessment of left atrial appendage flow velocity and its relation to spontaneous echocardiographic contrast in 89 cats with myocardial disease. J Vet Intern Med 2006;20:120–30.

[17] Kwon DH, Smedira NG, Popovic ZB, et al. Steep left ventricle to aortic root angle and hypertrophic obstructive cardiomyopathy: study of a novel association using three-dimensional multimodality imaging. Clin Cardiol 2009;32:397–402.

[18] Rishniw M, Thomas WP. Dynamic/right ventricular outflow obstruction: a new cause of systolic murmurs in cats. J Vet Intern Med 2002;16:547–52.

[19] Hatle L, Angelsen B. Doppler ultrasound in cardiology. Philadelphia: Lea & Febiger; 1985.

[20] Kofflard MJ, Ten Cate FJ, van der Lee C, van Domburg RT. Hypertrophic cardiomyopathy in a large community-based population: clinical outcome and identification of risk factors for sudden cardiac death and clinical deterioration. J Am Coll Cardiol 2003;41:994–6.
[21] Maron MS, Olivotto I, Betocchi S, et al. Effect of left ventricular outflow tract obstruction on clinical outcome in hypertrophic cardiomyopathy. N Engl J Med 2003;348:295–303.
[22] Sorajja P, Nishimura RA, Gersh BJ, et al. Outcome of mildly symptomatic or asymptomatic obstructive hypertrophic cardiomyopathy: a long-term follow-up study. J Am Coll Cardiol 2009;54:234–41.
[23] Rush JE, Freeman LM, Fenollosa NK, Brown DJ. Population and survival characteristics of cats with hypertrophic cardiomyopathy: 260 cases (1990–1999). J Am Vet Med Assoc 2002;220:202–7.
[24] Kitamura M, Shimizu M, Ino H, et al. Collagen remodelling and cardiac dysfunction in patients with hypertrophic cardiomyopathy: the significance of type III and VI collagens. Clin Cardiol 2001;24:325–9.
[25] Kittleson MD, Meur KM, Munro MJ, et al. Familial hypertrophic cardiomyopathy in Maine Coon cats: an animal model of human disease. Circulation 1999;99:3172–80.
[26] Liu SK, Roberts WC, Maron BJ. Comparison of morphologic findings in spontaneously occurring hypertrophic cardiomyopathy in humans, cats and dogs. Am J Cardiol 1993;72:944–51.
[27] Fuentes VL. Diastolic function: is it the key to successful management of many feline cardiomyopathies? J Feline Med Surg 2003;5:51–6.
[28] MacDonald KA, Kittleson MD, Garcia-Nolen T, et al. Tissue Doppler imaging and gradient echo cardiac magnetic resonance imaging in normal cats and cats with hypertrophic cardiomyopathy. J Vet Intern Med 2006;20:627–34.
[29] Koffas H, Dukes-McEwan J, Corcoran BM, et al. Pulsed tissue Doppler imaging in normal cats and cats with hypertrophic cardiomyopathy. J Vet Intern Med 2006;20:65–77.
[30] Koffas H, Dukes-McEwan J, Corcoran BM, et al. Colour M-mode tissue Doppler imaging in healthy cats and cats with hypertrophic cardiomyopathy. J Small Anim Pract 2008;49:330–8.
[31] Carlos Sampedrano C, Chetboul V, Gouni V, et al. Systolic and diastolic myocardial dysfunction in cats with hypertrophic cardiomyopathy of systemic hypertension. J Vet Intern Med 2006;20:1106–15.
[32] Chetboul V, Blot S, Carlos Sampedrano C, et al. Tissue Doppler imaging for detection of radial and longitudinal myocardial dysfunction in a family of cats affected by dystrophin-deficient hypertrophic muscular dystrophy. J Vet Intern Med 2006;20:640–7.
[33] Carlos Sampedrano C, Chetboul V, Mary J, et al. Prospective echocardiographic and tissue Doppler imaging screening of a population of Maine Coon cats tested for the A31P mutation in the myosin-binding protein C gene: a specific analysis of the heterozygous status. J Vet Intern Med 2009;23:91–9.
[34] Saxon B, Hendrick M, Waddle JR. Restrictive cardiomyopathy in a cat with hypereosinophilic syndrome. Can Vet J 1991;32:367–9.
[35] Pion PD, Kittleson MD, Rogers QR, et al. Myocardial failure in cats associated with low plasma taurine: a reversible cardiomyopathy. Science 1987;237:764–8.
[36] Sisson DD, Knight DH, Helinski C, et al. Plasma taurine concentrations and M-mode echocardiographic measures in healthy cats and in cats with dilated cardiomyopathy. J Vet Intern Med 1991;5:232–8.
[37] Harvey AM, Battersby IA, Faena M, et al. Arrhythmogenic right ventricular cardiomyopathy in two cats. J Small Anim Pract 2005;46:151–6.
[38] Gelberg HB. Purkinje fiber dysplasia (histiocytoid cardiomyopathy) with ventricular noncompaction in a Savannah kitten. Vet Pathol 2009;46:693–7.
[39] Disatian S, Bright JM, Boon J. Association of age and heart rate with pulsed wave Doppler measurements in healthy, nonsedated cats. J Vet Intern Med 2008;22:351–6.
[40] Santilli RA, Bussadori C. Doppler echocardiographic study of the left ventricular diastole in non-anesthetized healthy cats. Vet J 1998;156:203–15.

14 Pulmonary Arterial Hypertension

VALÉRIE CHETBOUL

Etiology and Pathogenesis of PAH, 230
Conventional Echocardiography and PAH, 231
Conventional Doppler and PAH, 234
New Imaging Techniques and PAH, 237

Pulmonary arterial hypertension (PAH) is defined by an increase in systolic (PAPs) and/or diastolic (PAPd) pulmonary artery pressure (PAP), which may lead to the development of right-sided congestive heart failure [1-5]. The normal PAP values in the awake dog range from 15 to 25 mm Hg in systole, 5 to 10 mm Hg in diastole, and 15 mm Hg for the mean PAP [1]. These values may rise moderately during physical exercise or at high altitude [1,5]. Systolic PAH is generally regarded as mild when the PAPs is ≤50 mm Hg, moderate when the PAPs is between 51 and 75 mm Hg, and severe when the PAPs is >75 mm Hg [3].

The increasingly widespread use of echo Doppler in veterinary medicine has led to a better understanding of PAH in carnivores over the past 15 years. The sensitivity and specificity of the different echo Doppler variables potentially modified by PAH have been studied recently, especially in dogs [3,4,6]. The noninvasive diagnosis of PAH is therefore established at an increasingly early stage. The echo Doppler examination (with tissue Doppler imaging [TDI] if necessary) has now largely replaced right heart catheterization, an "invasive" gold-standard technique used before to precisely measure the PAP.

After a brief paragraph on the etiology and pathophysiology of PAH, this chapter presents the main conventional echo Doppler changes associated with canine PAH, PAP quantification by Doppler techniques, and, finally, the contribution of new imaging techniques such as TDI and derived techniques (primarily strain imaging).

Etiology and Pathogenesis of PAH

In dogs, the PAH is rarely idiopathic (so-called "primary" PAH) [1,7,8]. In most cases, it is qualified as "secondary" because it is a complication of various parasitic, cardiac, vascular, or respiratory diseases. Different pathophysiologic mechanisms are involved in secondary PAH. It is possible to separate the causes of PAH into three major groups [1-4,6,9]:

1. *Increase of right cardiac output* associated with congenital left-to-right shunts ("hyperkinetic" PAHs) such as atrial septal defect, ventricular septal defect, and patent ductus arteriosus.
2. *Decrease of the diameter and/or the pulmonary artery density.* A major cause of this type of PAH is hypoxemia, leading to reflex pulmonary arterial vasoconstriction followed by vascular wall remodeling (hypertrophy of the tunica media and fibrosis of the tunica intima). This form of PAH (also called "precapillary") is mainly found with respiratory diseases (e.g., tracheal collapse, laryngeal paralysis, and chronic bronchitis), obesity, and chest wall deformities. In the case of pulmonary thromboembolism, the decrease in pulmonary arterial diameter is also involved in the development of PAH due to reflex vasoconstriction (dependent on thromboxane A2, histamine, and serotonin). Lastly, PAH associated with parasitic diseases falls into this category (angiostrongylosis or dirofilariasis).
3. *Increase in pulmonary venous pressure.* This type of PAH, also called "postcapillary," is associated with left-sided congenital or acquired cardiopathies accompanied by elevated left atrial pressure. These include, in decreasing order of frequency, degenerative mitral valve disease (DMVD), dilated cardiomyopathy, and, more rarely, aortic stenosis, mitral dysplasia, and valvular endocarditis (aortic and mitral). A study performed in our unit on 617 dogs with DMVD demonstrated that the prevalence of PAH associated with DMVD is far from negligible (14% in all classes combined), reaching more than 70% of the animals in International Small Animal Cardiac Health Council (ISACHC) class III [3]. This work has also shown that, as in humans [10], PAH can be present early on (at the asymptomatic stage), particularly in dogs with significant mitral systolic regurgitation in color Doppler mode. As a matter of fact, 29% of dogs with PAH in this study were in ISACHC class I (and half of them were not receiving any medical treatment) [3]. Finally, ruling in or out the presence of PAH in a dog with asymptomatic DMVD is important because the level of PAP can predict the risk of decompensation within a year [11].

The advantages of the echo Doppler examinations are not only to allow the diagnosis of PAH by unraveling its direct and indirect signs (see below), but also to identify the cause of PAH (Figure 14-1), whether cardiac (hyperkinetic or postcapillary PAH) or precapillary (pulmonary

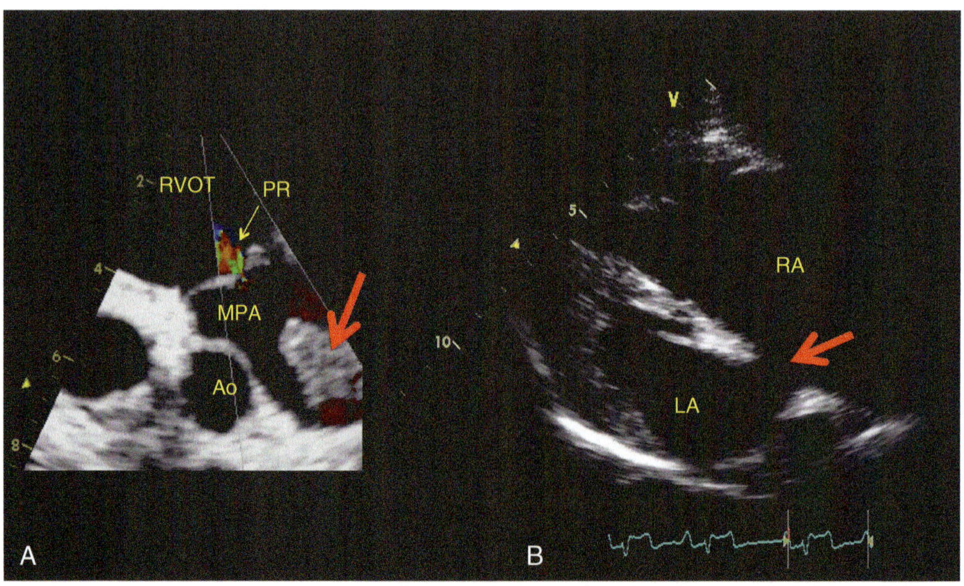

• **Fig. 14-1** Identification of the cause of pulmonary arterial hypertension (PAH) by echocardiographic examination. A, Left parasternal short axis transaortic view. A large hyperechoic thrombus *(red arrow)* can be seen in the main pulmonary artery (MPA) in this German Shorthaired Pointer with nephrotic syndrome, with a complaint of exercise intolerance and malaise. The systolic pulmonary arterial pressure (PAPs) is estimated at 150 mm Hg. Note that the pulmonic regurgitation (PR), in color Doppler mode, is characterized by an aliasing phenomenon (due to the increased velocity of the regurgitation secondary to the diastolic PAH). B, Right parasternal long axis 4 chambers view. In this 10-year-old German Shepherd with exercise intolerance for several years, the pulmonary hypertension (systolic pulmonary arterial pressure estimated at 85 mm Hg) was associated with the presence of a large (1.5 cm in diameter) atrial septal defect *(arrow)*. Note the marked right atrial dilatation. *Ao,* Aorta; *LA,* left atrium; *RA,* right atrium; *RVOT,* right ventricular outflow tract. (Photo credit: Valérie Chetboul.)

thromboembolism and dirofilariasis being the main examples).

Conventional Echocardiography and PAH

The presence of PAH and its severity can be evaluated indirectly by identifying bidimensional (2D) and time-motion (TM) echocardiographic anomalies, which can be isolated or variably combined. Some 2D and TM variables are even correlated to the PAP value [3,6,12-14]. The 2D and TM changes associated with PAH include the following:

1. First, a dilation of the main pulmonary artery (MPA) and its two branches, often associated with dilation of the right ventricular outflow tract (RVOT) (Figures 14-2 and 14-3). A positive correlation has been demonstrated between the degree of pulmonary arterial dilation (evaluated using the ratio between the main pulmonary artery and the aortic diameters: MPA/Ao) [3,6] and the PAPs value (in other words, the higher the PAPs, the greater the MPA/Ao). However, in a study performed in our unit on 105 either healthy dogs (n = 45) or dogs with PAH (n = 60), an increased MPA/Ao (>1.15) only allowed detection of PAH with 45% sensitivity.
2. To this MPA dilation is added a diastolic pulmonic valve doming (Figures 14-4 and 14-5). However, this pulmonic valvular prolapse is not pathognomonic for PAH (it can also be encountered in cases of patent ductus arteriosus or pulmonic stenosis) [12]. It is also not consistently present in PAH; in the previous study [6], it was observed in only 32% of the dogs presenting with mild PAH and in 61% of those with moderate or severe PAH.
3. Then, right ventricular hypertrophy and/or dilatation sets in, with a flattened septum or even a paradoxic septal motion, when the right intraventricular diastolic

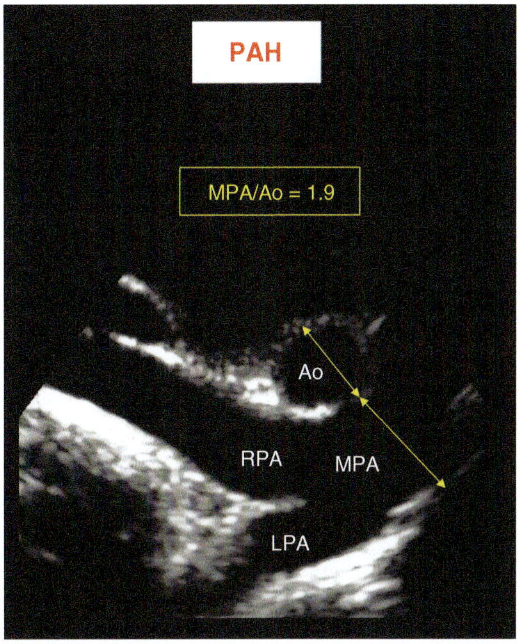

• **Fig. 14-3** Dilation of the main pulmonary artery (MPA) and its two branches in a Dachshund with pulmonary arterial hypertension (PAH), visualized using a "modified" right parasternal short axis transaortic view. The MPA/aorta ratio (MPA/Ao) is significantly increased (1.9; normal reference range = 0.8–1.15 [6]). In addition, note the abnormally clear view of both the right pulmonary artery (RPA) and the left pulmonary artery (LPA) due to their dilatation (diameter similar to that of the aorta). (Photo credit: Valérie Chetboul.)

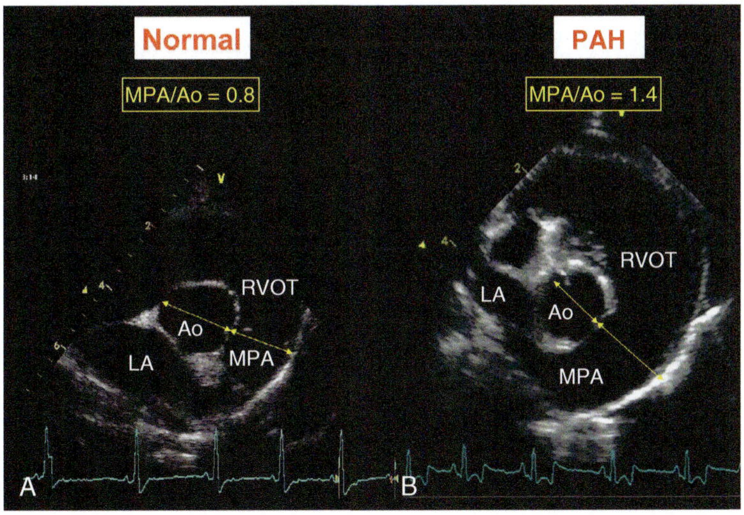

• **Fig. 14-2** Early indirect echocardiographic signs of pulmonary arterial hypertension (PAH): dilation of both the main pulmonary artery (MPA) and the right ventricular outflow tract (RVOT) (right parasternal short axis transaortic view). In comparison with a normal dog **(A)**, in which the MPA/aorta ratio (MPA/Ao) is in the normal reference range (0.8–1.15 [6]), the MPA/Ao in the dog with PAH **(B)** is elevated (1.4). RVOT dilation is also present. *LA,* Left atrium. (Photo credit: Valérie Chetboul.)

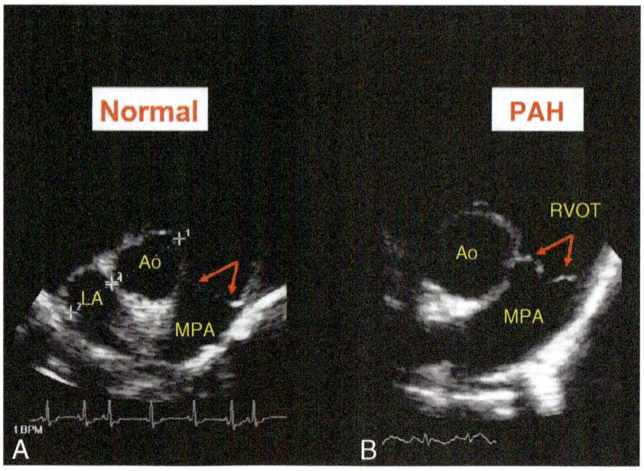

• **Fig. 14-4** Another indirect echocardiographic sign of pulmonary arterial hypertension (PAH): the modification of the shape of the pulmonic valves (right parasternal short axis transaortic view). In comparison with the normal dog (A), with straight pulmonic valve cusps in diastole *(arrows)*, note in the dog with PAH (B) their more rounded shape with diastolic doming *(arrows)* beyond the valvular annulus. *Ao,* Aorta; *LA,* left atrium; *MPA,* main pulmonary artery; *RVOT,* right ventricular outflow tract. (Photo credit: Valérie Chetboul.)

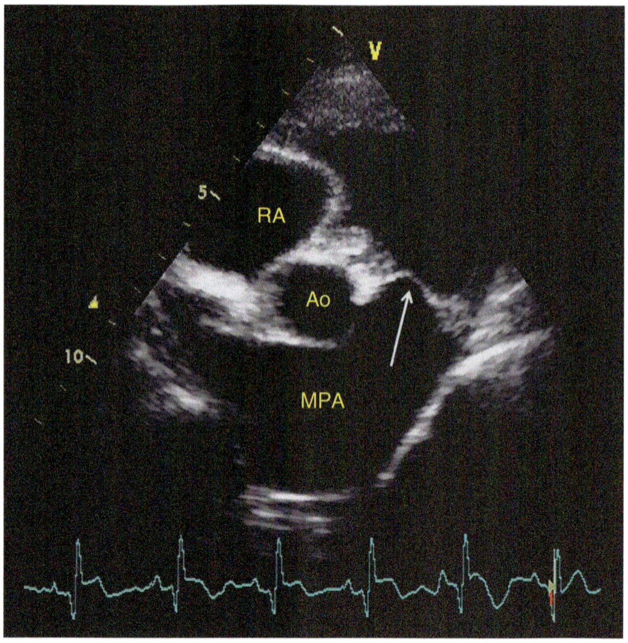

• **Fig. 14-5** Another example of marked diastolic pulmonic valve cusp doming *(arrow)* in a dog with pulmonary arterial hypertension (PAH) (right parasternal short axis transaortic view). *Ao,* Aorta; *MPA,* main pulmonary artery; *RA,* right atrium. (Photo credit: Valérie Chetboul.)

pressure becomes equal to or greater than the left intraventricular pressure, respectively (Figures 14-6 and 14-7; Videos 14-1 and 14-2). However, the absence of right ventricular changes in TM mode cannot exclude PAH. For example, in a study in 86 dogs with PAH secondary to DMVD [3], right cardiomegaly was found in approximately one third of the animals.

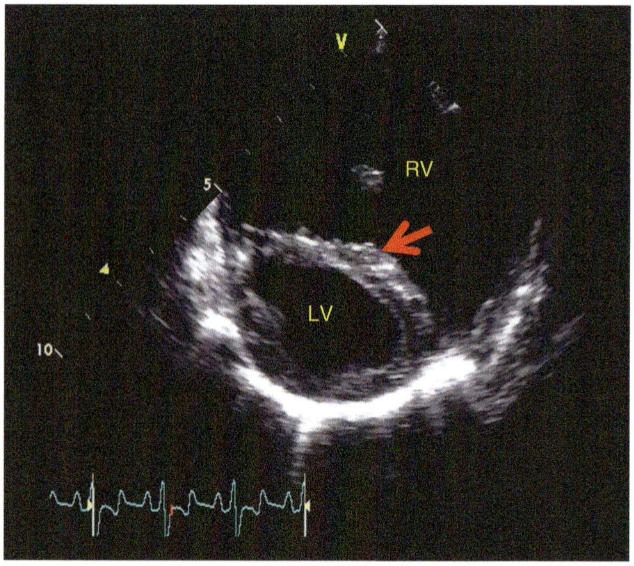

• **Fig. 14-6** Indirect echocardiographic sign of significant pulmonary arterial hypertension (PAH) in a dog (right parasternal short axis transventricular view): right ventricular dilation with interventricular septum flattening *(arrow)* and left ventricular cavity reduction. *LV,* Left ventricle; *RV,* right ventricle. (Photo credit: Valérie Chetboul.)

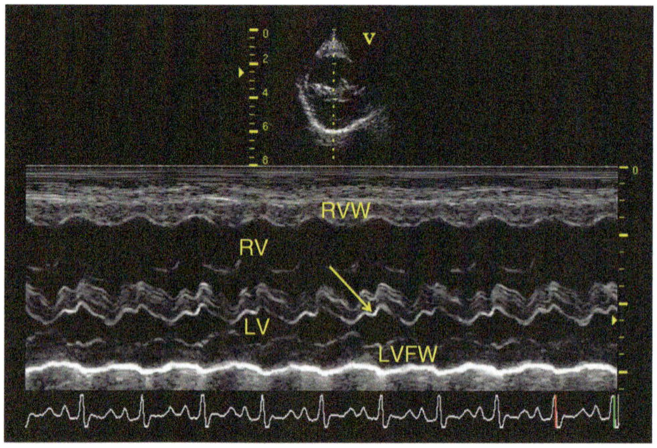

• **Fig. 14-7** Indirect echocardiographic sign of significant pulmonary artery hypertension (PAH) in time-motion (TM) mode (right parasternal short axis transventricular view) in a Pinscher. Note the hypertrophy and, more importantly, the dilation of the right ventricle (RV), the reduced left ventricular chamber, and the paradoxic septal motion *(arrow)* characterized by diastolic posterior motion of the interventricular septum toward the left ventricular free wall (LVFW). *LV,* Left ventricle; *RVW,* right ventricular wall. (Photo credit: Valérie Chetboul.)

4. The right ventricular modification can be accompanied by a decreased left ventricular cavity size secondary to preload decrease and flattening of the interventricular septum (see Figures 14-6 and 14-7).
5. Next, right atrial dilation appears (Figures 14-8 and 14-9) with possible systolic prolapse of the tricuspid valve (Figure 14-10). This right atrial dilation

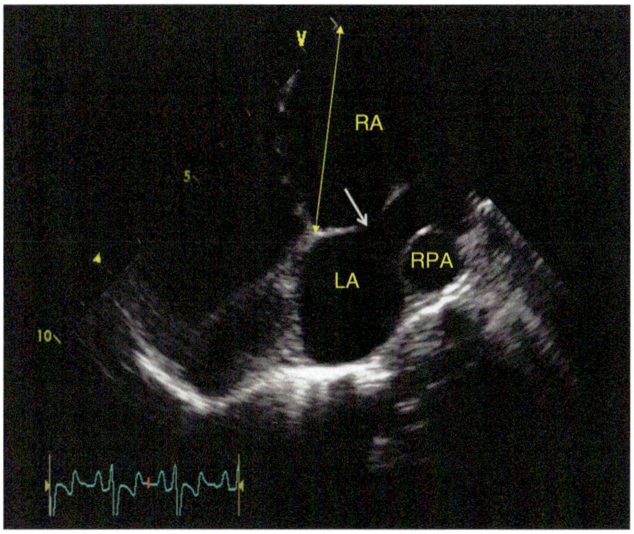

• **Fig. 14-8** Indirect echocardiographic sign of significant pulmonary arterial hypertension (PAH) (right parasternal long axis 4 chambers view): right atrial dilation. In this dog with PAH, the right atrial width at the level of the tricuspid annulus *(double arrow)* is greater than that of the left atrium (LA). In addition, note the abnormal shape of the interatrial septum *(arrow)* bulging into the LA as well as the dilated right pulmonary artery (RPA, transverse view). *RA,* Right atrium. (Photo credit: Valérie Chetboul.)

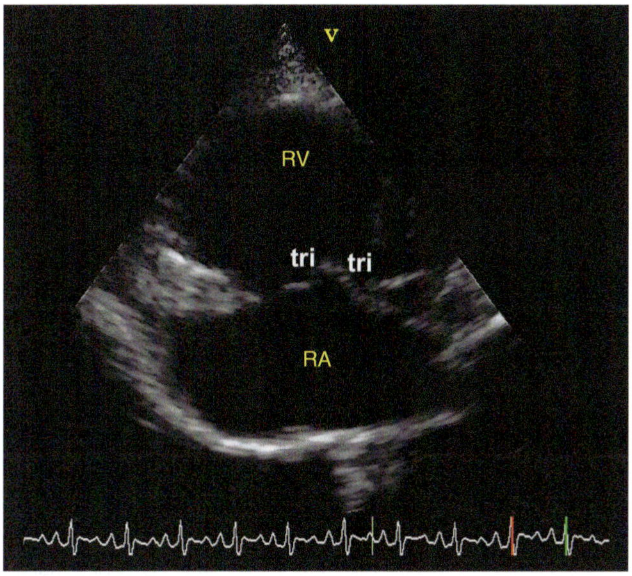

• **Fig. 14-9** Another example of right atrial dilation in a dog with pulmonary arterial hypertension (PAH) (left apical 4 chambers view). The width of the right atrium (RA), whose shape is abnormally flared, is greater than that of the right ventricle (RV). *tri,* Tricuspid valve leaflet. (Photo credit: Valérie Chetboul.)

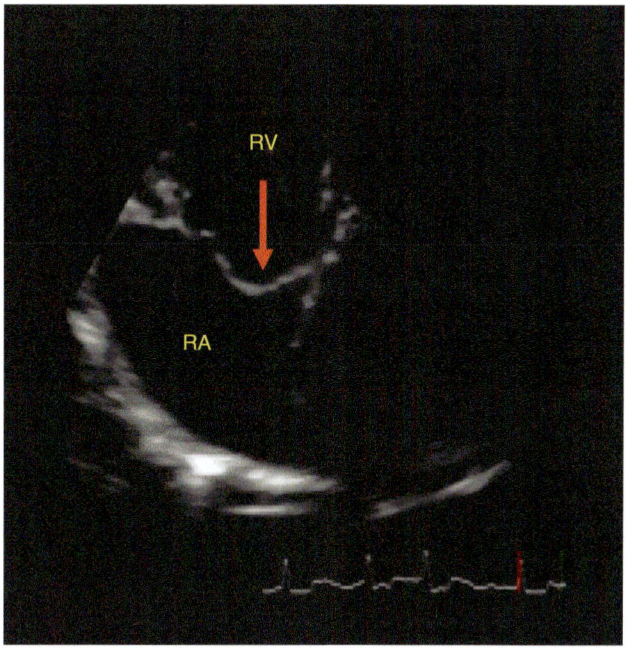

• **Fig. 14-10** Another indirect echocardiographic sign of pulmonary arterial hypertension (PAH) in a dog: systolic prolapse of the tricuspid leaflets toward the right atrium (RA) *(arrow)* (left apical 4 chambers view). In addition, note that the diameter of the distorted right atrial cavity is greater than that of the right ventricle (RV). (Photo credit: Valérie Chetboul.)

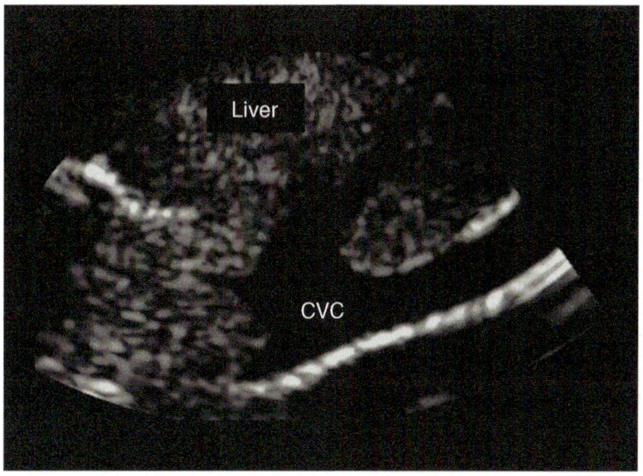

• **Fig. 14-11** Indirect echocardiographic signs of severe pulmonary arterial hypertension (PAH): the dilation of the caudal vena cava (CVC) and suprahepatic veins, preliminary phase prior to the appearance of ascites (same dog as in Figure 14-3). (Photo credit: Valérie Chetboul.)

is most often the result of significant tricuspid valve regurgitation.

6. The final phase is right-sided congestive heart failure (R-CHF), with dilation of the caudal vena cava and suprahepatic venous system prior to the appearance of ascites (Figure 14-11).
7. Additional potential echocardiographic changes associated with PAH are:
   a. A decrease in the anterior mitral leaflet ejection fraction (EF) slope due to the decrease in cardiac output (in TM mode).
   b. A systolic anterior motion of the mitral valve (2D and TM modes). However, this motion is not pathognomonic of PAH because it can be observed in other situations of right ventricular pressure overload (i.e., pulmonic stenosis).

Conventional Doppler and PAH

Conventional Doppler presents a dual advantage:

- Detection of indirect signs of PAH (complementary to those detected in 2D and TM modes), some Doppler variables being correlated to the PAP value.
- Quantification of PAPs and PAPd.

Indirect Doppler Signs of PAH

In addition to the high velocity and abnormal turbulent nature of the systolic tricuspid and diastolic pulmonic regurgitations (Videos 14-3 and 14-4) (see "Pulmonary arterial pressure estimation" below), indirect Doppler signs of PAH include several possible modifications of the systolic pulmonic flow velocity envelope [4,6,12,15]. These Doppler alterations can be isolated or variously combined.

1. The normal pulmonic flow is characterized by a symmetric V-shaped velocity envelope with a relatively rounded peak (Figure 14-12, *A*). With PAH, the shape of the envelope changes: the peak becomes more pointed and the acceleration time (AT) shortens, the maximal flow velocity being reached earlier (Figure 14-12, *B*). In addition to the AT shortening, a reduction of the ratio between the AT and the pulmonary ejection time (ET) is noted. These two indices (AT and AT/ET) enable us to predict the presence of PAH in the West Highland White Terrier (WHWT) with pulmonary interstitial fibrosis with reasonably good sensitivity and specificity: 88% and 80%, respectively, for an AT value of 58 ms (healthy WHWT: median = 73 ms, [53–104 ms]) and 73% and 87%, respectively, for an AT/ET ratio of 0.31 (healthy WHWT: median = 0.4 [0.28–0.55] [4]). In the WHWT, these two indices have also been shown to be negatively correlated with PAPs values. A similar negative correlation has been found in dogs with PAH secondary to DMVD [6]. In this latter study, however, an AT/ET ratio <0.3 (lower limit of the normal reference range) predicted the presence of PAH with a very low sensitivity (15% only) and 100% specificity [6]. However, the sensitivity was much higher (71%) with 71% specificity when using an AT/ET value <0.44 [6].
2. "Notching," resulting from the partial closure of the pulmonic valve cusps during systole, can also be observed on the spectral envelope of the pulmonic flow (Figure 14-13). However, the absence of this notching does not exclude PAH. With DMVD, for example, it is only encountered in 11% of dogs with mild PAH and in 38% of those with moderate or severe PAH [6].
3. PAH can also be accompanied by an increase in the index known as the "right Tei index" (Figure 14-14) [16]. This index of right myocardial performance is defined as follows (see Chapter 10):

   (Right isovolumetric contraction time +
   Right isovolumic relaxation time)/ET

   In a study focusing on PAH secondary to DMVD, the right Tei index was shown to be positively correlated to the PAPs value: mean ± standard deviation of 0.14 ± 0.10 (0.01–0.40) in healthy dogs versus 0.49 ± 0.31 (0.07–1.32) in those with significant PAH [6]. However, in this same study, a right Tei index >0.4 (upper limit of the normal reference range) predicted the presence of PAH with a weak sensitivity (43%) [6].
4. A decrease in the maximal velocity of the systolic pulmonic flow can be observed with significant PAH, sometimes with end-systolic flow direction reversal (backward instead of forward).

Finally, in addition to the above-mentioned Doppler changes, increase in left isovolumetric relaxation time and inversion of the mitral E and A waves may be seen when decreased left ventricular filling pressure and left diastolic dysfunction become present.

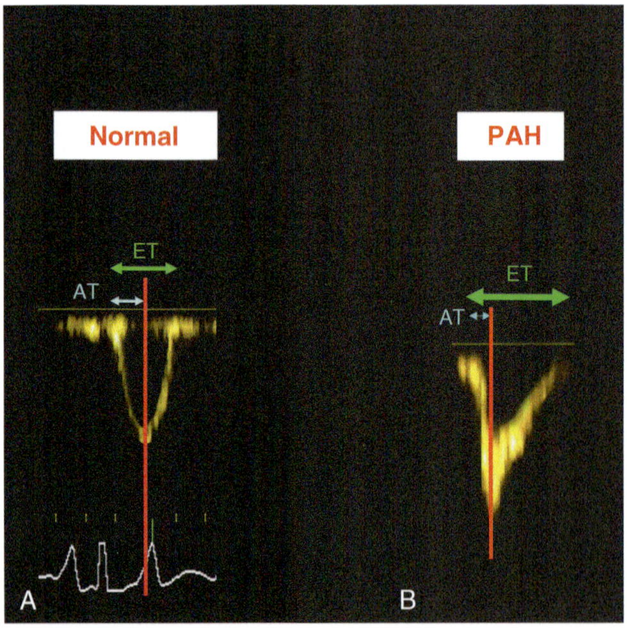

• **Fig. 14.12** Indirect Doppler sign of pulmonary arterial hypertension (PAH): modification of the shape of the transpulmonic flow spectral envelope in a dog. In the normal animal (**A**), the spectral envelope of the pulmonic flow is symmetric, characterized by an acceleration time (AT) equal to half of the ejection time (ET). In a dog with PAH (**B**), the curve is asymmetric, with an AT significantly less than half of ET (AT/ET = 0.2). (Photo credit: Valérie Chetboul.)

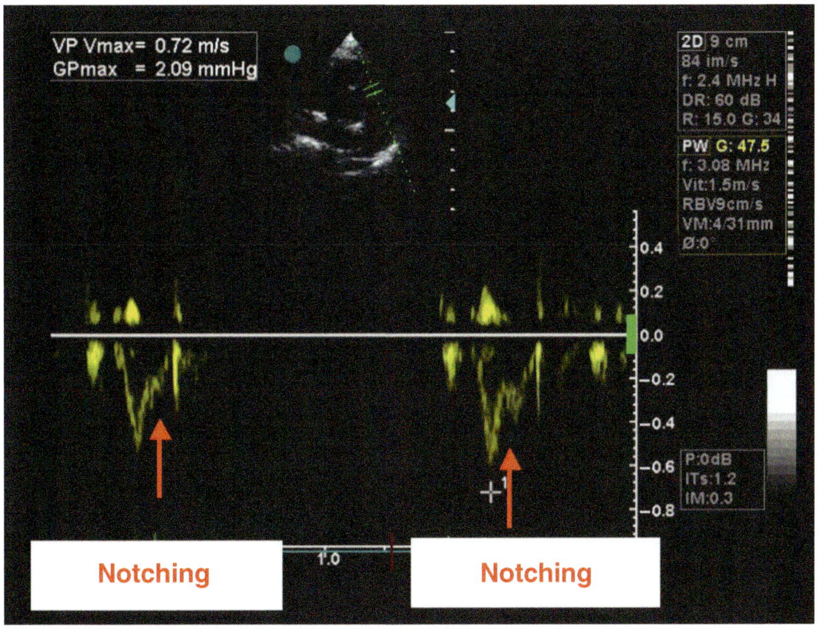

• **Fig. 14-13** Another example of modification of the pulmonic flow spectral envelope in a dog with pulmonary arterial hypertension (PAH). As in the example shown in Figure 14-12, *B*, the transpulmonic flow spectral envelope is asymmetric. In addition, notching appears in the ascending section of the envelope. (Photo credit: Valérie Chetboul.)

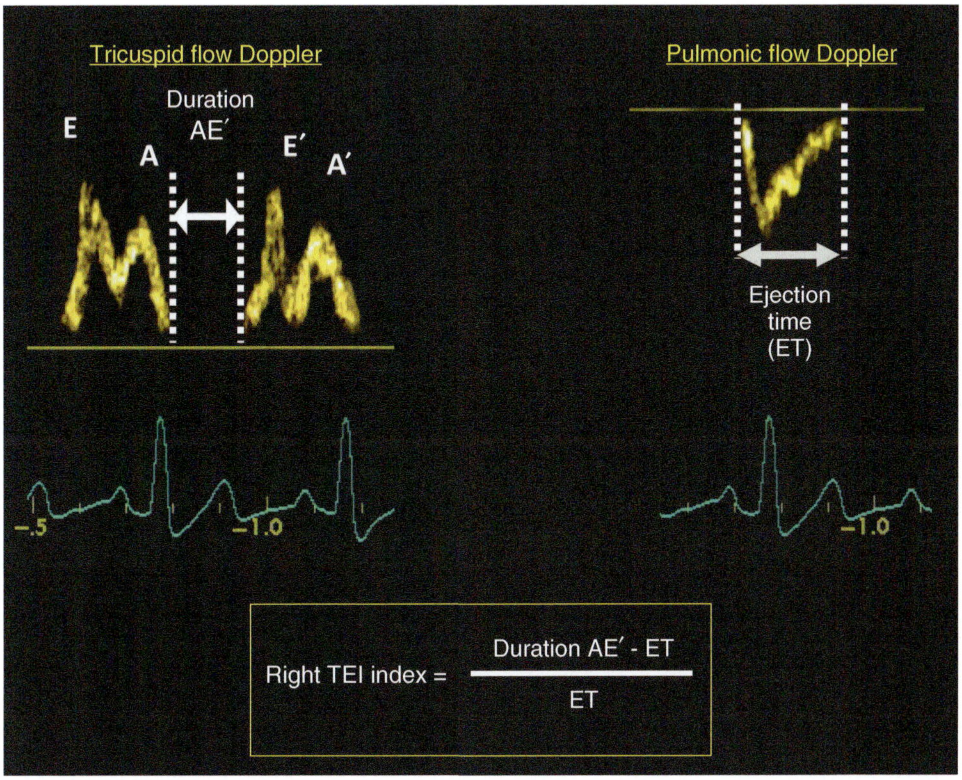

• **Fig. 14-14** Right Tei index calculation. The right Tei index is calculated from the pulsed wave Doppler spectral envelopes of the diastolic tricuspid *(left)* and systolic pulmonic flows *(right)*. The tricuspid Doppler signal reveals two diastolic waves for each cardiac cycle: E in early diastole and A in end-diastole for the first cycle; E′ and A′ for the second cycle. The distance between the end of the A wave (opening of the tricuspid valve) and the beginning of the E′ wave (opening of the tricuspid valve in the following cycle) is measured. The pulmonic Doppler signal is used to calculate the pulmonic ejection time (ET = flow duration, determined by the beginning and end of the spectral envelope). The difference between the AE′ duration and ET corresponds to the sum of the right isovolumetric times (contraction and relaxation). The right Tei index is defined as the ratio between this difference (AE′ − ET) and ET. In this example, note the transpulmonic flow anomaly (asymmetric spectral envelope with notching). (Photo credit: Valérie Chetboul.)

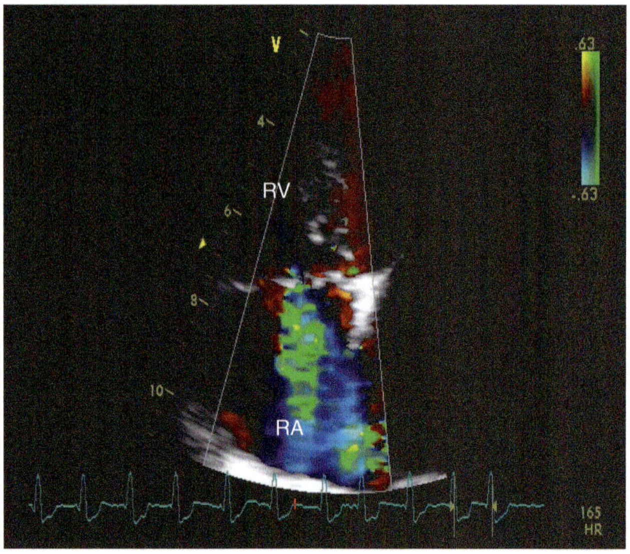

• **Fig. 14-15** Systolic pulmonary arterial pressure (PAPs) estimation (step 1). The condition necessary for calculation of the PAPs is the presence of systolic tricuspid regurgitation that will, in a first step, be identified in color Doppler mode by the operator, using a left apical 4 chambers view. The next step (see Figure 14-16) is to measure the maximal velocity of this regurgitant jet in continuous wave Doppler mode (after having verified the absence of pulmonic stenosis). In this American Staffordshire Terrier with advanced congenital mitral stenosis (right-sided congestive heart failure—ascites—complicated with atrial fibrillation), the tricuspid regurgitation is abnormal, characterized by the presence of turbulence and significant colorimetric extension (more than 60% of the right atrial atria, reaching the right atrial roof). *RA,* Right atrium; *RV,* right ventricle. (Photo credit: Valérie Chetboul.)

Pulmonary Arterial Pressure Estimation

PAPs Estimation

PAPs can be estimated by analyzing the maximal velocity of the systolic tricuspid regurgitation in continuous wave Doppler mode (Figures 14-15 and 14-16) [1-3,6,12]. When tricuspid regurgitation is present, the regurgitant jet flows from the right ventricle into the right atrium during systole. By measuring the maximal velocity of this regurgitation ($V_{tricuspid\ regurgitation}$), the systolic pressure gradient value ($\Delta P_{systolic}$) driving the latter can be calculated using the following formula (simplified Bernoulli equation):

$$\Delta P_{systolic} = P_{right\ ventricle\ systolic} - P_{right\ atrium} = 4\left(V_{tricuspid\ regurgitation}\right)^2$$

$$\text{or } P_{right\ ventricle\ systolic} = 4\left(V_{tricuspid\ regurgitation}\right)^2 + P_{right\ atrium}$$

where $P_{right\ atrium}$ is the right atrial pressure. In the absence of pulmonic stenosis, the PAPs and the right ventricular systolic pressure can be regarded as similar. Therefore:

$$PAPs \approx P_{right\ ventricle\ systolic} = 4\left(V_{tricuspid\ regurgitation}\right)^2 + P_{right\ atrium}$$

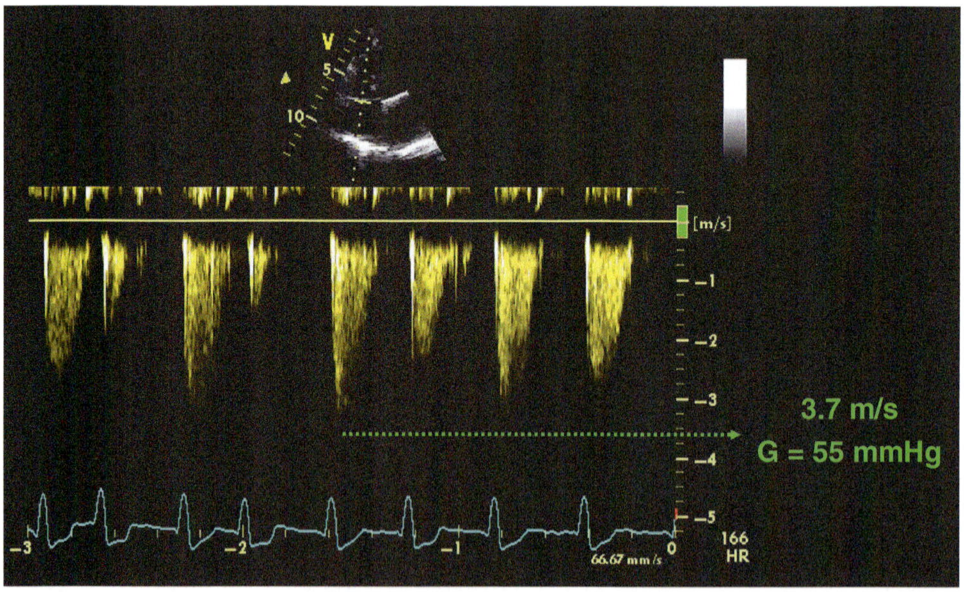

• **Fig. 14-16** Estimation of systolic pulmonary arterial pressure (PAPs) (phase 2): same animal as in Figure 14-15. The maximal velocity of the systolic tricuspid regurgitation is measured in continuous wave Doppler mode using a left apical 4 chambers view. Note that in this dog the spectral envelopes (negative because the regurgitant jet is moving away from the transducer) are variable from one cycle to another due to atrial fibrillation. The maximal velocity of the regurgitant jet is 3.7 m/s. According to the Bernoulli equation, the maximum systolic pressure gradient (G) between the right ventricle and right atrium driving this regurgitation is $4 \times 3.7^2 = 55$ mm Hg. The right atrial pressure can be estimated at 15 mm Hg because of the presence of ascites (right-sided congestive heart failure). The right ventricular systolic pressure (generally equivalent to the pulmonary arterial systolic pressure) is therefore very elevated, estimated at 55 + 15 = 70 mm Hg. More precisely, in this dog the maximal velocity of the systolic transpulmonic flow is 0.9 m/s, indicating that the maximal systolic pressure gradient between the main pulmonary artery and the right ventricle is 3 mm Hg. This means that the PAPs is 70 – 3 = 67 mm Hg. (Photo credit: Valérie Chetboul.)

The physiologic right atrial pressure is estimated at 5 mm Hg. It increases to 10 mm Hg when the right atrium is dilated and to 15 mm Hg when signs of R-CHF begin to appear.

This noninvasive method of PAPs quantification has been shown to be reliable in humans because the PAPs values thus obtained were comparable to those measured by catheterization [17].

PAPd Estimation

Estimation of PAPd is performed by analyzing the velocity of the diastolic pulmonic regurgitant jet in continuous wave Doppler mode (Figures 14-17 and 14-18) [1-3,6,12].

When pulmonic regurgitation is present, the regurgitant jet flows from the main pulmonary artery toward the right ventricle during diastole.

By measuring the velocity of this regurgitant jet in end-diastole ($V_{\text{pulmonic regurgitation}}$), the diastolic pressure gradient value ($\Delta P_{\text{diastolic}}$) driving the latter can be calculated using the following formula (simplified Bernoulli equation):

$$\Delta P_{\text{diastolic}} = \text{PAPd} - P_{\text{right ventricle}} = 4\left(V_{\text{pulmonic regurgitation}}\right)^2$$

where $P_{\textit{right ventricle}}$ is the right ventricular end-diastolic pressure. Therefore the PAPd is at least equal to $4\left(V_{\text{pulmonic regurgitation}}\right)^2$.

New Imaging Techniques and PAH

As detailed above, PAPs and PAPd can be determined using continuous Doppler analysis of the systolic tricuspid and diastolic pulmonic regurgitation flows. The condition necessary for these pressure calculations is the presence of these two regurgitations but they are not always present [18,19]. Indeed, in a study carried out in 86 dogs with PAH secondary to DMVD [3], PAPs could not be determined in 10% of the cases due to the absence of a tricuspid regurgitant jet important enough to be analyzed in continuous Doppler mode. This represents the main technical limitation of conventional Doppler. This limitation can be partly overcome by using TDI (Figures 14-19 and 14-20) and TDI-derived techniques such as strain imaging (Figure 14-21) [6,20-22]. Thus a study by our team using color 2D TDI has shown that PAH in dogs lead to systolic and diastolic longitudinal dysfunction of the right myocardial base characterized by:

- A decrease in the systolic S wave (Stdi)
- A decrease in the ratio of the early diastolic E and end-diastolic A waves (E/Atdi)
- An increase in the isovolumetric contraction and relaxation times
- An increase in the time-to-peak (time interval between the beginning of the QRS and the peak of the Stdi wave)

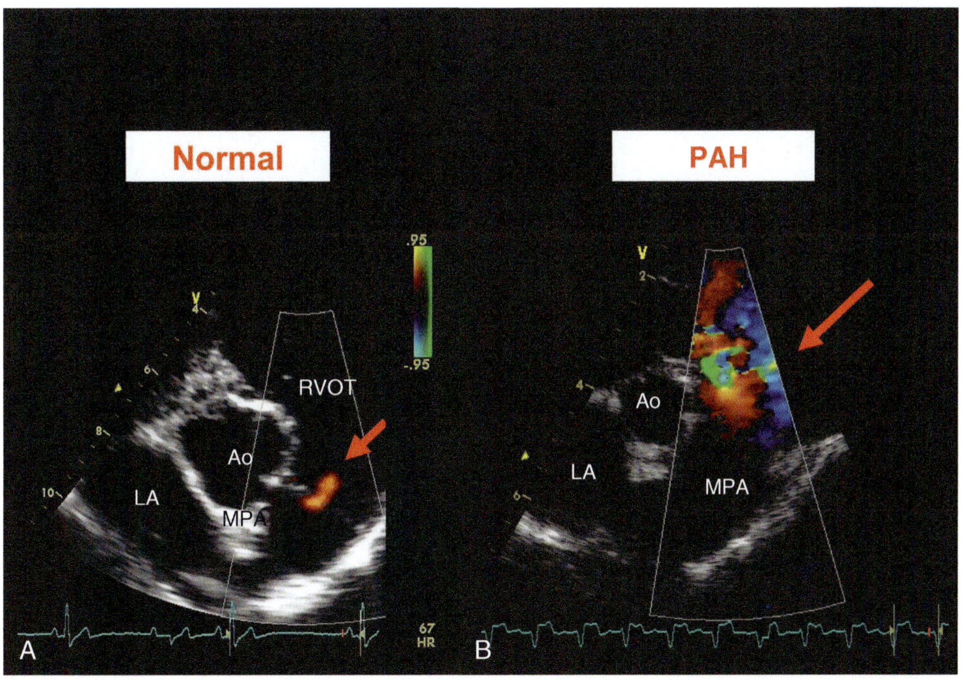

• **Fig. 14-17** Diastolic pulmonary artery pressure (PAPd) estimation (step 1). The condition necessary for calculation of the PAPd is the presence of a diastolic pulmonic regurgitation, which must be detected by the operator using the color Doppler mode *(arrows)* on a right parasternal short axis transaortic view. In a second step (see Figure 14-18), the maximal velocity of this regurgitant jet is measured using continuous wave Doppler mode. In comparison with a normal dog **(A)**, the diastolic pulmonic regurgitation in the dog with pulmonary arterial hypertension (PAH) **(B)** is abnormal and characterized by the presence of turbulence and significant colorimetric extension (occupying the entire right ventricular outflow tract [RVOT] and extending far beyond the anterior aortic wall in end-diastole). *Ao,* Aorta; *LA,* left atrium; *MPA,* main pulmonary artery. (Photo credit: Valérie Chetboul.)

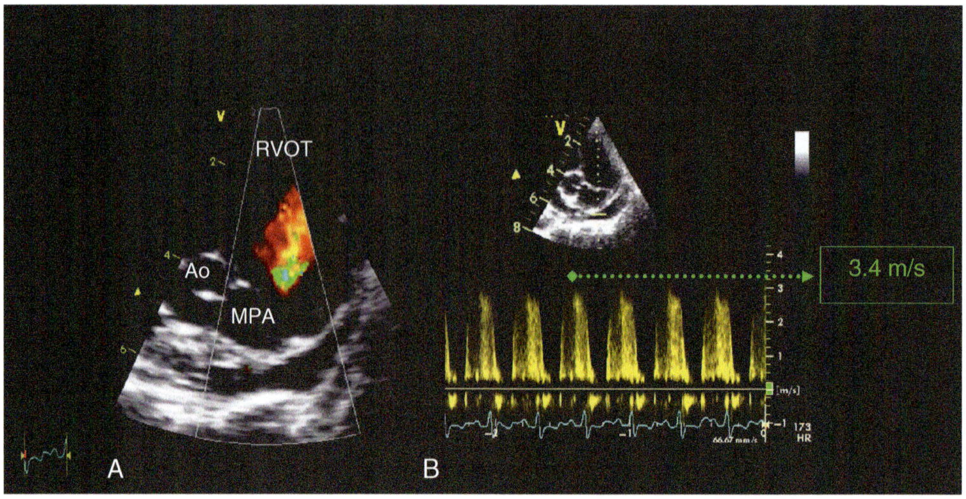

• **Fig. 14-18** Diastolic pulmonary artery pressure (PAPd) estimation (step 2). After detecting the diastolic pulmonic regurgitant jet in color Doppler mode (A) using a short right parasternal short axis transaortic view, the maximal velocity is measured in continuous wave Doppler mode (B). In this 3-month-old King Charles Spaniel with primary pulmonary artery hypertension (PAH), the maximum velocity of the regurgitant jet (positive spectral envelopes because the jet is moving toward the transducer) is 3.4 m/s. According to the Bernoulli equation, the maximum diastolic pressure gradient between the main pulmonary artery (MPA) and the right ventricle driving this regurgitation is $4 \times 3.4^2 = 46$ mm Hg. The PAPd is therefore very elevated because it is at least 46 mm Hg (to which needs to be added the right ventricular diastolic pressure, unknown). *Ao,* Aorta; *RVOT,* right ventricular outflow tract. (Photo credit: Valérie Chetboul.)

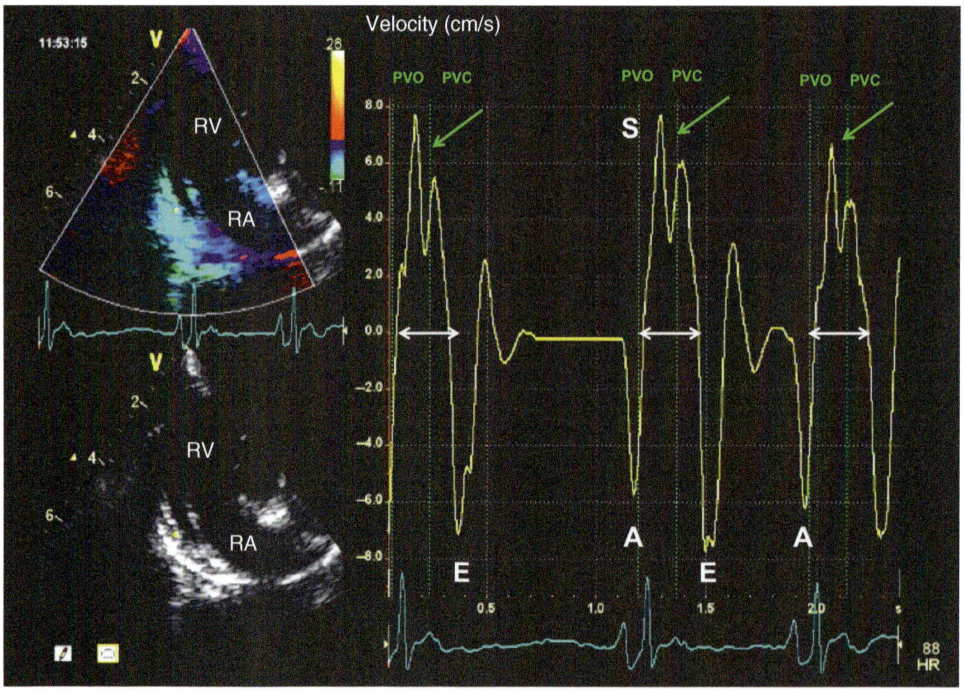

• **Fig. 14-19** Example of a systolic anomaly of the right ventricular wall longitudinal motion analyzed by color bidimensional (2D) tissue Doppler imaging (TDI) mode in a Yorkshire Terrier with pulmonary arterial hypertension (PAH) secondary to tracheal collapse. *Top left*, The color-coded myocardial velocities are superimposed in real time on the left parasternal long axis cross-section. Myocardial velocities are analyzed in one circular segment *(yellow)*, measuring 2 mm in diameter, located at the base of the right ventricular wall, with simultaneous recordings of electrical (electrocardiographic trace, *lower right*) and hemodynamic (*PVC,* pulmonic valve closure; *PVO,* pulmonic valve opening) events. The right basal longitudinal motion includes a systolic positive wave reaching its peak velocity in S and two negative E and A waves, in early diastole and end-diastole, respectively. Note that the closure of the pulmonic valve (*arrows*, PVC) occurs early—that is, before the end of the S wave (duration shown by the *double white arrows*)—thus confirming the early closure of the pulmonic valve cusps (explaining the splitting of the second heart sound detected on auscultation in this dog). Moreover, the aspect of the S wave is abnormal: biphasic aspect with a moderately decreased value (7.6 cm/s; normal value [21] = 12.5 ± 3.2 cm/s). *RA,* Right atrium; *RV,* right ventricle. (Photo credit: Valérie Chetboul.)

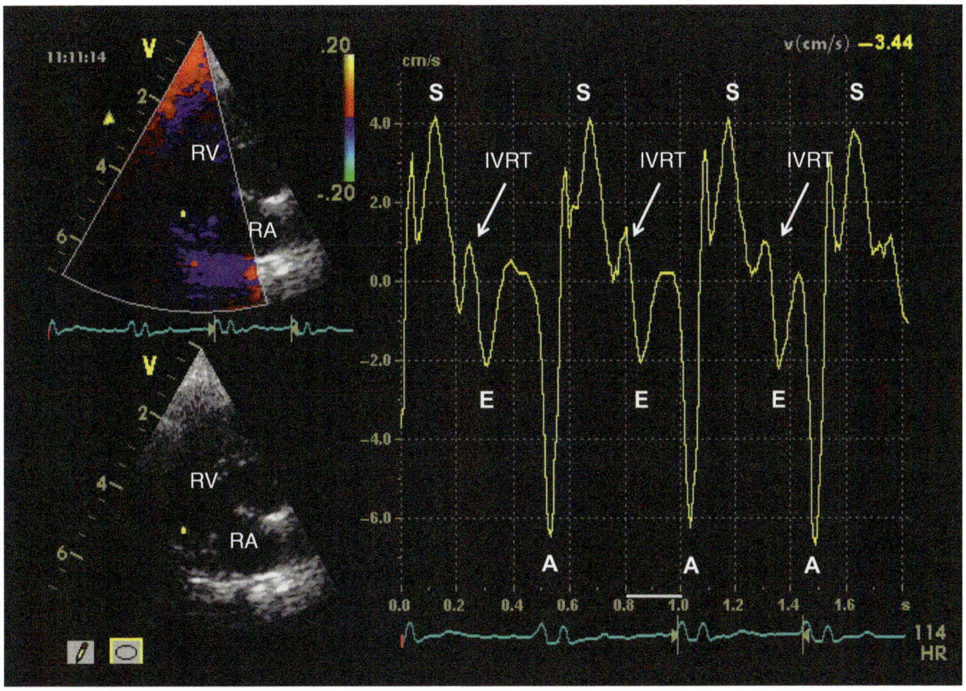

• **Fig. 14-20** Example of systolic and diastolic anomalies of the right ventricular wall longitudinal motion analyzed using color bidimensional (2D) tissue Doppler imaging (TDI) mode in another Yorkshire Terrier with pulmonary arterial hypertension (PAH) secondary to tracheal collapse. *Top left*, The color-coded velocities are superimposed in real time on the left apical 5 chambers cross-section. Myocardial velocities are analyzed in one circular segment *(yellow)*, measuring 2 mm in diameter, located at the base of the ventricular wall, concomitantly with an electrocardiographic trace *(lower right)*. The right basal longitudinal motion includes a positive systolic wave reaching its peak velocity in S and two negative E and A waves in early diastole and end-diastole, respectively. Note the inversion of the ratio of the diastolic E and A waves (E/A ratio = 0.32; normal reference range [21] = 1.6 ± 0.6), the decreased S wave (4.1 cm/s; normal value [21] = 12.5 ± 3.2 cm/s), and the presence of an abnormally well-identified isovolumetric relaxation period (IVRT, 75 ms), which is virtually nonexistent in normal dogs. *RA,* Right atrium; *RV,* right ventricle. (Photo credit: Valérie Chetboul.)

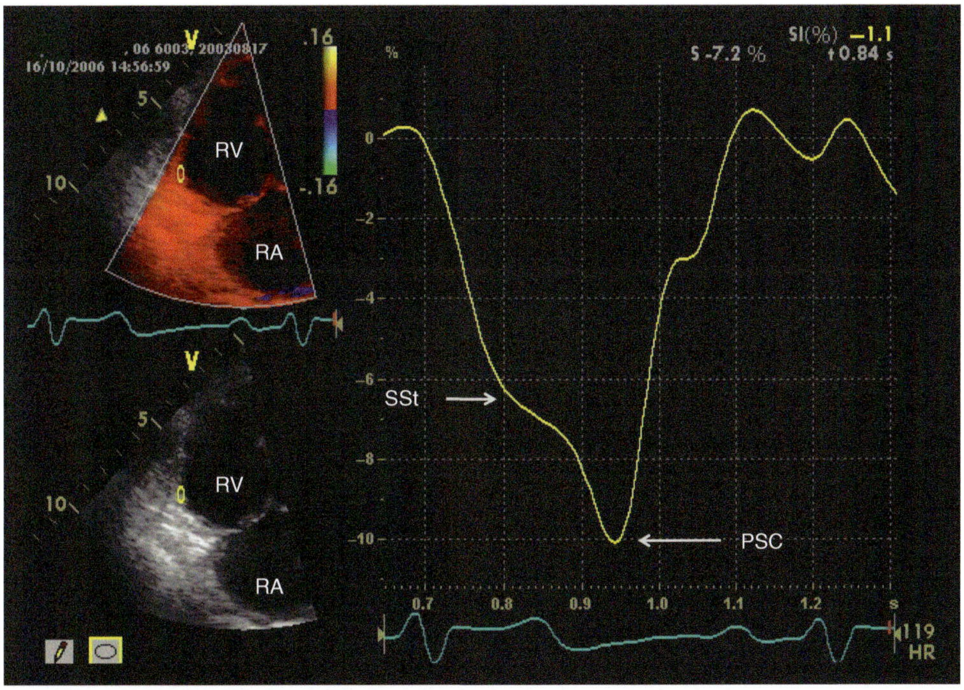

• **Fig. 14-21** Example of systolic and diastolic anomalies of the basal right ventricular wall longitudinal motion analyzed using strain imaging in a dog with pulmonary arterial hypertension (PAH) secondary to angiostrongylosis. The systolic longitudinal strain (SSt) is negative and then the curve goes back to baseline during diastole, confirming systolic shortening followed by regional diastolic elongation, respectively. The right longitudinal strain anomaly is twofold: the absolute value of the maximum systolic strain (SSt) is markedly reduced (SSt = −6.4%; normal value [21] = −9.5 ± 5.5%) and a postsystolic contraction (PSC) occurs following the T wave, during the diastolic phase, with a significantly greater amplitude than that of SSt (−10.2%). The corresponding color-coded velocities are superimposed in real time on the bidimensional (2D) image *(upper left)*. Size of the region of interest: 5 mm/3 mm. *RA,* Right atrium; *RV,* right ventricle. (Photo credit: Valérie Chetboul.)

- A decrease in the global TDI index of right myocardial function (Gtdi) defined using the following formula: Gtdi = Stdi × E/Atdi.

Stdi, E/Atdi, and Gtdi were negatively correlated with the value of the PAPs. Conversely, a positive correlation was observed between the PAPs and the time intervals calculated in TDI (the two isovolumetric times and the time to peak Stdi).

Finally, the sensitivity and specificity of these TDI variables have proven to be unquestionably superior to those of the aforementioned echo Doppler parameters, including the Tei index. Thus a Gtdi value <6.2 (lower limit of normal in the normal reference range) predicts the presence of PAH with 64% sensitivity and 100% specificity [6]. For any value <11.8, the sensitivity is 89% with a specificity of 93%.

REFERENCES

[1] Kittleson MD, Kienle RD. Pulmonary arterial and pulmonary arterial hypertension. In: Kittleson MD, Kienle RD, editors. Small animal cardiovascular medicine. Saint Louis: Mosby; 1998, p. 433–49.

[2] Johnson L, Boon J, Orton EC. Clinical characteristics of 53 dogs with Doppler-derived evidence of pulmonary hypertension: 1992–1996. J Vet Intern Med 1999;13:440–7.

[3] Serres FJ, Chetboul V, Tissier R, et al. Doppler echocardiography-derived evidence of pulmonary arterial hypertension in dogs with degenerative mitral valve disease: 86 cases (2001–2005). J Am Vet Med Assoc 2006;229:1772–8.

[4] Schober KE, Baade H. Doppler echocardiographic prediction of pulmonary hypertension in West Highland White terriers with chronic pulmonary disease. J Vet Intern Med 2006;20:912–20.

[5] Glaus T, Tomsa K, Hassig M, et al. Echocardiographic changes induced by moderate to marked hypobaric hypoxia in dogs. Vet Radiol Ultrasound 2004;45: 233–7.

[6] Serres F, Chetboul V, Gouni V, et al. Diagnostic value of echo-Doppler and tissue Doppler imaging in dogs with pulmonary arterial hypertension. J Vet Intern Med 2007;21:1280–9.

[7] Glaus TM, Soldati G, Maurer R, et al. Clinical and pathological characterisation of primary pulmonary hypertension in a dog. Vet Rec 2004;154:786–9.

[8] Kolm US, Amberger CN, Boujon CE, et al. Plexogenic pulmonary arteriopathy in a Pembroke Welsh Corgi. J Small Anim Pract 2004;45:461–6.

[9] Chin KM, Rubin LJ. Pulmonary arterial hypertension. J Am Coll Cardiol 2008;51:1527–38.

[10] Rosenhek R, Rader F, Klaar U, et al. Outcome of watchful waiting in asymptomatic severe mitral regurgitation. Circulation 2006;113:2238–44.

[11] Chetboul V, Serres F, Tissier R, et al. Association of plasma N-terminal pro-B-type natriuretic peptide concentration with mitral regurgitation severity and outcome in dogs with asymptomatic degenerative mitral valve disease. J Vet Intern Med 2009;23:984–94.

[12] Boon JA. Acquired heart disease. In: Boon JA, editor. Manual of veterinary echocardiography. Baltimore: The Williams & Wilkins Co; 1998, p. 261–382.

[13] Kellihan HB, Stepien RL. Pulmonary hypertension in dogs: diagnosis and therapy. Vet Clin North Am Small Anim Pract 2010;40:623–41.

[14] Stepien RL. Pulmonary arterial hypertension secondary to chronic left-sided cardiac dysfunction in dogs. J Small Anim Pract 2009;50 (Suppl.1):34–43.

[15] Uehara Y. An attempt to estimate the pulmonary artery pressure in dogs by means of pulsed Doppler echocardiography. J Vet Med Sci 1993;55:307–12.

[16] Baumwart RD, Meurs KM, Bonagura JD. Tei index of myocardial performance applied to the right ventricle in normal dogs. J Vet Intern Med 2005;19:828–32.

[17] Currie PJ, Seward JB, Chan KL, et al. Continuous wave Doppler determination of right ventricular pressure: a simultaneous Doppler-catheterization study in 127 patients. J Am Coll Cardiol 1985;6:750–6.

[18] Rishniw M, Erb HN. Prevalence and characterization of pulmonary regurgitation in normal adult dogs. J Vet Cardiol 2000;2:17–21.

[19] Nakayama T, Wakao Y, Takiguchi S, et al. Prevalence of valvular regurgitation in normal beagle dogs detected by color Doppler echocardiography. J Vet Med Sci 1994;56:973–5.

[20] Chetboul V. Advanced techniques in echocardiography in small animals. Vet Clin North Am Small Anim Pract 2010;40:529–43.

[21] Chetboul V, Carlos Sampedrano C, Gouni V, et al. Quantitative assessment of regional right ventricular myocardial velocities in awake dogs by Doppler tissue imaging: repeatability, reproducibility, effect of body weight and breed, and comparison with left ventricular myocardial velocities. J Vet Intern Med 2005;19:837–44.

[22] Chetboul V, Carlos Sampedrano C, Gouni V, et al. Ultrasonographic assessment of regional radial and longitudinal systolic function in healthy awake dogs. J Vet Intern Med 2006;20:885–93.

15 Dirofilariasis: Specific Bidimensional Aspects

ÉRIC DE MADRON

Echocardiographic Aspects of *Dirofilaria*, 242
Other Echocardiographic Anomalies Associated with Dirofilariasis, 242

Dirofilariasis is a parasitic infestation by nematodes transmitted by mosquitoes: *Dirofilaria immitis*. This parasitic infestation affects primarily domestic and wild canines but also may affect cats. L3-stage larvae are injected by mosquitoes and make their way to the pulmonary arteries, which they reach in their L4-stage larval form after 4 to 5 months. Their presence triggers arteritis, leading progressively to pulmonary arterial hypertension. When the parasitic burden is low, adult *Dirofilaria* are located in the distal pulmonary arteries. In this case, there is no detectable pulmonary hypertension, hence no echocardiographic anomalies. When the worm burden is more severe, the adult *Dirofilaria* increasingly colonize more proximal sections of pulmonary arteries, including the main pulmonary artery, and therefore may be visualized by echocardiography. Signs of pulmonary hypertension become visible (see Chapter 14). In cases of very serious infestation, the adult *Dirofilaria* can be found in the right cardiac cavities and even in the caudal vena cava, leading to a hemolytic syndrome called the caval syndrome.

Echocardiographic Aspects of *Dirofilaria*

Adult *Dirofilaria* cuticles are highly echogenic. *Dirofilaria* can be visualized with bidimensional (2D) echocardiography and appear as two parallel echogenic lines 2 mm apart, forming an "equal" sign (Figure 15-1) [1-4].

Depending on the severity of the infestation, the adult *Dirofilaria* can be identified in the right pulmonary artery (see Figure 15-1), the main pulmonary artery, the right ventricle, or the right atrium (Figure 15-2) [1-4].

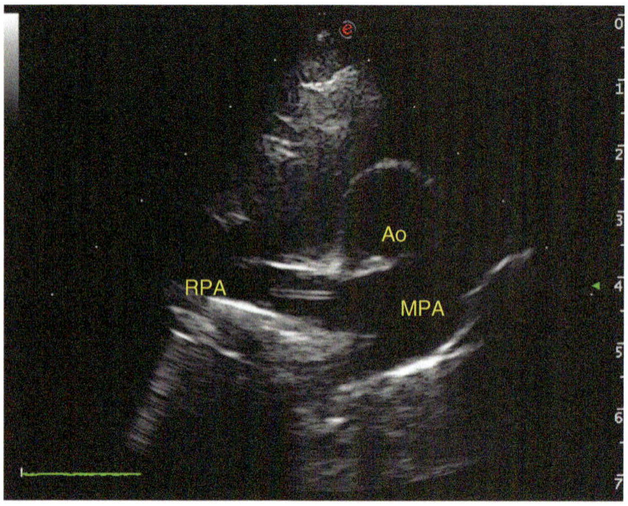

• **Fig. 15-1** Bidimensional (2D) echocardiogram (right parasternal short axis transaortic view) in a cat, revealing the presence of an adult *Dirofilaria* in the right pulmonary artery (RPA). *Ao,* Aorta; *MPA,* main pulmonary artery. (Photo credit: Claudio Bussadori.)

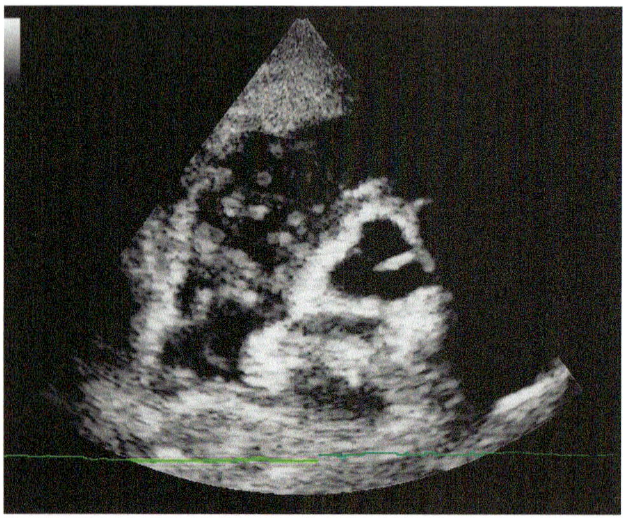

• **Fig. 15-2** Bidimensional (2D) echocardiogram (right parasternal short axis transaortic view) revealing multiple *Dirofilaria* echoes in the right atrium. (Photo credit: Claudio Bussadori.)

In severe cases with caval syndrome, the numerous adult *Dirofilaria* form a localized mass in the right atrium, which then moves into the right ventricular inflow tract in early diastole (Figure 15-3) [2].

In cats, in which the serologic diagnosis of dirofilariasis is more difficult, 2D echocardiography identification can be very useful. A good correlation has been shown between the number of *Dirofilaria* identified by echocardiography and that obtained at necropsy in experimentally infected cats. 2D echocardiography overestimates this number in 27% of cases, underestimates it in 53% of cases, and is correct in 22% of cases. False positives are possible, attributable to the fact that the chordae tendineae of the right ventricular papillary muscles can mimic the "equal" sign. Echocardiography allows the diagnosis of severe infestations (>11 adult worms) in 95% of cases and can distinguish infested and noninfested cats in 88% of cases [3].

Other Echocardiographic Anomalies Associated with Dirofilariasis

The presence of other echocardiographic anomalies depends on the degree of pulmonary arterial hypertension associated with the dirofilariasis. They include dilation of the main pulmonary artery, right ventricle, and right atrium. The interventricular septum can also become flattened and adopt a paradoxic motion [5].

The Doppler anomalies are those of pulmonary arterial hypertension (see Chapter 14).

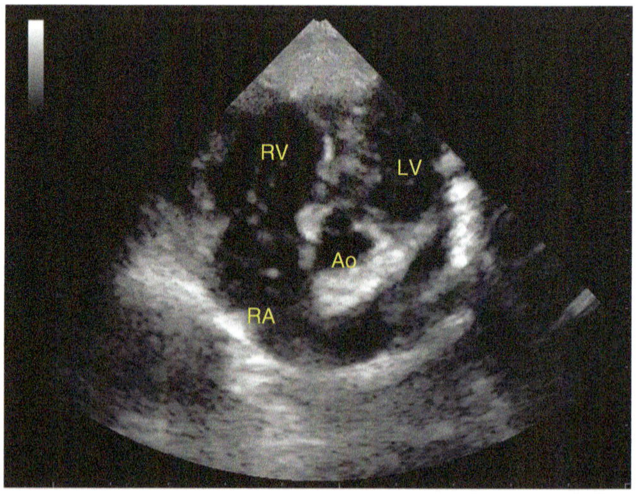

• **Fig. 15-3** Bidimensional (2D) echocardiogram (left apical 5 chambers view) displaying multiple echoes of adult *Dirofilaria* in the right atrium (RA) and right ventricle (RV). *Ao,* Aorta; *LV,* left ventricle. (Photo credit: Claudio Bussadori.)

REFERENCES

[1] Badertscher RR, Losonsky JM, Paul AJ, Kneller SK. Two-dimensional echocardiography in the diagnosis of dirofilariasis in nine dogs. J Am Vet Med Assoc 1988;193:843–6.

[2] Atkins CE, Keene BW, McGuirk SM. Pathophysiologic mechanism of cardiac dysfunction in experimentally induced heartworm caval syndrome in dogs: an echocardiographic study. Am J Vet Res 1988;49:403–10.

[3] Atkins CE, Arther RG, Ciszewski DK, et al. Echocardiographic quantification of *Dirofilaria immitis* infection in experimentally infected cats. Vet Parasitol 2008;158:164–70.

[4] Selzer BA, Newell SM, Mansour AR, McCall JW. Radiographic and 2-D echocardiographic findings in eighteen cats experimentally exposed to *D. immitis* via mosquito bites. Vet Radiol Ultrasound 1996;37:499–505.

[5] Lombard CW, Ackerman N. Right heart enlargement in heartworm infected dogs: a radiographic, electrocardiographic and echocardiographic correlation. Vet Radiol 1984;25:210–7.

16

Cardiac Manifestations of Systemic Diseases

VALÉRIE CHETBOUL AND ÉRIC DE MADRON

Systemic Arterial Hypertension, 246
Hyperthyroid Cardiopathy, 252
Anemia, 254

Systemic Arterial Hypertension

Systemic arterial hypertension (SHT) is defined by chronic systolic increase (>160 mm Hg) and/or chronic diastolic increase (>100 mm Hg) of the systemic arterial pressure. In the animal, SHT is most often secondary to another disorder (mainly chronic renal failure and endocrine diseases such as feline hyperthyroidism) [1-5]. These disorders can be directly responsible for cardiovascular lesions. Added to this are lesions resulting from SHT itself. The risk of end-organ damage, including the cardiovascular system, is considered to be significant when the arterial blood pressure is ≥180 mm Hg and ≥120 mm Hg in systole and diastole, respectively [1].

SHT is the main cardiovascular disorder in elderly cats. It is much less frequent in the dog. Functional and morphologic cardiovascular changes secondary to SHT observed by conventional echo Doppler and tissue Doppler have been thoroughly described in the feline species [6-12]. Fewer data are available for the canine species [13]. However, a number of particularities seem to differ between the two species. They are described separately in this chapter.

Feline Systemic Arterial Hypertension

Left Ventricular Remodeling (2D and TM Modes)

As in humans [14-16], left myocardial hypertrophy is the most frequent result of feline SHT [8-12]. The echocardiographic study conducted by Snyder et al, performed in 2001 on 19 hypertensive cats [8], demonstrated for the first time that these cats had significantly thicker septal and left ventricular free walls than normal cats. These results were later confirmed by our team, in a study including 58 hypertensive cats [10]. In this study, the 39 cats that underwent echocardiographic examination had significantly thicker septal and left ventricular free walls than the cats in the control group (in systole and diastole) as well as decreased systolic and diastolic left ventricular diameters. No correlation was observed between the degree of wall hypertrophy and the blood pressure value or the age of the animals. This study also confirmed for the first time that, as in humans [14], feline SHT is associated with different forms of left ventricular geometry (Figure 16-1). Six different categories of left ventricular geometry associated with feline SHT have thus been defined: (1) concentric hypertrophy, representing the most common type of remodeling (59%; Figure 16-2); (2) normal left ventricular geometry (15%); (3) concentric and symmetric left ventricular hypertrophy (26%); (4) asymmetric concentric left ventricular hypertrophy (33%) with free wall or septal predominance (23% and 10%, respectively); (5) eccentric left ventricular hypertrophy (13%); and (6) localized septal hypertrophy at the subaortic level (13%).

No difference of signalment (breed, sex), associated disorders (retinopathy and renal failure), or blood pressure levels were found between these different types of ventricular remodeling, with the exception of cats with eccentric hypertrophy (who were significantly younger than the

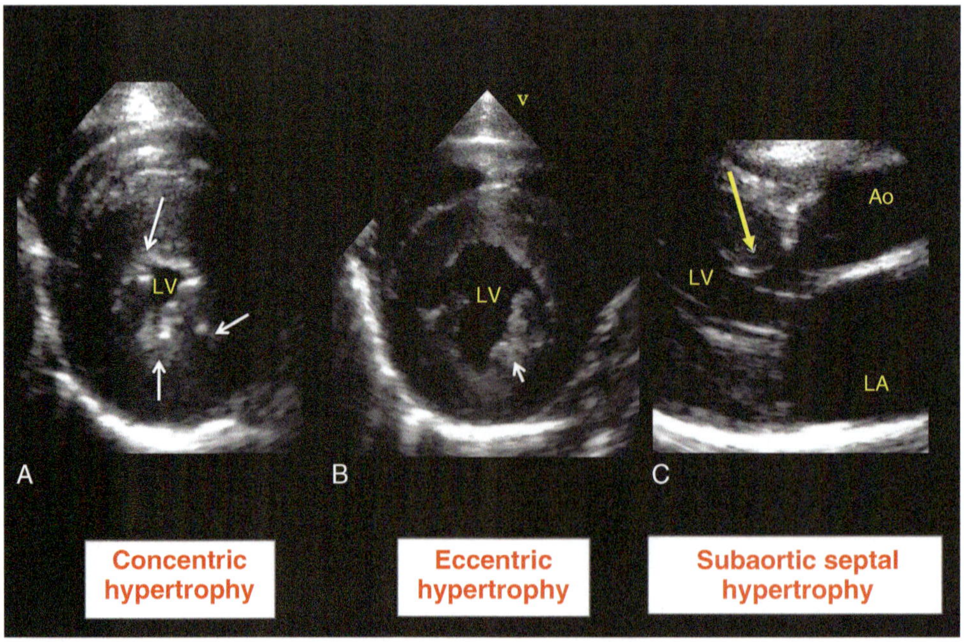

• **Fig. 16-1** The different types of left ventricular hypertrophy in the hypertensive cat. A and B, Left ventricular concentric and eccentric hypertrophy, respectively (right parasternal short axis transventricular views in diastole). The chamber is reduced in the first case and increased in the second. Note the subendocardial hyperechoic plaque (fibrosis) *(arrows)*. C, An example of subaortic septal hypertrophy *(arrow)* (right parasternal long axis 5 chambers view). *Ao,* Aorta; *LA,* left atrium; *LV,* left ventricle. (Photo credit: Valérie Chetboul.)

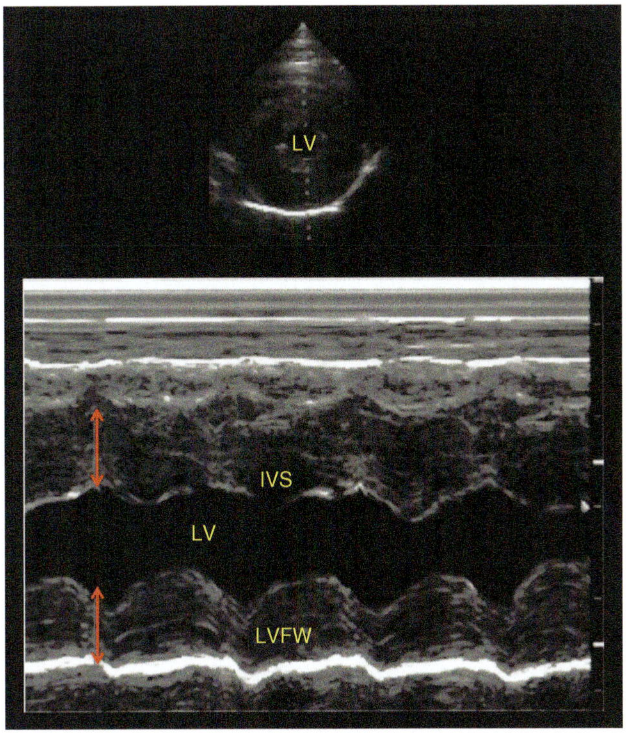

• **Fig. 16-2** Left ventricular concentric hypertrophy in a hypertensive cat. This transventricular time-motion (TM) echocardiogram confirms that the hypertrophy is concentric, involving the interventricular septum (IVS) and the left ventricular free wall (LVFW) simultaneously. The hypertrophy is considered to be symmetric because the ratio of the diastolic wall thicknesses (LVFW/IVS) ranges between 0.7 and 1.3 (LVFW in diastole = 6.5 mm; IVS in diastole = 7.8 mm; IVS/LVFW in diastole = 1.2). *LV,* Left ventricle. (Photo credit: Valérie Chetboul.)

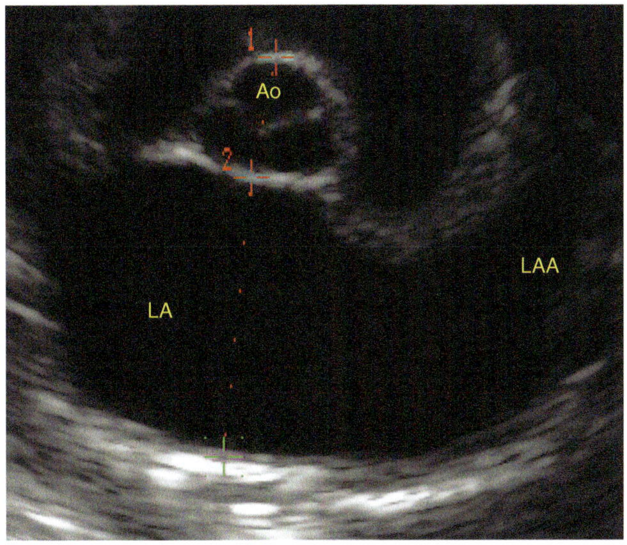

• **Fig. 16-3** Left atrial dilation in a hypertensive cat. This right parasternal short axis transaortic view confirms marked left atrial dilation (LA/Ao ratio = 2.4) with abnormal visualization of the left atrial appendage (LAA). *Ao,* Aorta; *LA,* left atrium. (Photo credit: Valérie Chetboul.)

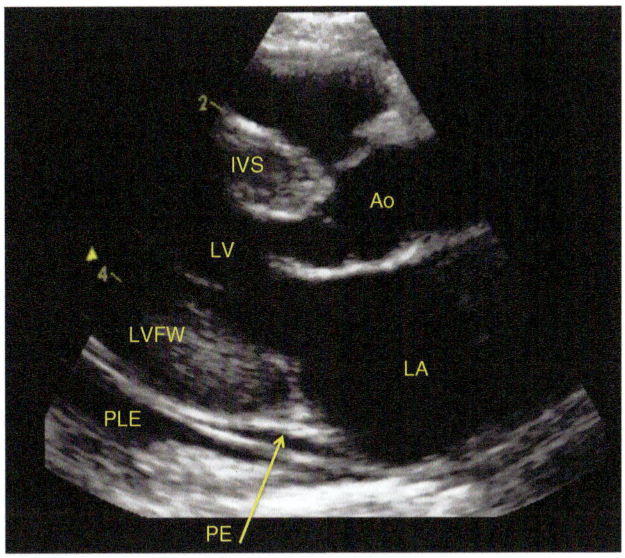

• **Fig. 16-4** Left atrial dilation and signs of congestive heart failure in a hypertensive cat. This right parasternal long axis 5 chambers view illustrates several anomalies: left atrial dilation (twice the aortic diameter); an anechoic space between the two pericardial layers, beneath the left ventricular free wall (LVFW), corresponding to pericardial effusion (PE); pleural effusion (PLE); and hyperechoic remodeling of the interventricular septum (IVS). *Ao,* Aorta; *LA,* left atrium; *LV,* left ventricle. (Photo credit: Valérie Chetboul.)

other hypertensive animals). This lack of difference is likely linked with the existence of numerous nonmechanical factors involved in hypertensive hypertrophy [17,18]. A subsequent retrospective study confirmed the high prevalence (70% in time-motion [TM] mode) and the diversity of left ventricular remodeling with feline SHT [11].

Finally, it is worth mentioning that the myocardial hypertrophy associated with SHT is often accompanied by a heterogeneous myocardial echostructure (see Figure 16-1), with the presence of hyperechoic plaques, indicating the presence of fibrotic zones, predominantly in the endocardial region. This hypertrophy can regress with antihypertensive treatment such as amlodipine [8].

Other Cardiovascular Changes Observed in Conventional Echo Doppler Examination

- Left atrial dilation and congestive heart failure are rarely associated with hypertensive left ventricular remodeling (Figures 16-3 and 16-4) [7,10]. These anomalies were observed in 28% (left atrial dilation) and 12% (congestive heart failure) of the cases in our study [10].
- Dilation of the ascending aorta is a frequent modification associated with feline SHT (Figure 16-5). Nelson et al [9] evaluated the aortic diameter of 15 hypertensive cats in four different areas (using a right parasternal long axis view): the aortic annulus, the sinuses of Valsalva, the tubular junction, and the proximal ascending aorta (diameters corresponding to A1, A2, A3, and A4; see Figure 16-5). The A3 and A4 diameters along with the A4/A1 and A3/A1 ratios were found to be significantly higher in hypertensive cats compared to a healthy feline control group. They were also positively correlated with the systolic arterial pressure value [9].

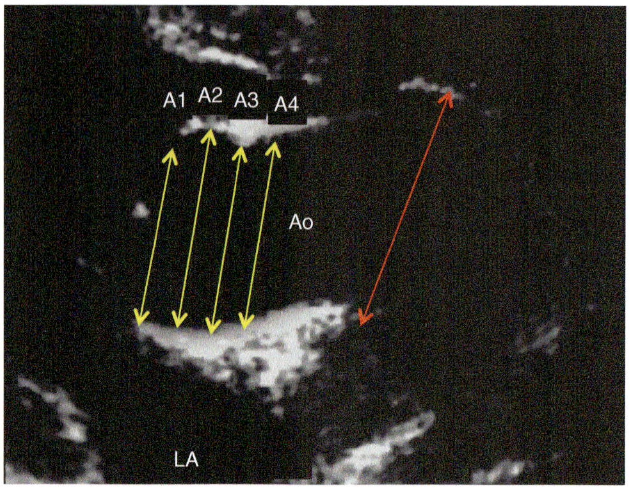

• **Fig. 16-5** Aortic dilation in a hypertensive cat. The four aortic diameters measured in the study by Nelson et al [9] are visible on this right parasternal long axis view: aortic annulus diameter (1), aortic diameter at the level of the sinuses of Valsalva (2), diameter at the sinotubular junction (3), and proximal aorta diameter (4). Note the abnormally rectilinear shape of the aorta due to the dilation of the artery in 3 and 4. Note also the abnormally clear view of the aortic arch due to its dilation *(double red arrow)*. *Ao,* Aorta; *LA,* left atrium. (Photo credit: Valérie Chetboul.)

- Rarely, the aortic dilation secondary to SHT may lead to functional aortic regurgitation due to valvular annulus dilation (Figure 16-6). Even more rarely, SHT can result in aortic wall dissection, as it does in humans [7].
- Alteration of the diastolic function is frequently associated with feline SHT [12]. Although better documented using tissue Doppler (see below), the hemodynamic modifications of this diastolic dysfunction can be detected using pulsed wave spectral Doppler. They include mitral E and A wave inversion (Figure 16-7) and lengthening of the isovolumic relaxation time [12].

Myocardial Dysfunction Analyzed Using Tissue Doppler

Myocardial tissue Doppler imaging (TDI) is a particular Doppler technique that consists of measuring the myocardial motion velocity throughout the entire cardiac cycle (see details in Chapter 4) [19]. Depending on the selected cross-section (right parasternal short axis transventricular or left apical), TDI enables analysis of the longitudinal and radial left myocardial function. This

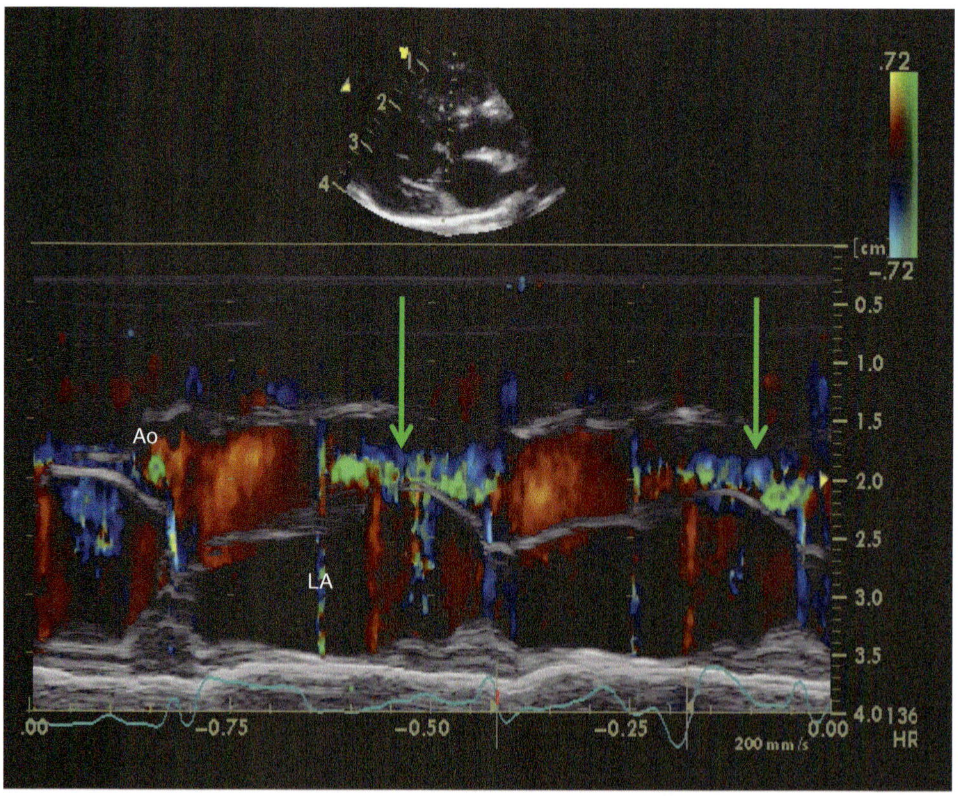

• **Fig. 16-6** Transaortic color time-motion (TM) view in a hypertensive cat. Note the presence of aortic regurgitation *(green arrows)* during the entire duration of ventricular diastole. *Ao,* Aorta; *LA,* left atrium. (Photo credit: Valérie Chetboul.)

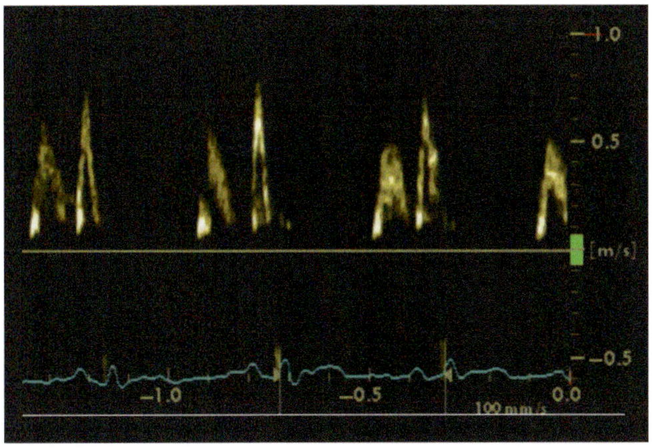

• **Fig. 16-7** Inversion of the mitral E and A waves in a hypertensive cat. The E/A ratio is <1 (0.75), indicating impaired diastolic function. (Photo credit: Valérie Chetboul.)

technique, validated in the awake cat in color bidimensional (2D) TDI mode [20,21], was used by our team to study regional myocardial dysfunction associated with feline SHT [12]. These changes appear to be similar to those associated with feline primary hypertrophic cardiomyopathy, concerning mainly the basal and apical longitudinal left ventricular free wall diastolic functions (Figure 16-8), the basal interventricular septum function (Figure 16-9), and to a lesser degree the left ventricular radial function [12]. This dysfunction is found not only in the hypertrophied left myocardial segments, but also in the segments having a normal thickness in TM mode. In this study [12], TDI was also able to demonstrate that SHT affects the left longitudinal systolic function (see Figure 16-8), despite the normal to increased shortening fractions. The systolic dysfunction associated with SHT was characterized by a significant decrease of left longitudinal systolic velocities and of the base-apex gradient in hypertensive cats compared to control cats. In addition, a particular longitudinal systolic and diastolic impairment appeared (see Figure 16-8): the presence of postsystolic contractions in hypertensive cats (80% and 71% of the cases at the base and apex, respectively) along with disappearance of the E wave in more than one third of them. None of these waves, though, was found in the study's 56 control group cats. Postsystolic contractions are now considered markers for myocardial segmental asynchrony and dysfunction. They are frequently found in myocardial ischemia in humans or experimentally [22,23]. Even though these contractions can be observed in one third of normal myocardial segments in humans, they are always more frequent and of greater amplitude during myocardial ischemia [23].

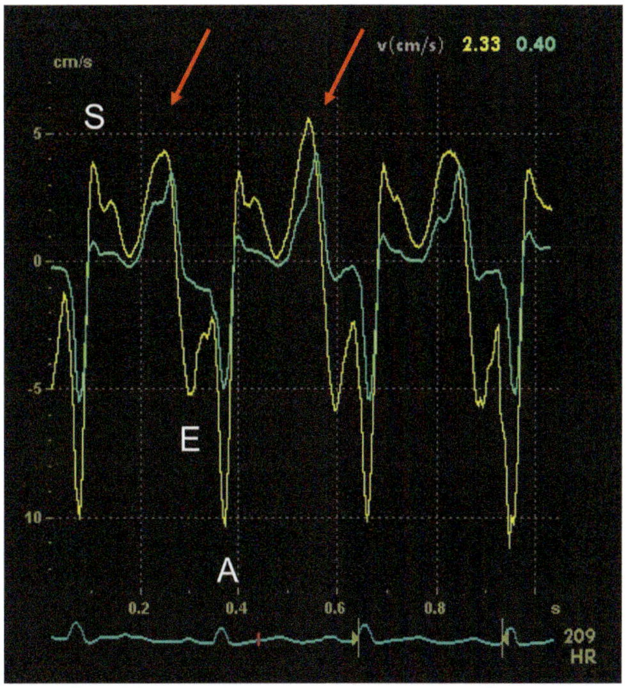

• **Fig. 16-8** Changes to the left longitudinal myocardial function analyzed using color bidimensional (2D) tissue Doppler imaging (TDI) in a hypertensive cat. The TDI analysis was performed using a left apical 4 chambers view on two circular segments of the left ventricular free wall each measuring 2 mm in diameter, one at the base *(yellow curve)* and one at the apex *(green curve)*. The different phases of the cardiac cycle are identified, including a positive S wave during systole and two negative waves, E and A, concomitant with early diastole and end-diastole, respectively. At the base as well as at the apex, the impaired diastolic function is characterized by an E/A ratio <1. In addition, the presence of another systolic and diastolic anomaly is added: the presence of a postsystolic contraction *(red arrows)* with a greater amplitude than S and intercalated between the latter and the E wave. (Photo credit: Valérie Chetboul.)

Canine Systemic Arterial Hypertension: Particularities

Few data on the cardiovascular consequences of SHT in dogs are available at this time. Only a few clinical cases or case series have been published, mostly focusing on renal function impairment during SHT or hypertensive endocrine diseases in dogs [24-34].

Our team recently performed a study in 58 dogs (30 with spontaneous SHT and 28 control dogs of the same age and weight) in order to better characterize the cardiovascular changes associated with canine SHT, using conventional echo Doppler and TDI. The results can be summarized as follows:

- A symmetric and concentric myocardial hypertrophy was found in almost half of the cases (47%; Figure 16-10). No other type of abnormal left ventricular geometry was observed.

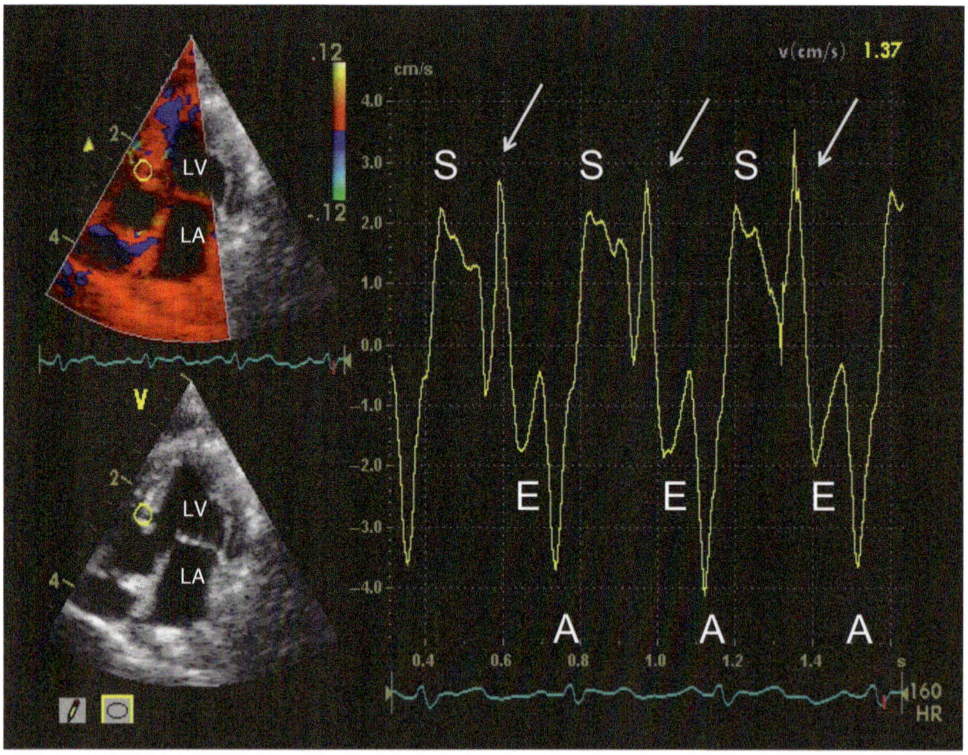

• **Fig. 16-9** Impairment of the septal longitudinal myocardial function analyzed using color bidimensional (2D) tissue Doppler imaging (TDI) in a hypertensive cat. The TDI analysis was performed in a circular segment measuring 2 mm in diameter located at the base of the interventricular septum, using a left apical cross-section. As in the cat in Figure 16-8, the diastolic function impairment is characterized by an E/A ratio <1 and the presence of a postsystolic contraction *(white arrows)* intercalated between the systolic S wave and the early diastolic E wave. *A,* End-diastolic wave; *LA,* left atrium; *LV,* left ventricle. (Photo credit: Valérie Chetboul.)

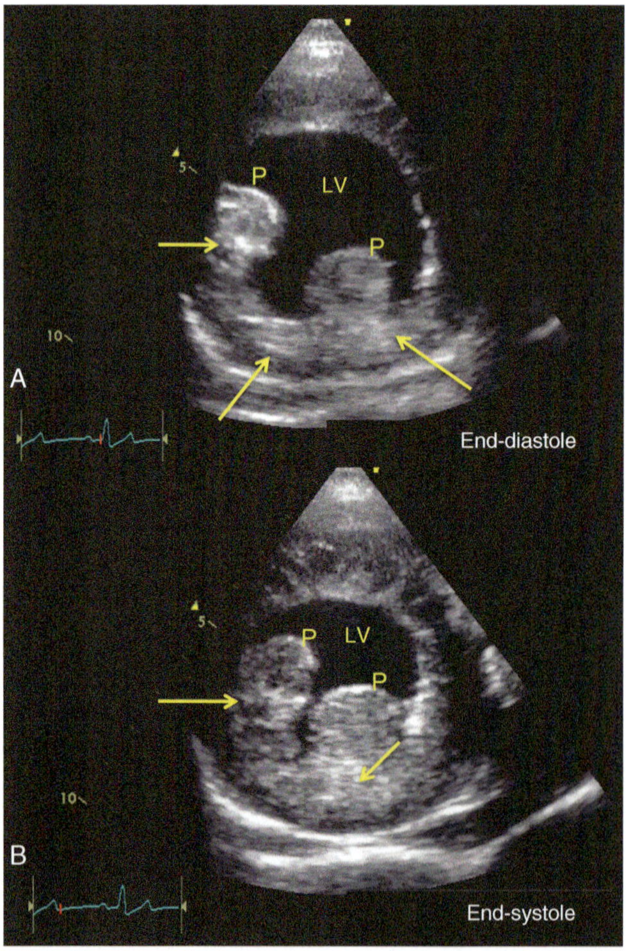

• **Fig. 16-10** Left ventricular concentric hypertrophy observed in (A) diastole and (B) systole on a right parasternal short axis transventricular cross-section in a hypertensive dog. Hyperechoic plaques *(arrows)* are observed in the left myocardium and within the hypertrophied papillary muscles (P). *LV,* Left ventricle. (Photo credit: Valérie Chetboul.)

- No hypertensive animals presented with left atrial dilation or signs of congestive heart failure.
- Aortic dilation with functional aortic regurgitation was detected using color Doppler in one third of the hypertensive dogs (Figures 16-11 to 16-13, Video 16-1).
- All of the hypertensive dogs that underwent a TDI exam had impaired longitudinal basal and apical diastolic function (Figure 16-14) with E and A wave inversion (early diastole and end-diastole, respectively), impaired basal septal longitudinal diastolic

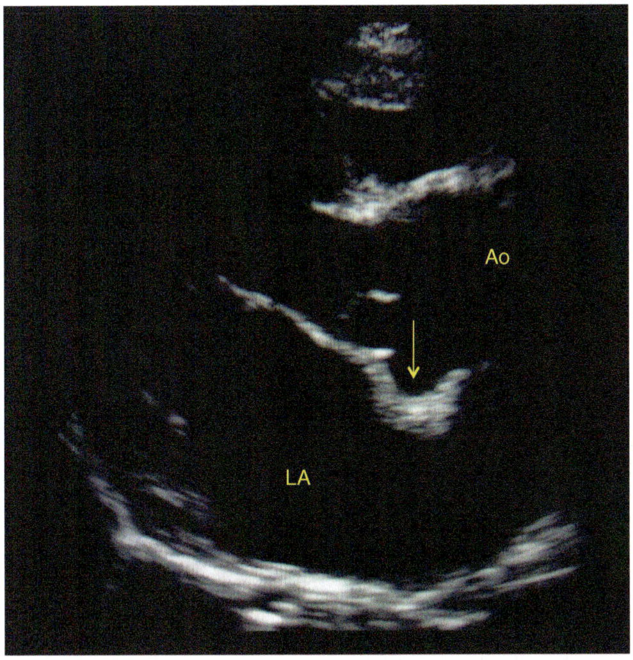

• **Fig. 16-11** Aortic and left coronary artery dilation *(arrow)* in a hypertensive dog (right parasternal long axis 5 chambers view). *Ao,* Aorta; *LA,* left atrium. (Photo credit: Valérie Chetboul.)

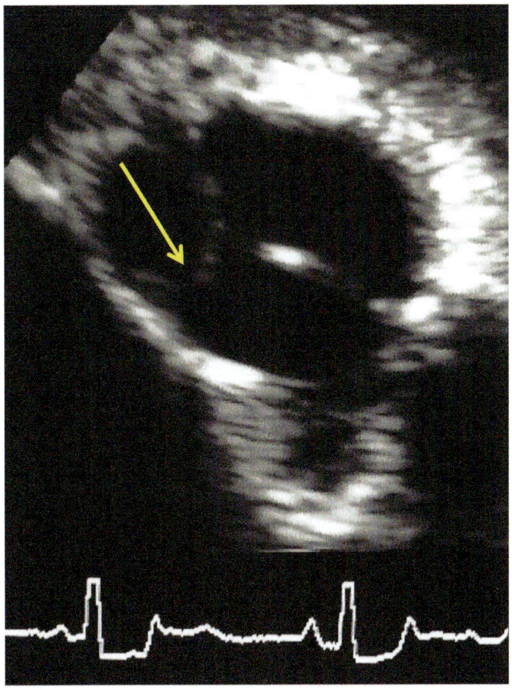

• **Fig. 16-12** Deformed aortic valve cusps closure line *(arrow)* associated with an aortic dilation in a hypertensive dog (right parasternal short axis transaortic view). (Photo credit: Valérie Chetboul.)

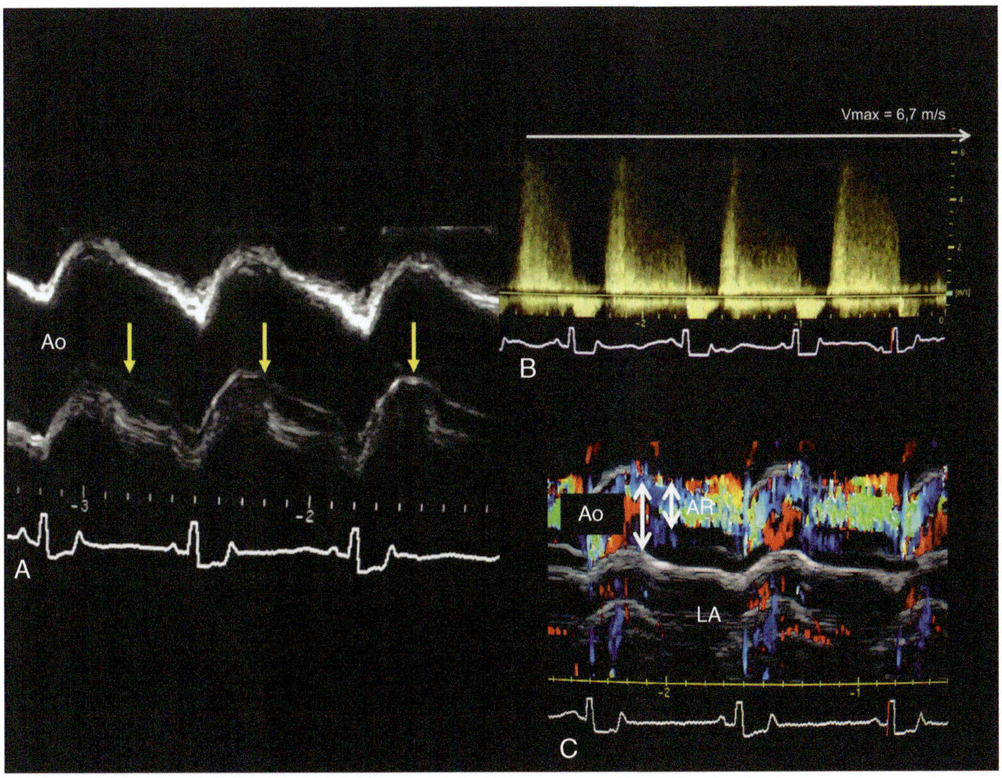

• **Fig. 16-13** Dissection and aortic regurgitation in a hypertensive dog. A, The arterial wall dissection is confirmed with the visualization on the transaortic time-motion (TM) view of two wall lines *(arrows)* moving in parallel. B, The diastolic aortic regurgitation maximum velocity (Vmax), measured using continuous wave Doppler, is elevated, indicating a markedly increased aorta–left ventricle pressure gradient (180 mm Hg) due to diastolic arterial hypertension. C, The color TM mode shows that the aortic regurgitation (AR) is both holodiastolic and significant (regurgitant jet height/aortic diameter = 70%). *Ao,* Aorta; *LA,* left atrium. (Photo credit: Valérie Chetboul.)

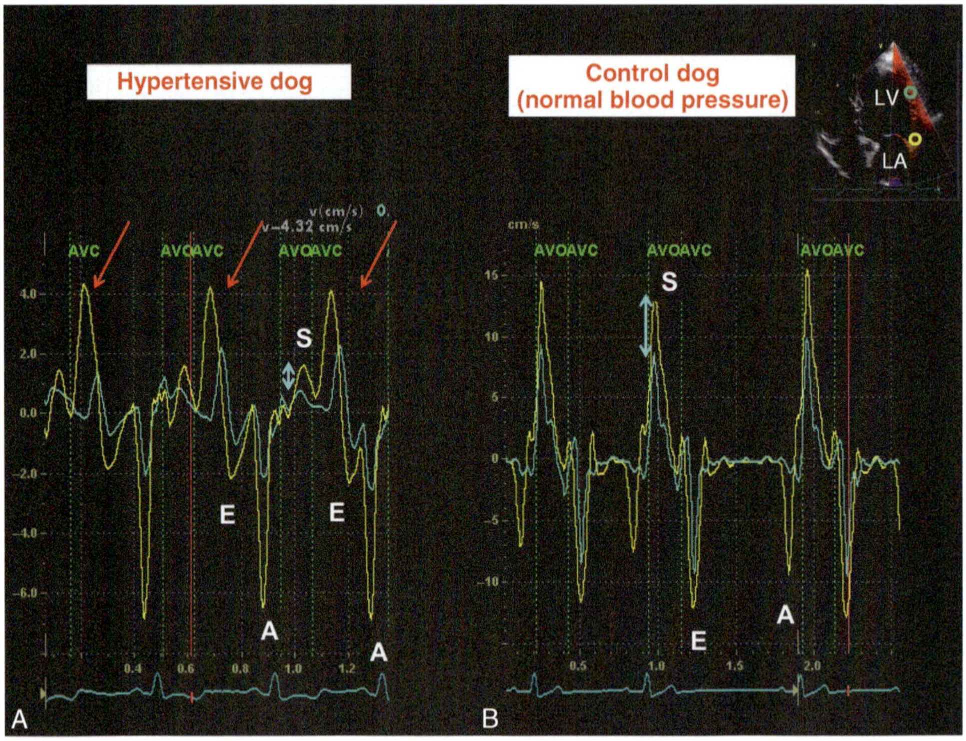

• **Fig. 16-14** Longitudinal left myocardial function impairment analyzed using color bidimensional (2D) tissue Doppler imaging (TDI) in a hypertensive dog (A), compared to a normotensive dog (B). In these two dogs, the right myocardial velocities are analyzed simultaneously in two circular segments of the left ventricular wall measuring 2 mm in diameter: a basal *(yellow)* and an apical segment *(green)*. The trace obtained shows that the basal segment moves more rapidly *(yellow curve)* than the apical segment *(green curve)* during systole and diastole, thus defining an intramyocardial velocity gradient throughout the cardiac cycle. In the hypertensive animal, the myocardial impairment is systolic and diastolic and characterized by a decrease in the systolic S wave, a decrease in the base-apex systolic gradient *(double blue arrow)*, and the presence of a postsystolic contraction with a greater amplitude than S *(red arrows)* and by early diastolic and end-diastolic wave inversion (E and A, respectively) with an E/A ratio <1. *AVC,* Aortic valve closure; *AVO,* aortic valve opening; *LA,* left atrium; *LV,* left ventricle. (Photo credit: Valérie Chetboul.)

(Figure 16-15), and subendocardial radial functions, independent of the presence of myocardial hypertrophy on TM mode.

- This was accompanied by a significant decrease in systolic velocities and base-apex systolic velocity gradients compared to control animals.
- Finally, postsystolic contractions during the left ventricular free wall longitudinal and radial motions were detected in 5% and 16% of the hypertensive dogs, respectively. In one animal, the longitudinal E wave had disappeared (see Figure 16-14; Figure 16-16). A longitudinal septal postsystolic contraction was detected in 8% of the hypertensive dogs. None of these waves was found in the 28 control dogs.

Therefore, as in cats, canine SHT is associated with myocardial systolic and diastolic dysfunction mostly affecting the longitudinal movement and frequent presence of postsystolic contractions. SHT is also frequently associated with myocardial hypertrophy. However, the latter has the particularity of being homogenous (no eccentric or subaortic segmental hypertrophy was found in this series). Finally, aortic regurgitation, rare in hypertensive cats, is a frequent complication in dogs with SHT.

Hyperthyroid Cardiopathy

Hyperthyroidism is mostly encountered in cats. This endocrine disease is a multisystemic disorder affecting both the energetic metabolism and the cardiovascular system. It leads to a metabolic and oxygen consumption increase as well as to peripheral vasodilation. The trophic effects of the thyroid hormone on cardiomyocytes lead to left ventricular hypertrophy. Adrenergic receptor sensitivity is increased, resulting in increased contractility. Cardiac output, heart rate, ejection fraction, and oxygen consumption all increase. With time, diastolic dysfunction sets in. These changes can lead to high cardiac output congestive heart failure [36].

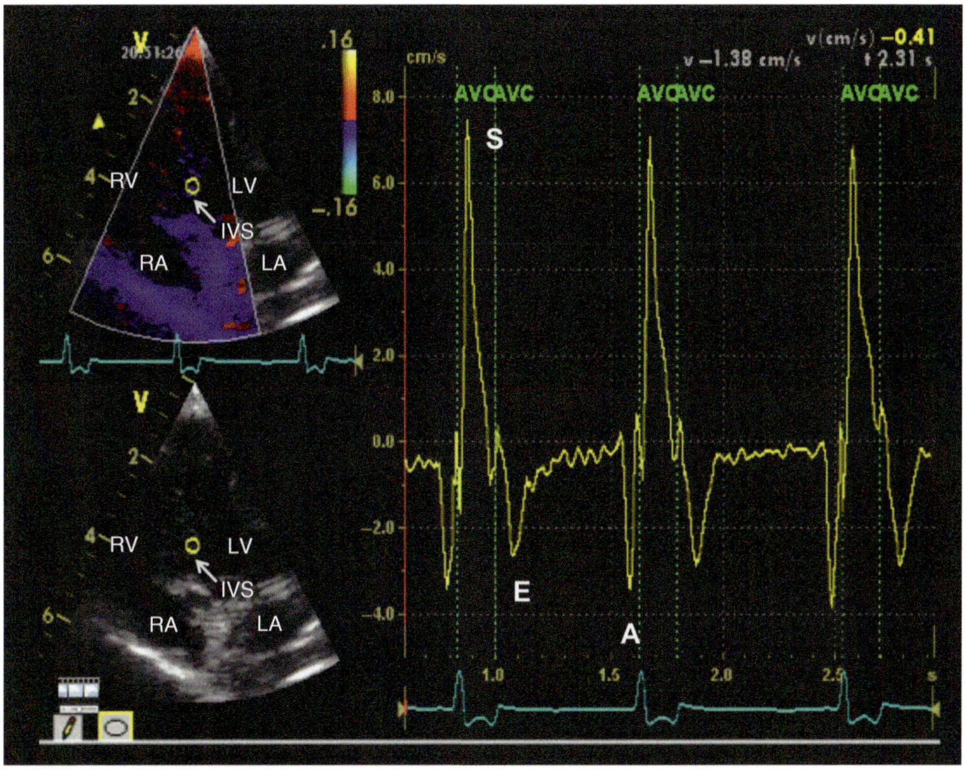

• **Fig. 16-15** Longitudinal septal function impairment analyzed using color bidimensional (2D) tissue Doppler imaging (TDI) in a hypertensive dog. Myocardial velocities are analyzed in a circular segment located at the base of the interventricular septum (IVS), measuring 2 mm in diameter. The myocardial change is diastolic and characterized by early diastolic and end-diastolic wave inversion (E and A, respectively) with an E/A ratio <1. *AVC,* Aortic valve closure; *AVO,* aortic valve opening; *LA,* left atrium; *LV,* left ventricle; *RA,* right atrium; *RV,* right ventricle; *S,* positive systolic wave. (Photo credit: Valérie Chetboul.)

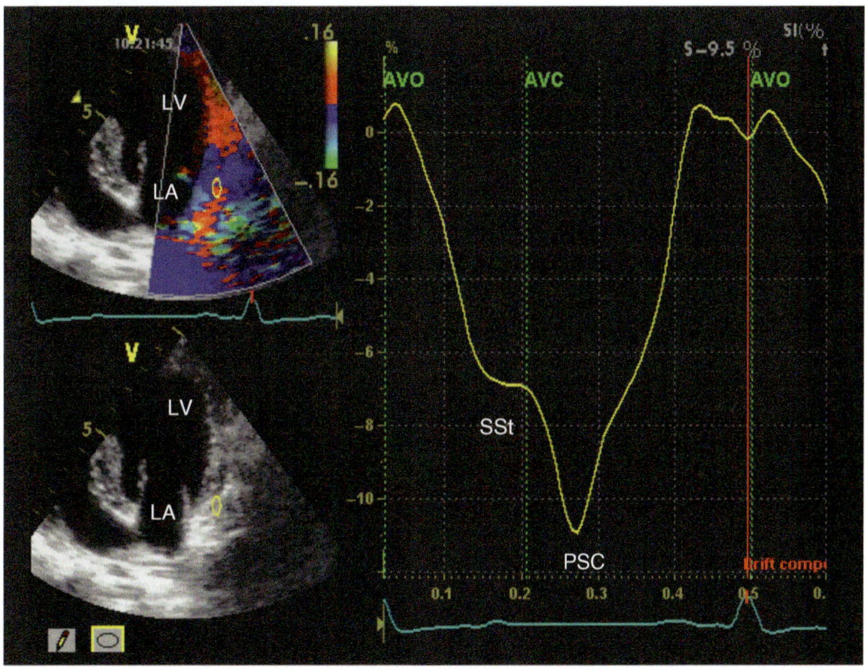

• **Fig. 16-16** Example of longitudinal myocardial function impairment analyzed at the left ventricular free wall base using strain imaging in a hypertensive dog. The longitudinal systolic strain is, as normally expected, negative but its absolute peak value (SSt) is decreased (7%; normal reference range = 19% to 35% [35]). In addition, prior to returning to the baseline, a postsystolic contraction (PSC) occurs after the closure of the aortic valve, with a greater amplitude (11.2%) than the SSt. Size of the region of interest: 5 mm/3 mm. *AVC,* Aortic valve closure; *AVO,* aortic valve opening; *LA,* left atrium; *LV,* left ventricle. (Photo credit: Valérie Chetboul.)

TM and 2d Echocardiographic Aspects

Echocardiographic changes are inconsistently present. They include left chamber dilation and septum and/or left ventricular free wall hypertrophy. Shortening fraction is sometimes increased (Table 16-1) [36,37].

Several studies have compared the echocardiographic parameters in hyperthyroid cats prior to and following radioiodine (^{131}I) treatment. In a study, only the left ventricular free wall thickness prior to treatment could be correlated to serum T4 concentration [38]. In 37% of cases, one or more parameters were abnormal before treatment [38]. In another study, pretreatment echocardiographic changes were minimal and most parameters remained within normal values (Figure 16-17). Cats with elevated levels of cardiac troponin I (cTnI) tended to have greater septal systolic and diastolic thicknesses than cats with normal cTnI levels [39].

The most frequent abnormalities—septal or free wall hypertrophy—tended to be reversible following treatment [38].

Decreased shortening fraction following treatment has been observed by several authors [38,39].

It is interesting to note that despite the normalization of certain parameters following treatment, some anomalies persisted in 32% of cases [38]. In this latter group, 45% of cats had normal echocardiograms prior to treatment. This indicates that some anomalies can appear even after treatment [38].

Doppler Echocardiography

In the first stages of hyperthyroid cardiopathy, there are no observable diastolic anomalies [40]. However, with lasting hyperthyroidism, the ensuing cardiac remodeling could affect diastolic function. Relaxation disturbances are then observed, characterized by inversion of the E/A ratio and an increase in isovolumic relaxation time (Figure 16-18).

In more advanced stages, a restrictive type of diastolic anomaly could appear. In this case, cardiac changes could become irreversible despite treatment of the hyperthyroidism.

TABLE 16-1 Echocardiographic Abnormalities Observed in 103 Hyperthyroid Cats [36]

Anomaly	Percentage of Cats (n = 103)
Left atrial dilation	67
LV dilation in diastole	45
Septal hypertrophy	39
LV free wall hypertrophy	71
SF increase (%)	20

LV, Left ventricle; *SF*, left ventricle shortening fraction.

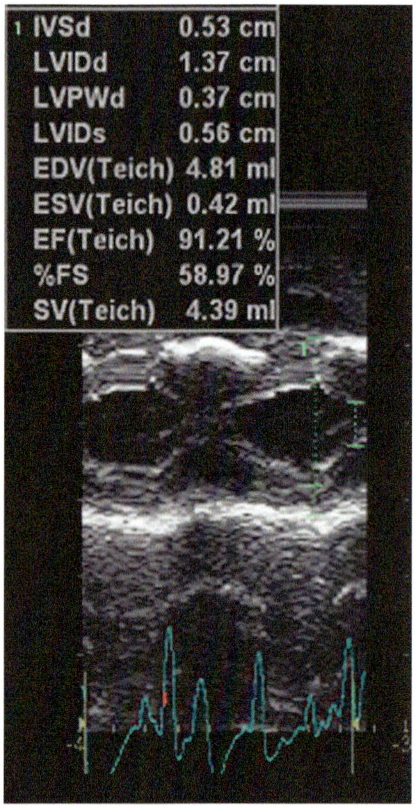

• **Fig. 16-17** Time-motion (TM) echocardiogram of the left ventricle of a hyperthyroid cat. The septal thickness is greater than that of the free wall. However, this thickness remains within the normal upper limits. The shortening fraction is normal (59%). (Photo credit: Éric de Madron.)

Anemia

Prolonged anemia can have significant cardiovascular consequences, leading to high cardiac output congestive heart failure [41]. First, blood viscosity is decreased. In addition, the increased tissue oxygen requirements result in arterial vasodilation. Afterload thus becomes significantly reduced. Furthermore, cardiac adrenergic stimulation is increased [41]. Anemia-induced cardiac changes are well documented in human patients suffering from chronic congenital anemia (thalassemia or sickle cell anemia) [42] or anemia secondary to renal failure [43,44]. One can observe an increase in the left ventricular end-diastolic diameter, left ventricular hypertrophy with increased ventricular mass, a hyperdynamic state with increased stroke volume, and

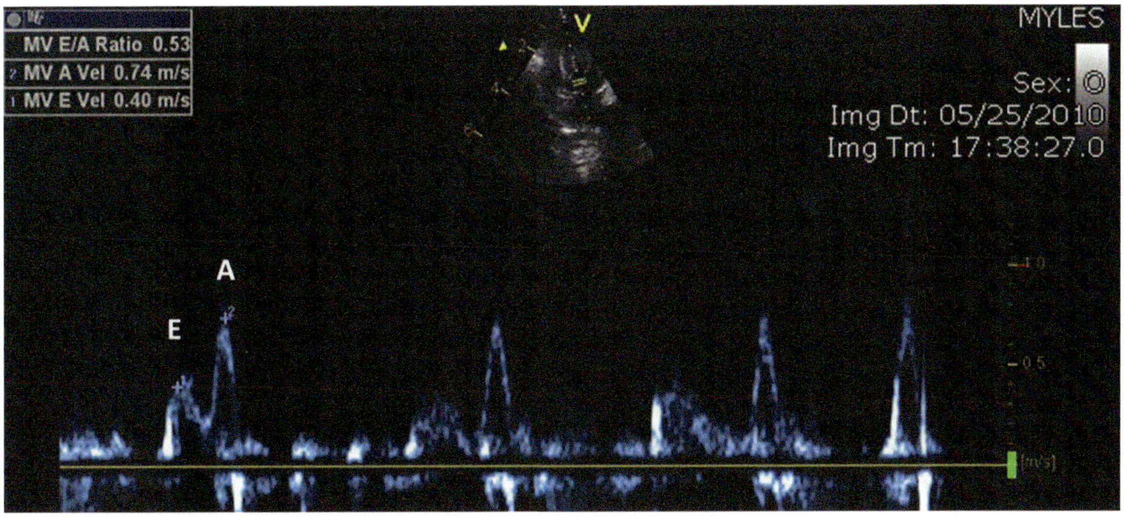

• **Fig. 16-18** Spectral Doppler of the transmitral flow in the same hyperthyroid cat as in Figure 16-17. Note the inversion of the E/A ratio, indicating delayed relaxation. (Photo credit: Éric de Madron.)

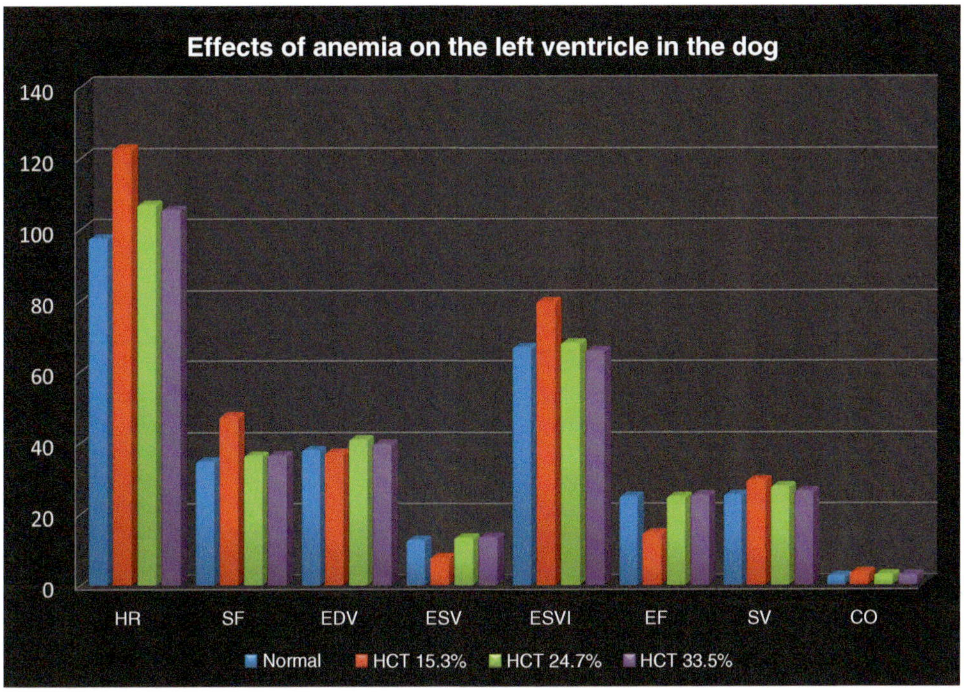

• **Fig. 16-19** The impact of anemia on the left ventricle in dogs. *CO,* Cardiac output; *EDV,* end-diastolic volume; *EF,* ejection fraction; *ESV,* end-systolic volume; *ESVI,* indexed end-systolic volume; *HCT,* hematocrit; *HR,* heart rate; *SF,* shortening fraction; *SV,* stroke volume. (Adapted from Spotswood TC, Kirberger RM, Koma LMPK, et al. Changes in echocardiographic variables of left ventricular size and function in a model of canine normovolemic anemia. Vet Radiol Ultrasound 2006;47:358–65.)

decreased aortic ejection acceleration time. Variable diastolic anomalies have also been observed [42-44]. These changes are reversible once the anemia has been corrected [43,44].

A study was performed in dogs with experimentally induced normovolemic anemia. A number of changes similar to the ones mentioned above were documented, such as a hyperdynamic state with increased shortening fraction and stroke volume, decreased end-systolic volume, and increased heart rate (Figure 16-19) [45].

REFERENCES

[1] Brown S, Atkins C, Bagley R, et al. Guidelines for the identification, evaluation, and management of systemic hypertension in dogs and cats. J Vet Intern Med 2007;21:542–58.

[2] Wehner A, Hartmann K, Hirschberger J. Associations between proteinuria, systemic hypertension and glomerular filtration rate in dogs with renal and nonrenal diseases. Vet Rec 2008;162:141–7.

[3] Finco DR. Association of systemic hypertension with renal injury in dogs with induced renal failure. J Vet Intern Med 2004;18:289–94.

[4] Syme HM, Barber PJ, Markwell PJ, et al. Prevalence of systolic hypertension in cats with chronic renal failure at initial evaluation. J Am Vet Med Assoc 2002;220:1799–804.

[5] Sennello KA, Schulman RL, Prosek R, et al. Systolic blood pressure in cats with diabetes mellitus. J Am Vet Med Assoc 2003;223:198–201.

[6] Littman MP. Spontaneous systemic hypertension in 24 cats. J Vet Intern Med 1994;8:79–86.

[7] Wey AC, Atkins CE. Aortic dissection and congestive heart failure associated with systemic hypertension in a cat. J Vet Intern Med 2000;14:208–13.

[8] Snyder PS, Sadek D, Jones GL. Effect of amlodipine on echocardiographic variables in cats with systemic hypertension. J Vet Intern Med 2001;15:52–6.

[9] Nelson L, Riedesel EA, Ware WA, Christensen WF. Echocardiographic and radiographic changes associated with systemic hypertension in cats. J Vet Intern Med 2002;16:418–25.

[10] Chetboul V, Lefebvre HP, Pinhas C, et al. Spontaneous feline hypertension: clinical and echocardiographic abnormalities, and survival rate. J Vet Intern Med 2003;17:89–95.

[11] Henik RA, Stepien RL, Bortnowski HB. Spectrum of M-mode echocardiographic abnormalities in 75 cats with systemic hypertension. J Am Anim Hosp Assoc 2004;40:359–63.

[12] Carlos Sampedrano C, Chetboul V, Gouni V, et al. Systolic and diastolic myocardial dysfunction in cats with hypertrophic cardiomyopathy or systemic hypertension. J Vet Intern Med 2006;20:1106–15.

[13] Misbach C, Gouni V, Tissier R, et al. Echocardiographic and tissue Doppler imaging alterations associated with spontaneous canine systemic hypertension. J Vet Intern Med 2011;25:1025–35.

[14] Ganau A, Devereux RB, Roman MJ, et al. Patterns of left ventricular hypertrophy and geometric remodeling in essential hypertension. J Am Coll Cardiol 1992;19:1550–8.

[15] Heesen WF, Beltman FW, May JF, et al. High prevalence of concentric remodeling in elderly individuals with isolated systolic hypertension. Hypertension 1997;29:539–43.

[16] Koren MJ, Devereux RB, Casale PN, et al. Relation of left ventricular mass and geometry to morbidity and mortality in uncomplicated essential hypertension. Ann Intern Med 1991;114:345–52.

[17] Devereux RB, Roman MJ. Left ventricular hypertrophy in hypertension: stimuli, patterns, and consequences. Hypertens Res 1999;22:1–9.

[18] Schlaich MP, Schmieder RE. Left ventricular hypertrophy and its regression: pathophysiology and therapeutic approach: focus on treatment by antihypertensive agents. Am J Hypertens 1998;11:1394–404.

[19] Chetboul V. Tissue Doppler imaging: a promising technique for quantifying regional myocardial function. J Vet Cardiol 2002;4:7–12.

[20] Chetboul V, Athanassiadis N, Carlos C, et al. Quantification, repeatability, and reproducibility of feline radial and longitudinal left ventricular velocities by tissue Doppler imaging. Am J Vet Res 2004;65:566–72.

[21] Chetboul V, Carlos Sampedrano C, Tissier R, et al. Quantitative assessment of velocities of the annulus of the left atrioventricular valve and left ventricular free wall in healthy cats by use of two-dimensional color tissue Doppler imaging. Am J Vet Res 2006;67:250–8.

[22] Ring M, Persson H, Mejhert M, et al. Post-systolic motion in patients with heart failure–a marker of left ventricular dyssynchrony? Eur J Echocardiogr 2007;8:352–9.

[23] Voigt JU, Lindenmeier G, Exner B, et al. Incidence and characteristics of segmental postsystolic longitudinal shortening in normal, acutely ischemic, and scarred myocardium. J Am Soc Echocardiogr 2003;16:415–23.

[24] Howard EB, Nielsen SW. Pheochromocytomas associated with hypertensive lesions in dogs. J Am Vet Med Assoc 1965;147:245–52.

[25] Littman MP, Robertson JL, Bovée KC. Spontaneous systemic hypertension in dogs: five cases (1981–1983). J Am Vet Med Assoc 1988;193:486–94.

[26] Ortega TM, Feldman EC, Nelson RW, et al. Systemic arterial blood pressure and urine protein/creatinine ratio in dogs with hyperadrenocorticism. J Am Vet Med Assoc 1996;209:1724–9.

[27] Struble AL, Feldman EC, Nelson RW, Kass PH. Systemic hypertension and proteinuria in dogs with diabetes mellitus. J Am Vet Med Assoc 1998;213:822–5.

[28] Jacob F, Polzin DJ, Osborne CA, et al. Association between initial systolic blood pressure and risk of developing a uremic crisis or of dying in dogs with chronic renal failure. J Am Vet Med Assoc 2003;222:322–9.

[29] Finco DR. Association of systemic hypertension with renal injury in dogs with induced renal failure. J Vet Intern Med 2004;18:289–94.

[30] Wehner A, Hartmann K, Hirschberger J. Associations between proteinuria, systemic hypertension and glomerular filtration rate in dogs with renal and non-renal diseases. Vet Rec 2008;162:141–7.

[31] Mishina M, Watanabe T. Development of hypertension and effects of benazepril hydrochloride in a canine remnant kidney model of chronic renal failure. J Vet Med Sci 2008;70:455–60.

[32] Simpson AC, McCown JL. Systemic hypertension in a dog with a functional thyroid gland adenocarcinoma. J Am Vet Med Assoc 2009;235:1474–9.
[33] Kang MH, Park HM. Hypertension after ingestion of baked garlic *(Allium sativum)* in a dog. J Vet Med Sci 2010;72:515–8.
[34] Bacic A, Kogika MM, Barbaro KC, et al. Evaluation of albuminuria and its relationship with blood pressure in dogs with chronic kidney disease. Vet Clin Pathol 2010;39:203–9.
[35] Chetboul V, Carlos Sampedrano C, Gouni V, et al. Ultrasonographic assessment of regional radial and longitudinal systolic function in healthy awake dogs. J Vet Intern Med 2006;20:885–93.
[36] Moise NS, Dietze AE, Mezza LE, et al. Echocardiography, electrocardiography and radiography in cats with dilatation cardiomyopathy, hypertrophic cardiomyopathy and hyperthyroidism. Am J Vet Res 1986;47:1476–86.
[37] Bond BR, Fox PR, Peterson ME, Skavaril RV. Echocardiographic findings in 103 cats with hyperthyroidism. J Am Vet Med Assoc 1988;192:1546–9.
[38] Weichselbaum RC, Feeney DA, Jessen CR. Relationship between selected echocardiographic variables before and after radioiodine treatment in 91 hyperthyroid cats. Vet Radiol Ultrasound 2005;46:506–13.
[39] Connolly DJ, Guitian J, Boswood A, et al. Serum troponin I levels in hyperthyroid cats before and after treatment with radioactive iodine. J Feline Med Surg 2005;7:289–300.
[40] Hadzović-Dzuvo A, Kucukalić-Selimović E, Nakas-Ićindić E, et al. Echocardiographic evaluation of cardiac function in female patients with thyroid disorders. Bosn J Basic Med Sci 2010;10:112–5.
[41] Rosenthal DS, Braunwald E. Hematological-oncological disorders and heart disease. In: Braunwald E, editor. Heart disease: a textbook of cardiovascular medicine. 4th ed. Philadelphia: WB Saunders; 1992, p. 1742–62.
[42] Al-Saad HI, Bou-Holaigah IH, Khan MN, et al. Left ventricular diastolic dysfunction in congenital chronic anaemias during childhood as determined by comprehensive echocardiographic imaging including acoustic quantification. Eur J Echocardiogr 2002;3:103–10.
[43] Satoh K, Masuda T, Ikeda Y, et al. Hemodynamic changes by recombinant erythropoietin therapy in hemodialyzed patients. Hypertension 1990;15:262–6.
[44] London GM, Pannier B, Guerin AP, et al. Alterations of left ventricular hypertrophy in and survival of patients receiving hemodialysis: follow-up of an interventional study. J Am Soc Nephrol 2001;12:2759–67.
[45] Spotswood TC, Kirberger RM, Koma LMPK, et al. Changes in echocardiographic variables of left ventricular size and function in a model of canine normovolemic anemia. Vet Radiol Ultrasound 2006;47:358–65.

17
Pericardial Diseases

ÉRIC DE MADRON

Pericardium Anatomy and Function, 260
Pericardial Effusions, 260
Constrictive Pericarditis, 268
Congenital Anomalies of the Pericardium, 269

Pericardium Anatomy and Function

Anatomy

The pericardium is composed of two serosal layers surrounding the heart. The fibrous external layer is attached cranially to the adventitia of the ascending aorta, main pulmonary artery, venae cavae, and pulmonary veins. It is attached caudally to the basal part of the diaphragm by the phrenopericardial ligament. The internal layer (epicardium) adheres to the myocardium. Normally, a small space is present between these two layers containing 0.5 to 15 mL of serous fluid. This fluid amount is regulated by osmosis, diffusion, and lymphatic drainage [1].

Function

Although the pericardium is not essential for good cardiac function, it prevents excessive cardiac cavity dilation, maintains the heart in a central position, helps to harmonize the stroke volumes of both ventricles, and protects the heart against infections and adhesions [2,3].

Intrapericardial Pressure and Ventricular Interdependence

The pericardium is not a highly compliant structure. Therefore any increase in intrapericardial liquid or in the volume of the intracardiac structures leads to a rapid rise of the intrapericardial pressure. Thus an acute increase of the right ventricular volume reduces left ventricle compliance [4]. The opposite is observed when cardiac filling is reduced with sodium nitroprusside. This is not the case when cardiac cavity dilation is progressive because the pericardium is able to stretch with time [5].

Echocardiography of the Normal Pericardium

On echocardiographic examination, the two pericardial layers appear as a single very echogenic structure surrounding the external surface of the myocardium. This hyperreflectivity comes from the epicardium. These two pericardial layers seem to be attached to the atrial walls but in reality they are not distinguishable from this very thin wall.

Pericardial Effusions

Pericardial disorders represent 1% of canine cardiopathies [6]. Pericardial effusions represent the most common manifestation of these disorders [6]. As they build up, these effusions lead to intrapericardial pressure elevation and collapse of the cardiac chambers, causing a syndrome called cardiac tamponade. The most common causes in dogs are hemorrhagic pericardial effusion secondary to intrapericardial tumors and idiopathic hemorrhagic pericarditis (Table 17-1) [7-11]. In cats, pericardial effusions are frequently associated with advanced cardiomyopathy. Another cause is feline infectious peritonitis (Table 17-2) [6-12].

Cardiac tumors are discussed in Chapter 18 [7].

TABLE 17-1 Etiology and Prevalence of 42 Cases of Pericardial Effusion in Dogs [7]

Etiology	Total (%)
Neoplasias	56
Right atrium hemangiosarcoma	33
Chemodectoma	12
Metastatic adenocarcinoma	5
Lymphosarcoma	2
Thymoma	2
Not determined	2
Idiopathic (hemorrhagic pericarditis)	19
Cardiopathy	14
Dilated cardiomyopathies	7
Degenerative mitral valve disease	5
Atrial wall tear	2
Miscellaneous	11
Traumatic	5
Infectious (coccidiomycosis)	2
Uremic	2

TABLE 17-2 Etiology and Prevalence of Pericardial Disease in Cats [6,12]

Etiology	Total (%)
Cardiopathy Hypertrophic cardiomyopathy Dilated cardiomyopathy Restrictive cardiomyopathy Mitral valve dysplasia Hyperthyroidism	25% [6]–77.5% [12]
Infectious disease Feline infectious peritonitis Systemic infections	3.4% [12]–28% [6]
Renal failure ± overhydration	3.4% [12]–11% [6]
Coagulopathy	0% [12]–11% [6]
Neoplasia Lymphosarcoma Metastasis	0% [12]–15% [6]
Iatrogenic	0% [12]–3% [6]
Pericardoperitoneal diaphragmatic hernia	0% [6]–0.7% [12]
Miscellaneous	0% [12]–1% [6]

Echocardiographic Characteristics of Pericardial Effusion

TM and 2D Echocardiography

Pericardial Effusion per se

Bidimensional (2D) echocardiography is the most sensitive technique for the detection of pericardial effusion, even subclinical [13,14]. Pericardial effusion appears as an anechoic space between the external pericardial and the epicardial layers (Figure 17-1) [13,14]. The importance of the space depends on the quantity of accumulated fluid. The best view with which to visualize this is the right parasternal long axis view (Video 17-1). In this view, small effusions appear as an anechoic space located between the external pericardial layer and the left ventricular free wall, the maximal accumulation being at the level of the atrioventricular groove (see Figure 17-1). More significant effusions lead to greater separation of the two pericardial layers and extension of the fluid toward the cardiac apex (Figure 17-2).

In the case of significant effusion, pericardial fluid is also visible around the right ventricle. Hemorrhagic effusions are sometimes characterized by the presence of hyperechoic microcavitation.

Pericardial and pleural effusions are easily differentiated using 2D echocardiography. Pericardial effusion narrows toward the atria whereas pleural effusion widens at the heart base (Figure 17-3).

Echocardiographic Signs of Cardiac Tamponade

Cardiac tamponade is the phenomenon that explains all symptoms associated with significant pericardial effusions. Under normal conditions, intrapericardial pressure oscillates between –4 and +4 mm Hg during the respiratory cycle. Right and left ventricular diastolic pressures exceed intrapericardial pressure by several millimeters of mercury [3,8]. The accumulation of pericardial fluid progressively increases the intrapericardial pressure (phase 1) [8]. Once this pressure equals the right ventricular and atrial diastolic pressures, the filling of these chambers becomes impeded

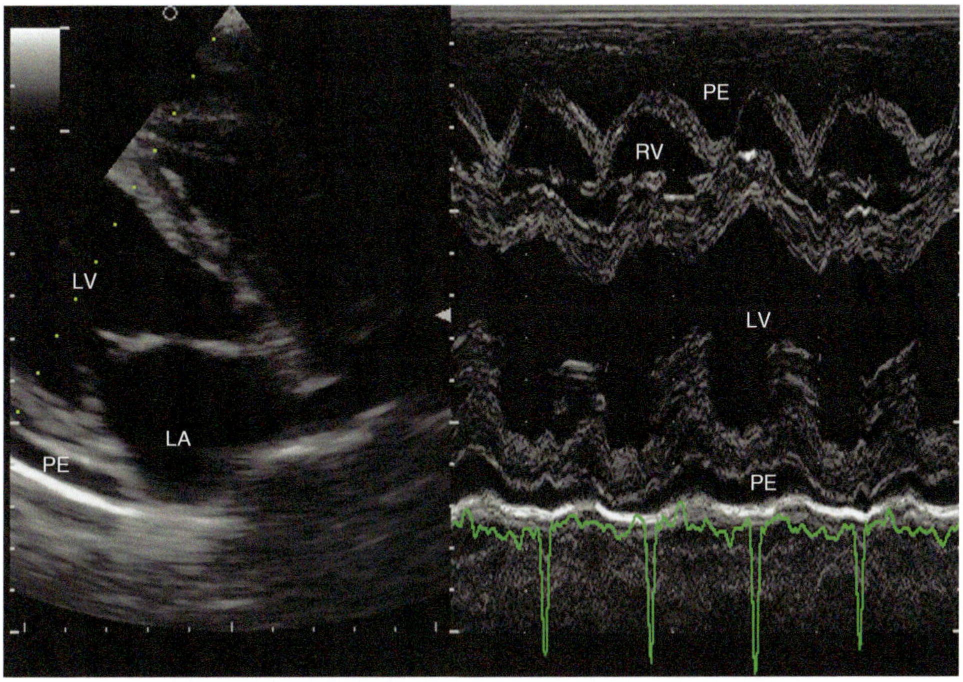

• **Fig. 17-1** Time-motion (TM) echocardiogram (transventricular view) in a dog with pericardial effusion. The effusion (PE) forms an anechoic space between the posterior edge of the left ventricular free wall and the external pericardial membrane as well as between the thoracic wall and the anterior edge of the right ventricular wall. Note the episodic collapse (during expiration) of the right ventricle (RV). *LA,* Left atrium; *LV,* left ventricle. (Photo credit: Éric de Madron.)

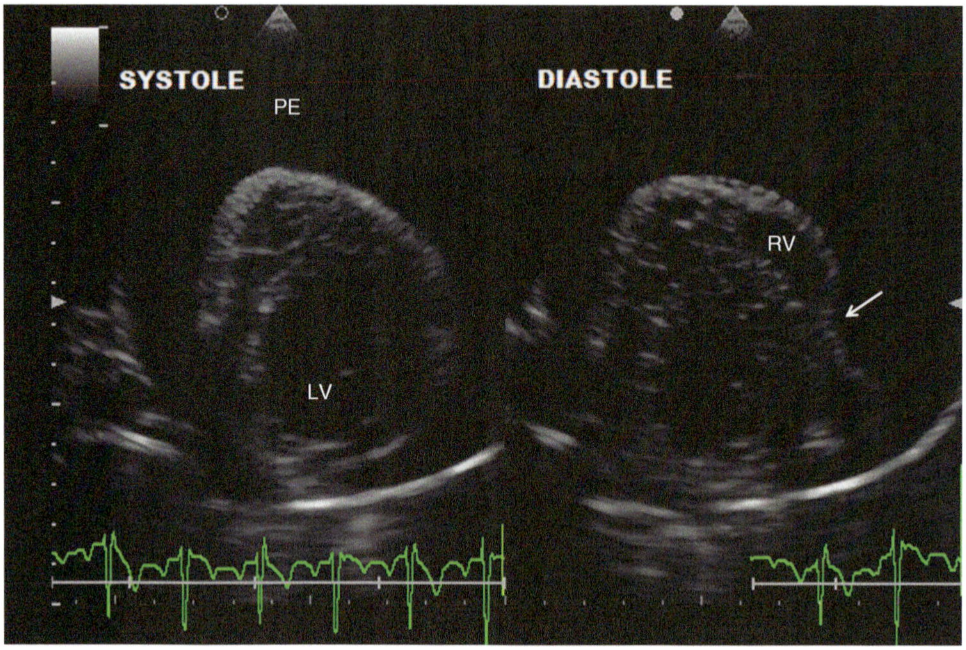

• **Fig. 17-2** Bidimensional (2D) echocardiogram (right parasternal long axis view) of a dog with severe pericardial effusion (PE). Note the right ventricular wall collapse *(arrow)*, visible only in diastole *(right image)*, indicating phase 2 tamponade. *LV,* Left ventricle; *RV,* right ventricle. (Photo credit: Éric de Madron.)

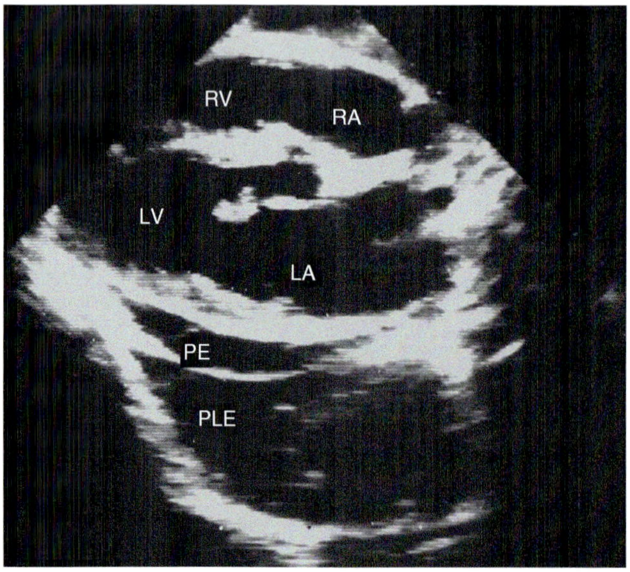

• **Fig. 17-3** Bidimensional (2D) echocardiogram of a dog with pericardial effusion (PE) and pleural effusion (PLE). PE narrows toward the atria, which is not the case for PLE. *LA,* Left atrium; *LV,* left ventricle; *RA,* right atrium; *RV,* right ventricle. (Photo credit: Éric de Madron.)

and the right cavities begin to collapse; this is phase 2 of cardiac tamponade (Figure 17-4; Videos 17-1 and 17-2) [8]. This leads to hypotension, ascites, and/or pleural effusion due to systemic venous hypertension (Figure 17-5).

When the right ventricular diastolic and intrapericardial pressures are equal to the left ventricle diastolic pressure, the cardiac flow decreases significantly, resulting in tachycardia and peripheral vasoconstriction; this is phase 3 of cardiac tamponade (Figure 17-6) [8]. At this time, cardiogenic shock occurs, leading to death [3,8].

In the case of cardiac tamponade, the ventricular stroke volume is strongly influenced by the phase of the respiratory cycle. During inspiration, intrapleural pressure becomes negative and intrapericardial pressure decreases, allowing better filling of the right ventricle. This increase in the right ventricular diastolic dimensions occurs to the detriment of the left ventricle. Therefore the left ventricular stroke volume decreases, resulting in a decrease of the systolic systemic arterial pressure by more than 10 mm Hg. The opposite phenomenon is observed

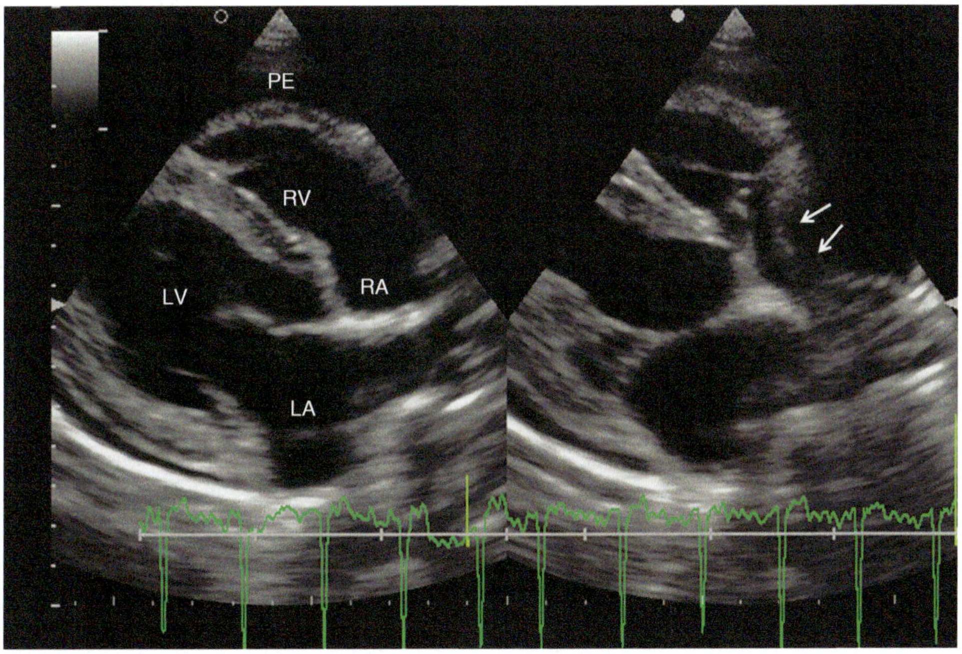

• **Fig. 17-4** Bidimensional (2D) echocardiogram (right parasternal long axis view) in a dog with pericardial effusion (PE). Note the anechoic space surrounding the heart. The right atrium wall (RA) collapses in systole *(arrows, right image)* indicating phase 2 cardiac tamponade. The hyperechoic external pericardial layer is visible at the bottom of the image. *LA,* Left atrium; *LV,* left ventricle; *RV,* right ventricle. (Photo credit: Éric de Madron.)

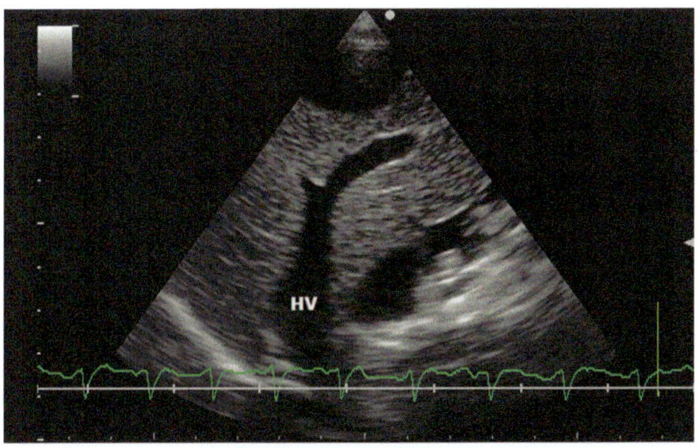

• **Fig. 17-5** Echogram of the liver in a dog presenting with cardiac tamponade. Note the congestion of the hepatic veins (HV) and the presence of ascites. (Photo credit: Éric de Madron.)

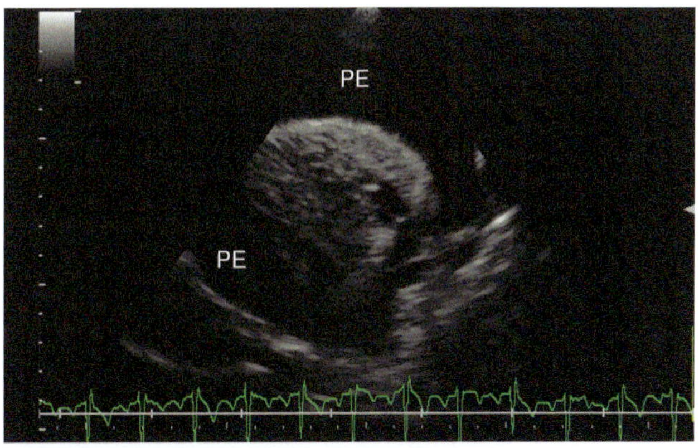

• **Fig. 17-6** Bidimensional (2D) echocardiogram (right parasternal long axis view) in a dog with pericardial effusion (PE). The PE is marked, leading to collapse of the right and left cavities, which become obliterated. This is phase 3 cardiac tamponade, requiring immediate pericardiocentesis. (Photo credit: Éric de Madron.)

during expiration. This exaggerated fluctuation of the pulse amplitude with respiration is referred to as *pulsus paradoxus* (Figure 17-7) [2,3,8].

The development of cardiac tamponade depends on the speed at which pericardial effusion forms. In the case of acute effusion, amounts of pericardial fluid as small as even 50 or 100 mL could be sufficient to create tamponade, because the pericardium has not had time to distend (see Figure 17-4). However, with chronic progressive effusions, the pericardium has time to stretch and large amounts of liquid (500 mL or more) can accumulate until a critical volume is reached. At that point, intrapericardial pressure will start to increase. Pressure increases very rapidly once critical volume is reached [3,8].

Although diagnosis of cardiac tamponade is first and foremost clinical, echocardiography is able to confirm its presence and detect its early signs. Tamponade is initially

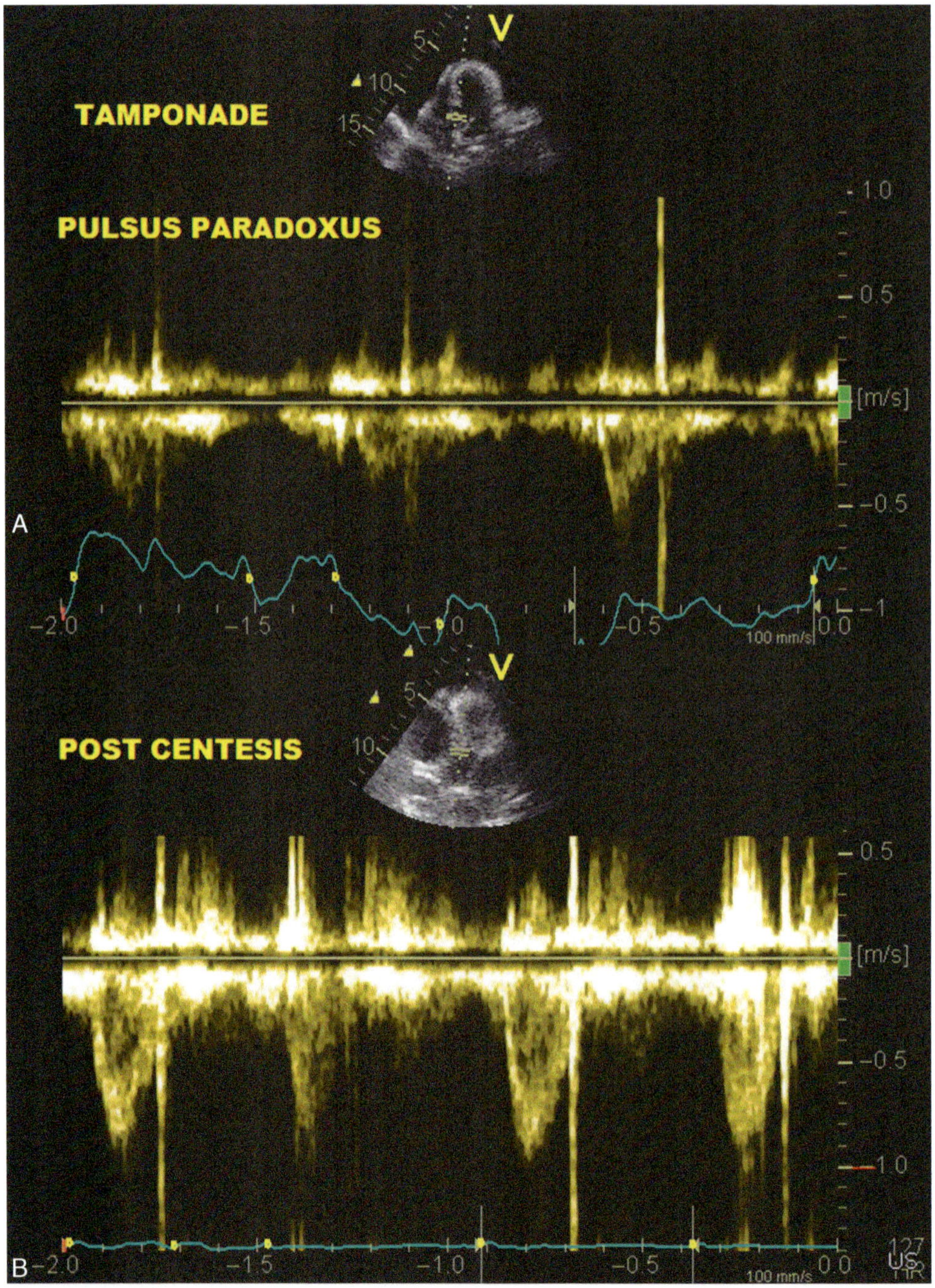

• **Fig. 17-7** A, Spectral Doppler of the aortic flow in a dog with cardiac tamponade. The amplitude of the flow is globally reduced and varies excessively with respiration. B, Spectral Doppler of the aortic flow in the same dog after pericardiocentesis. The amplitude of the flow has increased considerably, with much less variation with respiration. (Photo credit: Éric de Madron.)

characterized by the collapse and inversion of the right atrial free wall, beginning in end-diastole and ending during ventricular systole [2]. Once tamponade is established, the right ventricular wall collapses (see Figure 17-2) [15]. This collapse varies according to the phases of respiration (see Figure 17-1). The time-motion (TM) mode demonstrates that this right ventricular collapse worsens during expiration, when the intrapleural pressures transmitted to the pericardium increase. The opposite is the case for the left ventricle.

In severe cases, the left ventricular internal diameter is reduced (see Figure 17-6). The heart is animated by exaggerated movements and "dances" in the pericardial liquid.

The treatment is pericardiocentesis, which can be echo-guided.

Spectral and Tissue Doppler Echocardiography

In the case of cardiac tamponade, the mean mitral spectral velocity decreases and the mean tricuspid velocity increases significantly during inspiration [16]. Similarly, isovolumic relaxation time (IVRT) increases during inspiration [2] and the mitral flow propagation velocity decreases. These exaggerated respiratory variations disappear following pericardiocentesis (Figures 17-8 and 17-9).

The mitral annulus E′ wave is also reduced during tamponade.

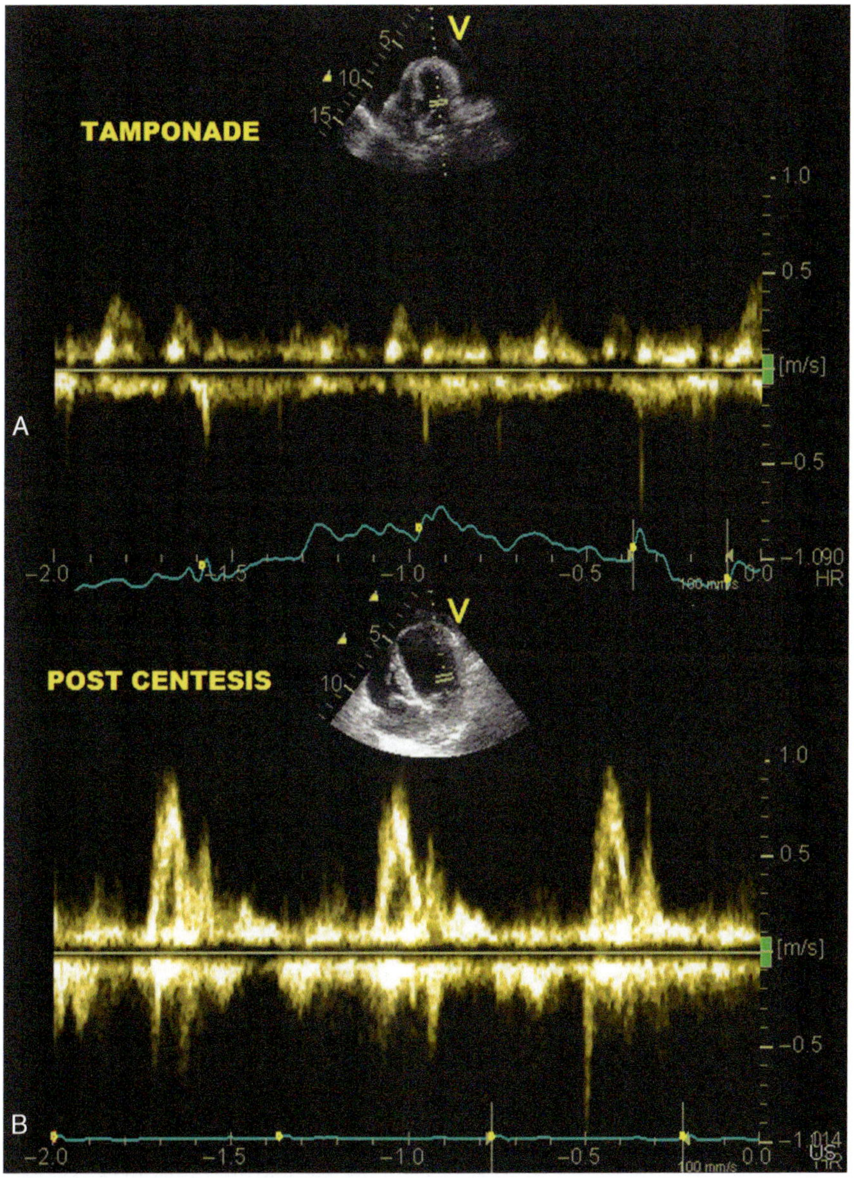

• **Fig. 17-8** A, Spectral Doppler of the mitral flow in a dog with cardiac tamponade. The mitral flow amplitude is globally greatly reduced. B, Spectral Doppler of the mitral flow in the same dog after pericardiocentesis. The amplitude of the flow has increased considerably. (Photo credit: Éric de Madron.)

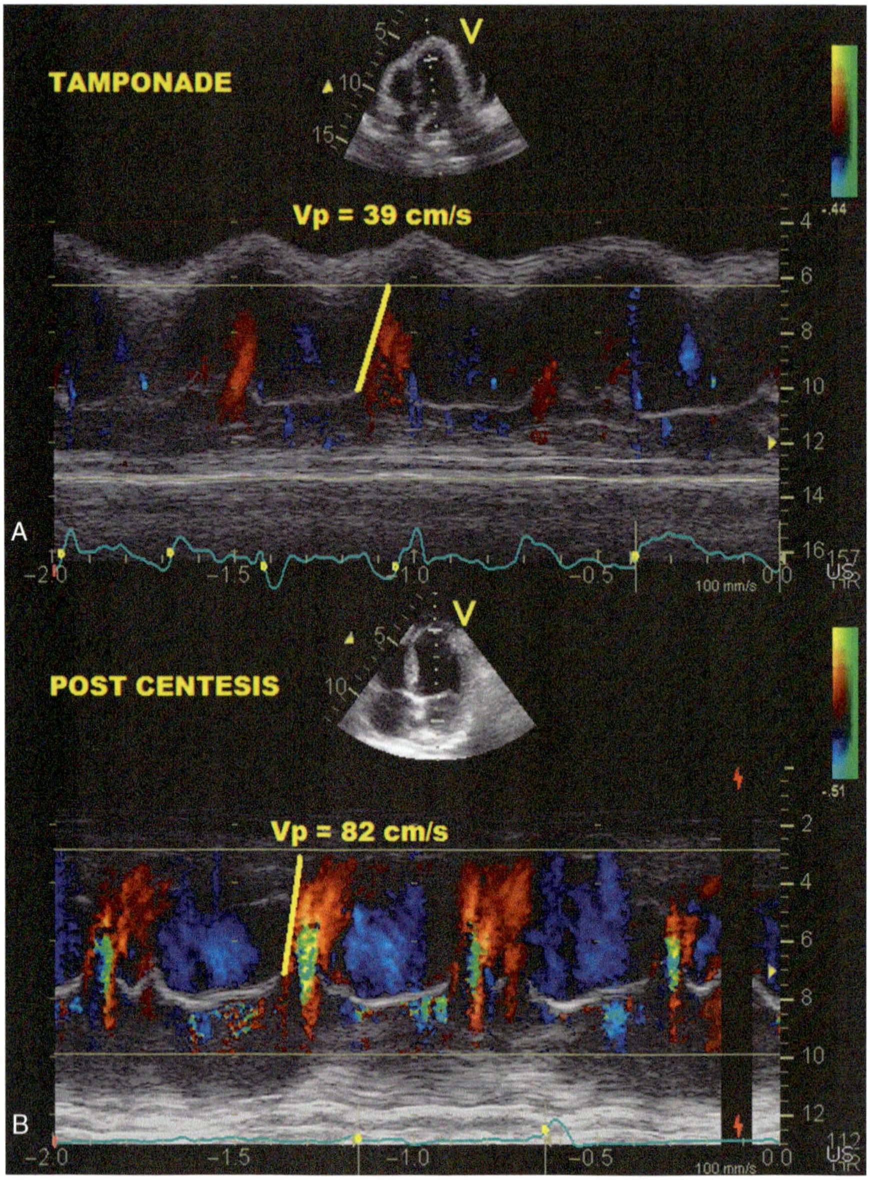

• **Fig. 17-9** A, Color Doppler time-motion (TM) of the mitral flow in a dog with cardiac tamponade. The mitral flow propagation velocity (Vp) is 39 cm/s. B, Color Doppler TM of the mitral flow in a dog following pericardiocentesis. The mitral flow propagation velocity has increased to 82 cm/s. (Photo credit: Éric de Madron.)

Identification of the Pericardial Effusion Etiology

Advanced Valvular or Myocardial Pathologies

Cats with hypertrophic or restrictive cardiomyopathy [12] and dogs with advanced degenerative mitral valve disease with pulmonary arterial hypertension can develop serous pericardial effusion as a result of increased diastolic pressure in the pericardial veins (Figures 17-10 and 17-11, Videos 17-3 and 17-4).

In this context, fluid overload could be a triggering factor [12]. Pericardial effusion is usually minimal to moderate. The underlying cardiomyopathy is easily identifiable. Pericardiocentesis is necessary only if signs of cardiac tamponade, such as right atrial wall collapse, are present.

Left Atrial Wall Rupture

In cases of mitral regurgitation, erosion of the left atrial wall by the regurgitant flow *(jet lesions)* can lead to a rupture of this wall, with acute intrapericardial hemorrhage [17-19]. On echocardiography, marked left atrial dilation can be noted, with a large mitral regurgitation jet documented by color Doppler (Figure 17-12, *B*), pericardial effusion with cardiac tamponade, and in some cases (but not all) an intrapericardial thrombus (Figure 17-12, *A*) [17,18].

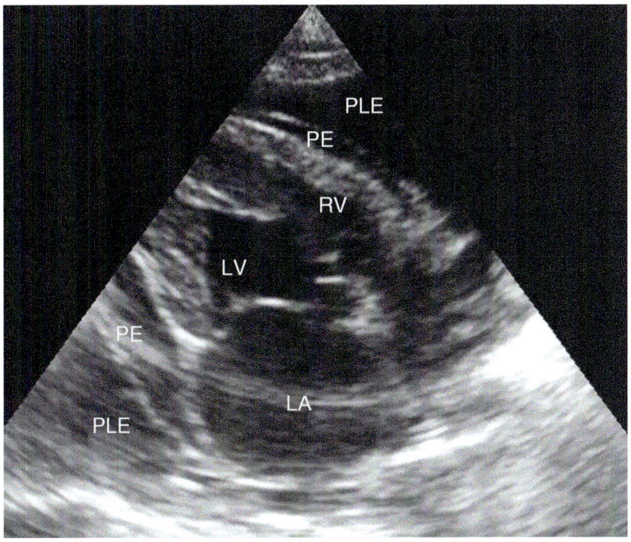

• **Fig. 17-10** Bidimensional (2D) echocardiogram (right parasternal long axis view) in a cat with restrictive cardiomyopathy. A small pericardial effusion (PE) is present along with pleural effusion (PLE). *LA,* Left atrium; *LV,* left ventricle; *RV,* right ventricle. (Photo credit: Éric de Madron.)

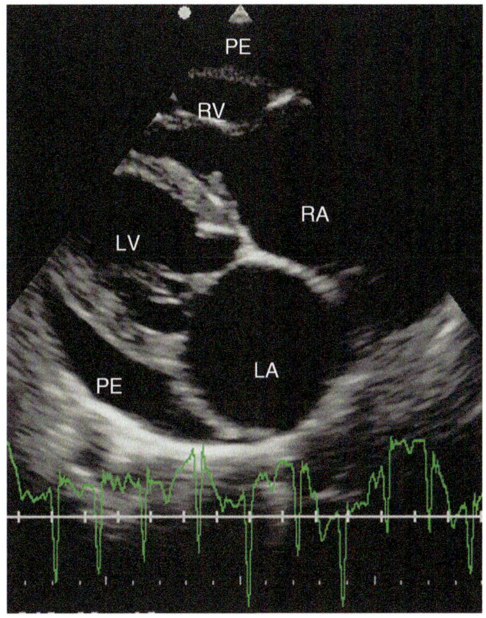

• **Fig. 17-11** Bidimensional (2D) echocardiogram (right parasternal long axis view) in a dog with advanced mitral regurgitation and pulmonary hypertension. Note the presence of pericardial effusion (PE). Both atria and the right ventricle (RV) are dilated. *LA,* Left atrium; *LV,* left ventricle; *RA,* right atrium. (Photo credit: Éric de Madron.)

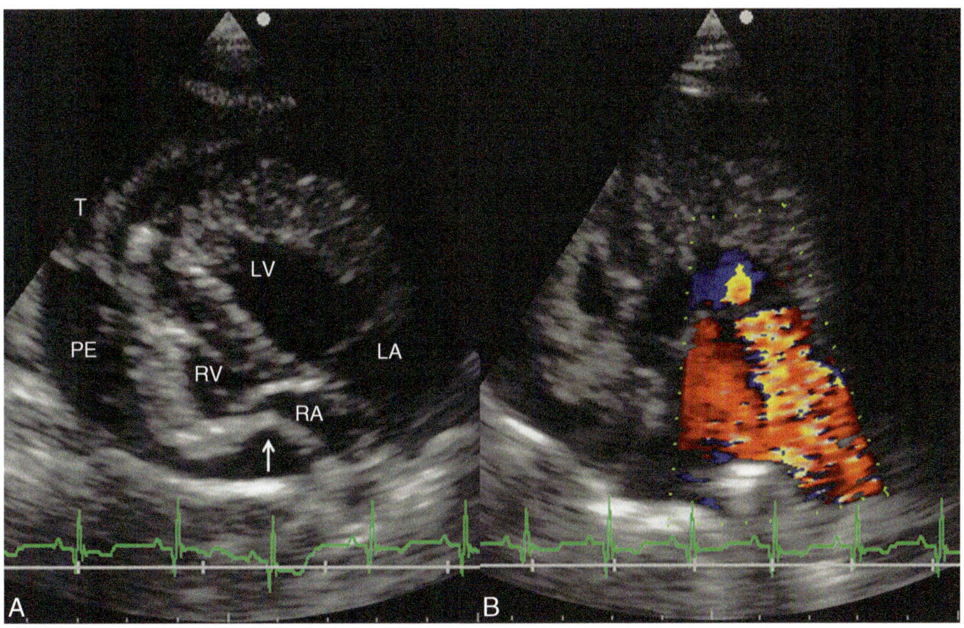

• **Fig. 17-12** A, Bidimensional (2D) echocardiogram (left apical 4 chambers view) in a dog with intrapericardial hemorrhage following left atrium wall rupture. The pericardial effusion (PE), right atrial wall collapse indicating cardiac tamponade, and presence of a thrombus (T) floating along the cardiac apex can be observed. B, 2D echocardiogram with color Doppler (left apical 4 chambers view) in the same dog showing the mitral regurgitation jet. It is large and lateral, which could explain the atrial endocardial erosion that led to the atrial wall tear. *LA,* Left atrium; *LV,* left ventricle; *RA,* right atrium; *RV,* right ventricle. (Photo credit: Éric de Madron.)

Hemorrhagic Pericarditis

Idiopathic hemorrhagic pericarditis mostly occurs in large middle-aged dogs, usually male [7-11]. It is characterized by inflammatory pericardial thickening and fibrosis of the parietal layer (and sometimes of the visceral layer). This inflammation is accompanied by neovascularization with fibrin deposits. This leads to intrapericardial hemorrhages, which can result in cardiac tamponade. The intrapericardial blood is generally noncoagulable due to coagulation factor consumption. As a result, intrapericardial thrombi are generally not visible.

Echocardiographically, idiopathic pericarditis is a diagnosis by exclusion. The absence of cardiac masses or advanced concomitant cardiopathy is the main echocardiographic criterion. The pericardial parietal layer can have a thickened appearance.

Pericardial Effusion Secondary to a Cardiac Tumor

Since 31% to 57% of pericardial effusions are cancerous in origin in dogs [7,9], a rigorous examination of all sites where these tumors tend to be located must be performed. A diagnosis of cardiac tumor is based on the detection of an intrapericardial mass [20]. The sites requiring thorough examination are the right atrial wall, right atrioventricular junction (right and left parasternal long axis views), right atrial appendage (oblique right parasternal short axis view, at the level of the heart base, or right parasternal long axis view: Videos 17-5 and 17-6) [21-23], and ascending aorta (cranial right and left parasternal long axis views) (see Chapter 18) [21-23].

Not all masses detected by echography are necessarily of tumoral origin. As a matter of fact, severe intrapericardial hemorrhages associated with some cases of pericarditis [24], left atrial wall ruptures secondary to degenerative mitral valve disease [17,18], could result in the formation of an intrapericardial thrombi floating in the pericardial sac or adhering to the epicardium (Figure 17-13). Intrapericardial cysts could also resemble hemangiosarcomas [25]. Fibrin masses can also form with irritating effusions, such as cholesterol-rich effusions [26].

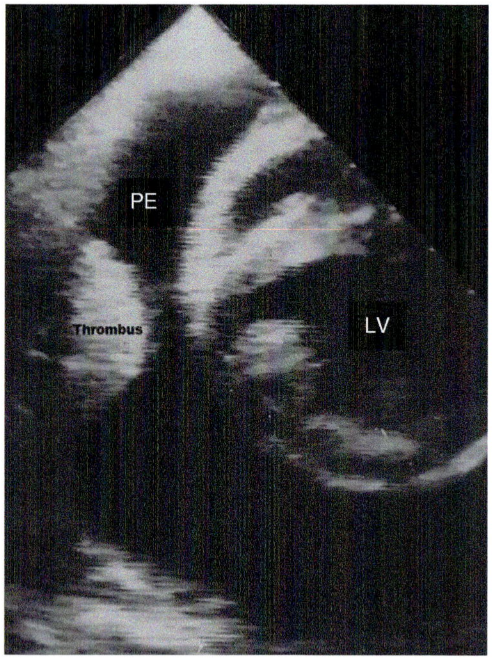

• **Fig. 17-13** Bidimensional (2D) echocardiogram (right parasternal short axis transventricular view) in a cat with severe hemorrhagic pericarditis. Pericardial effusion (PE) is present along with a hyperechoic thrombus adhered to the inner side of the parietal pericardial layer. *LV*, Left ventricle. (Photo credit: Éric de Madron.)

Constrictive Pericarditis

Constrictive pericarditis is characterized by a thickened, fibrous pericardium impeding the end-diastolic filling of the ventricles. Histologically, the disease is characterized by chronic and moderate inflammation of the pericardium. In most cases, only the parietal layer is affected but the visceral layer can also be involved in some cases. A small pericardial effusion is usually associated with this inflammation. Inflammatory granulomas are sometimes present, compressing the ventricular outflow tracts. Constrictive pericarditis is a rare condition in cats and dogs [27-29]. In most cases, the etiology remains unknown [27]. Identified causes include metallic foreign bodies, actinomycosis, and coccidioidomycosis. Idiopathic hemorrhagic pericarditis can sometimes evolve into constrictive pericarditis. Chylothorax is another etiology: the presence of chyle in the pleural space has an irritating effect on the pericardium and can induce constrictive pericarditis [30].

2D and TM Echocardiography

Constrictive pericarditis can be suspected when the combination of thickened pericardium, small pericardial effusion, and signs of cardiac tamponade are present. In the cases of constrictive pericarditis, the respiratory variations of the intrathoracic pressure are not transmitted by the pericardium. Therefore the diastolic right ventricular volume does not vary between inspiration and expiration [3]. Left atrial and ventricular diameters are normal. Sometimes an abnormally rigid left ventricular free wall during diastole can be detected in TM mode [13].

Doppler Echocardiography

Pericardial fibrosis leads to restrictive ventricular diastolic dysfunction. Ventricular filling can take place only in early diastole. As soon as ventricular volume expansion is checked by the inextensible pericardium, filling ceases and atrial and ventricular diastolic pressures equalize. Recordings of the ventricular diastolic pressure are characterized by an initial trough followed by a plateau (square root sign √) [3]. This is different from the type of diastolic dysfunction observed with tamponade, which mostly affects the initial relaxation, especially on inspiration (see above).

An increased mitral E wave with rapid acceleration and a reduced A wave can be observed [2]. Although the rigid pericardium isolates the heart from the respiratory fluctuations of the intrapleural pressure, the latter does affect the pulmonary venous flow. Therefore a significant decrease in the transmitral E wave amplitude and in the aortic and pulmonic systolic velocities can be observed during inspiration [2]. However, the increased left atrial pressure can mask these fluctuations by increasing the E wave amplitude [2].

The increased early diastolic filling is characterized by an increased mitral flow propagation velocity (Vp) measured by color TM mode of the mitral valve [31]. Improved diastolic function could be documented following pericardiectomy [31].

Congenital Anomalies of the Pericardium

Total or Partial Absence of the Pericardium

Total or partial absences of the pericardium are rare. They are mostly discovered at necropsy [8,32]. They are usually asymptomatic. In some cases of partial absence, however, part of the heart (in most cases the appendage) can get caught in the hole and become strangulated. Echocardiography reveals an exaggerated motion of the heart, abnormal septal motion, unusual echocardiographic windows, or a herniated cardiac structure.

Pericardoperitoneal Diaphragmatic Hernia (PPDH)

This is the most frequent congenital anomaly of the pericardium in dogs and cats. It originates either from a fusion defect between the lateral pleuroperitoneal layers and the sternal part of the diaphragm or from an abnormal development of the transverse septum [6,8]. The result is an abnormal communication between the peritoneal and pericardial cavities through which abdominal viscera can move. The degree of the hernia can vary from mild herniation of adipose tissue, without symptoms, to a major organ herniation such as liver, spleen, intestines, or stomach. This hernia can suddenly become accentuated by trauma [33]. PPDH can be associated with other congenital anomalies, such as umbilical hernias and sternal or cardiac anomalies. Echocardiography reveals the presence of portions of hepatic lobes, peritoneal fatty tissue, or intestinal loops within the pericardium [34].

Intrapericardial Cysts

These cysts are rare. They are the result of either incarceration of a portion of omentum in the pericardium associated with PPDH or a congenital anomaly [8, 25]. They are generally attached to the apical part of the pericardial parietal membrane by a fatty pedicle. On the macroscopic level, these cysts resemble in all points encysted hematomas. In a publication describing six cases of intrapericardial cysts [25], the authors report a symptomology similar to that of pericardial effusion.

Echography reveals an intrapericardial cystic mass compressing the cardiac cavities. However, this echographic aspect can be similar to that of a cardiac hemangiosarcoma [25].

REFERENCES

[1] Evans HE, Christensen GC. The heart and arteries. In: Miller's anatomy of the dog. 2nd ed. Philadelphia: WB Saunders; 1979, p. 632–56.

[2] Munt BI, Moss MD, Thompson CR. Pericardial disease. In: Otto CM, editor. The practice of clinical echocardiography. 3rd ed. Philadelphia: WB Saunders; 2007, p. 710–34.

[3] Lorell BH, Braunwald E. Pericardial diseases. In: Braunwald E, editor. Heart diseases: a textbook of cardiovascular medicine. 4th ed. Philadelphia: WB Saunders; 1992, p. 1465–516.

[4] Shirato K, Shabetai R, Bhargava V, et al. Alteration of the left ventricular diastolic pressure-segment length relation produced by the pericardium: effects of cardiac distension and after load reduction in conscious dogs. Circulation 1978;57:1191–8.

[5] Freeman G, Le WM. Pericardial adaptations during chronic cardiac dilation in dogs. Circ Res 1984;54:294–300.

[6] Reed JR. Pericardial diseases. In: Fox PR, editor. Canine and feline cardiology. New York: Churchill Livingstone; 1988, p. 495–518.

[7] Berg RJ, Wingfield W. Pericardial effusion in the dog: a review of 42 cases. J Am Anim Hosp Assoc 1984;20:721–30.

[8] Sisson D, Thomas WP. Pericardial disease and cardiac tumors. In: Fox PR, Sisson D, Moise NS, editors. Textbook of canine and feline cardiology. 2nd ed. Philadelphia: WB Saunders; 1999, p. 679–701.

[9] Stafford Johnson M, Martin M, Binns S, Day MJ. A retrospective study of clinical findings, treatment and outcome in 143 dogs with pericardial effusion. J Small Anim Pract 2004;45:546–52.
[10] Berg RJ, Wingfield WE, Hoopes PJ. Idiopathic hemorrhagic pericardial effusion in eight dogs. J Am Vet Med Assoc 1984;185:988–92.
[11] Gibbs C, Gaskell CJ, Darke PGG. Idiopathic pericardial haemorrhage in dogs: a review of fourteen cases. J Small Anim Pract 1982;23:483–500.
[12] Hall DJ, Shofer F, Meier CK, Sleeper MM. Pericardial effusion in cats: a retrospective study of clinical findings and outcome in 146 cats. J Vet Intern Med 2007;21:1002–7.
[13] Bonagura JD, Pipers FS. Echocardiographic features of pericardial effusion in dogs. J Am Vet Med Assoc 1981;179:49–56.
[14] Weyman AE. Cross-sectional echocardiography. In: Weyman AE, editor. Principles and practice of echocardiography. Philadelphia: Lea and Febiger; 1982, p. 480–92.
[15] Berry CR, Lombard CW, Hager DA, et al. Echocardiographic evaluation of cardiac tamponade in dogs before and after pericardiocentesis: four cases (1984–1986). J Am Vet Med Assoc 1998;192:1597–603.
[16] Pandian N, Wang S, McInerney K, et al. Doppler echocardiography in cardiac tamponade; abnormalities in tricuspid and mitral inflow response to respiration in experimental and clinical tamponade. J Am Coll Cardiol 1985;5:485.
[17] Sadanaga KK, MacDonald MJ, Buchanan JW. Echocardiography and surgery in a dog with left atrial rupture and hemopericardium. J Vet Intern Med 1990;4:216–21.
[18] Reineke EL, Burkett DE, Drobatz KJ. Left atrial rupture in dogs: 14 cases (1990–2005). J Vet Emerg Crit Care 2008;18:158–64.
[19] Buchanan JW, Kelly AM. Endocardial splitting of the left atrium in the dog with hemorrhage and hemopericardium. J Am Vet Radiol Soc 1964;5:28–39.
[20] Thomas WP, Sisson D, Bauer TG. Detection of cardiac masses in dogs by two-dimensional echocardiography. Vet Radiol 1984;25:65–72.
[21] De Madron É. Seven cases of pericardial effusion of cancerous foraging in the dog: clinical, electrocardiographic, radiographic and echocardiographic aspects. Prat Méd Chir Anim Comp 1990;25:59–69.
[22] De Madron É, Helfand SC, Stebbins KE. Use of chemotherapy for treatment of cardiac hemangiosarcoma in a dog. J Am Vet Med Assoc 1987;190:887–91.
[23] Thomas WP, Reed JR, Gomez JA. Diagnostic pneumopericardiography in dogs with spontaneous pericardial effusion. Vet Radiol 1984;25:2–16.
[24] De Madron É, Prymak C, Hendricks J. Idiopathic hemorrhagic pericardial effusion with organized thrombi in a dog. J Am Vet Med Assoc 1987;191:324–6.
[25] Sisson D, Thomas WP, Reed JR, et al. Intrapericardial cysts in the dog. J Vet Intern Med 1993;7:364–9.
[26] Macgregor JM, Rozanski EA, McCarthy RJ, et al. Cholesterol-based pericardial effusion and aortic thromboembolism in a 9-year-old mixed-breed dog with hypothyroidism. J Vet Intern Med 2004;18:354–8.
[27] Thomas WP, Reed JR, Bauer TG, Breznock EM. Constrictive pericardial disease in the dog. J Am Vet Med Assoc 1984;184:546–53.
[28] Bunch SE, Bolton GR, Hornbuckle WE. Pericardial effusion with restrictive pericarditis associated with congestive cardiomyopathy in a cat. J Am Anim Hosp Assoc 1981;17:739–45.
[29] Schwartz A, Wilson GP, Hamlin R, et al. Constrictive pericarditis in two dogs. J Am Vet Med Assoc 1971;159:763–80.
[30] Fossum TW, Mertens MM, Miller MW, et al. Thoracic duct ligation and pericardectomy for treatment of idiopathic chylothorax. J Vet Intern Med 2004;18:307–10.
[31] Woolley RM, Devine CB, French AT. Left ventricular flow propagation using color M-mode echocardiography in the diagnosis of effusive-constrictive pericardial disease. Vet Radiol Ultrasound 2006;47:366–9.
[32] Van der Gaag I, Van der Luer RJT. Eight cases of pericardial defects in the dog. Vet Pathol 1977;14:14–8.
[33] Evans SM, Biery DN. Congenital peritoneopericardial diaphragmatic hernia in the dog and cat; a literature review and 17 additional case histories. Vet Radiol 1980;21:108–16.
[34] Hay WH, Woodfield JA, Moon MA. Clinical, echocardiographic and radiographic findings of peritoneopericardial diaphragmatic hernia in two dogs and a cat. J Am Vet Med Assoc 1989;195:1245–8.

18 Cardiac Tumors

CLAUDIO BUSSADORI

Types of Tumors and Prevalence, 272

Goals of Echocardiography in Assessing Cardiac Tumors, 272

Specific Echocardiographic Presentation, 273

Types of Tumors and Prevalence

Cardiac tumors in animals are rare; the reported prevalence is 0.12% [1] to 0.19% [2] in dogs and 0.03% [1] in cats. They can be classified according to their origin (primary, secondary), their histologic characteristics (benign, malignant), or even their macroscopic appearance (dimension, form, location, mobility, attachment site).

In dogs, primary canine cardiac tumors mainly occur in large breeds [2], in middle-aged animals (with the exceptions of lymphomas, which appear more frequently in dogs from 7 to 15 years old) [3], and without obvious sex predisposition [2]. However, neutering seems to increase the risk of cardiac tumors in both sexes. In dogs, the most common primary cardiac tumors are right atrium hemangiosarcomas [3,4] and chemodectomas [5]. The frequency of hemangiosarcomas is almost 10 times that of chemodectomas [5]. Less common heart tumors include granular cell tumors [6], chondrosarcomas [7], osteosarcomas [8], fibromas [9], fibrosarcomas [10,11], cardiac lipomas [12], malignant mesenchymal tumors [13], lymphomas [14,15], rhabdomyosarcomas [16,17], neurofibromas [18], angiolipomas [19], myxomas [20-23], right atrial myxosarcomas [21,24,25], ectopic thyroid carcinomas [26-28], and pericardial mesothelioma (Figure 18-1) [1,5].

In cats, primary cardiac tumors reported are hemangiosarcomas [18,19,29], chemodectomas [18], angiolipomas [18], and ossifying endocardial myxoma of the right atrium [18,30].

Most of the literature refers to pathologic findings at necropsy [31]. According to these data, cardiac neoplasias seem to be very infrequent [32], with a very large variety of histologic types. However, the diagnosis of cardiac tumors is not that infrequent in daily echocardiography practice. In our institution, the prevalence of cardiac tumors in 5832 dogs referred for cardiac disease was 2.57%. We have also noticed, in contrast to the literature, that males are affected more frequently than females (74% males, 26% females). In our experience, heart base tumors (HBTs) were the most frequent, representing 38% of cardiac neoplasias. Histologically, almost all of these HBTs were confirmed to be chemodectoma. The second most commonly encountered tumors were hemangiosarcomas (HSAs, 31%), followed by heart wall neoplasias (9%), mesotheliomas (1%), lymphomas (1%), and ectopic thyroid tumors (1%). Nine percent of intracardiac neoplasias could not be classified because either histology was not available or their echocardiographic texture or location did not allow speculation regarding their nature.

Most of the affected dogs were mixed breed (23%), Boxers (15%), German Shepherds (13%), Yorkshire Terriers (5%), Labrador Retrievers (5%), English Bulldogs (4%), and others.

A breed predisposition has been reported for some of these tumors. Chemodectomas are more frequently found in brachycephalic breeds (Boxer, English Bulldog, Boston Terrier), while HSA is more prevalent in German Shepherds, American Cocker Spaniels, English Setters, Golden Retrievers, Labrador Retrievers, and Miniature Poodles [4,5].

Goals of Echocardiography in Assessing Cardiac Tumors

Nowadays, with the wide availability of echocardiography, the diagnosis of cardiac tumors is becoming more frequent [33]. Harmonic imaging and transesophageal echocardiography (TEE) have improved identification of cardiac tumors. In most cases, location, extension, and echocardiographic texture of these lesions are

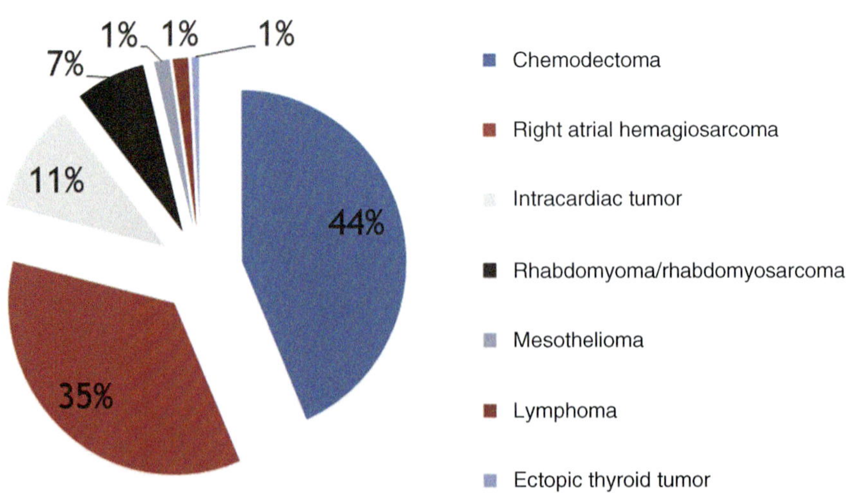

• **Fig. 18-1** Prevalence of cardiac tumors in dogs. (Claudio Bussadori, personal observations, 1997–2010.)

sufficient to identify the tumor type. Echocardiography is also useful to define the extension of the mass and the infiltration of myocardial tissue, to determine whether the mass is unifocal or multifocal, and to document the hemodynamic consequences of tumors invading cardiac cavities. Most intracavitary cardiac tumors can be visualized easily via transthoracic echocardiography (TTE), while TEE should be used to identify small masses if the acoustic window is inadequate and to study the relation of the tumor to other structures of the base of the heart. Contrast perfusion imaging may also help to differentiate a cardiac mass from adjacent myocardium: malignant and vascular tumors are hyperenhanced whereas stromal tumors and thrombi are hypoenhanced [34].

The hemodynamic consequences of cardiac tumors depend on their size and location [35,36]. Most intracardiac tumors are located in the right ventricle and may lead to an obstructive syndrome [36], resulting in weakness, syncope, or right heart failure [37]. Intramural cardiac tumors can trigger arrhythmias [17]. The most common symptoms reported in dogs with cardiac neoplasia (syncope, collapse, and exercise intolerance) are primarily related to cardiac tamponade [38]. In our experience, cardiac masses are associated with pericardial effusion (PE) in 54% of dogs. Eighty-nine percent of cardiac masses associated with PE were HSAs. Less frequently, large heart base tumors can also cause PE [39]. Right heart failure may sometimes result from vena cava compression [39].

Specific Echocardiographic Presentation

Hemangiosarcoma

Location

The most frequent sites for primary cardiac HSA are the right atrium and atrial appendage. Metastatic HSA could be identified as multifocal myocardial infiltrates. Primary or metastatic HSA appears as a heterogeneous mass with small hypoechoic cavities. Right atrial appendage HSA may grow into the pericardial space, creating a mass extending ventrally, and cranial to the right ventricular outflow tract. This mass may also extend dorsally, in contact with the aortic root and the main pulmonary artery. The external part of HSA facing the pericardial cavity frequently presents a floppy part, mostly composed of fibrin overlying the bleeding area. The mass eventually may disrupt the right atrial appendage trabeculae and invade part of the right atrial cavity and, albeit rarely, the tricuspid leaflets, the atrioventricular junction, and the coronary sinus. Some HSAs will expand into the right atrial chamber as a thin and pedunculated structure moving with the blood flow. Identification of this type of cardiac neoplasia requires careful bidimensional (2D) echocardiographic examination. Accurate recognition of the extent of myocardial infiltration is necessary to determine the feasibility of surgery and the overall prognosis. TEE is the gold-standard technique to define the extension of many cardiac tumors but in almost all cases of right atrial or right atrial appendage HSA, the quality of the images obtained by TTE is sufficient to assess the possibility of a surgical ablation of the atrial appendage [40]. It is better to perform this evaluation before draining any PE [38].

Views

The initial view used to look for a right atrial HSA is the right parasternal long axis view. From this view, the probe should be moved laterally and slightly counterclockwise in order to obtain an off-axis view where the right atrial appendage, the right atrium, part of the tricuspid valve, and both venae cavae are all visualized in the same plane. The probe then must be slightly inclined dorsally and cranially in order to visualize the typical mottled texture of the HSA and its degree of infiltration of the atrial and, in some cases, ventricular myocardium (Figures 18-2 and 18-3; Videos 18-1 to 18-4).

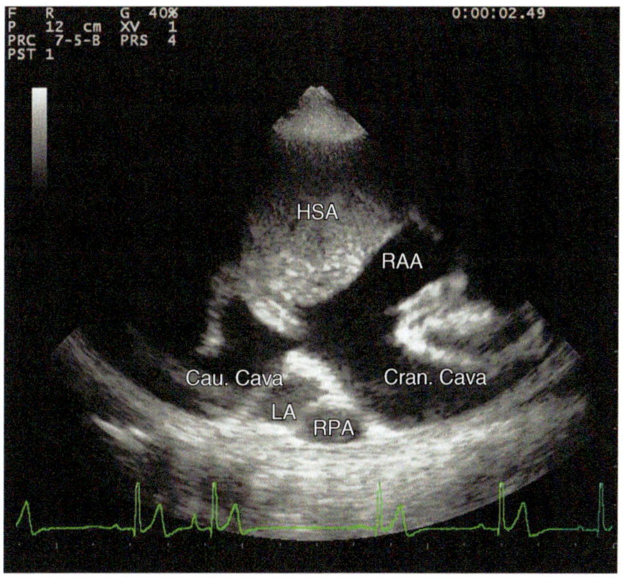

• **Fig. 18-2** Bidimensional (2D) echocardiogram (left cranial parasternal view optimized to visualize the junction of the two venae cavae in the right atrium) in a dog with hemangiosarcoma. The caudal (Cau. Cava) and cranial (Cran. Cava) venae cavae are visible, converging toward the right atrial cavity. Part of the left atrium (LA) and of the right pulmonary artery (RPA) are visible, medially. A heterogenic mass (HSA) originating from the right atrial appendage wall is invading the atrial appendage cavity (RAA) as well as part of the right atrial cavity. (Photo credit: Claudio Bussadori.)

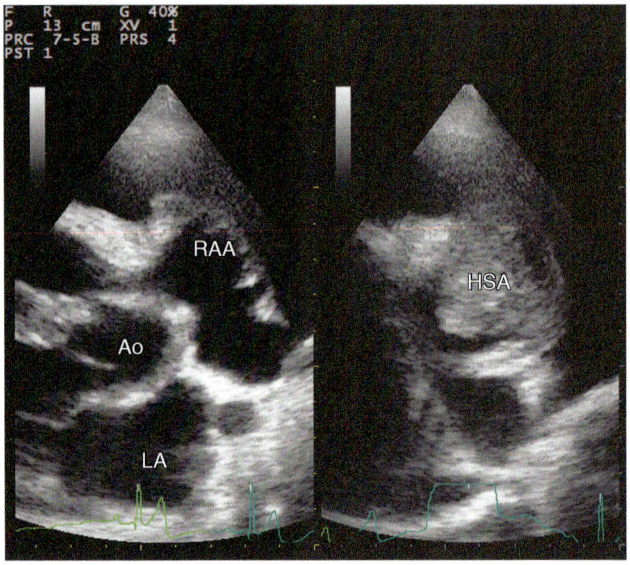

• **Fig. 18-3** Bidimensional (2D) echocardiogram (right parasternal long axis 5 chambers view) in a dog with hemangiosarcoma invading the right atrial lateral wall. These are two consecutive images. *Left,* A dorsomedial section of the right atrial appendage wall (RAA) is visible, apparently normal. *Right,* A more ventrolateral section of the right atrium wall is visible. A mass (HSA) is invading the neighboring structures, most notably the venae cavae and the atrioventricular junction. *Ao,* Aorta; *LA,* left atrium. (Photo credit: Claudio Bussadori.)

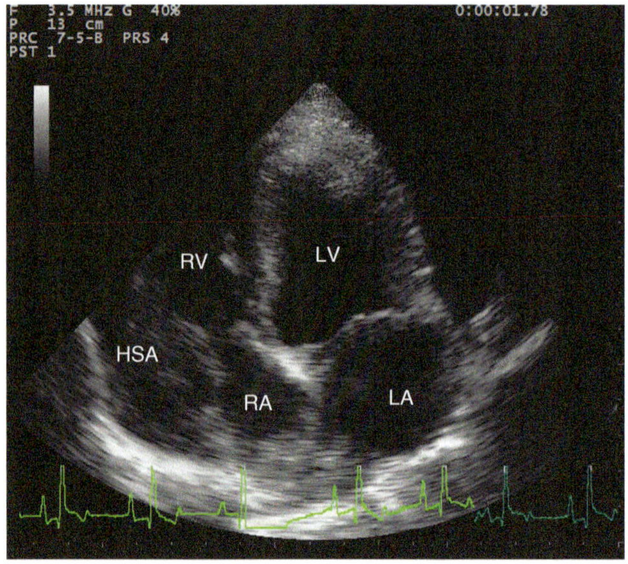

• **Fig. 18-4** Bidimensional (2D) echocardiogram (left apical 4 chambers view) in a dog with hemangiosarcoma invading the right atrial lateral wall. This view is slightly oblique in order to evaluate the relationship between the mass (HSA) and the atrioventricular junction. The echogenicity of the tumor is complex: hyperechoic with hypoechoic or anechoic zones. *LA,* Left atrium; *LV,* left ventricle; *RA,* right atrium; *RV,* right ventricle. (Photo credit: Claudio Bussadori.)

Evaluation of Myocardial Infiltration

Myocardial infiltration mostly occurs in the right atrial wall, but may also involve the right ventricular free wall. It may manifest as a heterogeneity of the atrial wall texture or sometimes just as an increased echogenicity. It is important to evaluate not only the degree of infiltration but also its potential extension into the venae cavae and the lateral atrioventricular junction in order to accurately determine the possibility of surgical intervention. This evaluation can be performed using the views mentioned above or even using a classical left apical 4 chambers view (Figure 18-4; see Videos 18-3 and 18-4).

Neoplastic Thrombosis

The presence of HSA can be favorable to thrombus formation. Therefore it is not uncommon to observe thrombi associated with HSA in the right atrium or right atrial appendage. This "neoplastic" thrombosis may lead to overestimation of tumor dimension. Differentiating thrombus from HSA is discussed below.

Before performing pericardiocentesis, it is extremely important to consider the benefit/risks ratio. Serious complications due to acute bleeding may occur once the fluid compressing the heart is drained. Unfortunately, there are no echocardiographic signs that can accurately predict this complication. However, the presence of anechoic irregularities on the external border of the mass, together with smoke and recent worsening of the symptoms, could be a predictor of acute relapse of tamponade after pericardiocentesis [15,38].

Differential Diagnosis

Organized Thrombus

Echocardiography is extremely valuable to distinguish HSA from an atrial thrombus or pericardial cyst. Typically, HSA disrupts the myocardial tissue and appears as a heterogeneous mass with small hypoechoic cavities. In contrast, an organized thrombus has a more regular shape with rounded and smooth borders and a center less echoic than its periphery (Figures 18-5 and 18-6).

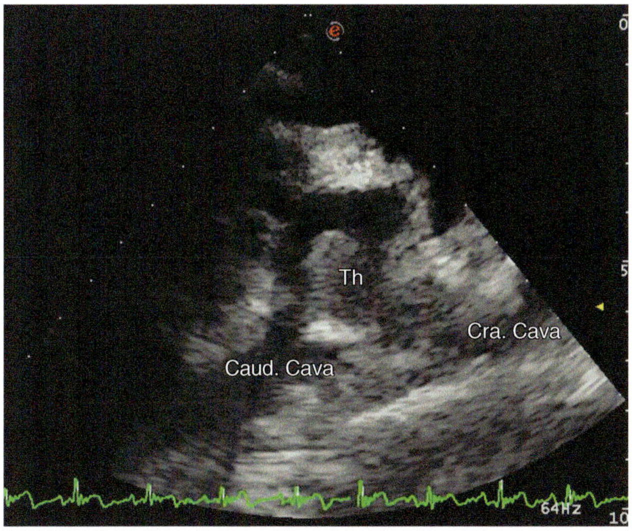

• **Fig. 18-5** Bidimensional (2D) echocardiogram (left cranial parasternal view optimized to visualize the junction of the venae cavae in the right atrium) in a dog with a recent thrombus (Th) originating from the cranial vena cava (Cra. Cava) and invading the right atrial cavity. *Caud. Cava,* Caudal vena cava. (Photo credit: Claudio Bussadori.)

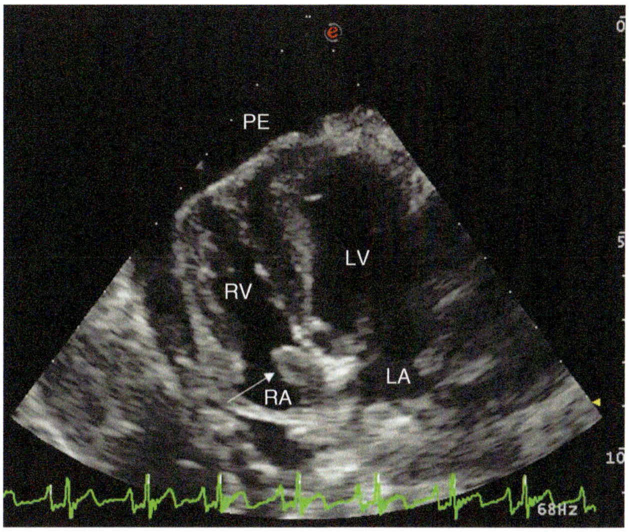

• **Fig. 18-6** Bidimensional (2D) echocardiogram (left apical 4 chambers view) in a dog with an organized thrombus *(arrow)* attached to the interatrial septum. Note the hypoechoic thrombus center. *LA,* Left atrium; *LV,* left ventricle; *PE,* pericardial effusion; *RA,* right atrium; *RV,* right ventricle. (Photo credit: Claudio Bussadori.)

Pericardial Cysts

Differentiating HSA from others cardiac diseases such as cardiac hemangioma or pericardial cyst has important prognostic and treatment implications [40]. Pericardial cysts result from defective embryologic development of the pericardium. Bidimensional echocardiographic examination reveals a round unilocular or multilocular hypoechoic or anechoic structure, with a well-defined capsule separating it from other cardiac structures. Pericardial cysts are usually located in the left or right costophrenic angles. In cats, the presence of a pericardial cyst compressing the right ventricle may lead to cardiac tamponade [41]. Some authors suggest that intrapericardial cysts in dogs can develop in association with, and possibly as a result of, congenital herniation and entrapment of omentum or a portion of the falciform ligament in the pericardial sac [42].

Heart Base Tumors

Heart base tumors (HBTs) are due to pathologic growth of masses originating from different tissues that are either normally or abnormally present in this anatomic region. The most frequent HBTs are chemodectomas. Other tumors in this area, less frequently encountered, are ectopic thyroid carcinomas [27] and lymphomas [5,14].

There are differences of echogenicity (homogenous or heterogenous tissue, degree of echogenicity), site of origin, dimensions, shape, location, contour (smooth or irregular), mobility, infiltration, single or multiple lesions, unilocular or multilocular structures, and growth type, which can help to differentiate these types of tumors. However, cytologic or histologic examination of the tumor is necessary to obtain a definitive diagnosis [43]. The different presentations of HBTs are summarized in Table 18-1.

Chemodectomas

Chemodectomas are primary cardiac tumors of chemoreceptor tissue, located around the carotid bifurcation, the aortic root, the main pulmonary arteries, and the jugular veins. Chemodectomas appear as soft nodular, encapsulated, homogeneous masses mainly growing at the base of the heart. These tumors are usually solitary but can sometimes, albeit rarely, be multiple. They can be associated with other endocrine tumors. They typically are locally invasive but can sometimes metastasize to other parenchymas. In many cases, chemodectomas are incidental findings discovered during a routine echocardiogram, because these tumors can remain asymptomatic for a long time until PE or signs related to compression of a structure at the base of the heart occur.

Location

Chemodectomas extend caudally toward the left atrium, laterally and to the right toward the right atrium and the venae cavae, and cranially around the pulmonary artery. Sometimes they encircle the pulmonary artery bifurcation.

Views

The extension of the tumor toward the left atrium can be studied from the right parasternal long axis (Figure 18-7; Video 18-5) and short axis (Figure 18-8; Video 18-6) views, as well as from the left cranial parasternal long axis view of the ascending aorta (Figure 18-9). The left apical 4 chambers view allows the evaluation of left atrial invasion as well as potential compression of the pulmonary veins (Figure 18-10; Video 18-7).

TABLE 18-1 Main Echographic Characteristics of Tumors in the Base of the Heart in Dogs

Characteristics	Chemodectoma	Ectopic Thyroid Tumors	Lymphoma
Site of origin	Base of the heart between the aortic root and the pulmonary artery	Base of the heart, cranial mediastinum	Pulmonary hilus
Extension	Dorsally, encircling the pulmonary arteries Ventrally, compressing the atria	Mediastinum, surrounding the mediastinal vessels	
Dimension	Variable (2 to 15 cm)	Frequently very large	Variable
Echogenicity	Homogeneous, hyperechoic	Homogeneous, hyperechoic	Homogeneous, hyperechoic
Aspect of the contours	Smooth	Smooth	Smooth
Mobility	None	None	None
Infiltration	Extremely rare	None	None
Single or multifocal mass	Single mass	Single mass	Single or multifocal mass
Growth speed	Very slow	Slow	Rapid

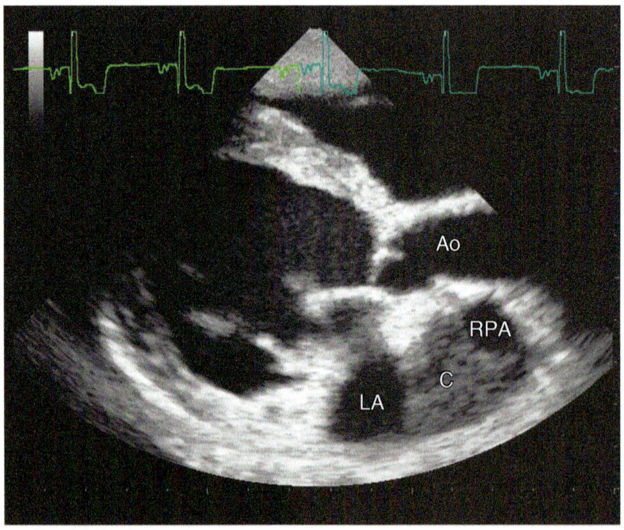

• **Fig. 18-7** Bidimensional (2D) echocardiogram (right parasternal long axis view) in a dog with a chemodectoma. One section of the chemodectoma (C) is visible, medial to the aortic root (Ao) and dorsal to the left atrium (LA). A transverse section of the right pulmonary artery (RPA) is visible, partially compressed by the tumor, between the aortic root and the chemodectoma. (Photo credit: Claudio Bussadori.)

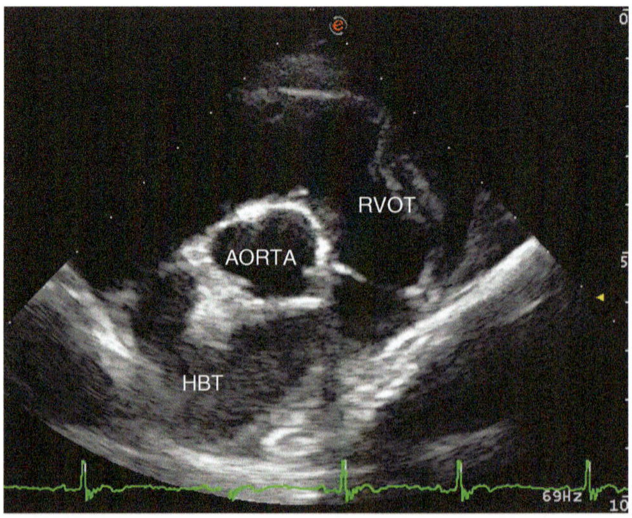

• **Fig. 18-8** Bidimensional (2D) echocardiogram (right parasternal short axis view of the base of the heart) in a dog with a heart base tumor. This view shows the extension of the mass (HBT) in the left atrium and pulmonary artery. Note also the protrusion in the right ventricle outflow tract (RVOT), due to the cranial extension of the mass, compressing this region of the heart. (Photo credit: Claudio Bussadori.)

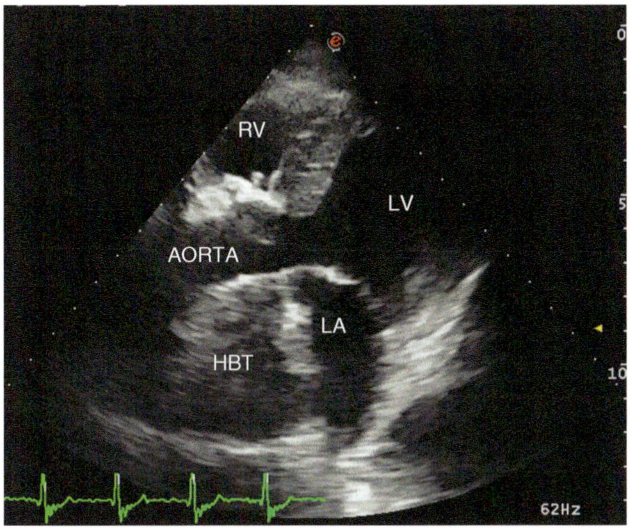

• **Fig. 18-9** Bidimensional (2D) echocardiogram (left cranial parasternal long axis view of the ascending aorta) in a dog with a chemodectoma (HBT), compressing the left atrium (LA). *LV,* Left ventricle; *RV,* right ventricle. (Photo credit: Claudio Bussadori.)

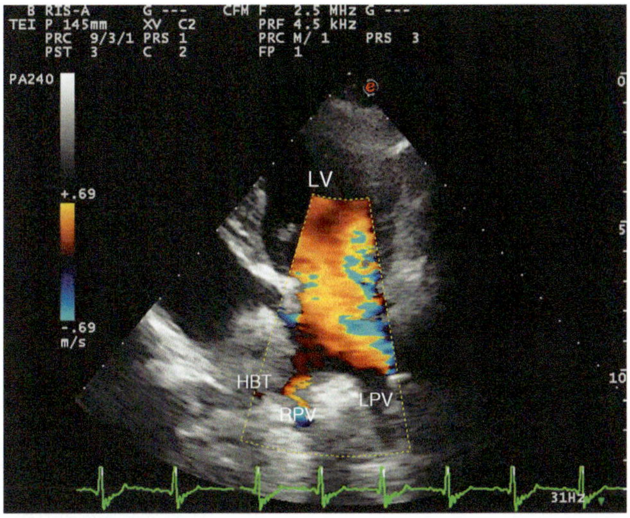

• **Fig. 18-10** Bidimensional (2D) echocardiogram in color Doppler mode (oblique left apical 4 chambers view) in a dog with a heart base tumor. A large mass (HBT) is visible, compressing both atria and obstructing the right pulmonary vein (RPV). *LPV,* Left pulmonary vein; *LV,* left ventricle. (Photo credit: Claudio Bussadori.)

The right and left parasternal short axis views are the best to evaluate the posterior contours and dimensions of the mass. The left cranial parasternal view optimized for the visualization of the pulmonary arteries bifurcation allows the study of the relationship between the mass and the pulmonary arteries (Figure 18-11).

Chemodectomas originating from chemoreceptor cells that migrated during fetal life may grow in unusual locations—that is, in the fold between the interatrial septum primum and secundum, leading to invasion of both atrial cavities (Figure 18-12).

Ectopic Thyroid Tumors

Tumors originating from thyroid cells could appear in various sites—in the neck, the cranial mediastinum, and the base of the heart—depending on the embryologic distribution of these cells [26]. Echocardiography can be helpful to evaluate ectopic thyroid tumors located at the heart base. Small ectopic thyroid tumors are usually located in the same position as small chemodectomas, between the

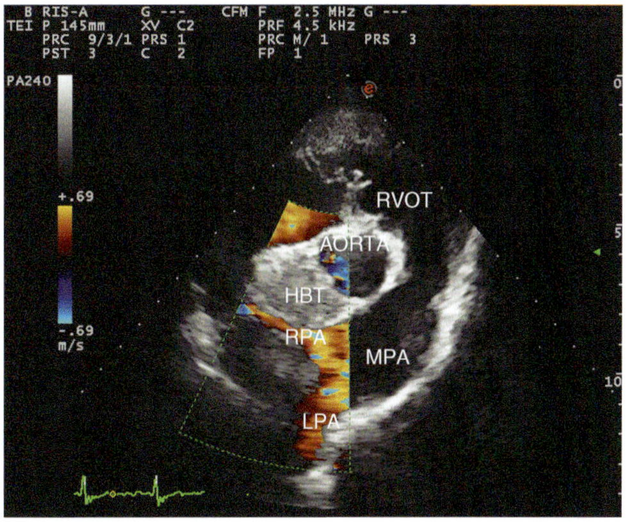

• **Fig. 18-11** Bidimensional (2D) echocardiogram in color Doppler mode (right parasternal short axis view at the base of the heart) in a dog with a heart base tumor. The degree of the severity of the pulmonary artery compression can be appreciated in this view: the right pulmonary artery (RPA) is strangled by the mass (HBT). The left pulmonary artery (LPA) is only partially compressed. *MPA,* Main pulmonary artery; *RVOT,* right ventricular outflow tract. (Photo credit: Claudio Bussadori.)

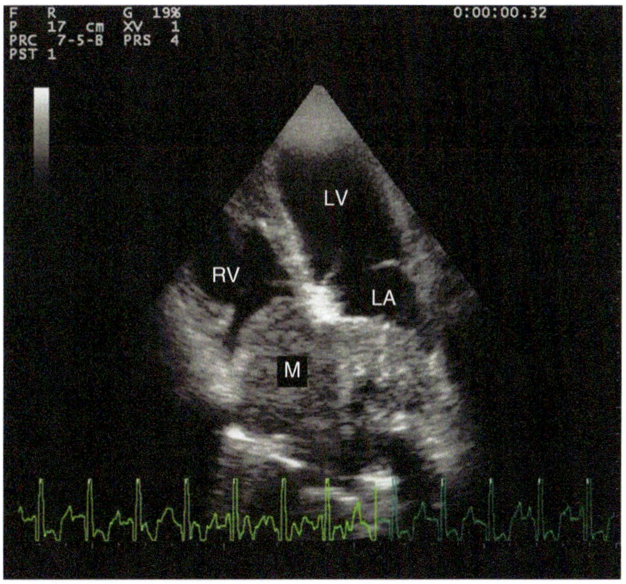

• **Fig. 18-12** Bidimensional (2D) echocardiogram (oblique left apical 4 chambers view) in a dog with a heart base tumor. A large mass (M), originating from the interatrial septum, is invading both atria. On this view, the mass seems to completely obliterate the right atrial cavity. *LA,* Left atrium; *LV,* left ventricle; *RV,* right ventricle. (Photo credit: Claudio Bussadori.)

aorta and the main pulmonary artery. At that stage, the two types of tumors share echocardiographic characteristics and cannot be differentiated. However, the growth pattern of ectopic thyroid tumors differs from that of chemodectomas: ectopic thyroid tumors tend to invade the dorsocranial mediastinum parallel to the ascending aorta, cranial mediastinal arteries, and cranial vena cava instead of wrapping around the main pulmonary artery and the pulmonary bifurcation. TTE and TEE are recommended to assess the presence of mediastinal vessels within the mass, in order to guide the surgical approach (Figure 18-13).

Lymphomas

Lymphomas involving lymph nodes located at the pulmonary hilus may result in a heart base mass, creating atrial compression and pericardial effusion [15]. Lymphomas differ from other heart base tumors in that they initially tend to be located dorsal to the left atrium. They then may expand either dorsally toward the carina or ventrally, compressing the left atrium and other cardiac structures. Compression of the right atrium and the venae cavae, as well as involvement of the aortic root and main pulmonary artery, are rare with lymphomas.

Intracardiac Tumors

Primary intracardiac tumors arise from the myocardial wall. Differentiating intracardiac thrombus from tumor using echocardiography can sometimes be challenging. In the dog, intracardiac thrombi are mostly observed in the context of a coagulation disorder. They are usually located in low blood flow areas: the right atrium or the main pulmonary artery. In most cases, it is possible to identify a thin anechoic border between the endocardium and the thrombus, even when the thrombus is strongly attached to the endocardium (Figures 18-14 and 18-15).

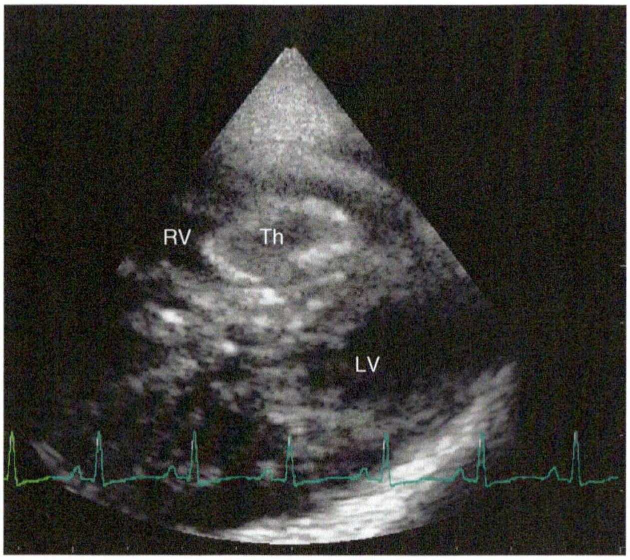

• **Fig. 18-14** Bidimensional (2D) echocardiogram (oblique left apical short axis view of the right and left ventricles) in a dog with an organized thrombus (Th) inside the right ventricular cavity. Note the hyperechoic borders of the thrombus and the distinct anechoic space between the thrombus and endocardium. *LV,* Left ventricle; *RV,* right ventricle. (Photo credit: Claudio Bussadori.)

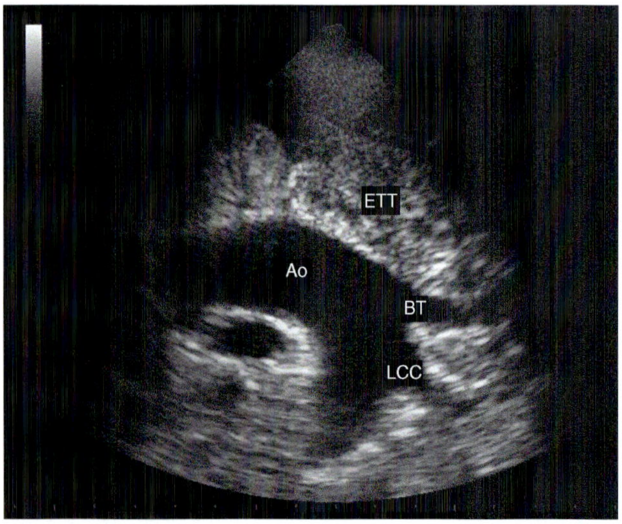

• **Fig. 18-13** Bidimensional (2D) echocardiogram (long axis view of the aortic arch) obtained by examining the cranial mediastinum in a dog with a large ectopic thyroid tumor (ETT). This tumor surrounds the aortic root (Ao). This creates an acoustic interface facilitating the visualization of the cranial mediastinal vessels, both compressed by the mass. *BT,* Brachiocephalic trunk; *LCC,* left common carotid artery. (Photo credit: Claudio Bussadori.)

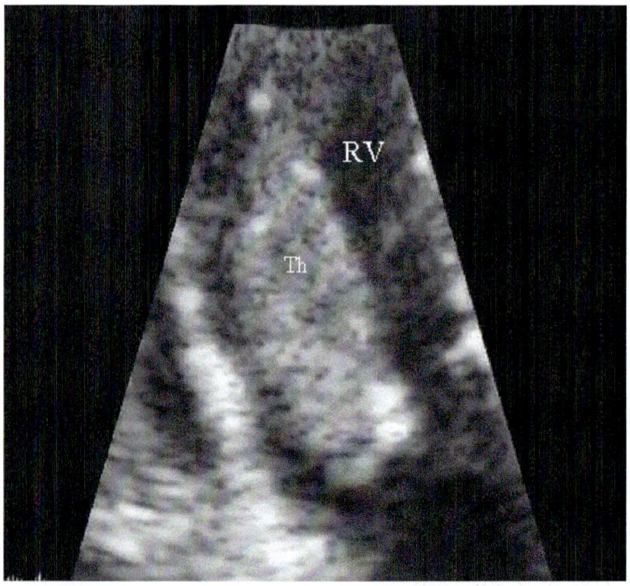

• **Fig. 18-15** Enlarged view of a thrombus (Th) within the right ventricular cavity. An anechoic line between the thrombus and the right ventricular wall is clearly visible. *RV,* Right ventricle. (Photo credit: Claudio Bussadori.)

Atrial Tumors

In humans, tumors located in the left or right atria are almost always myxomas or myxosarcomas. In dogs, atrial tumors are rare. Myxosarcomas are extremely rare [24]. Myxomas are more frequently encountered attached to the atrioventricular valvular leaflets (Figure 18-16) [20, 23].

A tumor can also come from another location (such as an adrenal gland) and invade the right atrium and sometimes the right ventricular cavity via the caudal vena cava.

In these cases, the neoplastic tissue grows inside the blood vessel and progresses as far as the right atrium without infiltrating the surrounding endothelium [44]. Other tumors such as sarcomas and carcinomas may also invade atrial cavities [37].

Myocardial Tumors

Rhabdomyosarcoma is the most frequently encountered tumor originating from the myocardial wall. This tumor disrupts the normal myocardial echocardiographic texture, resulting in hyperechoic focal lesions of various shapes and dimensions (Figure 18-17) [16,17]. Arrhythmias may result from invasion of the conduction tissue. Eventually, the mass may obstruct cardiac cavities, leading to weakness and syncope [11]. Low pulse repetition frequency (PRF) color flow Doppler may help to visualize the path of blood around the mass (Figure 18-18).

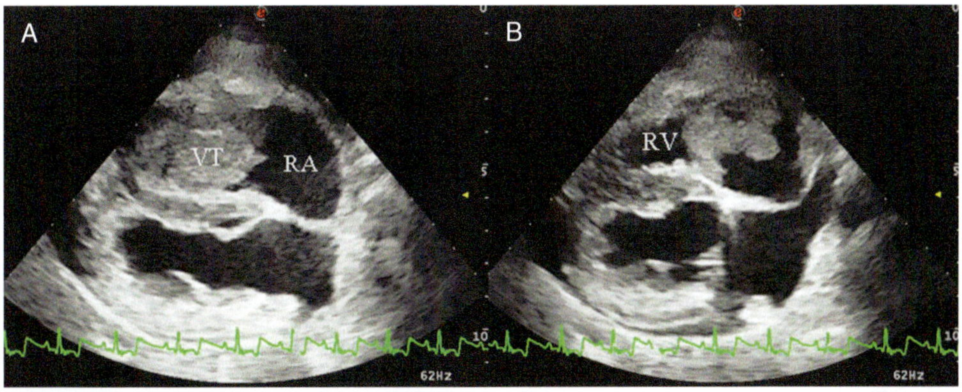

• **Fig. 18-16** Bidimensional (2D) echocardiogram (right parasternal long axis view) in a dog with a tricuspid valve tumor (VT). This valvular mass occupies the right ventricular inflow tract in diastole (A) and prolapses into the right atrium (RA) during systole (B). *RV,* Right ventricle. (Photo credit: Claudio Bussadori.)

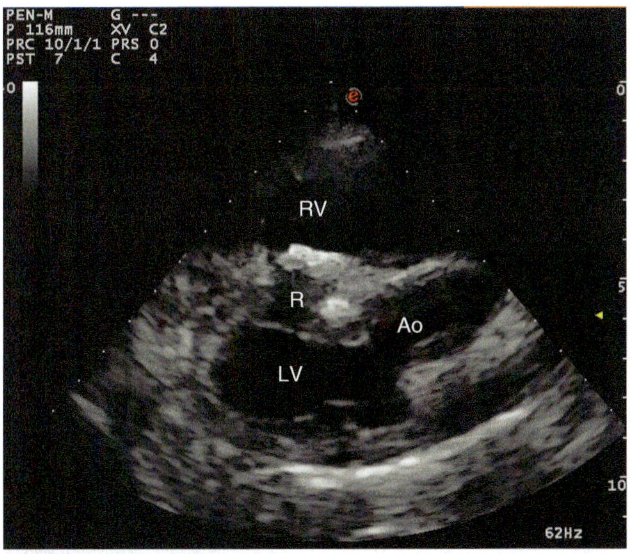

• **Fig. 18-17** Bidimensional (2D) echocardiogram (right parasternal long axis view) in a dog with septal rhabdomyosarcoma (R). Note the focal hyperechoic lesions and the heterogeneity of the interventricular septum due to tumor infiltration. *Ao,* Aorta; *LV,* left ventricle; *RV,* right ventricle. (Photo credit: Claudio Bussadori.)

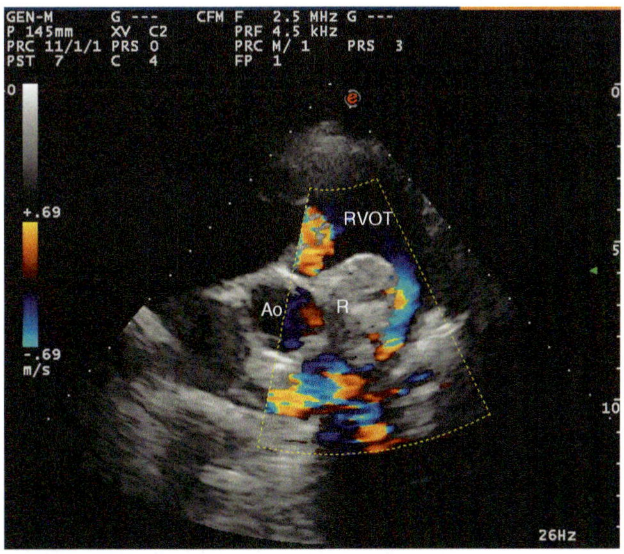

• **Fig. 18-18** Bidimensional (2D) echocardiogram (right parasternal short axis view at the base of the heart) in a dog with a rhabdomyosarcoma (R) originating from the interventricular septum. The mass invades and partially obstructs the right ventricular outflow tract (RVOT). *Ao,* Aorta. (Photo credit: Claudio Bussadori.)

Metastatic Tumors

Metastatic heart tumors are relatively frequent [18]. They reach the heart either by anatomic continuity or via the caudal vena cava, the lymphatic circulation, or the coronary arteries, leading to intramural metastases. In dogs and cats, cardiac metastases of HSA, lymphoma, melanoma, and carcinoma have been described mainly in the left ventricular free wall, while metastatic carcinomas may cause pericarditis with or without PE [3].

Intramural metastases appear as multiple disseminated nodules. Their texture is more heterogeneous than that of the surrounding normal myocardium. Sometimes it is possible to observe the absence of systolic contraction of the myocardial segment invaded by a metastasis. Epicardial metastases may result in acute pericardial tamponade when rupturing.

Mesothelioma

Mesothelioma is a rare malignant diffuse neoplasm [38], usually causing intracavitary hemorrhagic effusion in older dogs and cats. A juvenile form of mesothelioma has been documented in a 7-week-old puppy [45] and an 11-month-old dog [46].

The neoplastic process occurs from the ectodermic cells originating from, in decreasing order of frequency [47], the pleura [48], the peritoneum [49], the pericardium, and the testicular tunica vaginalis [50].

Cough, dyspnea, tachypnea, and weakness are the clinical signs most frequently detected and are related to PLE or PE. The presence of chronic pericardial tamponade is a common cause of ascites [51].

In the early stages, mesothelioma cannot be visualized by ultrasonography or even by computed tomography [51], due to the lack of organization of the neoplastic cells in a distinct mass and the absence of significant cavity effusion. A diffuse thickening of the affected surface could be the only echographic sign of the presence of this tumor.

In more advanced stages, the neoplasia may organize in polypoid formations or isolated nodules on the pleura [52] or even involve the entire mesothelium (Figure 18-19). Chronic tamponade may be present, causing ascites [53].

Several cavities can be involved at the same time [54] but distant metastases are rare. In male dogs, especially in German Shepherds, mesothelioma is associated with a fibrous thickening of the peritoneum or the pleura (sclerosing mesothelioma) [55,56].

In cats, mesothelioma occurs in the thoracic or abdominal cavity and is usually associated with pleural or peritoneal effusions [57].

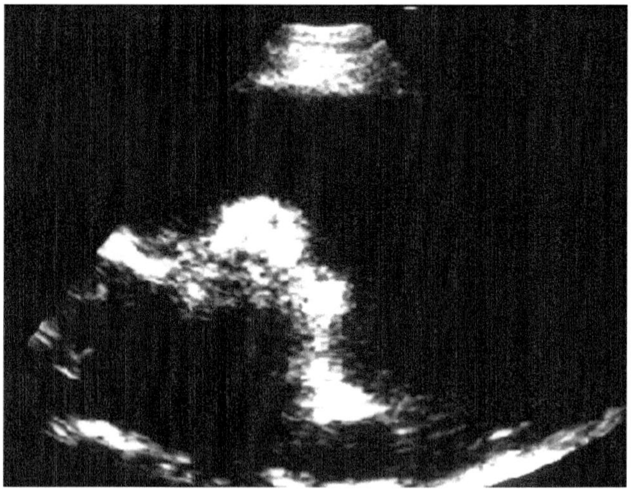

• **Fig. 18-19** Echographic view of the pericardiophrenic ligament, deformed by large hyperechoic nodules in a dog with thoracic mesothelioma. Note the large amount of pleural effusion around the ligament. (Photo credit: Claudio Bussadori.)

REFERENCES

[1] Ware W. Cardiac neoplasia. In: Kirk RW, Bonagura JD, editors. Kirk's current veterinary therapy XII: small animal practice. Philadelphia: W.B. Saunders; 1995.
[2] Detweiler DK, Patterson DF. The prevalence and types of cardiovascular disease in dogs. Ann N Y Acad Sci 1965;127:481–516.
[3] Walter JH, Rudolph R. Systemic, metastatic, eu- and heterotrope tumours of the heart in necropsied dogs. Zentralbl Veterinarmed A 1996;43:31–45.
[4] Kleine LJ, Zook BC, Munson TO. Primary cardiac hemangiosarcomas in dogs. J Am Vet Med Assoc 1970;157:326–37.
[5] Ware WA, Hopper DL. Cardiac tumors in dogs: 1982-1995. J Vet Intern Med 1999;13:95–103.
[6] Sanford SE, Hoover DM, Miller RB. Primary cardiac cell tumor in a dog. Vet Pathol 1984;21:489–94.
[7] Dupuy-Mateos WP, Blunden AS, White RN. Primary cardiac chondrosarcoma in a paced dog. Vet Rec 2008;163:272–3.
[8] Schelling SH, Moses BL. Primary intracardiac osteosarcoma in a dog. J Vet Diagn Invest 1994;6:396–8.
[9] Lombard C. Primary fibroma in the right atrium of a dog. J Small Anim Pract 1980;21:439–48.
[10] Madarame H, Sato K, Ogihara K, et al. Primary cardiac fibrosarcoma in a dog. J Vet Med Sci 2004;66:979–82.
[11] Atkins C. Diagnosis of intracardiac fibrosarcoma using two-dimensional echocardiography. Vet Radiol 1984;20:131–7.
[12] Brambilla P. Primary cardiac lipoma in a dog. J Vet Intern Med 2006;20:691–3.
[13] Machida N, Kobayashi M, Tanaka R, et al. Primary malignant mixed mesenchymal tumour of the heart in a dog. J Comp Pathol 2003;128:71–4.
[14] Ogilvie G. Malignant lymphoma with cardiac and bone involvement in a dog. J Am Vet Med Assoc 1989;194:793–6.
[15] MacGregor JM, Faria ML, Moore AS, Tobias AH. Cardiac lymphoma and pericardial effusion in dogs: 12 cases (1994–2004). J Am Vet Med Assoc 2005;1:1449–53.
[16] Zaher A, Radi AM. Canine cardiac rhabdomyoma. Toxicol Pathol 2009;37:348–50.
[17] Krotje LJ, Ware WA, Niyo Y. Intracardiac rhabdomyosarcoma in a dog. J Am Vet Med Assoc 1990;197: 368–71.
[18] Aupperle H, Marz I, Ellenberger C, et al. Primary and secondary heart tumours in dogs and cats. J Comp Pathol 2007;136:18–26.
[19] Liggett AD, Frazier KS, Styer EL. Angiolipomatous tumors in dogs and a cat. Vet Pathol 2002;39:286–9.
[20] Akkoc A, Ozyigit MO, Cangul IT. Valvular cardiac myxoma in a dog. J Vet Med A Physiol Pathol Clin Med 2007;54:356–8.
[21] Adissu HA, Wood GA, Caswell JL. Cardiac myxosarcoma with adrenal adenoma and pituitary hyperplasia resembling carney complex in a dog. Vet Pathol 2010;47:354–7.
[22] Darke PG, Gordon LR. Cardiac myxoma in a dog. Vet Rec 1974;95:565–7.
[23] Machida N, Hoshi K, Kobayashi M, et al. Cardiac myxoma of the tricuspid valve in a dog. J Comp Pathol 2003;129:320–4.
[24] Briggs OM, Kirberger RM, Goldberg NB. Right atrial myxosarcoma in a dog. J S Afr Vet Assoc 1997;68:144–6.
[25] Foale RD, White RA, Harley R, Herrtage ME. Left ventricular myxosarcoma in a dog. J Small Anim Pract 2003;44:503–7.
[26] Holscher M. Ectopic thyroid tumor in a dog: thyroglobulin, calcitonin and neuron-specific enolase immunocytochemical studies. Vet Pathol 1986;23:778–9.
[27] Stephens L. Ectopic thyroid carcinoma with metastases in a beagle dog. Vet Pathol 1982;19:669–75.
[28] Bracha S, Caron I, Holmberg DL, et al. Ectopic thyroid carcinoma causing right ventricular outflow tract obstruction in a dog. J Am Anim Hosp Assoc 2009;45:138–41.
[29] Merlo M, Bo S, Ratto A. Primary right atrium haemangiosarcoma in a cat. J Feline Med Surg 2002;4:61–4.
[30] Campbell MD, Gelberg HB. Endocardial ossifying myxoma of the right atrium in a cat. Vet Pathol 2000;37:460–2.
[31] Gamlem H, Nordstoga K, Arnesen K. Canine vascular neoplasia: a population-based clinicopathologic study of 439 tumours and tumour-like lesions in 420 dogs. APMIS 2008;116:41–54.
[32] Bonnett BN, Egenvall A. Hedhammar Å, Olson P. Mortality in over 350,000 insured swedish dogs from 1995-2000: I. Breed-, gender-, age- and cause-specific rates. Acta Vet Scand 2005;46:105–20.
[33] Bussadori CB, Quintavalla C, Pradelli D, Marconato L. Diagnostic imaging for the identification of cardiac tumours in humans and dogs. Proceedings 13th Ljudevit Jurak International Symposium on Comparative Pathology. Zagreb 2002. Acta Clinica Croatica 2002;41:155.
[34] Kirkpatrick JN. Differential diagnosis of cardiac masses using contrast echocardiographic perfusion imaging. J Am Coll Cardiol 2004;43:1412–9.
[35] Ehrhart N, Ehrhart EJ, Willis J, et al. Analysis of factors affecting survival in dogs with aortic body tumors. Vet Surg 2002;31:44–8.

[36] Fernandez-del Palacio MJ, Talavera Lopez J, Bayon del Rio A, et al. Left ventricular outflow tract obstruction secondary to hemangiosarcoma in a dog. J Vet Intern Med 2006;20:687–90.

[37] Warman SM, McGregor R, Fews D, Ferasin L. Congestive heart failure caused by intracardiac tumours in two dogs. J Small Anim Pract 2006;47:480–3.

[38] MacDonald KA, Cagney O, Magne ML. Echocardiographic and clinicopathologic characterization of pericardial effusion in dogs: 107 cases (1985–2006). J Am Vet Med Assoc 2009;15:1456–61.

[39] Dunning D, Monnet E, Orton EC, Salman MD. Analysis of prognostic indicators for dogs with pericardial effusion: 46 cases (1985–1996). J Am Vet Med Assoc 1998;212:1276–80.

[40] Clifford CA, Mackin AJ, Henry CJ. Treatment of canine hemangiosarcoma: 2000 and beyond. J Vet Intern Med 2000;14:479–85.

[41] Less RD, Orton EC. Intrapericardial cyst causing cardiac tamponnade in a cat. J Am Anim Hosp Assoc 2000;36:115–9.

[42] Sisson D. Intrapericardial cyst in a dog. J Vet Intern Med 1993;7:364–9.

[43] Noszczyk-Nowak A, Nowak M, Paslawska U, et al. Cases with manifestation of chemodectoma diagnosed in dogs in department of internal diseases with horses, dogs and cats clinic, veterinary medicine faculty, university of environmental and life sciences, Wroclaw, Poland. Acta Vet Scand 2010;52:35–42.

[44] Pradelli D, Quintavalla C, Domenech O, Bussadori C. Tumour thrombus: direct endoluminal caudal caval vein-right atrium extension in a dog affected by adrenal neoplasia. Vet Res Commun 2003;27:787–9.

[45] Leisewitz AL, Nesbit JW. Malignant mesothelioma in a seven-week-old puppy. J South Afr Vet Assoc 1992;63:70–3.

[46] Kim JH, Choi YK, Yoon HY, et al. Juvenile malignant mesothelioma in a dog. J Vet Med Sci 2002;64:269–71.

[47] Reggeti F, Brisson B, Ruotsalo K, et al. Invasive epithelial mesothelioma in a dog. Vet Pathol 2005;42:77–81.

[48] Espino L, Vasquez S, Faílde D, et al. Localized pleural mesothelioma causing cranial vena cava syndrome in a dog. J Vet Diagn Invest 2010;22:309–12.

[49] Morini M, Morandi F, Burdisso R, Marcato PS. Deciduoid peritoneal mesothelioma in a dog. Vet Pathol 2006;43:198–201.

[50] Vascellari M, Carminato CA, Camali G, et al. Malignant mesothelioma of the tunica vaginalis testis in a dog: histological and immunohistochemical characterization. J Vet Diagn Invest 2011;23:135–9.

[51] Stepien RL, Whitley NT, Dubielzig RR. Idiopathic or mesothelioma-related pericardial effusion: clinical findings and survival in 17 dogs studied retrospectively. J Small Anim Pract 2000;41:342–7.

[52] Echandi RL, Morandi F, Newman SJ, Holford A. Imaging diagnosis canine thoracic mesothelioma. Vet Radiol Ultrasound 2007;48:243–5.

[53] Brower A, Herold LV, Kirby BM. Canine cardiac mesothelioma with granular cell morphology. Vet Pathol 2006;43:384–7.

[54] Sato T, Miyoshi T, Shibuya H, et al. Peritoneal biphasic mesothelioma in a dog. J Vet Med A Physiol Pathol Clin Med 2005;52:22–5.

[55] Schoning P, Layton CE, Fortney WD, et al. Sclerosing peritoneal mesothelioma in a dog evaluated by electron microscopy and immunoperoxidase techniques. J Vet Diagn Invest 1992;4:217–20.

[56] Geninet C, Bernex F, Rakotovao F, et al. Sclerosing peritoneal mesothelioma in a dog–a case report. J Vet Med A Physiol Pathol Clin Med 2003;50:402–5.

[57] Weiss AT, Da Costa AB, Klopfleisch R. Predominantly fibrous malignant mesothelioma in a cat. Vet Med Intern 2010;2010:396794 (epub).

PART V

Congenital Cardiopathies

19 Congenital Cardiopathies, 285

20 Echocardiographic Evaluation of Congenital Cardiopathies Before and After Intervention, 323

19 Congenital Cardiopathies

CLAUDIO BUSSADORI IN COLLABORATION WITH DANITZA PRADELLI

Left Ventricular Outflow Tract Obstructions/Subaortic Stenosis, 286
Pulmonic Stenosis, 291
Patent Ductus Arteriosus, 298
Ventricular Septal Defect, 303
Atrial Septal Defect, 305
Mitral Valve Dysplasia, 308
Tricuspid Valve Dysplasia, 310
Tetralogy of Fallot, 312
Cor Triatriatum, 313
Endocardial Cushion Defect, 316

Congenital heart diseases (CHDs) include all cardiac diseases present at birth. In dogs, the most commonly encountered CHDs are subaortic stenosis [1], pulmonic stenosis, and patent ductus arteriosus [2]. All CHDs should be considered "progressive," as their hemodynamic characteristics may change during the patient's life. Some of them, such as severe tetralogy of Fallot, could lead to early death while others may remain asymptomatic for years. Echocardiography is particularly useful in identifying congenital malformations and deciding on the most appropriate medical, interventional, or surgical treatment [3].

Left Ventricular Outflow Tract Obstructions/Subaortic Stenosis

Left ventricular outflow tract (LVOT) obstructions may present as a supravalvular, valvular, or subvalvular lesion. These congenital obstructions have been described in cats but remain extremely rare in this species [4,5]. Subaortic obstructions, also called subaortic stenosis (SAS), are most commonly encountered in dogs [6]. Males seem to be particularly predisposed, according to some studies [7, 8]. SAS may present as a single anomaly or in association with other lesions such as pulmonic stenosis. In our experience, SAS represents 21.3% of reported CHDs [9]. A genetic transmission of SAS has been documented in the Newfoundland [9] and is strongly suspected in other canine breeds. In Italy, a mandatory CHD screening, performed on Boxers over a period of 6 years, revealed that 165 of 1283 dogs (12.9%) had a CHD [6]. Of these, 8.5% had isolated SAS and 1% had SAS associated with pulmonic stenosis [7].

Anatomopathology

The primary lesion of SAS is the abnormal presence of endocardial tissue upstream of the aortic valve causing obstruction of the LVOT [10]. Sometimes the anterior (septal) mitral leaflet may be involved. The characteristics of the lesion can vary according to the breed. For instance, Boxers and Dogues de Bordeaux frequently present with an abnormal proliferation of tissue and hypoplasia of the aortic annulus and root hypoplasia [11,12] whereas the SAS lesion in Newfoundlands, German Shepherds, and Rottweilers is localized to the subvalvular region, with a normal aortic annulus and a poststenotic dilation of the aortic root. In the latter breeds, when the lesion is severe, the endocardial proliferation also may spread into the left ventricular cavity, the papillary muscles, and the chordae tendineae [13].

Recently, a study conducted on Boxers demonstrated the influence of the angle between the aorta and interventricular septum on the growth of anomalous endocardial tissue [14]. The shear stress is increased when the angle is steeper (<140 degrees), causing endocardial proliferation [14], thus predisposing the Boxer to the development and progression of SAS (Figure 19-1).

In most dogs, the degree of obstruction remains stable throughout the animal's lifetime. However, in some cases, the abnormal turbulent blood flow and architecture of the LVOT, as well as the impaired mitral leaflets motion, cause further proliferation of endocardial tissue, increasing resistance and the pressure gradient even in

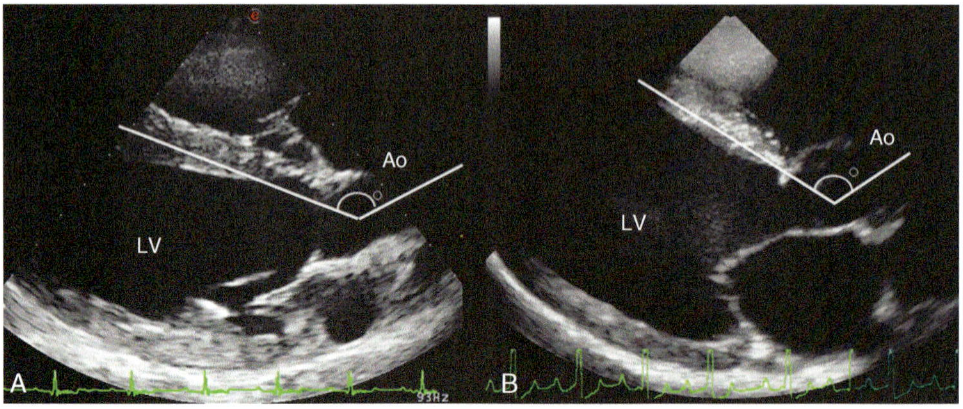

• **Fig. 19-1** Right parasternal long axis 5 chambers views showing the aortoseptal angle in **(A)** a normal dog and **(B)** in a Newfoundland with subaortic stenosis (SAS). *Ao,* Aorta; *LV,* left ventricle. (Photo credit: Claudio Bussadori.)

adulthood (Figure 19-2). This is why young animals with mild SAS should be reevaluated echocardiographically within the first 2 years of life, because of the potential worsening of the outflow obstruction.

Echocardiographic Aspects

Transthoracic echocardiography (TTE) is an irreplaceable tool to assess the severity and classify the different types of SAS. Transesophageal echocardiography (TEE) can also be helpful to better evaluate the type and grade of SAS when the quality of TTE exam is poor or when there is no evidence of subvalvular obstruction despite an elevated peak systolic aortic velocity [15].

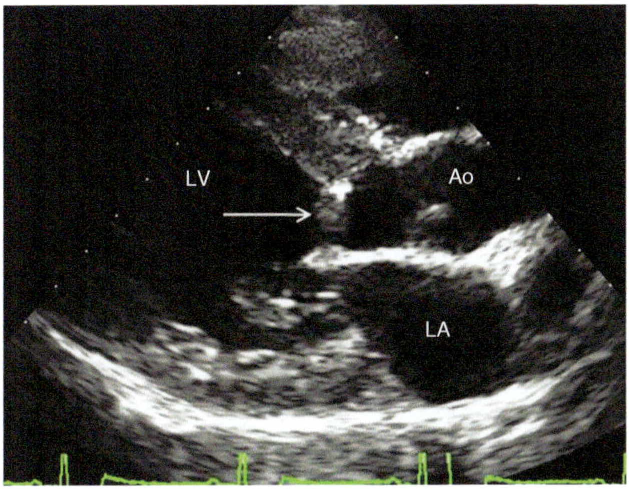

• **Fig. 19-2** Right parasternal long axis 5 chambers view in an adult dog with congenital subaortic stenosis (SAS). An endocardial proliferation *(arrow)* formed in adulthood and is now aggravating the obstruction created by the underlying congenital lesion. *Ao,* Aorta; *LA,* left atrium; *LV,* left ventricle. (Photo credit: Claudio Bussadori.)

Bidimensional and TM Echocardiographic Characteristics

Types of Subaortic Stenosis

According to the Pyle-Patterson classification [16], SAS lesions can be classified as one of three types (Figure 19-3):

- *Type 1* is characterized by the presence of small nodules (1 to 2 mm) on the endocardial surface of the interventricular septum, right below the aortic valve. These lesions are too small to create any obstruction detectable by Doppler echocardiography. However, their identification by bidimensional (2D) echocardiography is extremely important for breed screening purposes. Furthermore, follow-up on type 1 SAS is important because of the potential progression of the disease.
- *Type 2* is characterized by a narrow membrane of thickened endocardium extending partially along the LVOT. In most cases, the ridge originates from the base of the anterior leaflet of the mitral valve and extends transversally across the interventricular septum beneath the left coronary cusp of the aortic valve (Video 19-1).
- *Type 3* is characterized by the presence of a "tunnel" lesion: a fibrous band or collar raised 1 to 2 mm above

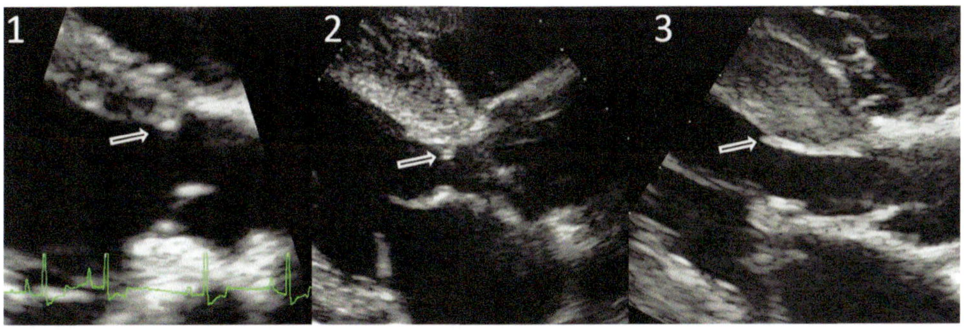

• **Fig. 19-3** Right parasternal long axis 5 chambers view displaying three variations of subaortic stenoses *(arrows)*. (Photo credit: Claudio Bussadori.)

the endocardial surface, starting from the aortic valve cusps, extending toward the interventricular septum, and involving the anterior mitral valve leaflet, thus completely encircling the LVOT. The ventricular surfaces of the aortic valve leaflets are also thickened.

In our experience, types 1 and 2 SAS are the most frequently observed forms, together representing 85% of SAS cases diagnosed in the dog [9].

Echocardiographic Aspects

The dimension and morphology of the aortic annulus and aortic valvular cusps are evaluated from the right parasternal long axis 5 chambers and the right parasternal short axis transaortic views. The aortic valve leaflets may be mildly to severely thickened and have a normal to reduced mobility. The abnormal fibrous tissue may not only be limited to the LVOT but also involve parts of the papillary muscles, the base of left ventricular septum, other areas of the endocardium, and the mitral valve leaflets. This finding is associated with a poorer prognosis, due to the ensuing profound impairment of the heart function (Figure 19-4).

The sphericity of the left ventricle may also be increased, especially in end-stage SAS where afterload mismatch is present (see below) (Figure 19-5).

The left parasternal cranial long axis view optimized for the aortic root or the right parasternal long axis 5 chambers view angled craniodorsally can be used to evaluate the

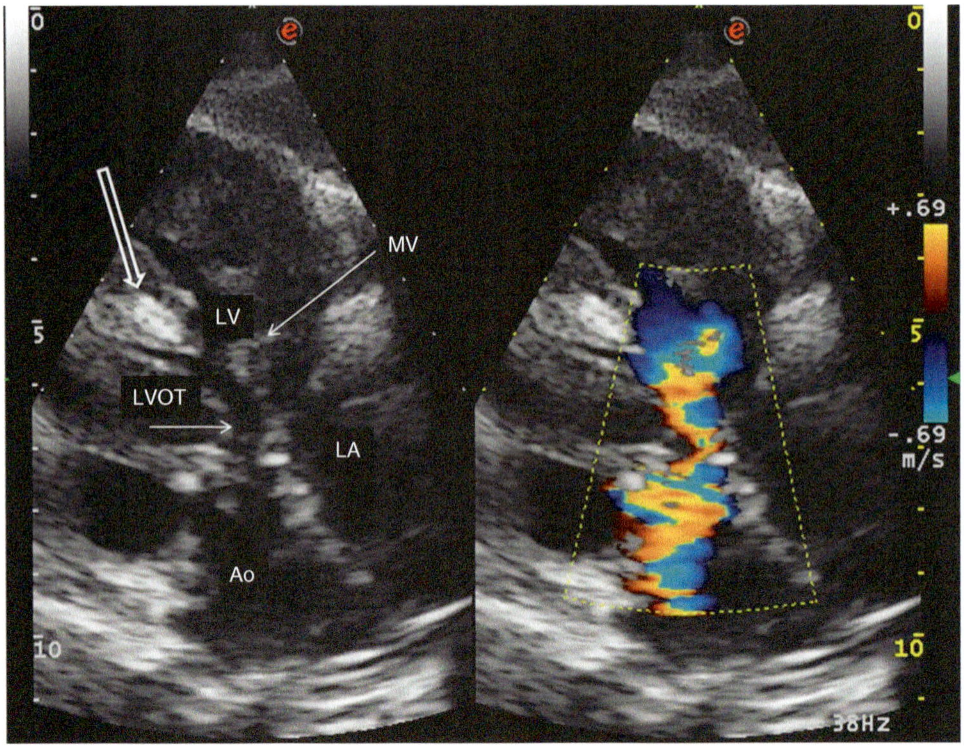

• **Fig. 19-4** Subxyphoid view with *(right)* and without *(left)* color Doppler in a Labrador puppy. The left ventricle outflow tract (LVOT) is strangled by a "tunnel" subaortic stenosis (SAS). Poststenotic dilation of the ascending aorta (Ao) is present. The thickened endocardium also affects the mitral valve (MV), creating mild mitral stenosis. The large openwork arrow points to the subendocardial fibrosis infiltrating the anterior papillary muscle. *LA,* Left atrium; *LV,* left ventricle. (Photo credit: Claudio Bussadori.)

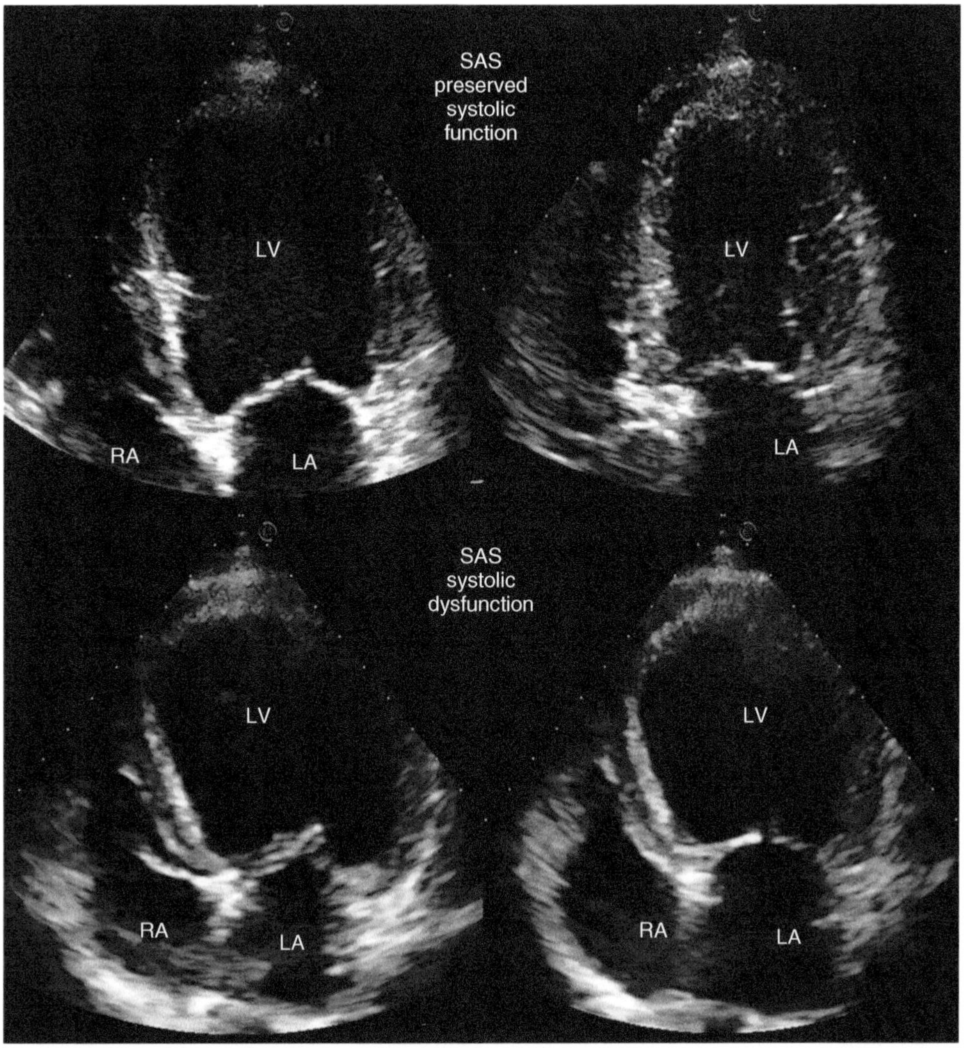

• **Fig. 19-5** Diastolic *(left)* and systolic *(right)* left apical 4 chambers views in a dog with subaortic stenosis (SAS). At the time of the first examination *(top)*, the left ventricular systolic function and geometry are still normal. Two years later *(bottom)*, the left ventricle (LV) has become more spherical and the systolic function has declined. *LA,* Left atrium; *RA,* right atrium. (Photo credit: Claudio Bussadori.)

aortic root morphology and obtain aortic measurements at the level of the sinuses of Valsalva and the sinotubular junction. It is best to perform measurements from inner edge to inner edge (Figure 19-6) [17,18].

The use of M-mode allows quantitative measurements of the septal and left ventricular free wall thicknesses. Usually the degree of the hypertrophy correlates with the severity of SAS, except in cases of "afterload mismatch," where the degree of hypertrophy becomes insufficient.

Afterload Mismatch

In the natural history of SAS, chronic left ventricular pressure overload results in concentric ventricular hypertrophy. This hypertrophy impedes the myocardial perfusion [19], leading to fibrosis, left ventricular diastolic dysfunction, myocardial ischemia, and arrhythmias

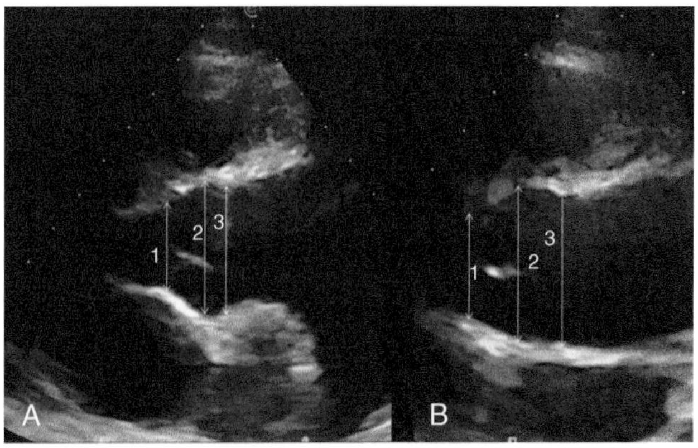

• **Fig. 19-6** Right parasternal long axis view with craniodorsal angulation (A) and left parasternal aortic long axis view (B) illustrating the poststenotic dilation of the ascending aorta associated with this subaortic stenosis (SAS). Note the different aortic diameters at the aortic root (1), sinuses of Valsalva (2), and sinotubular junction (3) levels. (Photo credit: Claudio Bussadori.)

[20]. At some point, the increased wall stress can no longer be compensated for by the hypertrophy, which becomes eccentric. The left ventricle becomes spherical and irreversible systolic dysfunction starts. This is called "afterload mismatch." The rightward displacement of the septum leads to right ventricular diastolic dysfunction. This may result in ascites, even in the absence of significant tricuspid regurgitation or pulmonary hypertension.

Afterload mismatch represents the final evolution of SAS and is associated with a poor prognosis, the survival time usually not exceeding 6 months.

Spectral Doppler

Spectral Doppler is helpful in the evaluation of aortic transvalvular flow. The best alignment with the aortic flow can be obtained using a subxyphoid view [21,22], with the dog in right lateral recumbency [23]. The standing position can also be used. Analysis of the transaortic flow is also often performed using a left apical 5 chambers view, with the animal standing or in lateral recumbency. Spectral pulsed wave and color Doppler examinations of the LVOT and aorta reveal a broad systolic turbulent jet (Video 19-2). Continuous wave (CW) Doppler examination allows the measurement of the peak aortic velocity and gradient (Figure 19-7), used to assess the severity of the stenosis [21,24,25]. The instantaneous peak gradient calculated by CW Doppler is usually significantly higher than the peak-to-peak gradient measured by cardiac catheterization. This can be explained by the fact that these two peaks do not occur simultaneously. Both the CW Doppler instantaneous peak gradient and the catheter-derived peak-to-peak gradient are universally considered markers of SAS severity. However, the mean pressure gradient has been shown to be more reliable and the agreement between mean gradient measured by Doppler and by catheterization is much higher [26-28]. For this reason, many echocardiography laboratories associated with interventional cardiology centers use mean gradient rather than peak gradient as an indicator of stenosis severity.

Based on the Doppler-derived maximal aortic pressure gradient, SAS could be classified as follows:

- Mild SAS: aortic peak gradient <40 to 50 mm Hg
- Moderate SAS: aortic peak gradient of 50 to 80 mm Hg
- Severe SAS: aortic peak gradient >80 mm Hg

In cases of end-stage aortic stenosis with afterload mismatch, one may observe a decrease in the anterograde systolic aortic velocity, indicating decreased systolic function, and a restrictive transmitral diastolic profile due to the increased left ventricular diastolic pressure (Figure 19-8).

In the long term, the impact of the high-velocity blood flow on the aortic valve leaflets provokes thickening of the latter and sometimes lesions that can become a suitable substrate for developing aortic valvular endocarditis [29-32]. The consequences of aortic endocarditis depend

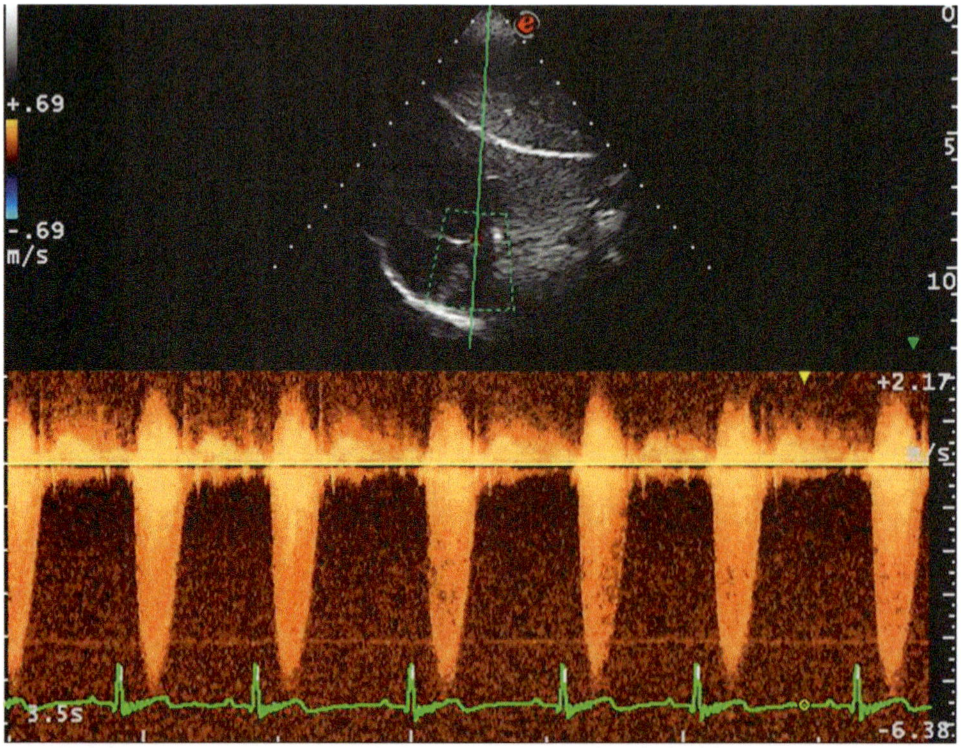

• **Fig. 19-7** Subxyphoid view allowing good alignment of the Doppler cursor with the ascending aorta and the aortic flow, here revealing severe subaortic stenosis (SAS) (the maximum velocity is 5.5 m/s, indicating a gradient of 121 mm Hg). (Photo credit: Claudio Bussadori.)

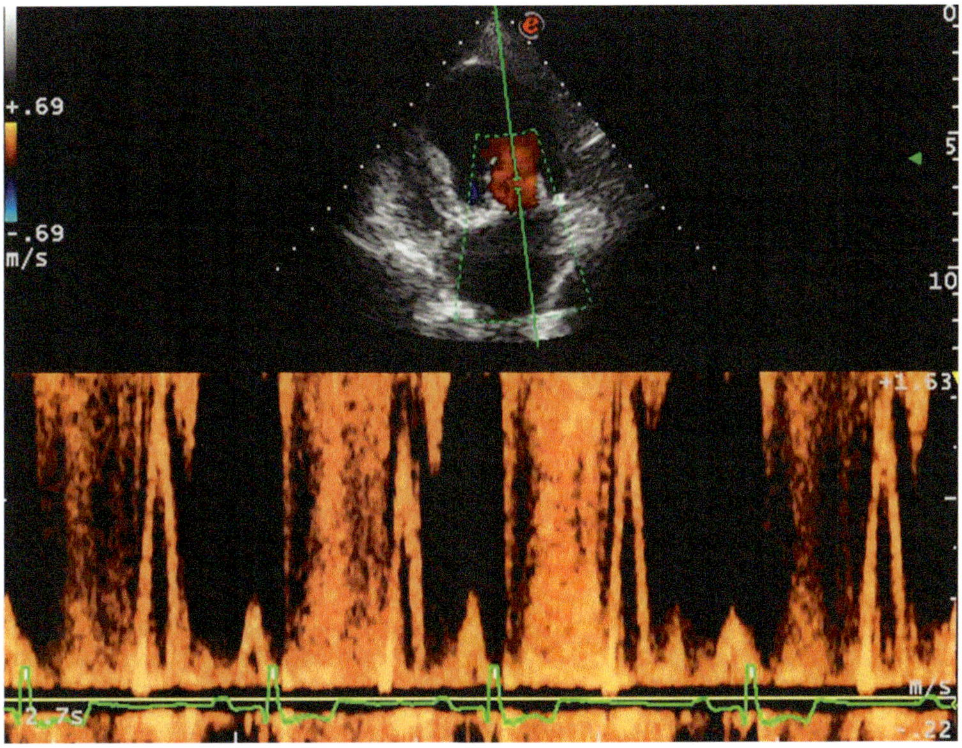

• **Fig. 19-8** Pulsed wave Doppler of the transmitral flow in a Boxer with severe subaortic stenosis (SAS) and afterload mismatch. The pattern of the diastolic mitral flow, with an elevated E/A ratio, indicates restrictive physiology. The deceleration time of the E wave is very short, indicating elevated ventricular diastolic pressure. (Photo credit: Claudio Bussadori.)

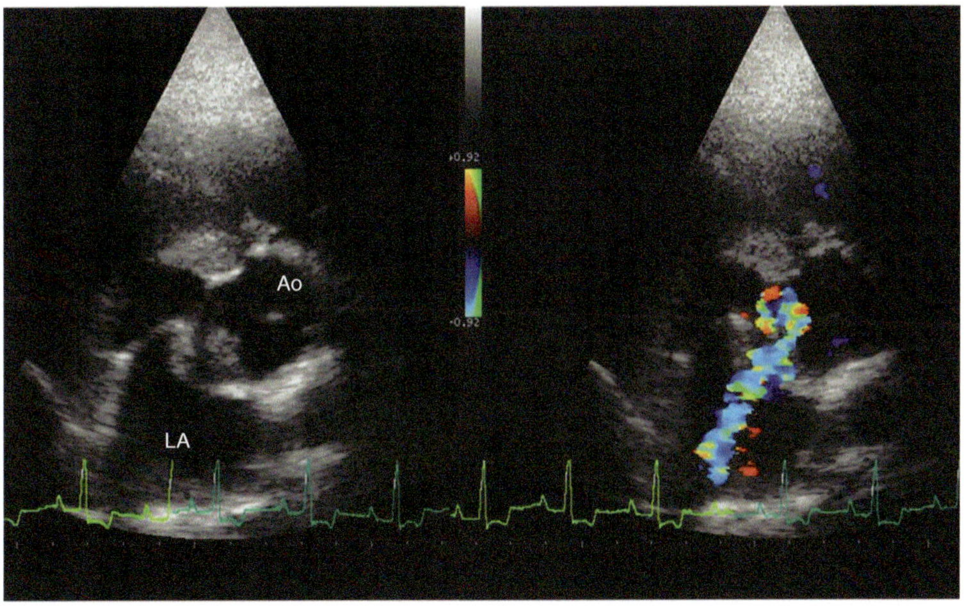

• **Fig. 19-9** Right parasternal long axis view of the aortic root with *(right)* and without *(left)* color Doppler in a Rottweiler with subaortic stenosis (SAS) and sinus of Valsalva endocarditis. The destruction of this region has created a fistula between the aorta (Ao) and the left atrium (LA), with significant regurgitation directly into the left atrium. (Photo credit: Claudio Bussadori.)

on the severity and the extension of the lesion and most often include aortic regurgitation and worsening of the stenosis. In more serious cases, the inflammatory process may involve surrounding structures such as the sinuses of Valsalva (Figure 19-9) [33].

Pulmonic Stenosis

Pulmonic stenosis (PS) is one of the most frequent congenital cardiopathies in dogs [34]. In our study, its prevalence was 32.1% [9]. It is rarely reported in cats [35-39].

In most cases, PS is an isolated lesion. However, it sometimes may be associated with other congenital cardiac malformations, such as atrial septal defect or interventricular septal defect, or be part of a complex malformation such as tetralogy of Fallot. It can also be associated with severe SAS (especially in Boxers) [7,9]. PS can be valvular, supravalvular, or subvalvular.

Anatomopathology

Valvular Pulmonic Stenosis

Two echocardiographic types of valvular PS in dogs can be encountered: type A and type B.

Type A valvular PS is characterized by an annulus of normal dimensions and a lack of division of the two valvular leaflets. The valve behaves as a diaphragm, adopting in systole a dome-shaped appearance moving toward the main pulmonary artery.

Type B valvular PS is characterized by a hypoplastic pulmonic valve annulus and thickening of valvular leaflets, which may not necessarily be fused.

Type A is the most common form and does not seem to have any particular breed predisposition [25]. Type B PS is found more often in brachycephalic breeds like English and French Bulldogs (the latter often showing extremely severe forms). In Boxers, type B PS is less frequent than type A PS. Type B PS can sometimes be associated with SAS [7].

In Pitbulls and American Staffordshire Terriers, severe PS can be associated with foci of endocardial fibroelastosis, appearing as hyperechoic endocardial areas with variable infiltrations of the endocardium and subendocardium. These lesions are associated with severe right ventricular diastolic dysfunction and refractory ventricular tachyarrhythmias leading to right heart failure or sudden death.

Supravalvular Pulmonic Stenosis

Supravalvular PS is characterized by a narrowing of the main pulmonary artery and its distal portions. This lesion is very rare in dogs [40]. In English and French Bulldogs, this stenosis can be located at the sinotubular junction (Figure 19-10). In this malformation, the main pulmonary artery adopts an hourglass shape. Stenosis of the pulmonary branches is frequently observed in children as part of a complex congenital heart disease such as tetralogy of Fallot but may be seen in dogs as an isolated disease (Figure 19-11).

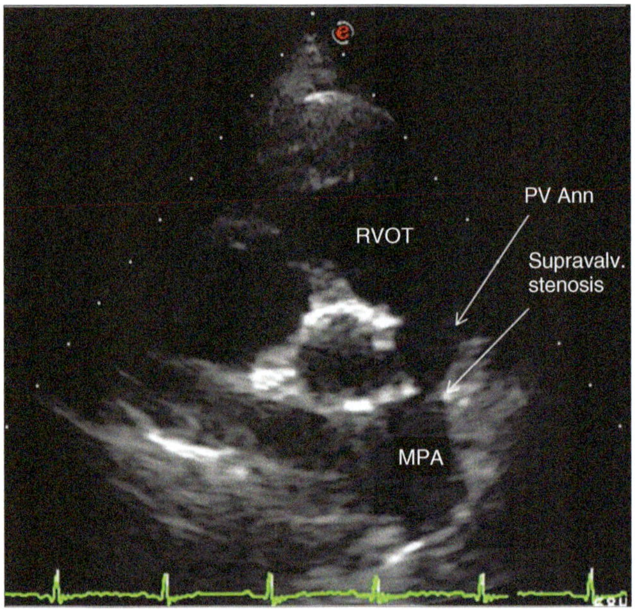

• **Fig. 19-10** Right parasternal short axis view of the base of the heart in an English Bulldog with supravalvular pulmonic stenosis (PS). The stenosis (Supravalv. stenosis) is visible below the pulmonic valvular annulus (PV Ann). Poststenotic dilation of the main pulmonary artery (MPA) is visible, giving it an hourglass appearance. *RVOT,* Right ventricular outflow tract. (Photo credit: Claudio Bussadori.)

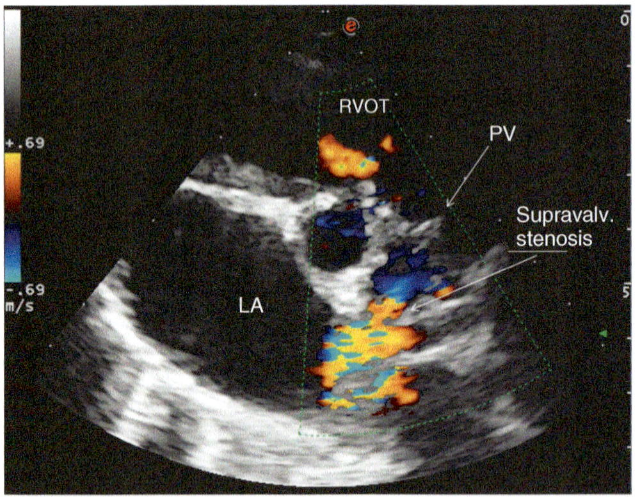

• **Fig. 19-11** Right parasternal short axis view of the base of the heart in color Doppler mode in a young Labrador with supravalvular pulmonic stenosis (PS). Aliasing is present downstream of the pulmonic valve (PV), at the level of the supravalvular stenosis (Supravalv. stenosis). *LA,* Left atrium; *RVOT,* right ventricular outflow tract. (Photo credit: Claudio Bussadori.)

Subvalvular Pulmonic Stenosis

Subvalvular PS can be caused by a number of obstructive anomalies. Severe hypertrophy and narrowing of the right ventricular outflow tract (RVOT) associated with severe annular hypoplasia must be distinguished from severe infundibular hypertrophy secondary to valvular PS. The latter form adds a dynamic obstruction to the fixed one caused by the valvular PS. Subvalvular obstruction can also be caused by the presence of an isolated fibrous ring localized under the valvular ostium (Figure 19-12).

Severe subvalvular obstructions can be caused by a double-chambered right ventricle. In this malformation, the right ventricular cavity is divided into two parts by an abnormal muscular, fibromuscular, or fibrous band, sometimes with thick endocardial proliferation on its rim. The right ventricular cavity thus becomes divided into a proximal "high-pressure" chamber and distal "low-pressure" chamber [41,42]. The location of this band may vary but is usually downstream of the tricuspid septal leaflet, connecting the ventricular septum to the anterior wall of the right ventricle (Figure 19-13) [43].

Pulmonic Stenosis Associated with a Coronary Anomaly

Another cause of PS, observed mostly in English Bulldogs [44,45] but sometimes in other breeds, is the coronary artery malformation type R2A, characterized by an aberrant coronary artery encircling the pulmonary artery

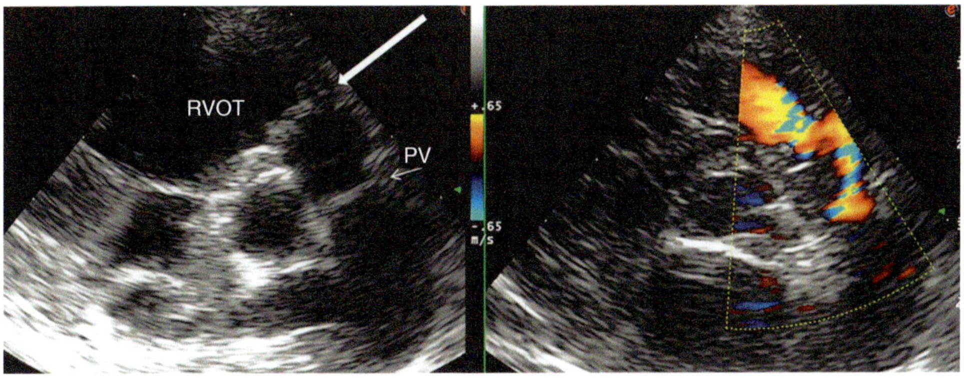

• **Fig. 19-12** Right parasternal short axis parasternal view of the heart base with *(right)* and without *(left)* color Doppler in a dog with a subvalvular diaphragm *(large arrow)* obstructing the right ventricular outflow tract (RVOT) as well as valvular pulmonic stenosis (PS) *(small arrow)*, as indicated by the domed appearance of the pulmonic valve (PV) in systole *(left)*. The image on the right is taken in diastole and shows a pulmonic regurgitation flow going through the malformed valve and the subvalvular diaphragm. (Photo credit: Claudio Bussadori.)

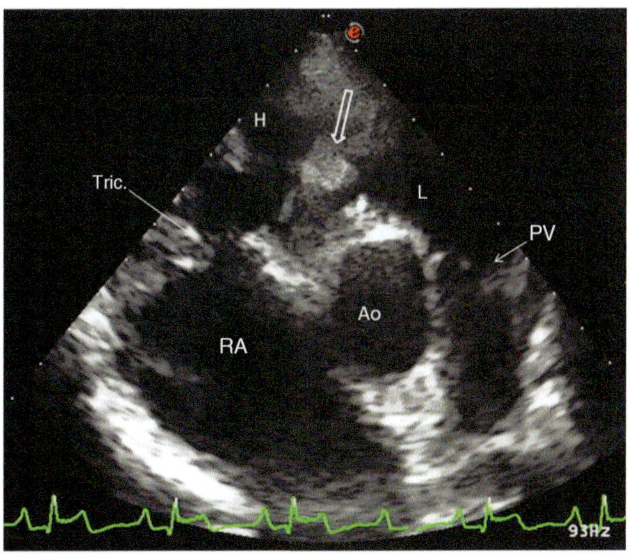

• **Fig. 19-13** Right parasternal short axis view of the base of the heart in a dog with a double-chambered right ventricle. The *openwork arrow* indicates abnormal fibromuscular tissue connecting the right ventricular anterior papillary muscle to the conal septum. Only a narrow passage exists between the filling cavity and the right ventricular outflow tract. The pressure in the filling cavity (H) is then elevated, while the pressure in the outflow tract (L) is low. The tricuspid (Tric.) and pulmonic valves (PV) are normal. The right atrium (RA) is dilated. *Ao*, Aorta. (Photo credit: Claudio Bussadori.)

(Figure 19-14) [46]. Histologic examination suggests that the underlying cause of this syndrome is a malformation of the left aortic sinus of Valsalva with inversion of the proximal segment of the left main coronary artery [45]. It is important to recognize this type of PS, since balloon valvuloplasty should not be performed in these animals (see Chapter 20).

Echocardiographic Aspects

Bidimensional and TM Echocardiographic Characteristics

Evaluation of the Valvular Apparatus

The morphologic evaluation of the pulmonic valvular apparatus and of the main pulmonary artery includes assessment of the valvular thickening and the fusion and mobility of the leaflets as well as identification of any fixed supravalvular or subvalvular obstruction. The examination begins with a right parasternal short axis transaortic view, on which the pulmonic valve annulus, the valvular leaflets, the RVOT, and the main pulmonary artery can be studied. The pulmonic and aortic annuli must be measured, for comparison, from inner edge to inner edge, right below the insertion point of the valvular leaflets in end-systole. The RVOT, pulmonic valve annulus, main pulmonary artery, and its bifurcation into the two pulmonary arteries are usually more visible using a left cranial parasternal short axis view (Figure 19-15).

This view also allows the acquisition of good cine-loops of the RVOT flow to look for possible dynamic stenosis.

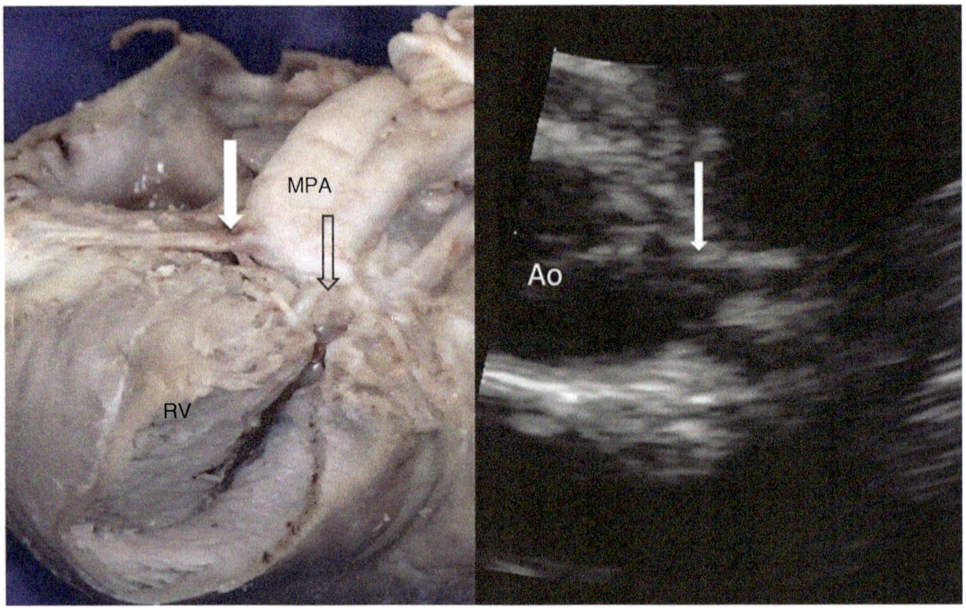

• **Fig. 19-14** Anatomic specimen and zoom of an echocardiographic view of the cardiac base in an American Staffordshire Terrier puppy with a type R2A coronary anomaly. The abnormal coronary artery *(solid arrows)* surrounds and strangles the pulmonic valve annulus *(openwork arrow)*. *Ao,* Aorta; *MPA,* main pulmonary aorta; *RV,* right ventricle. (Photo credit: Claudio Bussadori.)

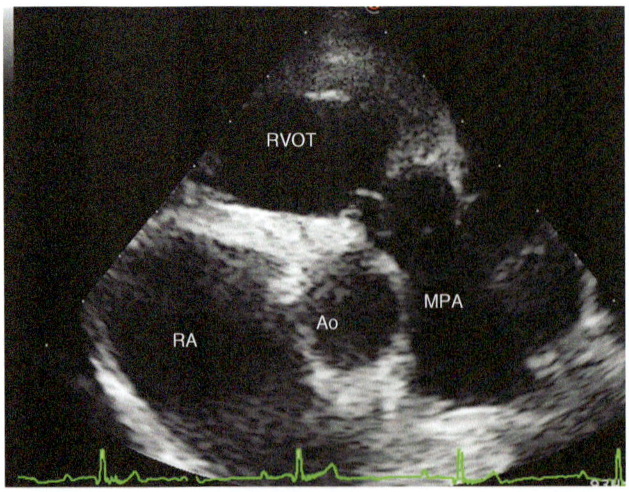

• **Fig. 19-15** Standard left cranial parasternal view for the evaluation of the right ventricular outflow tract (RVOT), the pulmonic valve, and the main pulmonary artery (MPA). *Ao,* Aorta; *RA,* right atrium. (Photo credit: Claudio Bussadori.)

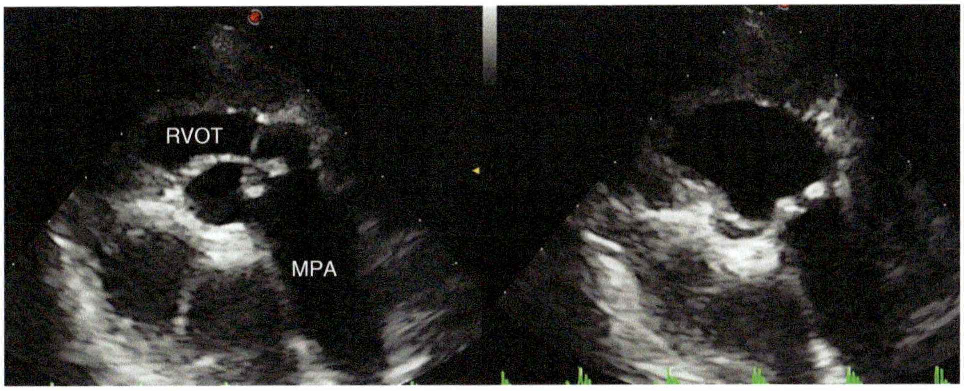

• **Fig. 19-16** Left cranial parasternal short axis view in a dog with type A valvular pulmonic stenosis (PS). The view on the left is taken in diastole. The view on the right is frozen in systole and demonstrates the domed appearance of the moderately thickened pulmonic valve cusps. *MPA,* Main pulmonary artery; *RVOT,* right ventricular outflow tract. (Photo credit: Claudio Bussadori.)

The 2D echocardiographic examination of the pulmonic valvular apparatus enables distinction between type A and type B PS [25].

Type A Pulmonic Stenosis. It is characterized by the lack of separation of the two valvular leaflets, which remain fused and move in systole like a diaphragm, with a dome-shaped appearance toward the main pulmonary artery (systolic doming effect) (Figure 19-16). The annulus has a normal size, with an aortic annulus/pulmonic valve annulus ratio <1.2. The main pulmonary artery and the proximal right and left pulmonary arteries are frequently dilated.

Type B Pulmonic Stenosis. It is characterized by severely thickened, poorly mobile leaflets, generally without fusion of the commissures. In more severe cases, this type of valvular stenosis is frequently associated with hypoplasia of the pulmonary annulus and an aortic annulus/pulmonic valve annulus ratio >1.5 (Figure 19-17) [47,48].

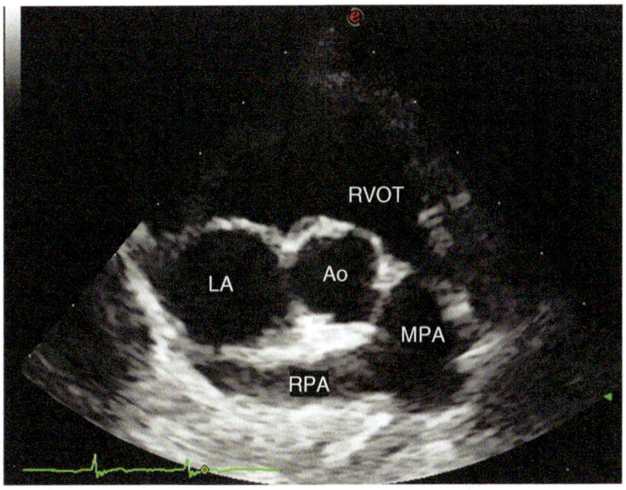

• **Fig. 19-17** Right parasternal short axis view of the base of the heart in an English Bulldog with type B valvular pulmonic stenosis (PS). The pulmonic valve annulus is hypoplasic. The pulmonic valve cusps are thickened. The main pulmonary artery (MPA) is dilated. *Ao,* Aorta; *LA,* left atrium; *RPA,* right pulmonary artery; *RVOT,* right ventricular outflow tract. (Photo credit: Claudio Bussadori.)

The echocardiographic examination needs to focus on the morphologic evaluation of the pulmonic valve and the main pulmonary artery, the assessment of right ventricular remodeling, and the right ventricular inflow and outflow characteristics.

Right Ventricular Hypertrophy

The degree of right ventricular hypertrophy as well as the right ventricular function can be assessed by both M-mode and 2D echocardiography. In the presence of PS, the inflow tract (better visualized using the right parasternal long axis and apical 4 chambers views) and the outflow tract walls are thickened and may be hypokinetic (Figure 19-18). In advanced cases, the chronic pressure overload leads to systolic dysfunction, with decreased motion and thickness of the right ventricular wall and progressive dilation of the right ventricular cavity (Figure 19-19).

Paradoxic Movement of the Interventricular Septum

The paradoxic systolic movement of the interventricular septum results from its exaggerated displacement toward the left ventricle during systole. It is caused by the increased systolic right ventricular pressure, reducing the

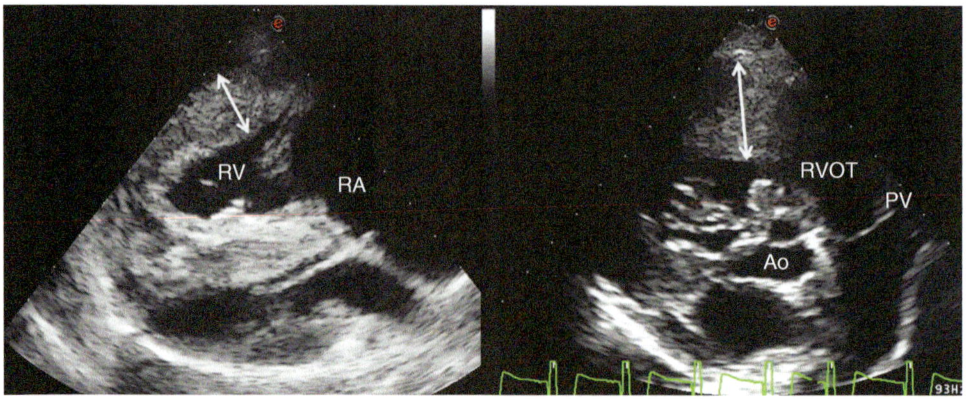

• **Fig. 19-18** Right parasternal long axis 4 chambers view *(left)* and right parasternal short axis view of the heart base *(right)* in a dog with severe pulmonic stenosis (PS). The right ventricular free wall is hypertrophied at the level of the inflow *(left)* and outflow tracts *(right, arrows)*. *Ao,* Aorta; *PV,* pulmonic valve; *RA,* right atrium; *RV,* right ventricle; *RVOT,* right ventricular outflow tract. (Photo credit: Claudio Bussadori.)

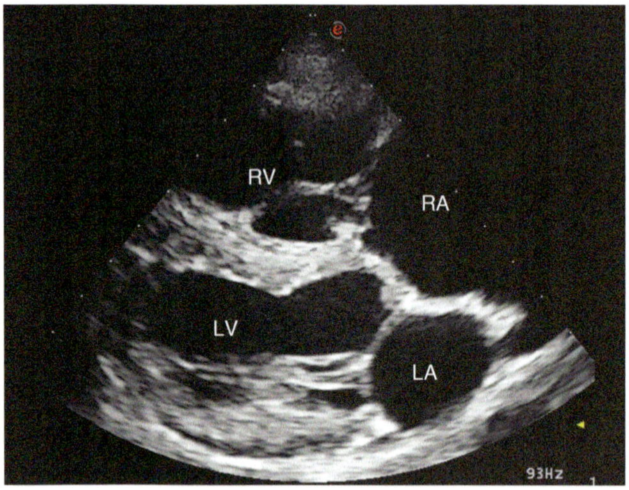

• **Fig. 19-19** Right parasternal long axis 4 chambers view in a 7-year-old Cocker Spaniel with severe pulmonic stenosis (PS). The right ventricular cavity is dilated. *LA,* Left atrium; *LV,* left ventricle; *RA,* right atrium; *RV,* right ventricle. (Photo credit: Claudio Bussadori.)

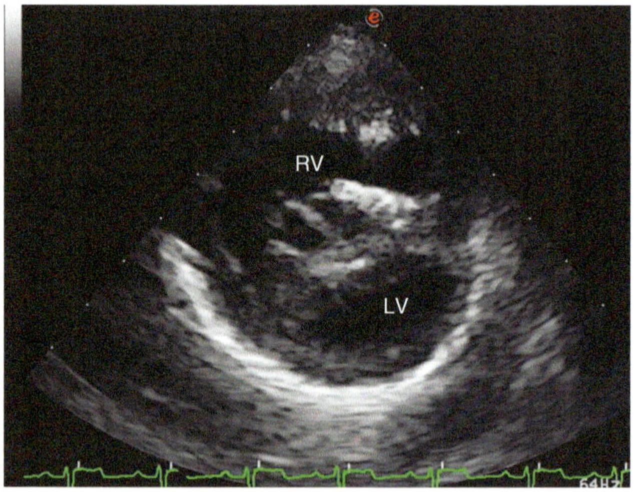

• **Fig. 19-20** Right parasternal short axis transventricular view in a dog with severe pulmonic stenosis (PS). The septum is flattened in systole. The geometry of the left ventricle (LV) is altered and its internal diameter is reduced. *RV,* Right ventricle. (Photo credit: Claudio Bussadori.)

pressure gradient between the two ventricles. The septal curvature radius is thus decreased, leading to its flattening. This flattening of the septum may be best appreciated on a right parasternal short axis view (Figure 19-20). In time-motion (TM) mode, the septum moves posteriorly, increasing the systolic diameter of the right ventricle and accentuating the decrease of the left ventricular systolic diameter (Figure 19-21). Dilation of the main pulmonary artery with hypertrophy of the right ventricle and paradoxic septal motion also can be seen in cases of pulmonary arterial hypertension. Evaluation of the pulmonic valvular morphology and documentation of an outflow obstruction by Doppler will allow one to easily distinguish the two conditions [49].

Doppler Characteristics

Color Doppler helps to locate the obstruction site of the RVOT (Video 19-3).

Spectral Doppler analysis of the pulmonic flow, mostly performed by CW Doppler, allows the measurement of the maximum and mean pressure gradients through the stenosis. Based on these pressures gradients, three levels of PS severity have generally been agreed upon:

- Mild PS: peak gradient <50 mm Hg
- Moderate PS: peak gradient of 50 to 80 mm Hg
- Severe PS: peak gradient >80 mm Hg

The dynamic subvalvular component of the global pressure gradient can be derived from careful analysis of the CW signal of the pulmonic flow. It appears as a bright shape superimposed on the signal of the fixed obstruction, starting after the onset of the main signal and peaking late, thus adopting the shape of a knife blade (Figure 19-22).

The presence of any tricuspid regurgitation (TR) should be documented because TR may worsen the prognosis, especially if it is significant. TR and severe stenosis are

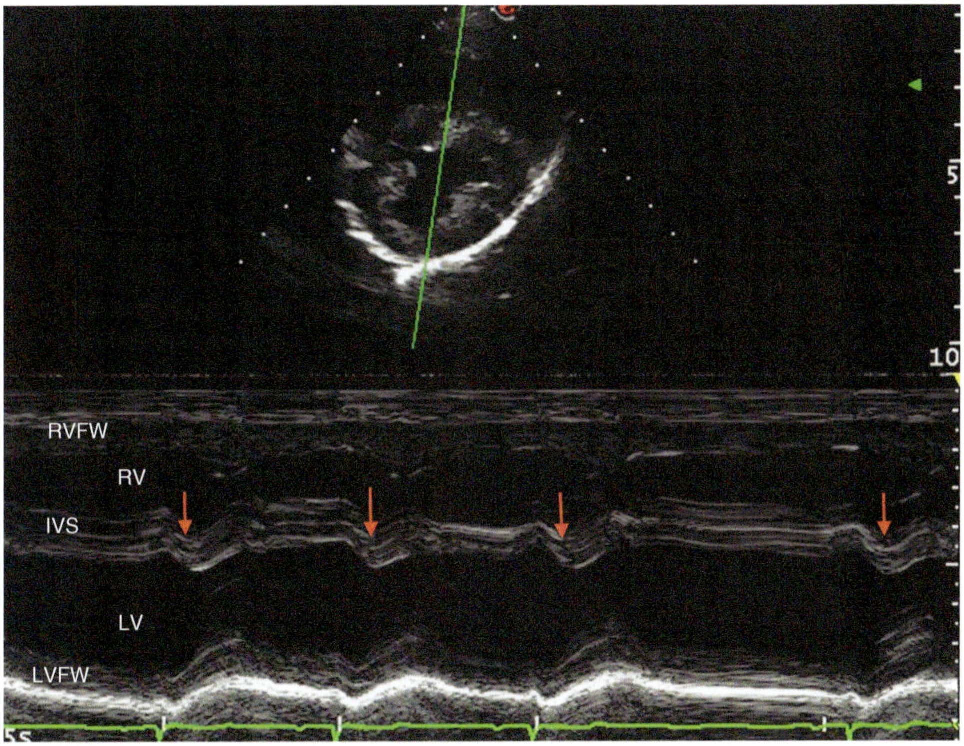

• **Fig. 19-21** Time-motion (TM) echocardiogram (transventricular view) in a dog with severe pulmonic stenosis (PS). The elevated right ventricular systolic pressure pushes the septum toward the left ventricle (LV), exaggerating its systolic posterior motion *(arrows)*. *IVS,* Interventricular septum; *LVFW,* left ventricular free wall; *RV,* right ventricle; *RVFW,* right ventricular free wall. (Photo credit: Claudio Bussadori.)

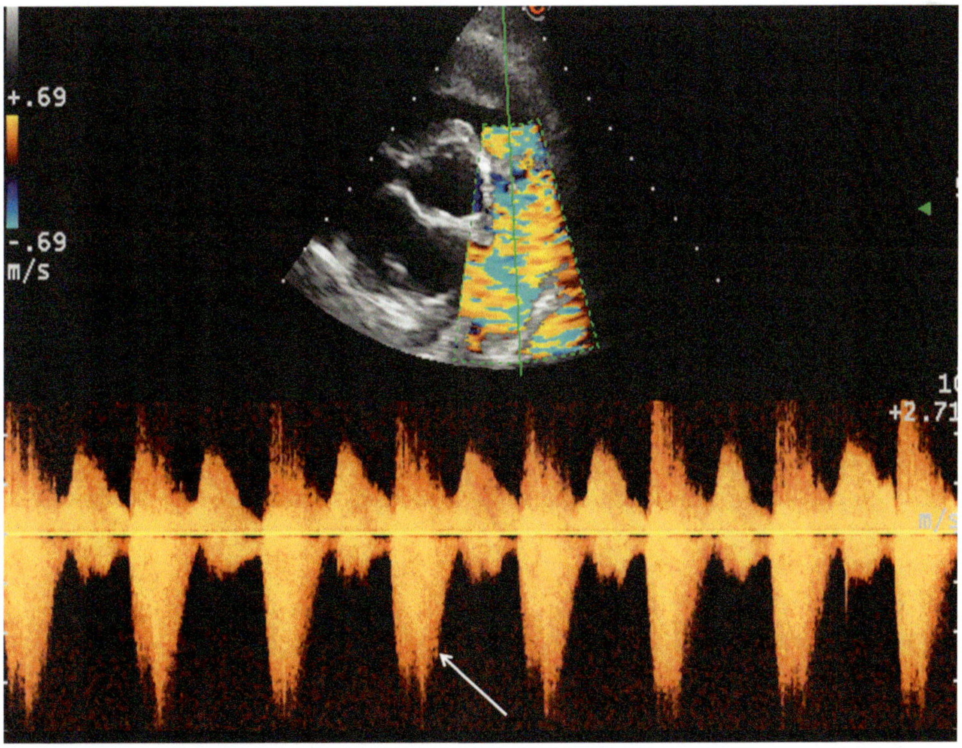

• **Fig. 19-22** Right parasternal short axis view of the base of the heart, with color and continuous wave spectral Doppler of the pulmonic flow in a dog with pulmonic stenosis (PS). The *arrow* indicates the "blade-like" aspect of the dynamic valvular stenosis superimposed on the fixed valvular obstruction signal. (Photo credit: Claudio Bussadori.)

independent predictors of cardiac death. Pressure gradients >60 mm Hg are associated with an increased risk of cardiac death, with 86% sensitivity and 71% specificity. These animals may benefit from pulmonic valve dilation [50-53].

Patent Ductus Arteriosus

Patent ductus arteriosus (PDA) results from the nonclosure of the ductus arteriosus after birth, leading to shunting of blood from the descending aorta into the pulmonary artery. It is a very common CHD in dogs [2,54] but extremely rare in cats [55,56]. It is usually an isolated defect. A polygenic type of inheritance has been shown in Miniature Poodles [57]. It is more often seen in German Shepherds and other Shepherd breeds, Collies, Newfoundlands, and Yorkshire Terriers but also may be found in mixed-breed dogs [9]. It is extremely rare in brachycephalic breeds [9]. Females are more predisposed to PDA than males [9]. Rarely, PDA can be associated with other congenital cardiopathies such as PS, left ventricle hypoplasia, and atrioventricular valve dysplasia [58]. The most common association observed in our laboratory is PDA and SAS in Newfoundlands.

The clinical signs depend on the amount of shunting. Dogs with small size PDA may remain asymptomatic for years whereas dogs with large size PDA may go into congestive heart failure before adulthood. Mitral regurgitation (MR) secondary to the mitral valve annulus dilation may eventually complicate PDA. In some dogs, the direction of the shunting could be reversed from left-to-right to right-to-left due to the presence of pulmonary hypertension (reverse PDA). The venous blood thus ejected in the descending aorta may lead to poor oxygenation of the lower extremity of the body, with weakness of the hind legs and cyanosis of the genital membranes.

Anatomopathology

The ductus arteriosus is an important channel in the fetal circulation. It extends from the bifurcation of the pulmonary artery to the area between the arch and the descending aorta, downstream of the origin of the left subclavian artery. The pulmonary extremity of the ductus arteriosus is wrapped into the reflection of the pericardium. During intrauterine life, the ductus allows the passage of blood coming from the main pulmonary artery directly into the aorta, the lung vasculature being nonpatent. The ductus normally closes spontaneously within the first days of life, when the pulmonary vascular resistance drops. The ductus closure is initiated by the rise in arterial oxygenation. Initially, the muscular fibers of the ductal wall contract, then postnatal intimal proliferation and the formation of thrombus occlude the ductal lumen. Ultimately, this vessel involutes progressively into a fibrous ligament [59-61]. If the ductus does not close, a left-to-right shunt is established leading to pulmonary overcirculation and left ventricular volume overload. During the perinatal period, adaptative mechanisms to this volume overload lead to marked ventricular hypertrophy and hyperplasia of myocardial cells [62]. This phenomenon of postnatal cell proliferation allows animals affected with PDA to develop an extraordinary degree of left ventricular dilatation, not seen in any other acquired left ventricular volume overload situation [63].

Echocardiographic Aspects

The goal of echocardiography in evaluating a patient with PDA is not only to confirm the diagnosis, but also to identify any other cardiovascular-associated pathologies, to evaluate the impact of the volume overload, to evaluate the anatomy of the PDA in order to plan the surgical or transcatheter occlusion, and to evaluate the possible need for other postoperative treatment.

Bidimensional and TM Echocardiography

Based on its ductal dimension, PDA can be classified into three broad categories:

- Small size PDA: The diameter of the ductal pulmonary ostium is <3 mm in small dogs and <4.5 to 5 mm in large dogs. Mild or moderate left ventricular dilatation may be observed, depending on the age of the dog. The systolic function remains normal.
- Medium size PDA: The diameter of the ductal pulmonary ostium is ≈4 mm in small dogs and ≈5 to 6 mm in large dogs. The left ventricular dimensions are generally increased (i.e., an end-diastolic volume index [EDVI] >150 mL/m^2 and an end-systolic volume index [ESVI] >60 mL/m^2). The mitral annulus is dilated and a central jet of MR may be observed. The main pulmonary artery appears dilated.
- Large size PDA: The diameter of the ductal pulmonary ostium is >5 mm in small dogs and >6 to 7 mm in large dogs. There is severe left ventricular remodeling, with an EDVI >200mL/m^2 and an ESVI >100 mL/m^2, and a change in geometry, with increased sphericity and volume/mass ratio. The ejection fraction is decreased. On the right parasternal long axis 4 chambers view, the first noticeable change is the increased left atrial and left ventricular inflow and outflow tract sizes (Video 19-4). Mitral annulus dilation gives the anterior mitral leaflet an elongated appearance (Figure 19-23). This may result in MR and marked left atrial dilation in severe cases.

On the right parasternal short axis view of the heart base, the dilation of the main pulmonary artery as well as the ostium of the PDA can be seen (Figure 19-24).

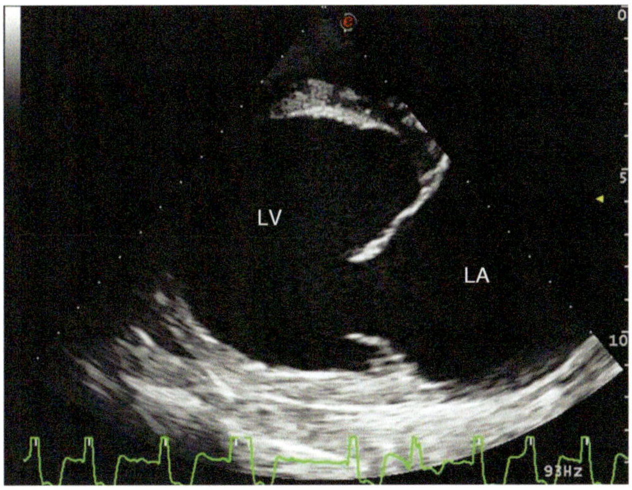

• **Fig. 19-23** Right parasternal long axis 4 chambers view in a dog with a patent ductus arteriosus (PDA) and significant left-to-right shunt. The left ventricle (LV) is spherical and markedly dilated. The left atrium (LA) is equally dilated. (Photo credit: Claudio Bussadori.)

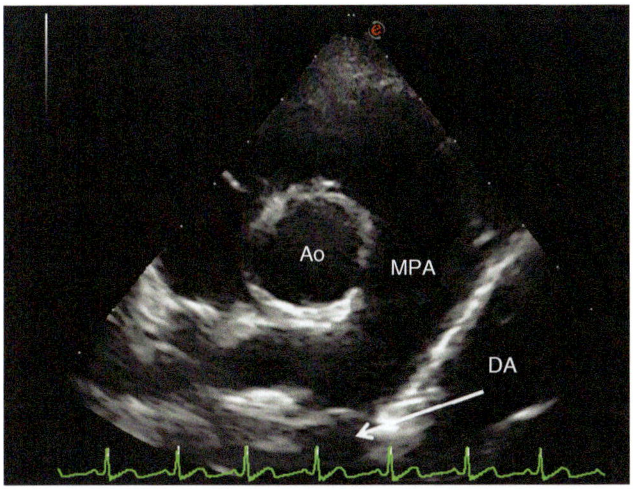

• **Fig. 19-24** Right parasternal short axis view of the base of the heart in a dog with a patent ductus arteriosus (PDA). The main pulmonary artery (MPA) is dilated. The PDA ampulla is visible *(arrow)*. *Ao,* Aorta. (Photo credit: Claudio Bussadori.)

The left cranial parasternal short axis view allows better visualization of the ductus, which may be seen in its entirety by directing the ultrasound beam slightly dorsally with respect to the pulmonary bifurcation (Figure 19-25). The shape of the ductus arteriosus is extremely variable: cylindrical, hourglass-shaped, funnel-shaped with narrowing at the pulmonary extremity, or with an aneurysmal dilation. This view should be used to obtain the most reliable measurements of the diameters of the ductal ostium and ampulla and to assess any aneurysmal dilation of the PDA. The PDA ostium must be well identified to accurately measure its diameter. A very common mistake with TTE is to measure the ductal ampulla instead of the ostial diameter, leading to overestimation of the occluding device size. In some cases, the length of

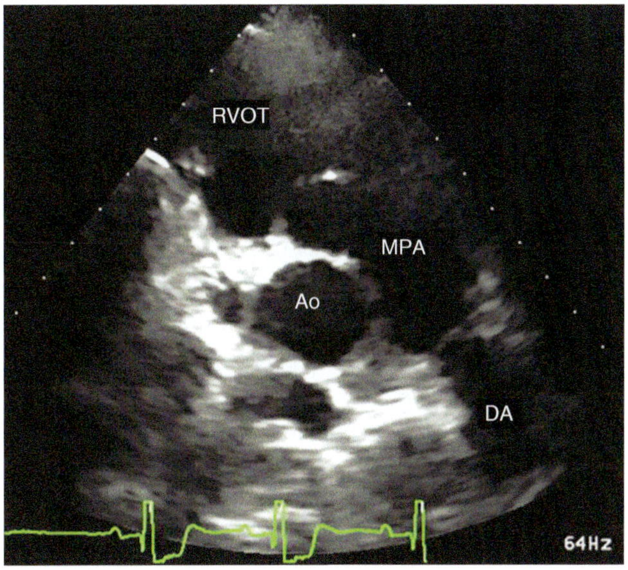

• **Fig. 19-25** Left cranial parasternal short axis view directed so as to visualize the patent ductus arteriosus (PDA) and its minimal diameter. *Ao,* Aorta; *MPA,* main pulmonary artery; *RVOT,* right ventricular outflow tract. (Photo credit: Claudio Bussadori.)

the ductus can also be measured. However, angiographic measures are more reliable [64]. All of these measures are necessary to select the best surgical or interventional closure option [65]. This view also allows the best possible alignment with the ductal flow for spectral and color Doppler studies. A more elongated view of the PDA can be obtained by rotating the probe 180 degrees counterclockwise from this view (Figure 19-26).

TM mode measurements used in PDA staging are end-systolic and end-diastolic left ventricular internal dimensions and the shortening fraction (SF). In the early stages of left-to-right shunting, the SF remains within the normal reference range, because systolic and diastolic diameters increase together. The SF decreases with the development of left ventricular systolic dysfunction (Figure 19-27). The degree of cardiac remodeling depends on the ductal ostium diameter and its relationship to the animal's size, as well as on the age of the animal prior to PDA closure. Within certain ductal sizes, the patient is able to adapt to the conditions caused by the increased pulmonary circulation. However, this does not occur when the duct is particularly large [66,67]. This cardiopathy will evolve progressively toward systolic dysfunction with symptoms of left-sided congestive heart failure or toward Eisenmenger syndrome (reverse PDA) (see below) [68,69].

Doppler Echocardiography

Spectral Doppler

The best alignment with the PDA flow can be obtained from both the right and the left parasternal views. Continuous Doppler allows measurement of the duration of the flow, its peak velocity, and variations during systole

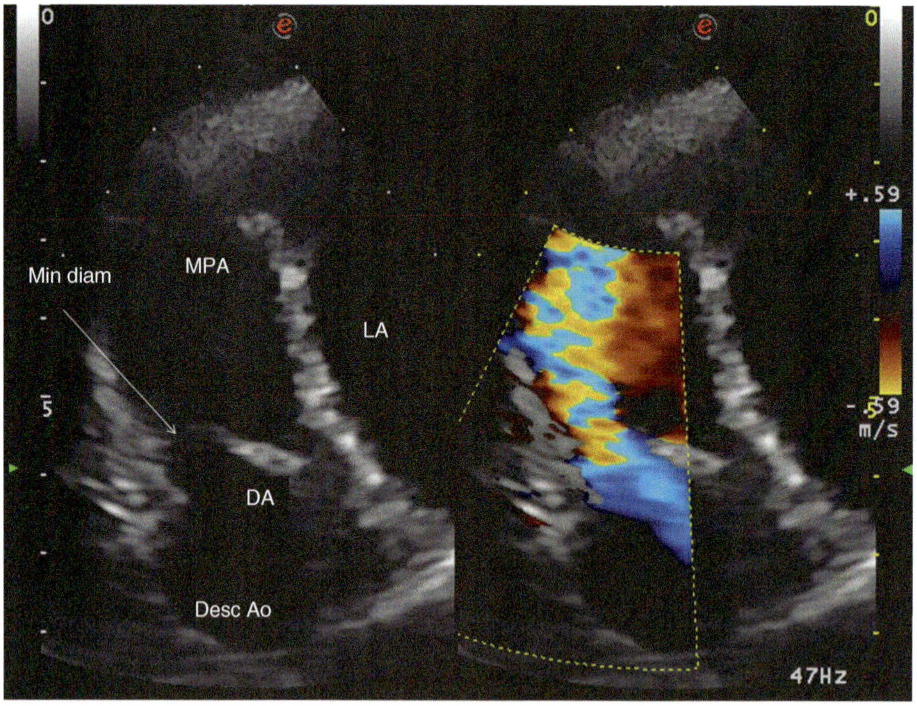

• **Fig. 19-26** Left cranial parasternal views of the cardiac base without *(left)* and with *(right)* color Doppler obtained by rotating the probe by 180 degrees in a counterclockwise fashion from the left cranial short axis position. The minimum diameter (Min diam) of the patent ductus arteriosus (PDA) is clearly visible. *Desc Ao,* Descending aorta; *LA,* left atrium; *MPA,* main pulmonary artery. (Photo credit: Claudio Bussadori.)

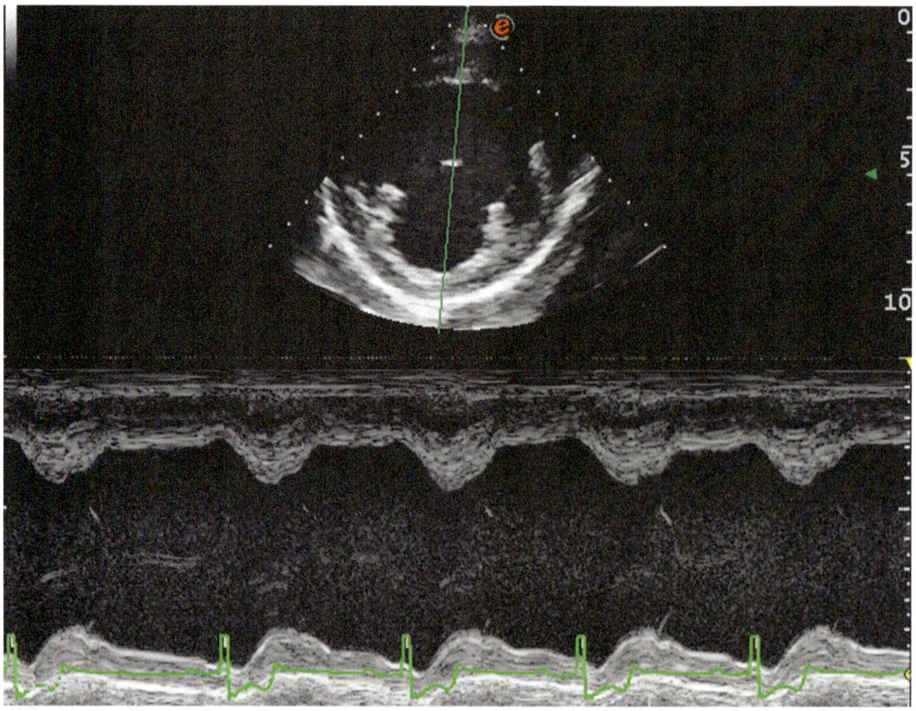

• **Fig. 19-27** Time-motion (TM) echocardiogram (transventricular view) in a dog with patent ductus arteriosus (PDA) and significant left-to-right shunt. Note the marked left ventricular dilation and moderate reduction of the contractility. (Photo credit: Claudio Bussadori.)

and diastole. The peak transductal flow velocity is governed by the gradient between aorta and pulmonary artery. In the absence of pulmonary hypertension or systolic dysfunction of the left ventricle, peak velocity will be around 4.5 m/s with a peak gradient around 80 mm Hg (Figure 19-28). The recording of lower peak velocities may be due to inadequate alignment of the ultrasound beam with the shunting flow, severe left ventricular dysfunction, or increased pulmonary artery pressure.

Pulsed wave Doppler allows quantification of the flow through the different valves and calculation of the pulmonic-to-systemic stroke volume ratio (Qp/Qs). In the case of a PDA, the Qp/Qs is measured differently than in other congenital cardiopathies: the Qp is obtained from the aortic systolic flow and the Qs from the systolic flow at the pulmonic valve annulus. This is because the only way to measure the pulmonary blood flow distal to the PDA is to measure it after its return to the heart via the pulmonary veins, therefore at the aortic level. The stroke volumes through the aortic or pulmonic valves are calculated by multiplying the velocity-time integral of the spectral Doppler envelope of the valvular flow by the area of the valve annulus (obtained by 2D echocardiography).

Color Doppler

Color Doppler is useful to identify transductal flow and possible pulmonic or mitral regurgitation. The turbulent high-velocity PDA flow is readily visible coming from the ductus toward the main pulmonary artery (Video 19-5). There is aliasing, creating a mosaic. The extension of the jet can give a semiquantitative indication of how much flow goes through the shunt. Therefore small "flames" of color indicate a ductus with a small PDA flow whereas an important dispersion of the mosaic effect in the main pulmonary artery indicates a large left-to-right shunt.

Pulmonary Arterial Hypertension: Reverse PDA

In a case of very large PDA, remodeling with severe hypertrophy of the smooth muscles of small pulmonary arteries occurs during the first months of life in order to protect pulmonary alveoli from volume overload. This results in a precapillary pulmonary hypertension and subsequent inversion of the shunt, which becomes right-to-left [69]. This reversal of flow due to the establishment of pulmonary hypertension is called Eisenmenger syndrome. The pulmonary hypertension in PDA with Eisenmenger syndrome should not be confused with postcapillary

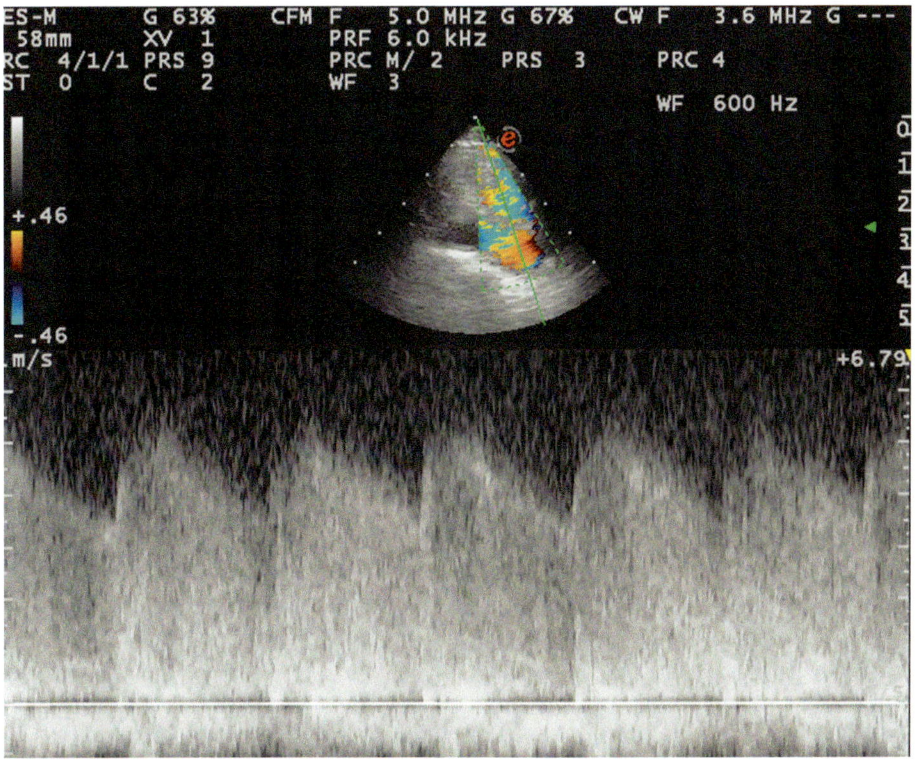

• **Fig. 19-28** Continuous spectral Doppler of a patent ductus arteriosus (PDA) flow recorded from a left cranial parasternal short axis view. The maximum pressure gradient between the aorta and the pulmonary artery is 100 mm Hg. (Photo credit: Claudio Bussadori.)

pulmonary hypertension that can be observed in some adult subjects with large PDA and severe chronic volume overload. In the latter case, the echocardiographic changes are still related to left ventricular volume overload with evidence of moderate pulmonary hypertension such as flattening of the interventricular septum, reduction of the aortopulmonary gradient, and TR. A complete reversal of the shunt in this situation is extremely rare. The echocardiographic pattern of reverse PDA always includes severe right ventricular hypertrophy with a normal or only mildly dilated left ventricle. The pulmonary artery is always dilated and the ductus is large, short, and without narrowing at the pulmonary extremity. Ductal flow is sometimes identifiable using low pulse repetition frequency (PRF) because of its low velocity (Figure 19-29). CW spectral Doppler easily identifies the pulmonic (Figure 19-30) and tricuspid regurgitant flows. With analysis of the latter, systolic, diastolic, and mean pulmonary pressures can be estimated. Echocardiographic confirmation of the presence of reverse PDA can be obtained by contrast echocardiography. In this particular condition, the blood flows through the PDA shunt from the main pulmonary artery into the descending aorta. The injection of an agitated saline solution in a peripheral vein results in micro-bubbles, which can be seen first in the right atrium and right ventricle, then in the pulmonary artery, and finally in the abdominal aorta. A specific contrast agent is not necessary, since it will not go through the lungs. In our laboratory, we use a mixture of 50% saline and 50% colloid solution

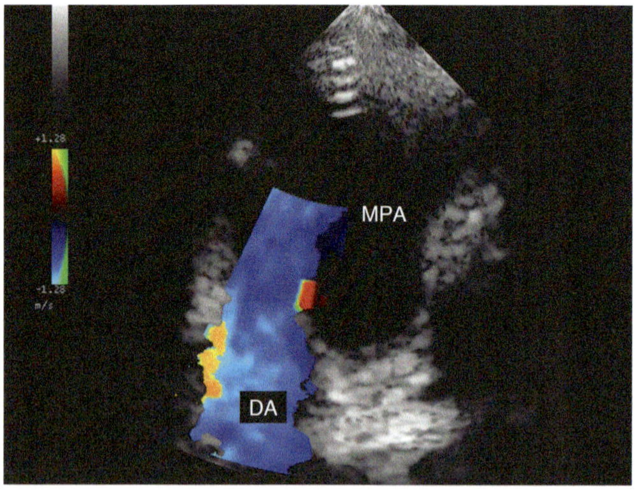

• **Fig. 19-29** Left cranial parasternal view with color Doppler in a dog with a very large patent ductus arteriosus (PDA) and Eisenmenger syndrome. A systolic flow traveling from the main pulmonary artery (MPA) toward the descending aorta is visible through the canal. (Photo credit: Claudio Bussadori.)

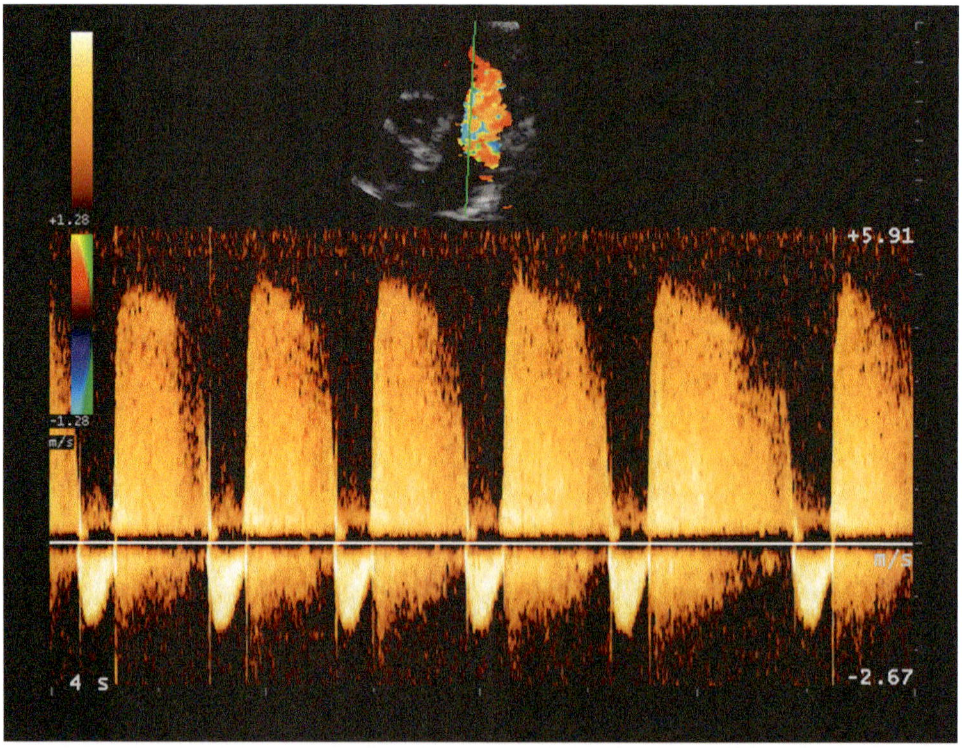

• **Fig. 19-30** Continuous wave spectral Doppler of a pulmonic regurgitation flow in a dog with reverse patent ductus arteriosus (PDA). The pulmonary regurgitation flow velocity is very elevated due to severe pulmonary arterial hypertension. (Photo credit: Claudio Bussadori.)

(Pentaspan ND®), using two syringes connected to a three-way stopcock, itself connected to a venous catheter (Figure 19-31). Once the solution is vigorously mixed, it is injected and bubbles can be identified in the abdominal aorta (Figure 19-32).

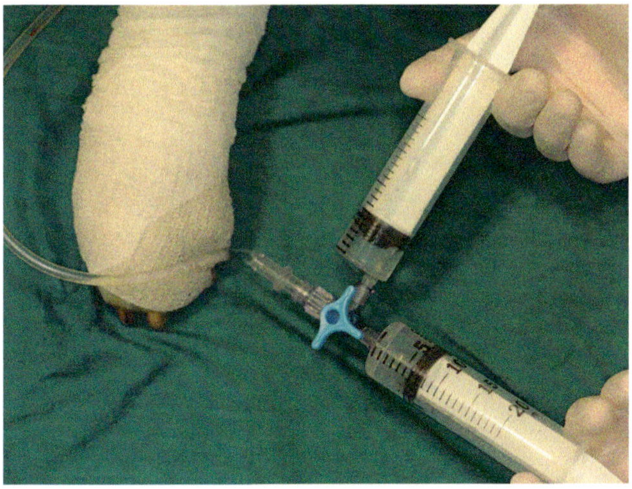

• **Fig. 19-31** The saline and colloid solution must be vigorously mixed prior to injection. (Photo credit: Claudio Bussadori.)

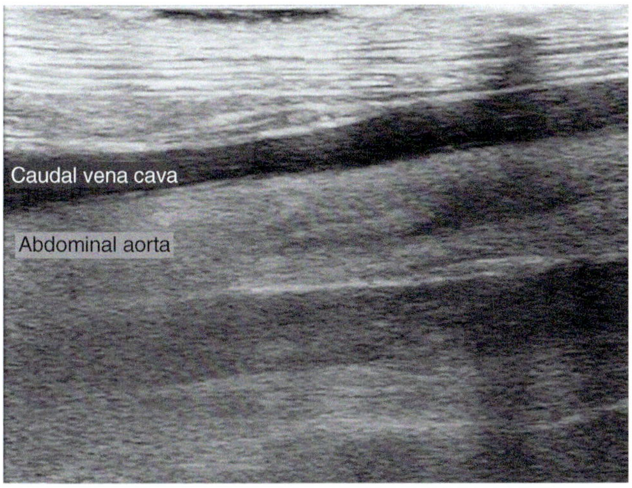

• **Fig. 19-32** Opacification of the abdominal aorta following the injection of the saline and colloid solution mixture in the cephalic vein in a dog with reverse patent ductus arteriosus (PDA). (Photo credit: Claudio Bussadori.)

Ventricular Septal Defect

Ventricular septal defect (VSD) is a congenital cardiac malformation characterized by an abnormal communication between the two ventricular chambers due to the presence of one or more holes in the ventricular septum [70].

A genetic transmission of VSD in dogs and cats has not been established. There is no sex predisposition. Breeds of dogs considered at risk are West Highland White Terriers, Lakeland Terriers, English Bulldogs, and English Springer Spaniels [71]. Sometimes VSD can be associated with other congenital cardiopathies, such as SAS, PDA, or double-chambered right ventricle, or be a part of a complex congenital malformation such as tetralogy of Fallot. In cats, VSD is one of the most common congenital heart malformations [71,72].

The amount of blood flow being shunted from the left ventricle into the right ventricle, and from there into the pulmonary artery, depends on the size of the ventricular communication, the pressure gradient that exists between the two communicating chambers, and afterload. The resistance to blood flow in a small (also called "restrictive") VSD limits the amount of left-to-right shunting and its hemodynamic impact. Conversely, a large (nonrestrictive) VSD does not create a resistance to the flow, allowing a large amount of left-to-right shunting, which will increase the right ventricular systolic load, leading to increased pulmonary flow. As a result, the left ventricular diastolic load will rise. In some cases, the increased pulmonary pressure results in a hypertrophic reaction of the pulmonary arteriole muscles, increasing the resistance to the vascular bed (Eisenmenger syndrome). Severe defects are rarely diagnosed in veterinary medicine, probably because puppies that are affected die within the first weeks of life due to left-sided congestive heart failure.

Anatomopathology

VSDs can be classified according to their position on the ventricular septum.

- Perimembranous VSDs (also called subaortic or infracristal VSDs) are located near the fibrous portion (next to the fibrous trigone of the heart formed by the aorta and the atrioventricular valves). This is the most common type encountered in dogs.
- Membranous VSDs (also called malalignment VSDs) result from the abnormal alignment of the infundibulum and the muscular septa (as in tetralogy of Fallot).
- Inlet VSDs are localized near the entrance of the ventricle, next to the mitral and tricuspid septal leaflets.
- Conal septum VSDs (also called subpulmonic, infundibular supracristal, ventricular outlet, subarterial doubly committed, or septal cone VSDs) are localized in the outlet portion of the septum, extending up to the semilunar valve (aortic and pulmonic). The right coronary aortic cusp may prolapse into the defect, causing aortic valve insufficiency and dilation of the sinus of Valsalva.
- Muscular-type VSDs are localized on the trabecular portion of the ventricular septum. These VSDs can be

of different sizes and can be classified according to their location as apical, anterior muscular, and midmuscular. Sometimes muscular VSDs have multiple channels.

Echocardiographic Aspects

The goals of echocardiography, when evaluating a VSD, are to identify the defect, define its size and extension, determine the direction of the shunt, evaluate the hemodynamic consequences and ventricular remodeling, and quantify the shunt.

Bidimensional and TM Echocardiography

The right parasternal long axis view optimized for the left ventricular outflow tract is the best view to see perimembranous, infracristal, and muscular VSD; their anterior extension; and the pseudoaneurysmal membrane that, in some cases, partially closes the defect (Figure 19-33) [73-75].

The inflow muscular VSD, localized between the mitral and tricuspid septal leaflets, is better visualized from the right parasternal long axis and short axis and apical 4 chambers views (Figure 19-34).

The right parasternal short axis view at the level of the heart base allows good visualization of perimembranous and subaortic defects (Figure 19-35).

Muscular defects of the trabeculae, located in the mid or apical septum, are better visualized from a right parasternal short axis view at the apical level of the ventricular septum (Figure 19-36).

TM mode measurements performed in affected patients may reveal an increased EDVI, depending on the severity of left volume overload. The SF increases in the initial stages, then declines with progressive left ventricular dysfunction.

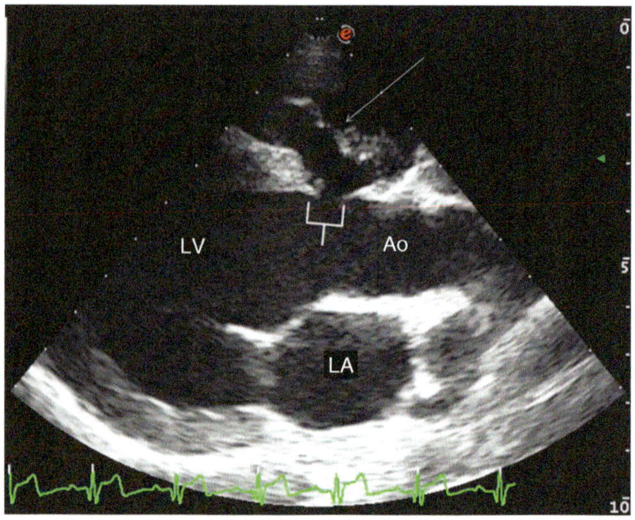

• **Fig. 19-33** Right parasternal long axis 5 chambers view in a dog with a perimembranous ventricular septal defect (VSD). The communication is clearly visible *(brackets)*. A pseudoaneurysmal tissue is floating in the right ventricle *(arrow)*. *Ao,* Aorta; *LA,* left atrium; *LV,* left ventricle. (Photo credit: Claudio Bussadori.)

Doppler Echocardiography

Color Doppler

The color Doppler may facilitate the localization of small VSD that are difficult to identify with 2D echocardiography (Video 19-6). It also helps to identify the borders of the defect. Finally, it allows proper orientation of the CW Doppler cursor in order to get good flow alignment and accurate measurement of the peak transventricular pressure gradient.

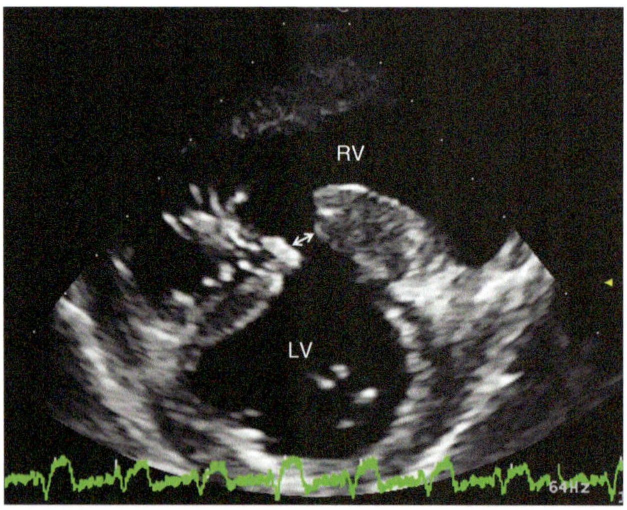

• **Fig. 19-34** Right parasternal short axis transventricular view in a dog with muscular ventricular septal defect (VSD) *(double arrow)* at the level of the left ventricular inflow tract. *LV,* Left ventricle; *RV,* right ventricle. (Photo credit: Claudio Bussadori.)

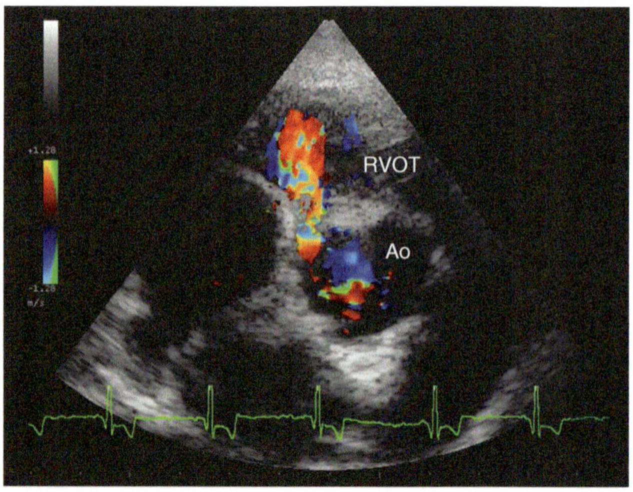

• **Fig. 19-35** Right parasternal short axis transaortic view in color Doppler mode in a dog with a perimembranous ventricular septal defect (VSD). The turbulent flow traveling from the aorta (Ao) into the right ventricular outflow tract (RVOT) through the defect is visible. (Photo credit: Claudio Bussadori.)

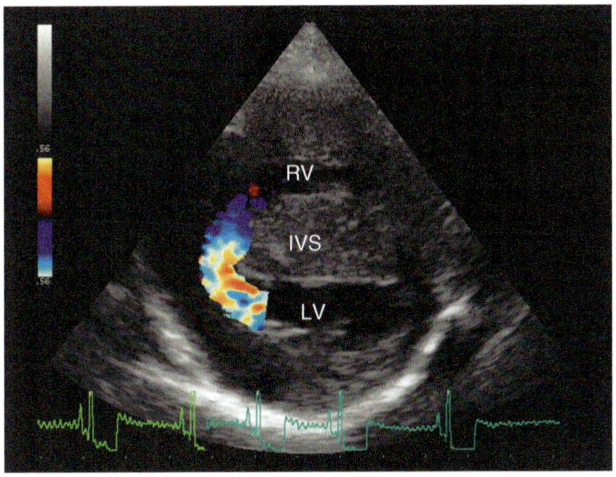

• **Fig. 19-36** Right parasternal short axis view (apical level) in color Doppler mode in a dog with a muscular ventricular septal defect (VSD). The color Doppler suggests a right-to-left shunt. The interventricular septum (IVS) is hypertrophied and flattened during systole due to a concomitant pulmonic stenosis. The right ventricular wall is hypertrophied. *LV,* Left ventricle; *RV,* right ventricle. (Photo credit: Claudio Bussadori.)

Spectral Doppler

Proper alignment with the VSD flow can be obtained from the right parasternal long axis and short axis views depending on the anatomic location of the defect. These views are best to measure flow velocity through the defect. The normal pressure gradient between the two ventricles through a small VSD is about 100 mm Hg, which means a peak velocity of approximately 4.5 to 5 m/s (Figure 19-37). A lower peak velocity may result from pulmonary hypertension due to Eisenmenger syndrome or right ventricular hypertension secondary to pulmonic stenosis. With large, nonrestrictive VSD, the pressure gradient between the two ventricles drops and is associated with a lower peak velocity.

The Qp/Qs ratio can be evaluated using pulsed Doppler. The aortic and pulmonic annulus areas and the spectral envelopes of the aortic and pulmonic systolic flows allow calculation of the corresponding stroke volumes. The VSD is considered small if Qp/Qs is equal to 1.5, moderate if Qp/Qs is between 1.5 and 2.5, and large if Qp/Qs exceeds 2.5. The amount of pulmonary hypertension in large defects can be calculated by subtracting the pressure gradient of the shunt flow through the VSD to the arterial systemic pressure. For instance, a shunt pressure gradient of 60 mm Hg and a systolic arterial pressure of 120 mm Hg indicate moderate pulmonary hypertension (right ventricular systolic pressure estimated at 60 mm Hg).

Atrial Septal Defect

Atrial septal defects (ASDs) are abnormal communications between the right and left atria. They have long been considered rare in veterinary medicine [76,77].

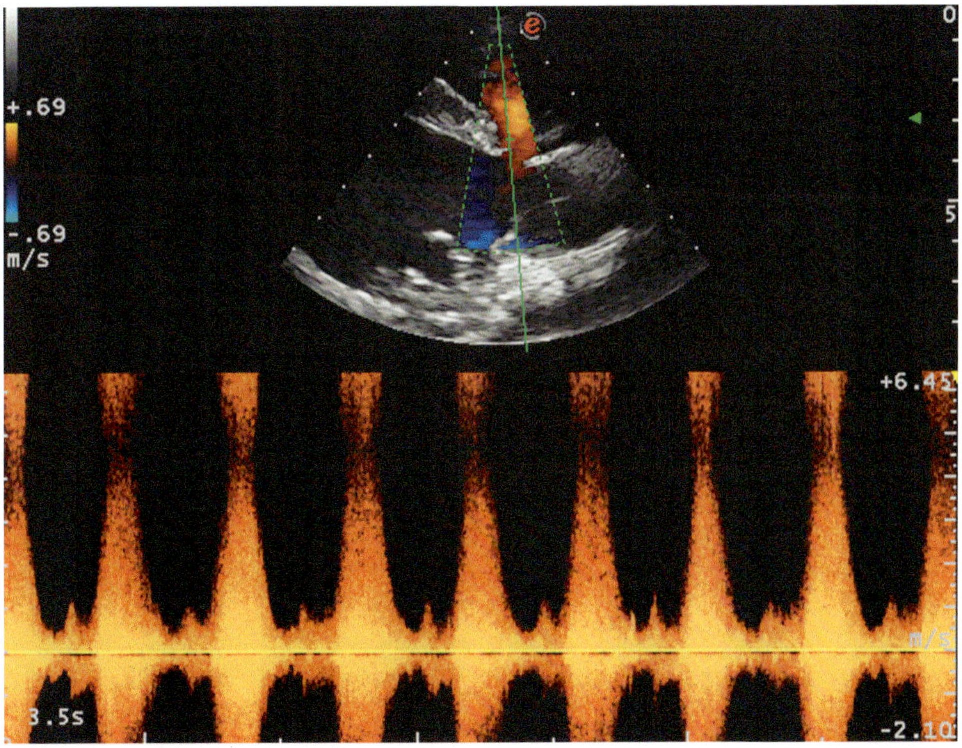

• **Fig. 19-37** Spectral continuous wave Doppler of a ventricular septal defect flow with left-to-right shunt. The maximum velocity reaches 4.5 m/s. (Photo credit: Claudio Bussadori.)

However, small ASDs may be largely underdiagnosed because they are not associated with heart murmurs or significant hemodynamic anomalies.

Anatomopathology

These defects can be located on different parts of the interatrial septum.

- The septum primum ASDs (ASD-OS1) are located underneath the fossa ovalis and usually originate from a fusion defect of the endocardial cushions.
- The septum secundum ASDs (ASD-OS2) are the most commonly encountered ASD, representing two thirds of all ASDs. They are located in the area delimited by the fossa ovalis. They are completely surrounded by atrial tissue. These ASDs can be closed by interventional closure procedure.
- The patent foramen ovale (PFO) is a very small defect located at the level of the junction between the septum secundum and septum primum, cranially to the entrance of coronary sinus in the right atrium. The conformation of the defect is similar to a tunnel between the septum primum and septum secundum. In humans, PFO may be present in 25% of the normal population. In animals, the prevalence of this defect is unknown. It has no hemodynamic significance.
- The sinus venosus ASDs are located near the ostia of the cranial vena cava and the pulmonary veins. This type of defect is rare in animals. It may be associated with an anomalous pulmonary venous return, with one or two pulmonary veins entering directly or through the cranial vena cava into the right atrium.
- The coronary sinus ASD results from the absence of separation between the coronary sinus and the left atrium. A variable segment of the portion of the coronary sinus (CS) traveling around the left atrium is unroofed, thus communicating with the latter chamber. This may be associated with a persistent left cranial vena cava.

Echocardiographic Aspects

Echocardiographic diagnosis of ASD is relatively simple but some views may be misleading. It is best to combine several views to define localization, size, and involvement of other structures adjacent to the ASD.

Bidimensional Echocardiography

From the right parasternal long axis 4 chambers view, the interatrial septum is perpendicular to the ultrasound beam. Therefore this view is ideal to visualize the thicker septal wall and the thin membrane of the fossa ovalis. Dilation of the right atrium and right ventricle may be present if the shunting through the ASD is significant.

For sinus venosus ASD, the right parasternal long axis view is the most useful. It will require small adjustments of the imaging plane angle to optimize visualization of the atrial roof and the abnormal communication. With this type of ASD, it is important to properly assess the connection of the pulmonary veins to the left atrium to rule out a potential anomalous pulmonary venous return, a common complication of this disease (Figure 19-38).

If an ASD is suspected on the right parasternal long axis 4 chambers view, it must be confirmed on a right parasternal short axis view of the base of the heart. This last view allows a more precise measurement of ASD-OS2 size in dogs and cats (Figure 19-39) [78].

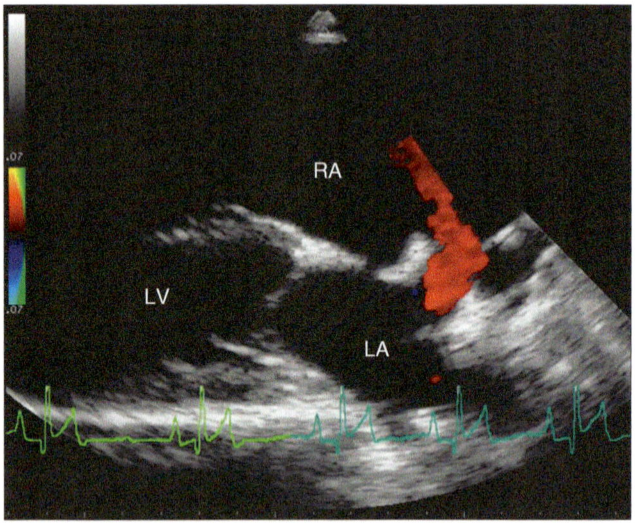

• **Fig. 19-38** Right parasternal long axis 4 chambers view in color Doppler mode in a dog with a sinus venosus atrial septal defect (ASD). The left-to-right shunt is visible. *LA,* Left atrium; *LV,* left ventricle; *RA,* right atrium. (Photo credit: Claudio Bussadori.)

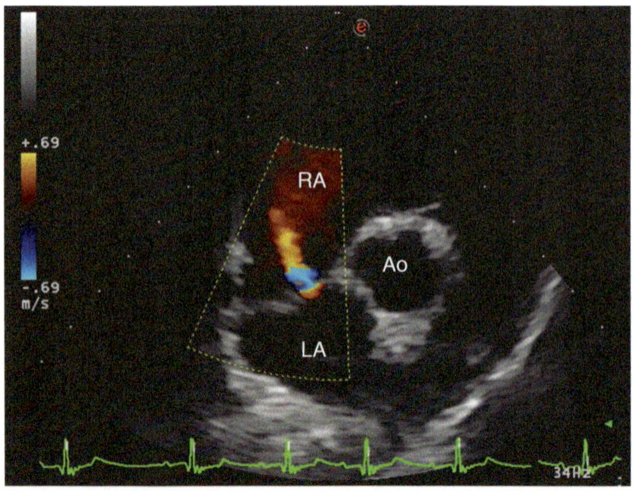

• **Fig. 19-39** Right parasternal short axis transaortic view using color Doppler in a dog with a septum secundum atrial septal defect (ASD-OS2). The left-to-right shunt is visible. *Ao,* Aorta; *LA,* left atrium; *RA,* right atrium. (Photo credit: Claudio Bussadori.)

On the left parasternal apical 4 chambers views, the very thin fossa ovalis may not be seen (echo dropout) due to the fact that the ultrasound beam is parallel to the interatrial septum. This could potentially lead to a false positive diagnosis of ASD.

Unroofed CS may be visualized using the right parasternal long axis view. Since a persistent left cranial vena cava draining into the coronary sinus is frequently associated with this defect, one of the most common clues is a dilated CS. The CS wall discontinuity allowing communication with the left atrium should be identified. When a persistent left cranial vena cava is present, a micro-bubble study may confirm the diagnosis: after injection of the saline solution described earlier into the left cephalic vein, bubbles appear first in the left atrium and immediately after in the right atrium.

Doppler Echocardiography

When using the right parasternal long axis 4 chambers view, the ultrasound beam is parallel to the blood flow crossing the defect and gives good spectral and color Doppler signals. This will allow confirmation of the diagnosis of ASD and give information about direction, velocity, and size of the interatrial shunt (Figure 19-40).

By positioning the sample volume of the pulsed wave Doppler across the ASD, one can record the typical ASD flow pattern, characterized by an almost continuous flow, with the highest velocities recorded in late systole (Figure 19-41). In the absence of other concomitant pathologies that could affect right ventricular afterload, the shunt direction is left-to-right. With large ASD, the peak and mean velocities of the pulmonic flow are increased due to the larger volume of blood crossing the valve, a phenomenon called "relative pulmonic stenosis" [79].

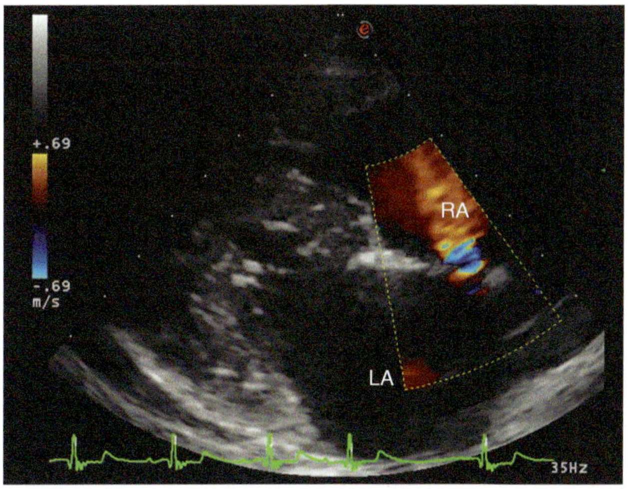

• **Fig. 19-40** Oblique right parasternal long axis 4 chambers view in color Doppler mode in a dog with a septum secundum atrial septal defect (ASD-OS2). The left-to-right shunt is visible. *LA*, Left atrium; *RA*, right atrium. (Photo credit: Claudio Bussadori.)

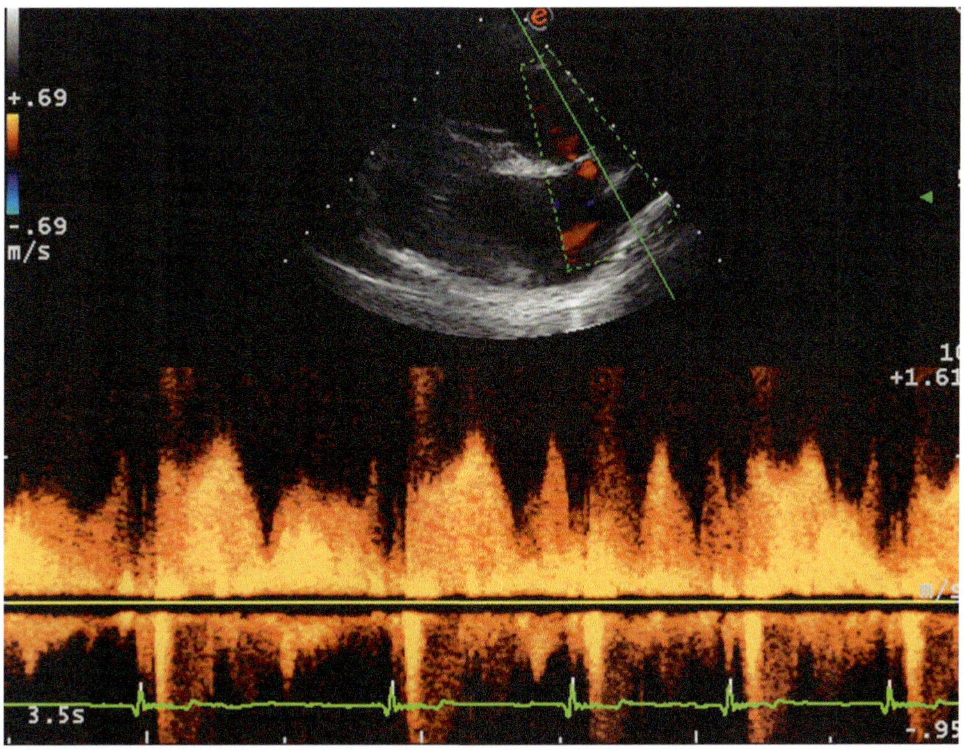

• **Fig. 19-41** Pulsed spectral Doppler in a dog with a septum secundum atrial septal defect (ASD-OS2). The sample volume is placed on the right side of the interatrial septum. A nearly continuous flow is recorded with the maximum velocity in end-systole. (Photo credit: Claudio Bussadori.)

Mitral Valve Dysplasia

Mitral valve dysplasia (MVD) is a congenital anomaly of the mitral valve apparatus. It usually leads to MR. Mitral stenosis (MS) and left ventricular outflow obstruction due to systolic anterior motion (SAM) of the mitral septal leaflet are encountered more rarely [80]. A combination of all of these functional anomalies is frequently seen, leading to pulmonary venous congestion and left-sided congestive heart failure. Giant breed dogs (Great Dane, German Shepherd, Bull Terrier [81], Golden Retriever [82], Newfoundland, Dalmatian [83]) are predisposed to MVD [9].

MVD is usually a single defect but can be associated with other cardiopathies such as SAS, tricuspid valve dysplasia, PDA, and VSD. The severity of the clinical symptoms is directly correlated to the severity of the MR and inversely correlated to atrial compliance. MVD should be suspected in giant breed dogs that develop heart failure before 1 year of age.

Anatomopathology

The mitral valve malformations may involve valve leaflets, chordae tendineae, mitral annulus, and papillary muscles [84]. Affected valve leaflets are thickened and sometimes elongated. The chordae tendineae either could be thickened and elongated as well or could be shorter than normal, sometimes even missing, with the mitral valve leaflet inserted directly on the papillary muscle. Papillary muscles may be misaligned, atrophic, or hypertrophied, thus contributing to the abnormal closure of the valve during systole (Figure 19-42).

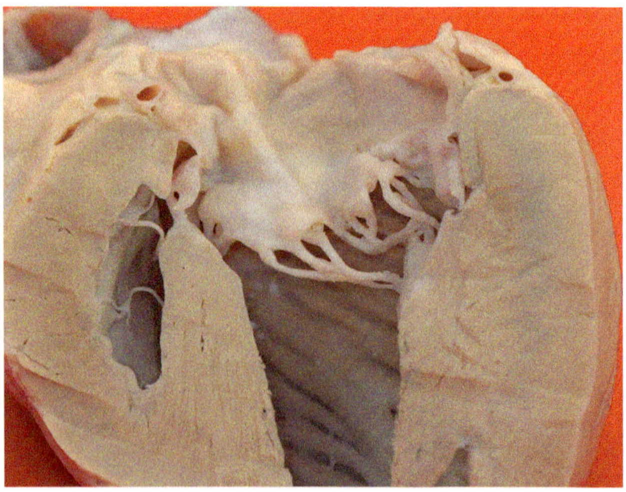

• **Fig. 19-42** Pathologic specimen of the heart of a German Shepherd with mitral valve dysplasia (MVD) with severe mitral regurgitation (MR). The papillary muscles are displaced dorsally and the chordae tendineae are thickened and elongated. (Photo credit: Claudio Bussadori.)

Echocardiographic Aspects

Bidimensional and TM Echocardiography

The mitral valve apparatus morphologic anomalies and the mitral valve leaflets motion are best evaluated using the right parasternal long axis and left apical 4 chambers views (Figure 19-43). In both views, the abnormal thickening of mitral leaflets and chordeae tendineae should be easily identified. Mitral leaflets do not join the mitral annular plane in diastole, creating a tent-shaped area (Figure 19-44), which increases with the severity of left ventricular dilation [85]. The presence of a SAM of the

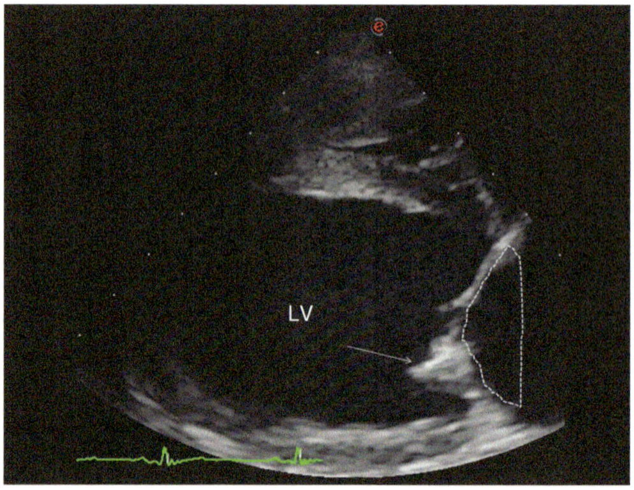

• **Fig. 19-43** Right parasternal long axis 4 chambers view in a dog with mild mitral valve dysplasia (MVD). The mitral valve posterior leaflet is thickened *(arrow)*. The dysplastic leaflets do not come back to the mitral annulus plane in systole, giving the mitral valve a tent shape *(area bordered by dotted line)*. *LV,* Left ventricle. (Photo credit: Claudio Bussadori.)

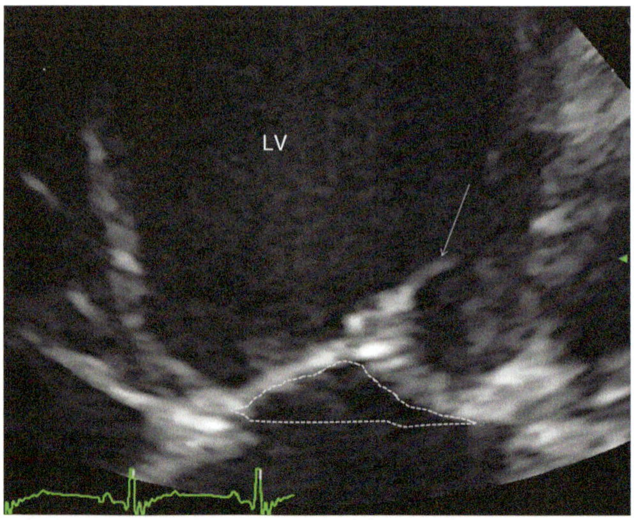

• **Fig. 19-44** Apical 4 chambers view, with zoom on the mitral valve, in the same dog as in Figure 19-43. The arrow indicates excessively shortened chordae tendineae preventing proper leaflet coaptation. The tenting of the mitral valve is indicated by the area bordered by the dotted line. *LV,* Left ventricle. (Photo credit: Claudio Bussadori.)

anterior mitral valve leaflet should be assessed on the right parasternal long axis 5 chambers view. Mitral valve stenosis should be suspected if a poor opening of the mitral leaflets in diastole is observed (Figure 19-45).

The left atrium is dilated due to either MR or MS. The left ventricle becomes dilated if there is a predominant MR.

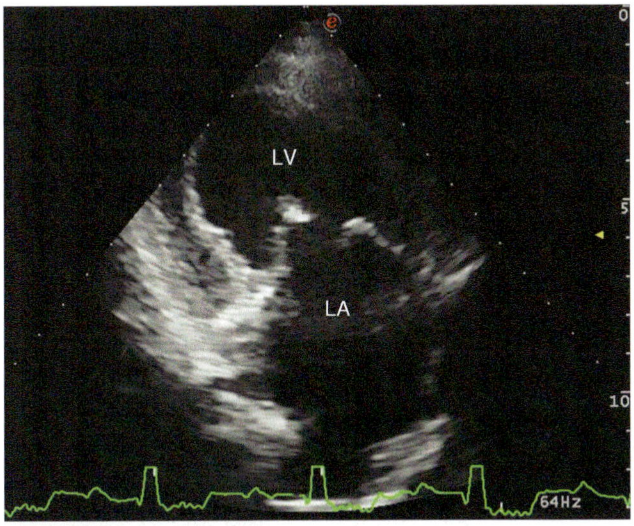

• **Fig. 19-45** Oblique apical 2 chambers view in early diastole in a dog with mitral valve dysplasia (MVD) with predominant stenosis. The opening of the leaflets in diastole remains incomplete, with a domed aspect. *LA,* Left atrium; *LV,* left ventricle. (Photo credit: Claudio Bussadori.)

The SF and the EDVI are increased in the case of predominant MR without systolic dysfunction. The septal motion appears exaggerated. In the presence of systolic dysfunction, the SF and ejection fraction will decline and the ESVI will increase.

Doppler Echocardiography

The mitral flow characteristics can be studied using the apical 4 chambers view, which allows the best alignment with the diastolic transmitral flow and the regurgitant jet. The MR can be documented by CW Doppler (Video 19-7).

The pulsed spectral Doppler of the diastolic mitral flow typically shows a tall E wave, due to the increased preload and elevated left atrial pressure. In the case of MS, the deceleration of the E wave is delayed and the A wave is increased (Figure 19-46). The A wave amplitude decreases when the left ventricular end-diastolic pressure increases. The E/A ratio decreases. The shallower the E wave deceleration slope, the more severe the stenosis. In humans, this is quantified by the measurement of the pressure half-time (Pt1/2), which is the time necessary for the pressure to decrease by one half (Dt) or for the Vmax to decrease to a velocity that is equal to the peak velocity divided by $\sqrt{2}$ (=1.4) (corresponding to 0.71 Vmax). A correlation between the Pt1/2 and the opening area of the mitral valve has been established. The longer the Pt1/2, the tighter the stenosis. An equivalent of this

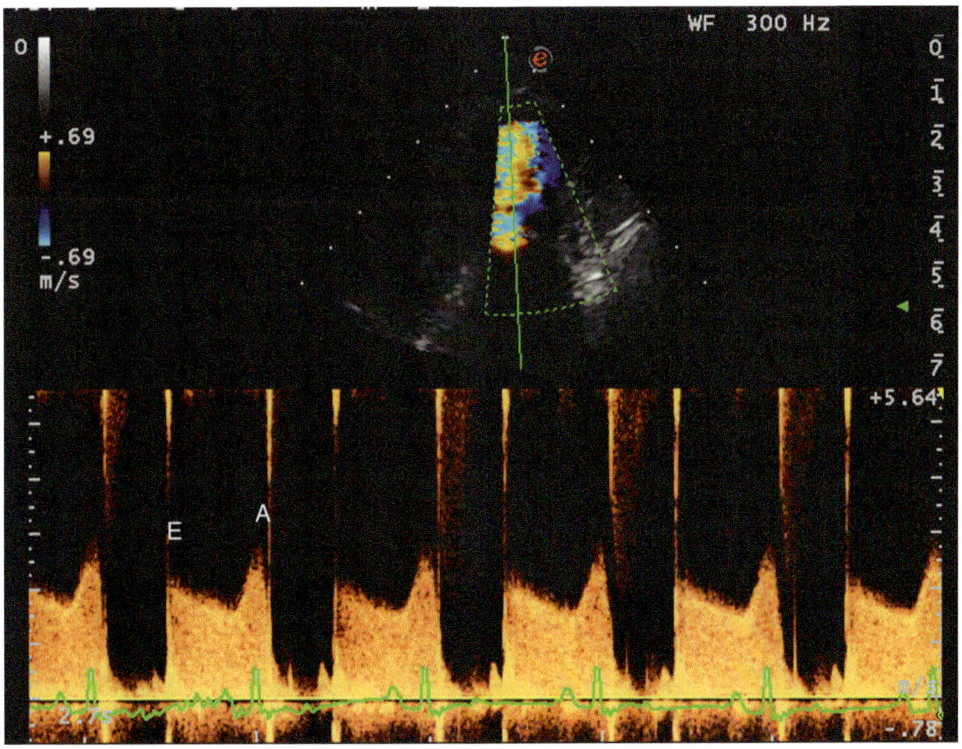

• **Fig. 19-46** Continuous wave spectral Doppler of the diastolic transmitral flow in a dog with mitral valve dysplasia (MVD) and severe stenosis. The deceleration slope of the early diastolic E wave is reduced and the E/A ratio is inversed. (Photo credit: Claudio Bussadori.)

measurement has not been established in dogs, so the evaluation remains subjective.

With MS, the acceleration and the turbulent character of the transmitral diastolic flow can be identified using color Doppler (Figure 19-47; Video 19-8).

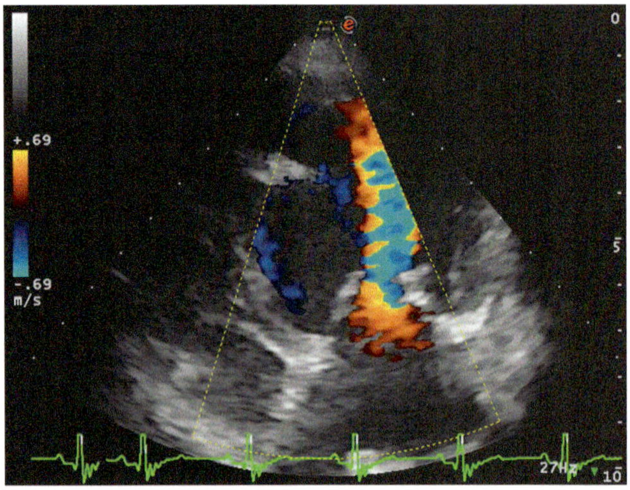

• **Fig. 19-47** Apical 4 chambers view in color Doppler mode in a dog with mitral valve dysplasia (MVD) with combined stenosis and regurgitation. The high velocity and turbulence of the diastolic flow are the result of stenosis. (Photo credit: Claudio Bussadori.)

Tricuspid Valve Dysplasia

Tricuspid valve dysplasia (TVD) is a congenital anomaly of the tricuspid valve apparatus. Valvular anomalies can lead to TR (more common) or stenosis (rare). It is not a very common CHD in cats [86] or dogs [87]. In our experience, the incidence of TVD is only 3.1% of the CHDs referred to our laboratory. It is more frequently observed in Labrador Retrievers, Boxers, German Shepherds, English Bulldogs [9,88], and Bullmastiffs [89]. In Labrador Retrievers, a hereditary transmission has recently been documented [90]. The clinical picture will depend on the type of lesion and the possible presence of other congenital or noncongenital pathologies that can contribute to further hemodynamic alterations. In Labrador Retrievers, the association of TVD with anomalous atrioventricular muscular fibers is frequently seen, creating the anatomic substrate for reentrant tachyarrhythmias. This may result in a severe tachycardia-induced cardiomyopathy with dilation of the four chambers and hypokinesia that may partially hide echocardiographic signs of TVD. In humans and in dogs, a particular form of TVD also called "Ebstein anomaly" has been described [91]. It is characterized by a very distal insertion of the three tricuspid leaflets in the right ventricular chamber, creating an "atrialized" right ventricle [92,93]. In non-Labrador breeds, the association with other CHD is uncommon [2,9,94-96].

Anatomopathology

The malformations of the tricuspid valve apparatus, such as those described in MVD, can involve the tricuspid valve leaflets, chordae tendineae, and papillary muscles. The valve leaflets can be thickened, shortened, or longer than normal or present fenestrations. In dogs, short or even absence of the chordae tendineae is frequent (Figure 19-48). The tricuspid valve leaflets are then attached directly to the papillary muscles.

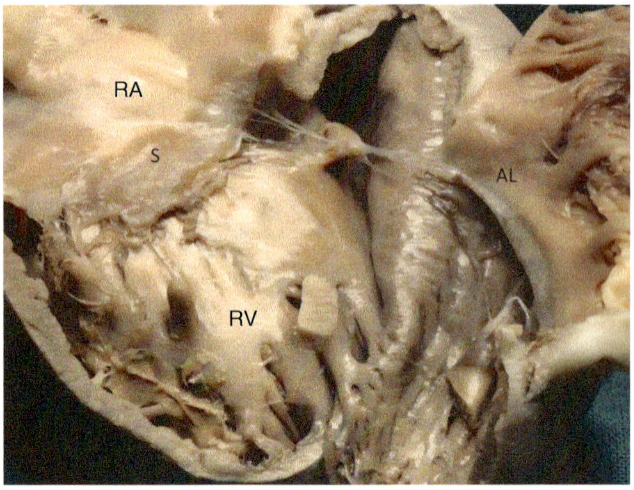

• **Fig. 19-48** Heart of a dog with severe tricuspid valve dysplasia (TVD) (anatomic specimen). The septal (S) and anterior lateral (AL) leaflets are hypoplastic and the chordae tendineae are shortened. *RA,* Right atrium; *RV,* right ventricle. (Photo credit: Claudio Bussadori.)

Echocardiographic Aspects

Bidimensional Echocardiography

The best views to evaluate the tricuspid valve apparatus are the right parasternal long axis 4 chambers (Figure 19-49) and left apical 4 chambers views (Figure 19-50). Normally, the septal insertion of the tricuspid valve is slightly lower than that of the mitral insertion. The insertion of the two valves on the septum forms the "crus cordis." In TVD, this distance is a bit more accentuated but not as marked as in Ebstein anomaly. The anomalies may affect all of the tricuspid valve leaflets, which can be thickened, fenestrated, or less mobile. The chordae tendineae are usually shorter than normal or absent. In the rare instance of tricuspid stenosis, the motion of the leaflets is greatly restricted and the valve orifice appears reduced. The optimal view to see this is the apical 4 chambers view (Figure 19-51). With severe TR, the right atrium and right ventricle appear dilated and the interventricular septum may be displaced toward the left ventricle in diastole, due to right ventricular volume overload (Figure 19-52).

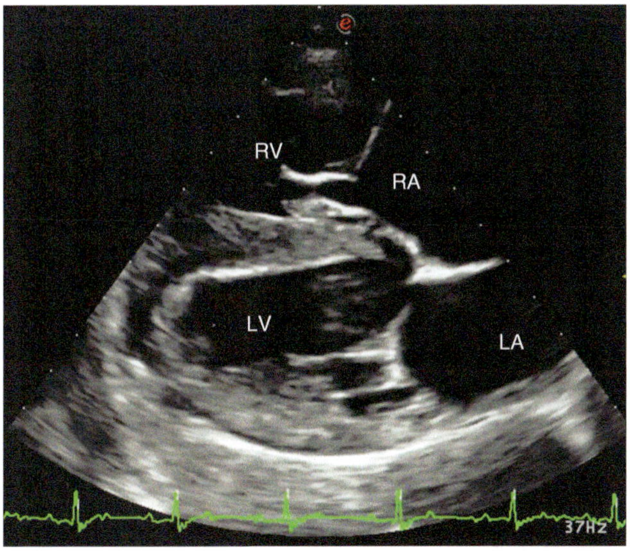

• **Fig. 19-49** Right parasternal long axis 4 chambers view in a dog with tricuspid valve dysplasia (TVD). The right cavities are dilated. The noncoaptation of the tricuspid leaflets is visible. *LA,* Left atrium; *LV,* left ventricle; *RA,* right atrium; *RV,* right ventricle. (Photo credit: Claudio Bussadori.)

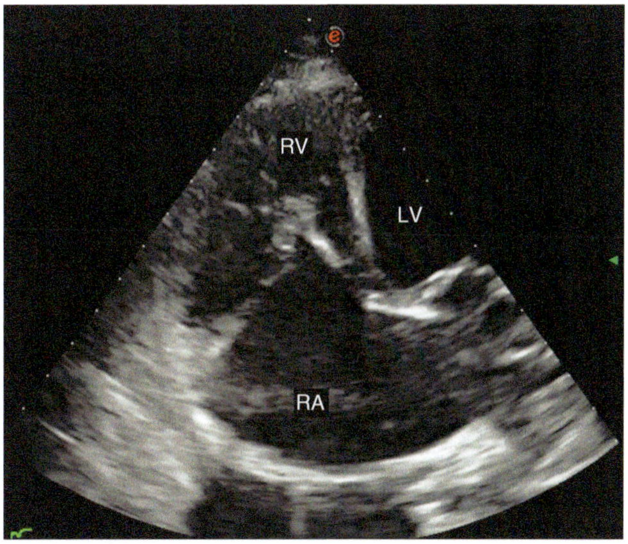

• **Fig. 19-50** Apical 4 chambers view centered on the right cavities of a dog with tricuspid valve dysplasia. The elongated tricuspid leaflets and the very short chordae tendineae lead to a displacement of the leaflet coaptation point in the right ventricular cavity. *LV,* Left ventricle; *RA,* right atrium; *RV,* right ventricle. (Photo credit: Claudio Bussadori.)

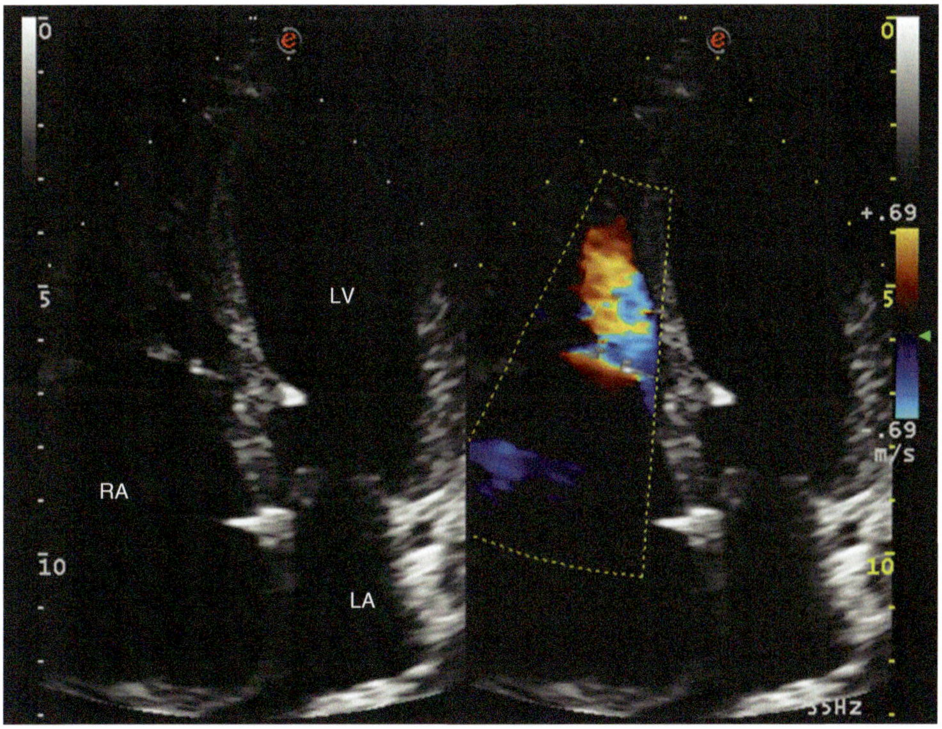

• **Fig. 19-51** Apical 4 chambers views without *(left)* and with *(right)* color Doppler in a dog with severe tricuspid valve dysplasia (TVD) and tricuspid stenosis. The color Doppler facilitates the visualization of the stenotic valve orifice. *LA,* Left atrium; *LV,* left ventricle; *RA,* right atrium. (Photo credit: Claudio Bussadori.)

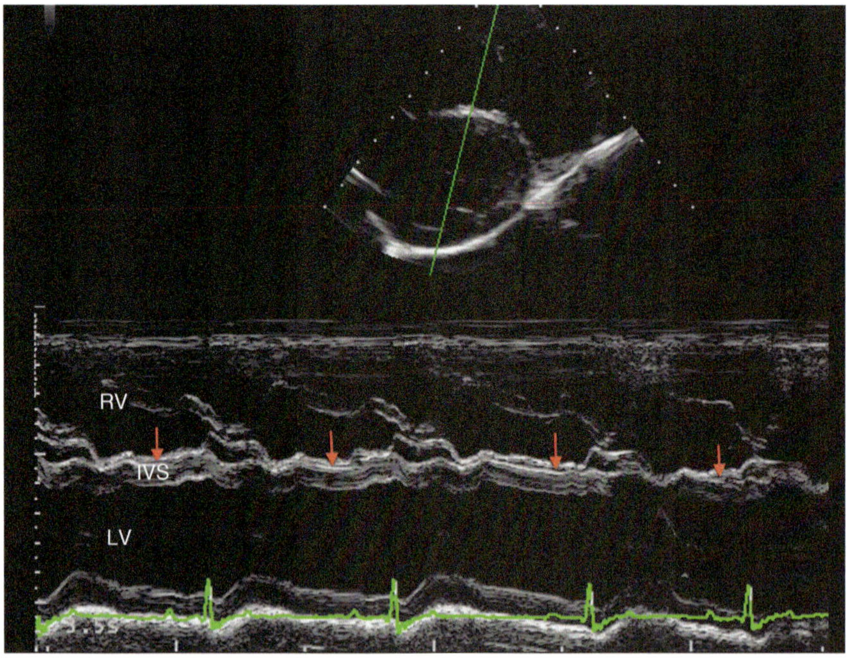

• **Fig. 19-52** Transventricular time-motion (TM) echocardiogram in a dog with tricuspid valve dysplasia (TVD). The septal movement is paradoxic in diastole *(arrows)* due to the right ventricular volume overload. *IVS,* Interventricular septum; *LV,* left ventricle; *RV,* right ventricle. (Photo credit: Claudio Bussadori.)

Doppler Echocardiography

The acceleration of the diastolic tricuspid flow can be documented using both color and spectral Doppler modes (Video 19-9). In cases of predominant stenosis, higher diastolic velocities and a typical pattern of stenosis such as increased pressure half-time can be observed. The retrograde systolic flow of TR usually does not exceed 3.5 m/s. Semiquantitative evaluation of the TR can be performed using color Doppler. The depth of the regurgitant colorimetric area is correlated with the severity of the valvular dysplasia (Figure 19-53). In the case of an associated PFO, a small interatrial right-to-left shunt may be observed once the right atrial pressure exceeds that of the left atrium.

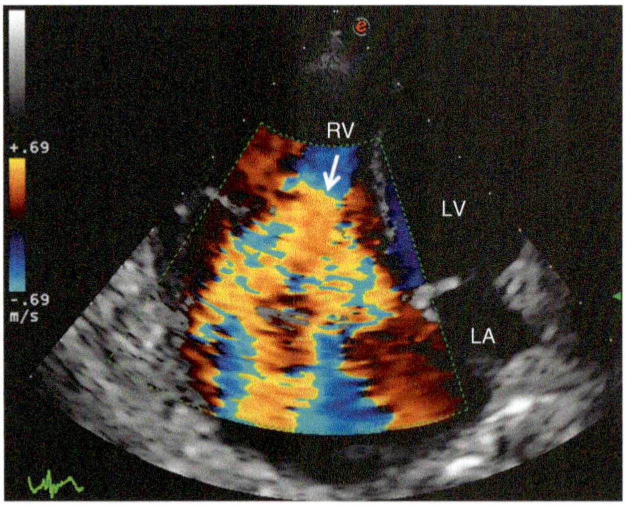

• **Fig. 19-53** Apical 4 chambers view centered on the right cavities, in color Doppler mode, in a dog with tricuspid valve dysplasia (TVD). Severe tricuspid regurgitation is present. The turbulence begins at the level of the inadequate coaptation of the tricuspid leaflets *(arrow)*. *LA,* Left atrium; *LV,* left ventricle; *RV,* right ventricle. (Photo credit: Claudio Bussadori.)

Tetralogy of Fallot

Tetralogy of Fallot (ToF) is a complex congenital heart malformation due to an anterior deviation of the outflow septum. The result is a large malalignment VSD associated with hypoplastic pulmonic valve annulus and main pulmonary artery, rudimentary pulmonic valve leaflets, and infundibular hypertrophy. The resulting increase in the right ventricular pressure leads to a right-to-left shunt through the VSD from the right ventricle directly into the aorta. The pulmonary flow may be greatly reduced by the combination of the right-to-left shunt and the outflow obstruction.

Tetralogy of Fallot is rare in both dogs and cats: in a series of 967 consecutive cases of CHD, the reported prevalence was 1% [9]. A hereditary origin was documented in the Keeshond [57,97]. No particular predisposition in sex or breed has been shown. The clinical picture is determined by the hemodynamic alterations, which depend on the degree of the right ventricular outflow obstruction and the systemic vascular resistance. In forms of ToF where the PS is mild, the right-to-left shunt may occur only at exercise, when the systemic vascular resistance drops. This may lead to exercise intolerance. These patients may survive up to 6 to 8 years of age. With severe obstruction, the right-to-left shunt becomes permanent, leading to cyanosis, polycythemia, and sudden death at an early age due to arterial thromboembolism or tachyarrhythmias.

Anatomopathology

The four major anatomic anomalies of ToF are PS, often associated with hypoplasia of the main pulmonary trunk; a large membranous VSD; right ventricular hypertrophy; and dextroposition or overriding of aorta over the VSD.

Echocardiographic Aspects

Bidimensional Echocardiography

The right ventricular hypertrophy can be clearly appreciated using the right parasternal long axis 4 chambers view. The VSD and the overriding aorta can be seen by gently switching to a right parasternal long axis 5 chambers view (Video 19-10). The large membranous VSD is also visible on the right parasternal short axis view at the level of the heart base, where the characteristics of the right ventricular outflow obstruction, including the hypoplasia of the main pulmonary artery, are best assessed (Figure 19-54).

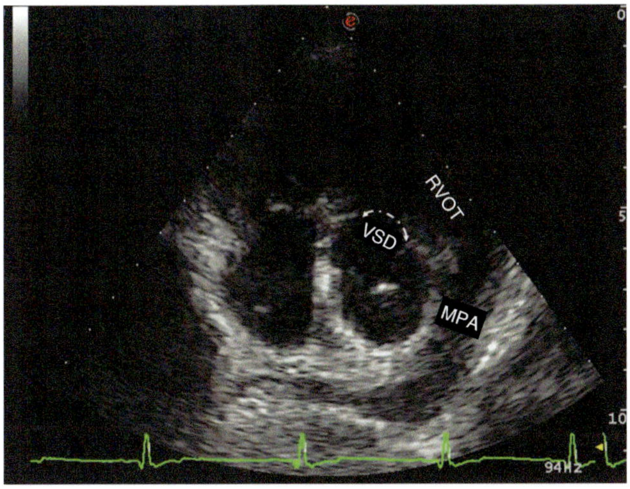

• **Fig. 19-54** Right parasternal short axis view of the base of the heart in a dog with tetralogy of Fallot (ToF). A large ventricular septal defect (VSD) and main pulmonary artery (MPA) hypoplasia are visible. *RVOT,* Right ventricular outflow tract. (Photo credit: Claudio Bussadori.)

Doppler Echocardiography

Color flow Doppler is quite useful to visualize the direction of the flow through the VSD (Figure 19-55). Both the PS and shunt pressure gradients can be quantified with continuous Doppler. These gradients are usually not very elevated since the right ventricular pressure is equal to or slightly higher than the left ventricular pressure.

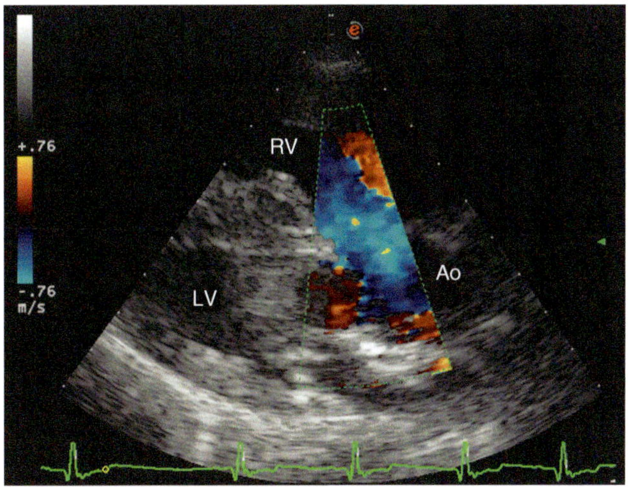

• **Fig. 19-55** Right parasternal long axis 5 chambers view in color Doppler mode in a dog with tetralogy of Fallot (ToF). Blood flow moving from the right ventricular outflow tract directly into the aorta (Ao) can be seen. *LV,* Left ventricle; *RV,* right ventricle. (Photo credit: Claudio Bussadori.)

Cor Triatriatum

Cor triatriatum is characterized by an abnormal atrial septation, creating a cranial and a caudal atrial chamber. The anomalous partitioning may affect the left atrium (cor triatriatum sinister, or CTS) or the right atrium (cor triatriatum dexter, or CTD). CTS results from the abnormal insertion of the pulmonary veins into the left atrium, leading to intraatrial obstruction. CTD results from the persistence of the embryonic right sinus venosus valve.

Cor triatriatum is an extremely uncommon CHD in dogs and cats. There is no recognized breed or sex predisposition. CTS has been described in cats [98-102] while CTD has been reported in different breeds of dogs [103-105] (Chow Chow, Cocker Spaniel, English Bulldog [106], German Shepherd Mix [107], Pyrenees, Akita [108], German Shorthair Pointer, Golden Retriever, Greyhound, Rottweiler) and in mixed breeds. In dogs, the age at diagnosis ranged from 8 weeks to 7 years [109].

The functional consequences of cor triatriatum depends on the size of the hole in the membrane dividing the affected atria. If the hole is small, the resistance to blood flow will increase pressure in the upstream chamber, which will result in dilation of the pulmonary (CTS) or caval (CTD) veins [110,111]. This will result in pulmonary congestion in the lungs and pulmonary edema in the case of CTS [99] or abdominal distension by ascites in the case of CTD [112]. Ebstein anomaly may be associated with cor triatriatum [113]. In humans, the diagnosis of CTS may be delayed by the presence of an associated ASD. This association is extremely rare in dogs and cats. Only one case of a cat with CTS and incomplete atrioventricular septal defect was reported [101].

This cardiac pathology should be considered as a differential diagnosis in kittens with signs of pulmonary edema [99] and in young dogs with abdominal distension.

Anatomopathology

Cor Triatriatum Sinister

CTS is the result of noninclusion of common pulmonary veins in the left atrium. This leads to the partitioning by an intraatrial membrane of the left atrium into two cavities: cranial and caudal. In humans, this membrane can have multiple fenestrations [117-119]. In animals, a single hole is usually present [106]. Of course, the absence of any perforation would be lethal during the fetal stage of life [120].

Cor Triatriatum Dexter

During the normal embryologic development of the heart, the sinus venosus represents a receiving chamber for the blood coming from the right and left common cardinalis veins and the developing caudal vena cava to the primitive atrium. Parts of the right sinus valve may remain as ridges bordering the opening of the caudal vena cava into the right atrium (Eustachian valve) and of the coronary sinus (Thebesian valve). CTD is caused by the persistence on the right side of the embryonic right sinus venosus valve [114]. It is characterized by a partition of the right atrium by a perforated fibromuscular diaphragm or septum. The tricuspid valve is connected to the cranial chamber while the caudal vena cava and the coronary sinus drain into the caudal chamber [107]. The fossa ovalis is located in the cranial chamber of the right atrium. The case of a puppy with triple right atria, where the cranial and caudal venae cavae emptied not only into separate chambers but also into a third ventral one, has been described [115].

A variant of CTD is called the Chiari network. This septation is a membrane with numerous fenestrations, not impeding blood flow [116].

Echocardiographic Aspects

Cor Triatriatum Sinister

The anomalous membrane within the left atrium can be easily visualized using the right parasternal long axis 4 chambers view. It appears as a linear structure located above the mitral valve. Examination of the interatrial septum should be performed carefully in order to detect any ASD, including a Doppler search of any anomalous ASD flow. Both left and right parasternal 4 chambers views allow good visualization of the abnormal membrane upstream of the mitral valve (Figure 19-56; Video 19-11). A turbulent blood flow within the left atrial cavity can be

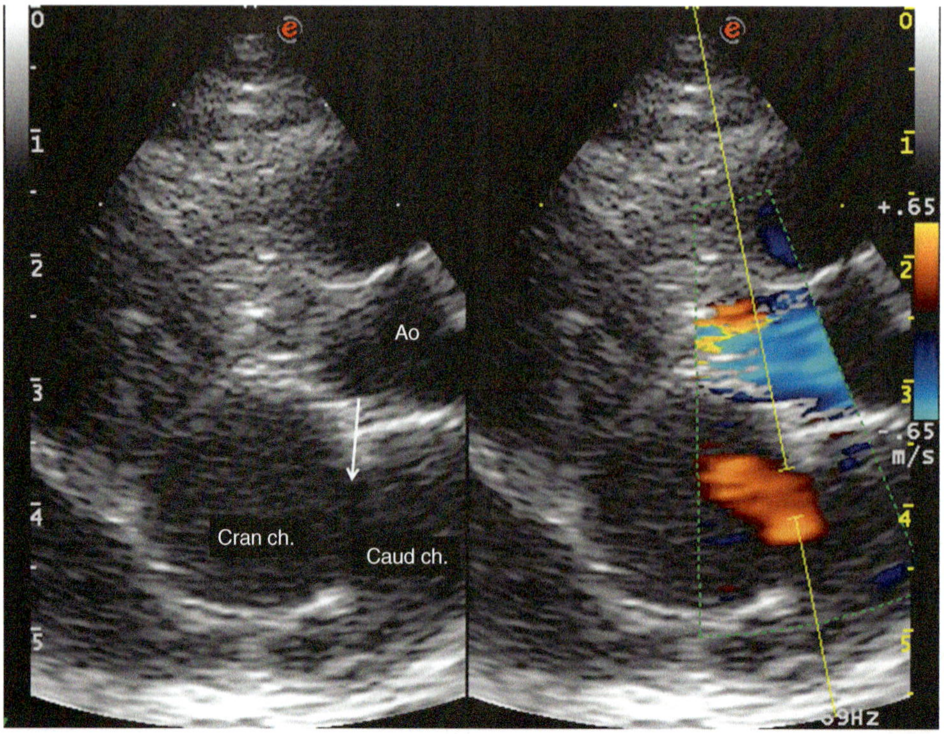

• **Fig. 19-56** Oblique left parasternal view without *(left)* and with *(right)* color Doppler in a cat with cor triatriatum sinister (CTS). The *arrow* indicates the location of the intraatrial membrane separating the caudal (Caud ch.) and cranial (Cran ch.) cavities. On the right image, the intraatrial flow is visible at the level of the membrane. *Ao,* Aorta. (Photo credit: Claudio Bussadori.)

detected using color Doppler (Figure 19-57; Video 19-12). The apical 4 chambers view allows the best alignment with the blood flow through the membrane perforation. This allows estimation of the intraatrial pressure gradient. CTS should be differentiated from supravalvular mitral stenosis by carefully observing the position of the obstructing membrane. A case of supravalvular mitral stenosis has been reported in a 3-year-old cat, in which the dividing membrane was located immediately above the mitral valve, distal to the left atrial appendage, and connected to the markedly enlarged proximal left atrial chamber [80].

Cor Triatriatum Dexter

On the right parasternal long axis 4 chambers view as well as the apical 4 and 5 chambers views, the right atrium appears partitioned by an incomplete or fenestrated septum (Figure 19-58) [121].

Typically, the caudal vena cava and coronary sinus drain into the caudal chamber. However, the case of a dog in which the caudal vena cava opened into the caudal chamber, while the coronary sinus opened into the cranial chamber, has been described [104]. In another case report, the fossa ovalis was located in the caudal chamber of the right atrium, with incomplete intraatrial septation at the level of the intervenous tubercle [122]. Both the opening of the coronary sinus and the fossa ovalis were located in the cranial chamber [122]. All vessels draining in the caudal chambers are easy to see echocardiographically because of their various degrees of dilatation. Anatomic variations of CTD include division of the right atrium by

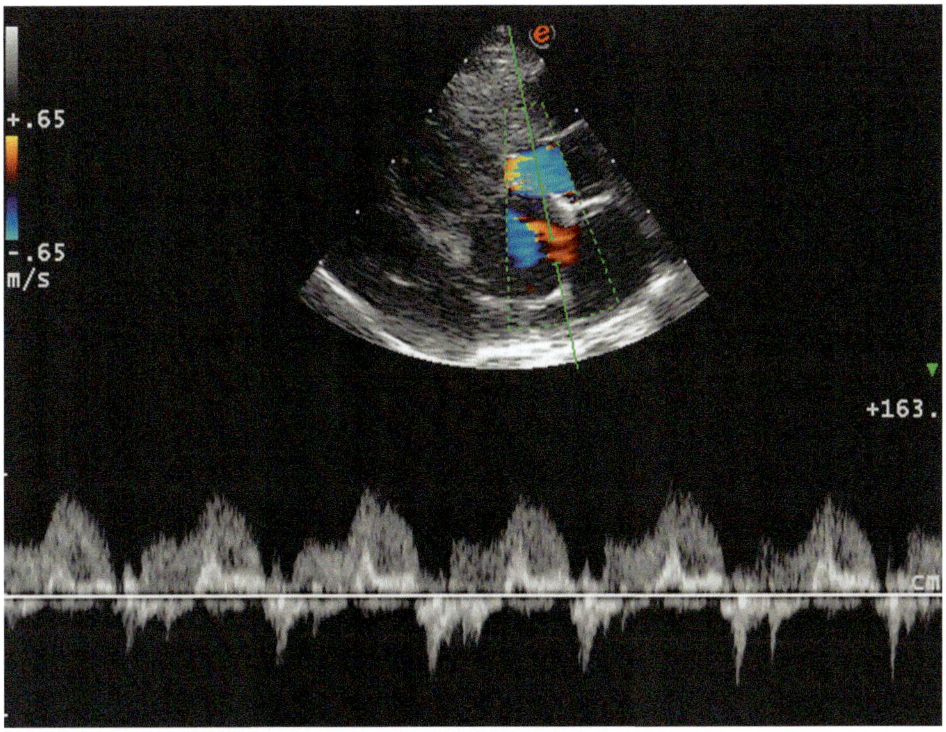

• **Fig. 19-57** Pulsed spectral Doppler of the intraatrial flow at the level of the intraatrial membrane in the same cat as in Figure 19-56. The flow is holodiastolic with a peak velocity in end-diastole. This indicates delayed ventricular relaxation due to concomitant hypertrophic cardiomyopathy. (Photo credit: Claudio Bussadori.)

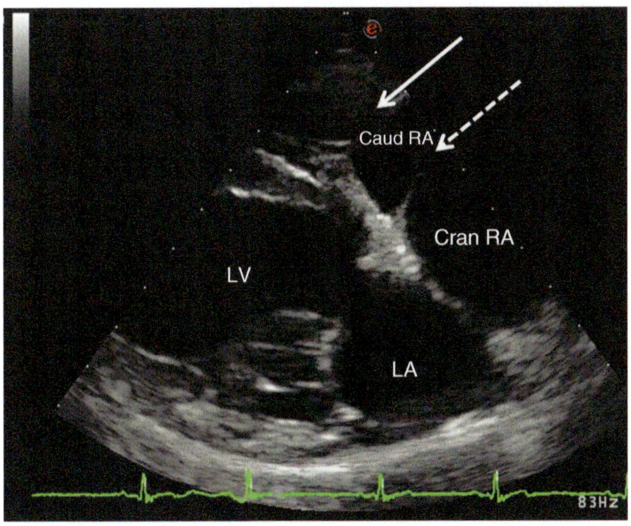

• **Fig. 19-58** Right parasternal long axis 4 chambers view in a dog with cor triatriatum dexter (CTD). The *solid arrow* indicates the tricuspid valve and the *dotted arrow* indicates the intraatrial membrane. *Caud RA,* Caudal right atrial chamber; *Cran RA,* cranial right atrial chamber; *LA,* left atrium; *LV,* left ventricle. (Photo credit: Claudio Bussadori.)

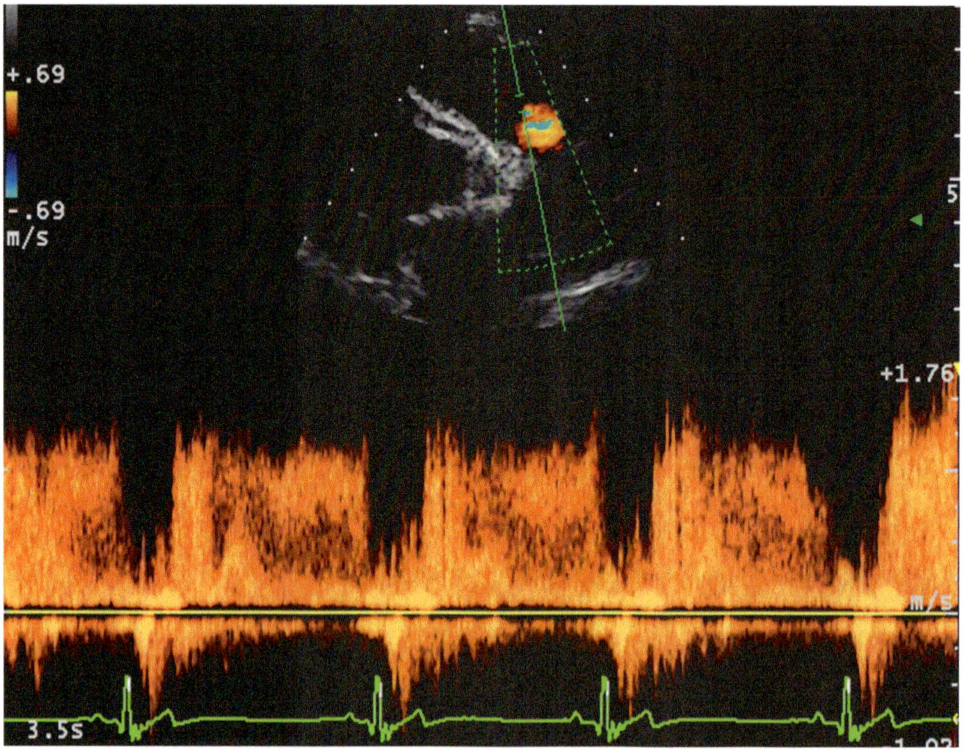

• **Fig. 19-59** Pulsed wave spectral Doppler of the intraatrial diastolic flow moving through the intraatrial membrane in a dog with cor triatriatum dexter (CTD). (Photo credit: Claudio Bussadori.)

both perforated and imperforated septa [123]. The imperforated septa are associated with anomalous collateral vessels usually connecting the caudal vena cava to the azygos vein or the vertebral venous circulation [124].

Spectral and color Doppler modes confirm the presence of obstruction to the blood flow between the cranial and caudal chambers: a turbulent intraatrial flow is recorded and the intraatrial pressure gradient can be measured. The pressure is normal in the cranial chamber and increased in the caudal chamber (Figure 19-59).

Endocardial Cushion Defect

The term *endocardial cushion defect* refers to a group of cardiac abnormalities ranging from ASD-OS1 [125-127] to complete atrioventricular (AV) canal defects with large ASD and VSD resulting in complete communication between all four cardiac chambers [128,129]. The latter is also called common AV canal. In the embryo, cardiac valves originate from precursor structures called endocardial cushions. After cardiac looping, endocardial swellings ("cushions") form and become populated by valve precursor cells formed by epithelial-mesenchymal transition. Epithelial-mesenchymal transformation in the AV canal and outflow tract is a crucial process that regulates initial valve formation, in which a subpopulation of endocardial cells invades the extracellular matrix as a result of regional interaction between the myocardium and endocardium. These mesenchymal cushions are at the origin of the valves and septa and develop into mature structures through complicated remodeling processes regulated mainly by bone morphogenetic protein (BMP) and transforming growth factor-β (TGF-β) [130-133]. Proper cushion formation is required for normal cardiac development, including chamber formation and septation.

Endocardial cushion defects have been reported in both cats and dogs [126,134-136], without any apparent breed or sex predisposition. In our experience, this disease is more frequently seen in cats than in dogs.

Anatomopathology

Complete Atrioventricular Defect

The complete AV canal is characterized by an atrioventricular communication with the interposition of a common atrioventricular valve. This common valve has five leaflets. All four cardiac cavities are connected (Figures 19-60 and 19-61) [129].

Three types of complete endocardial cushion defects can be distinguished: A, B, or C, depending on how the anterior leaflet of the common AV valve is connected to the ventricular chambers [137].

- In type A, the anterior leaflet is mostly connected to the left ventricle and the chordae tendineae are attached to the septal crest and right medial papillary muscle (Video 19-13).
- In type B, the anterior leaflet extends more into the right ventricle and is attached to an anomalous right papillary muscle originating from the trabecula septomarginalis.
- In type C, the anterior leaflet is floating but mostly located on the right side.

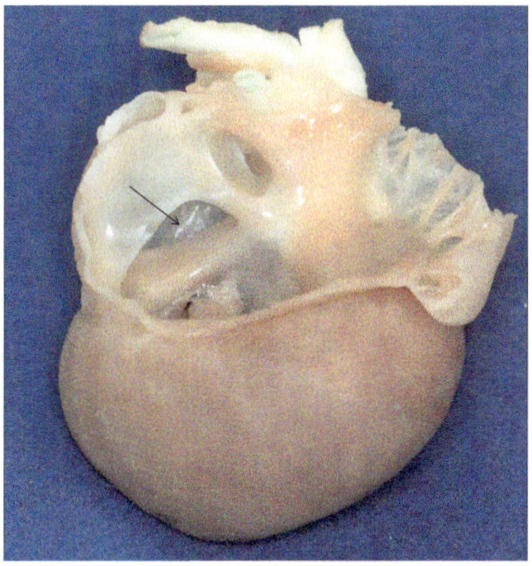

• **Fig. 19-60** Heart (anatomic specimen) of a 60-day-old kitten with a complete atrioventricular (AV) canal (viewed from the left). The left atrium is open. The *arrow* points at a large atrial septal defect (ASD). Part of the anterior leaflet of the only AV valve is also visible. (Photo credit: Claudio Bussadori.)

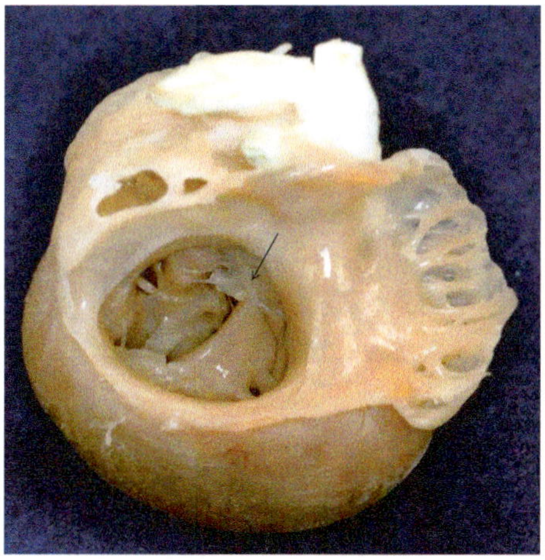

• **Fig. 19-61** Heart (anatomic specimen) of a 60-day-old kitten with a complete atrioventricular (AV) canal (dorsal view). The left atrium is open. The *arrow* indicates the single AV anterior valve leaflet. (Photo credit: Claudio Bussadori.)

Partial Atrioventricular Defect

Partial AV canal is characterized by ASD-OS1, VSD, and mitral valve malformation with regurgitation.

A band of myocardium connects the anterior leaflet to the posterior leaflet. This creates a three-leaflets valve in the left atrioventricular orifice. The discontinuity between the anterior and posterior leaflets constitutes what is inappropriately called "mitral cleft," through which MR occurs (Video 19-14). This MR, always present in a case of partial AV canal, helps to differentiate this CHD from an isolated ASD-OS1. In this last type of endocardial cushion defect, the VSD may be very small and hemodynamically not significant. From a pathophysiologic point of view, this type could be assimilated to a simple ASD-OS1 with a much better prognosis than complete AV canal.

Echocardiographic Aspects

Bidimensional Echocardiography

The predominant echocardiographic features of complete endocardial cushion defect include absence of atrioventricular septum and valvular malformation, a cleft anterior mitral leaflet, or a common atrioventricular valve [135]. The presence of a single common atrioventricular valve is well documented using the left parasternal apical 4 chambers and oblique views (Figure 19-62). A typical "goose neck" deformity of the LVOT can also be seen using a right parasternal long axis 5 chambers view (Figure 19-63) [138]. This deformation, referring to the angiocardiographic appearance initially described, results

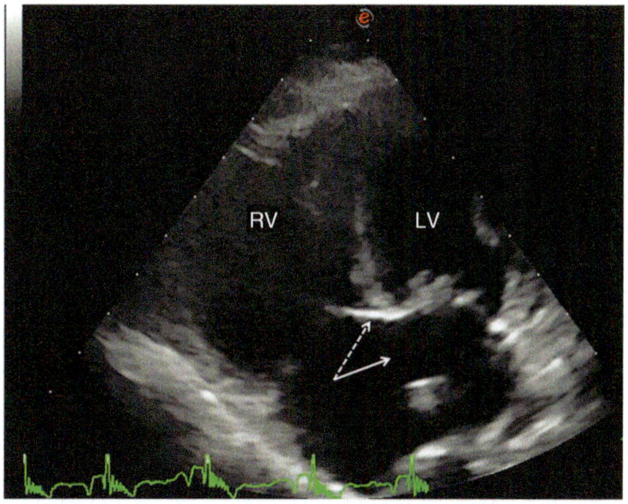

• **Fig. 19-62** Apical 4 chambers view in a case of partial atrioventricular (AV) defect. The *solid arrow* indicates a large septum primum atrial septal defect (ASD-OS1). The *dotted arrow* indicates a single AV valve. *LV,* Left ventricle; *RV,* right ventricle. (Photo credit: Claudio Bussadori.)

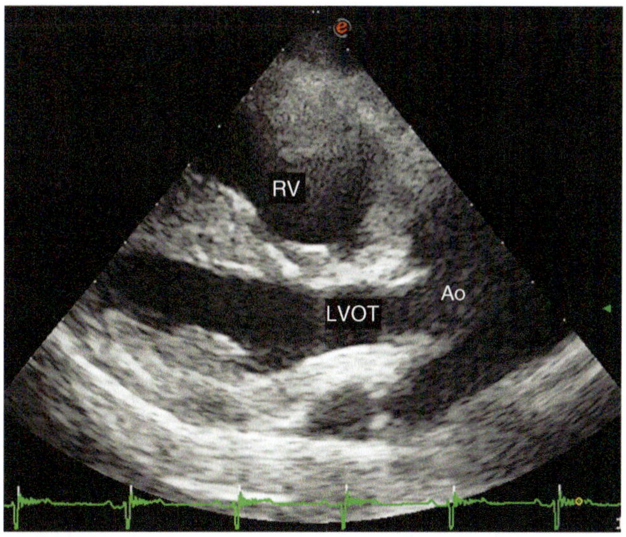

• **Fig. 19-63** Right parasternal long axis 5 chambers view in a puppy with a partial atrioventricular (AV) defect. The left ventricle outflow tract (LVOT) is elongated and takes the shape of a "goose neck." *Ao,* Aorta; *RV,* right ventricle. (Photo credit: Claudio Bussadori.)

from the abnormal anterior and apical displacement of the mitral valve, encroaching on the posterior and medial walls of the outflow tract, thus narrowing and elongating the lumen [139]. The causes of this deformity are probably more complex than abnormal position and attachment of the mitral valve; left ventricular geometry factors also may be involved [138]. In rare occasions, this "goose neck" deformation could lead to subaortic stenosis.

Doppler Echocardiography

Spectral and color Doppler interrogation allow the qualitative assessment of the respective atrioventricular flows and the assessment of the direction of the interatrial or interventricular shunts (Figure 19-64).

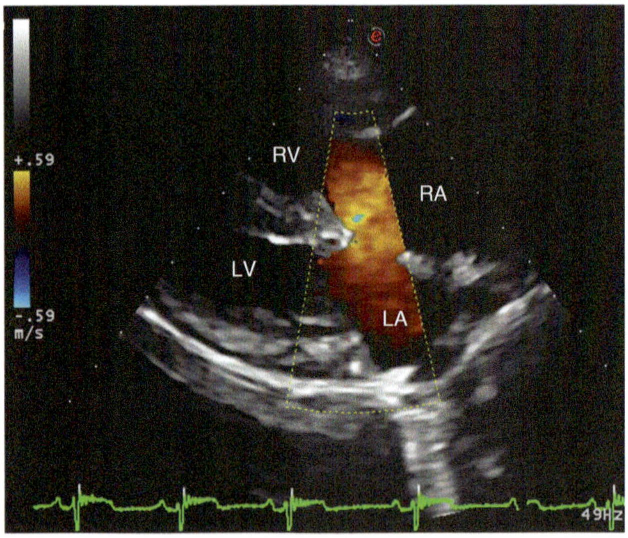

• **Fig. 19-64** Right parasternal long axis 5 chambers view in color Doppler mode in a cat with partial atrioventricular (AV) canal. The left-to-right interatrial shunt is clearly visible. *LA,* Left atrium; *LV,* left ventricle; *RA,* right atrium; *RV,* right ventricle. (Photo credit: Claudio Bussadori.)

The magnitude of the left-to-right intracardiac shunt can be estimated by measuring the pulmonary to systemic stroke volume ratio (Qp/Qs) from Doppler-derived pulmonic and aortic blood flow signals. Some authors suggest that dogs with a partial AV canal and concurrent mild MR may not exhibit any clinical signs during the first years of life, even in cases with a Qp/Qs ratio >2 [140].

REFERENCES

[1] Chetboul V, Trollé JM, Nicolle A, et al. Congenital heart diseases in the Boxer dog: a retrospective study of 105 cases (1998–2005). J Vet Med A Physiol Pathol Clin Med 2006;53:346–51.
[2] Baumgartner C, Glaus TM. Congenital cardiac diseases in dogs: a retrospective analysis. Schweiz Arch Tierheilkd 2003;145:527–33.
[3] Oyama MA, Sisson DD. Evaluation of canine congenital heart disease using an echocardiographic algorithm. J Am Anim Hosp Assoc 2001;37:519–35.
[4] Stephien RL, Bonagura JD. Aortic stenosis: clinical findings in six cats. J Small Anim Pract 1991;32:341–50.
[5] Lui S. Supravalvular aortic stenosis with deformity of the aortic valve in a cat. J Am Vet Med Assoc 1968;152:55–9.
[6] Heiene R, Indrebø A, Kvart C, et al. Prevalence of murmurs consistent with aortic stenosis among Boxer dogs in Norway and Sweden. Vet Rec 2000;147:152–6.
[7] Bussadori C, Pradelli D, Borgarelli M, et al. Congenital heart disease in Boxer dogs: results of 6 years of breed screening. Vet J 2009;18:187–92.
[8] Bussadori C, Quintavalla C, Capelli A. Prevalence of congenital heart disease in Boxers in Italy. J Vet Cardiol 2001;3:7–11.
[9] Oliveira P, Domenech O, Silva J, et al. Retrospective review of congenital heart disease in 976 dogs. J Vet Intern Med 2011;25:477–83.
[10] Freedom RM, Yoo SJ, Russell J, et al. Thoughts about fixed subaortic stenosis in man and dog. Cardiol Young 2005;15:186–205.
[11] Höllmer M, Willesen JL, Jensen AT, Koch J. Aortic stenosis in the Dogue de Bordeaux. J Small Anim Pract 2008;49:432–7.
[12] Bussadori C. Echo patterns in Boxers with subaortic stenosis. In: Proceedings for the Annual Forum of the American College of Veterinary Internal Medicine. Seattle, WA, USA; May 24 to 28, 2000, p. 86–87.
[13] Bussadori C. Breed related echocardiographic prognostic indicator in pulmonic and subaortic stenosis. In: Proceedings of the 16th ACVIM FORUM. San Diego, CA; 1998, p. 140–142 .
[14] Quintavalla C, Guazzetti S, Mavropoulou A, et al. Aorto-septal angle in Boxer dogs with subaortic stenosis: an echocardiographic study. Vet J 2010;185:332–7.
[15] Quintavalla C, Pradelli D, Domenech O, et al. Trans-esophageal echocardiography of the left ventricular outflow tract, aortic valve and ascending aorta in Boxer dogs with heart murmurs. Vet Radiol Ultrasound 2006;47:307–12.
[16] Pyle RL, Patterson DF, Chacko S. The genetics and pathology of discrete subaortic stenosis in the Newfoundland dog. Am Heart J 1976;92:324–34.
[17] Lai W, Mertens L, Cohen M, Geva T. Echocardiography in pediatric and congenital heart disease: from fetus to adult. Chichester, UK: John Wiley & Sons; 2009.

[18] Lang RM, Bierig M, Devereux RB, et al. Recommendations for chambre quantification: a report from the American Society of Echocardiography Guidelines and Standards Committee and the Chambre Quantification Writing Group, developed in conjunction with the European Association of Echocardiography, a branch of the European Society of Cardiology. J Am Soc Echocardiogr 2005;18:1440–63.

[19] Falk T, Jönsson L, Pedersen HD. Intramyocardial arterial narrowing in dogs with subaortic stenosis. J Small Anim Pract 2004;45:448–53.

[20] Hernandez JL, Bélanger MC, Benoit-Biancamano MO, et al. Left coronary aneurysmal dilation and subaortic stenosis in a dog. J Vet Cardiol 2008;10:75–9.

[21] Riesen SC, Doherr MG, Lombard CW. Comparison of Doppler-derived aortic velocities obtained from various transducer sites in healthy dogs and cats. Vet Radiol Ultrasound 2007;48:570–3.

[22] Lehmkuhl LB, Bonagura JD. Comparison of transducer placement sites for Doppler echocardiography in dogs with subaortic stenosis. Am J Vet Res 1994;55:192–8.

[23] Abbott JA, MacLean HN. Comparison of Doppler-derived peak aortic velocities obtained from subcostal and apical transducer sites in healthy dogs. Vet Radiol Ultrasound 2003;44:695–8.

[24] Kienle RD, Thomas WP, Pion PD. The natural clinical history of canine congenital subaortic stenosis. J Vet Intern Med 1994;8:423–31.

[25] Bussadori C, Amberger C, Le Bobinnec G, Lombard CW. Guidelines for the echocardiographic studies of suspected subaortic and pulmonic stenosis. J Vet Cardiol 2000;2:15–22.

[26] Stamm RB, Martin RP. Quantification of pressure gradients across stenotic valves by Doppler ultrasound. J Am Coll Cardiol 1983;2:707–18.

[27] Zhang Y, Myhre E, Nitter-Hauge S. Noninvasive quantification of the aortic valve area in aortic stenosis by Doppler echocardiography. Eur Heart J 1985;6:992–8.

[28] Zhang Y, Nitter-Hauge S. Determination of the mean pressure gradient in aortic stenosis by Doppler echocardiography. Eur Heart J 1985;6:999–1005.

[29] MacDonald K. Infective endocarditis in dogs: diagnosis and therapy. Vet Clin North Am Small Anim Pract 2010;40:665–84.

[30] Perez C, Fujii Y, Fauls M, et al. Fatal aortic endocarditis associated with community-acquired *Serratia marcescens* infection in a dog. J Am Anim Hosp Assoc 2011;47:133–7.

[31] Brown VA. Aortic valvular endocarditis in a dog. Can Vet J 2004;45:682–4.

[32] Peddle G, Sleeper MM. Canine bacterial endocarditis: a review. J Am Anim Hosp Assoc 2007;43:258–63.

[33] Sykes JE, Kittleson MD, Chomel BB, et al. Clinicopathologic findings and outcome in dogs with infective endocarditis: 71 cases (1992–2005). J Am Vet Med Assoc 2006;(228):1735–47.

[34] Tidholm A. Retrospective study of congenital heart defects in 151 dogs. J Small Anim Pract 1997;38:94–8.

[35] Schrope DP. Primary pulmonic infundibular stenosis in 12 cats: natural history and the effects of balloon valvuloplasty. J Vet Cardiol 2008;10:33–43.

[36] Schrope DP, Kelch WJ. Clinical and echocardiographic findings of pulmonary artery stenosis in seven cats. J Vet Cardiol 2007;9:83–9.

[37] Hopper BJ, Richardson JL, Irwin PJ. Pulmonic stenosis in two cats. Aust Vet J 2004;82:143–8.

[38] Johnson MS, Martin M. Balloon valvuloplasty in a cat with pulmonic stenosis. J Vet Intern Med 2003;17:928–30.

[39] Keirstead N, Miller L, Bailey T. Subvalvular pulmonary stenosis in a kitten. Can Vet J 2002;43:785–6.

[40] Anderson M. What is your diagnosis? Right-sided cardiomegaly associated with supravalvular pulmonic stenosis. J Am Vet Med Assoc 1992;200:2013–4.

[41] Fukushima R, Tanaka R, Suzuki S, et al. Epidemiological and morphological studies of double-chambered right ventricle in dogs. J Vet Med Sci 2011;73:1287–93.

[42] Koffas H, Fuentes VL, Boswood A, et al. Double chambered right ventricle in 9 cats. J Vet Intern Med 2007;21:76–80.

[43] Minors SL, O'Grady MR, Williams RM, O'Sullivan ML. Clinical and echocardiographic features of primary infundibular stenosis with intact ventricular septum in dogs. J Vet Intern Med 2006;20:1344–50.

[44] Buchanan JW. Pulmonic stenosis caused by single coronary artery in dogs: four cases (1965–1984). J Am Vet Med Assoc 1990;196:115–20.

[45] Buchanan JW. Pathogenesis of single right coronary artery and pulmonic stenosis in English Bulldogs. J Vet Intern Med 2001;15:101–4.

[46] Fonfara S, Martinez Pereira Y, Swift S, et al. Balloon valvuloplasty for treatment of pulmonic stenosis in English Bulldogs with an aberrant coronary artery. J Vet Intern Med 2010;24:345–9.

[47] Locatelli C, Domenech O, Silva J, et al. Independent predictors of immediate and long-term results after pulmonary balloon valvuloplasty in dogs. J Vet Cardiol 2011;13:21–30.

[48] Bashore TM. Adult congenital heart disease: right ventricular outflow tract lesions. Circulation 2007;115:1933–47.

[49] Paige CF, Abbott JA, Pyle RL. Systolic anterior motion of the mitral valve associated with right ventricular systolic hypertension in 9 dogs. J Vet Cardiol 2007;9:9–14.

[50] Francis AJ, Johnson MJ, Culshaw GC, et al. Outcome in 55 dogs with pulmonic stenosis that did not undergo balloon valvuloplasty or surgery. J Small Anim Pract 2011;52:282–8.
[51] Tobias AH, Stauthammer CD. Minimally invasive per-catheter occlusion and dilation procedures for congenital cardiovascular abnormalities in dogs. Vet Clin North Am Small Anim Pract 2010;40:581–603.
[52] Johnson MS, Martin M, Edwards D, et al. Pulmonic stenosis in dogs: balloon dilation improves clinical outcome. J Vet Intern Med 2004;18:656–62.
[53] Ristic JM, Marin CJ, Baines EA, Herrtage ME. Congenital pulmonic stenosis a retrospective study of 24 cases seen between 1990–1999. J Vet Cardiol 2001;3:13–9.
[54] Broaddus K, Tillson M. Patent ductus arteriosus in dogs. Compend Contin Educ Vet 2010;32:E1–14.
[55] Jones CL, Buchanan JW. Patent ductus arteriosus: anatomy and surgery in a cat. J Am Vet Med Assoc 1981;179:364–9.
[56] Summerfield NJ, Holt DE. Patent ductus arteriosus ligation and pulmonary artery banding in a kitten. J Am Anim Hosp Assoc 2005;41:133–6.
[57] Patterson DF. Lesion-specific genetic factors in canine congenital heart diseases: patent ductus arteriosus in Poodles, defects of the conotruncal septum in the Keeshond. Birth Defects Orig Artic Ser 1978;14:315–47.
[58] García-Rodríguez MB, Ríos Granja MA, Pérez García C, Gonzalo Orden JM. Complex cardiac congenital defects in an adult dog: an ultrasonographic and magnetic resonance imaging study. Can Vet J 2009;50:933–5.
[59] Slomp J, van Munsteren JC, Poelmann RE, et al. Formation of intimal cushions in the ductus arteriosus as a model for vascular intimal thickening: an immunohistochemical study of changes in extracellular matrix components. Atherosclerosis 1992;93:25–39.
[60] de Reeder EG, Poelmann RE, van Munsteren JC, et al. Ultrastructural and immunohistochemical changes of the extracellular matrix during intimal cushion formation in the ductus arteriosus of the dog. Atherosclerosis 1989;79:29–40.
[61] de Reeder EG, Gittenberger-de Groot AC, van Munsteren JC, et al. Distribution of prostacyclin synthase, 6-keto-prostaglandin f1 alpha, and 15-hydroxy-prostaglandin dehydrogenase in the normal and persistent ductus arteriosus of the dog. Am J Pathol 1989;135:881–7.
[62] Smolich JJ. Ultrastructural and functional features of the developing mammalian heart: a brief overview. Reprod Fertil Dev 1995;7:451–61.
[63] Buchanan JW, Patterson DF. Etiology of patent ductus arteriosus in dogs. J Vet Intern Med 2003;17:167–71.
[64] Saunders AB, Miller MW, Gordon SG, Bahr A. Echocardiographic and angiographic comparison of ductal dimensions in dogs with patent ductus arteriosus. J Vet Intern Med 2007;21:68–75.
[65] Van Israel N, French AT, Dukes-McEwan J, Corcoran BM. Review of left-to-right shunting patent ductus arteriosus and short term outcome in 98 dogs. J Small Anim Pract 2002;43:395–400.
[66] Aramaki Y, Chimura S, Hori Y, Eguchi T. Therapeutic changes of plasma n-terminal pro-brain natriuretic peptide concentrations in 9 dogs with patent ductus arteriosus. J Vet Med Sci 2011;73:83–8.
[67] Van Israel N, French AT, Dukes-McEwan J, Welsh EM. Patent ductus arteriosus in the older dog. J Vet Cardiol 2003;5:13–21.
[68] Patterson DF, Pyle RL, Buchanan JW, et al. Hereditary patent ductus arteriosus and its sequelae in the dog. Circ Res 1971;29:1–13.
[69] Cote E, Ettinger SJ. Long-term clinical management of right-to-left ("reversed") patent ductus arteriosus in 3 dogs. J Vet Intern Med 2001;15:39–42.
[70] Dirven MJ, Szatmari V, Cornelissen JM, van den Ingh TS. Case report: double-chambered right ventricle (DCRV), ventricular septal defect, and double caudal vena cava in a cat. Tijdschr Diergeneeskd 2010;135:180–8.
[71] Buchanan JW. Prevalence of cardiovascular disorders. In: Fox PR, Sisson DD, Moise NS, editors. Textbook of canine and feline cardiology. 2nd ed Philadelphia: WB Saunders Company; 1999, p. 458–63.
[72] Riesen SC, Kovacevic A, Lombard CW, Amberger C. Prevalence of heart disease in symptomatic cats: an overview from 1998 to 2005. Schweiz Arch Tierheilkd 2007;149:65–71.
[73] Thomas WP. Echocardiographic diagnosis of congenital membranous ventricular septal aneurysm in the dog and cat. J Am Anim Hosp Assoc 2005;41:215–20.
[74] Rausch WP, Keene BW. Spontaneous resolution of an isolated ventricular septal defect in a dog. J Am Vet Med Assoc 2003;223:219–20.
[75] Quintavalla C, Mavropoulou A, Buratti E. Aortic endocarditis associated with a perforated septal membranous aneurysm in a Boxer dog. J Small Anim Pract 2007;48:330–4.
[76] Boujon C, Amberger C, Lombard C. Right ventricular aneurysm and atrial septal defect in a cat. J Vet Cardiol 2004;6:44–8.
[77] Chetboul V, Charles V, Nicolle A, et al. Retrospective study of 156 atrial septal defects in dogs and cats (2001–2005). J Vet Med A Physiol Pathol Clin Med 2006;53:179–84.

[78] Lee SA, Lee SG, Moon HS, et al. Isolation, characterization and genetic analysis of canine GTA4 gene in a family of Doberman Pinschers with an atrial septal defect. J Genet 2007;86:241–7.
[79] Gordon SG, Nelson DA, Achen SE, et al. Open heart closure of an atrial septal defect by use of an atrial septal occluder in a dog. J Am Vet Med Assoc 2010;236:434–9.
[80] Fine DM, Tobias AH, Jacob KA. Supravalvular mitral stenosis in a cat. J Am Anim Hosp Assoc 2002;38:403–6.
[81] Behr L, Chetboul V, Sampedrano CC, et al. Beating heart mitral valve replacement with a bovine pericardial bioprosthesis for treatment of mitral valve dysplasia in a bull terrier. Vet Surg 2007;36:190–8.
[82] White RN, Boswood A, Garden OA, Hammond RA. Surgical management of subvalvular aortic stenosis and mitral dysplasia in a Golden Retriever. J Small Anim Pract 1997;38:251–5.
[83] Atwell RB, Sutton RH. Atrioventricular valve dysplasia in Dalmatians. Aust Vet J 1998;76:249.
[84] Domanjko-Petric A. What is your diagnosis? Mitral and tricuspid dysplasia. J Small Anim Pract 2004;45:83–4.
[85] Karaca O, Avci A, Guler GB, et al. Tenting area reflects disease severity and prognosis in patients with non-ischaemic dilated cardiomyopathy and functional mitral regurgitation. Eur J Heart Fail 2011;13:284–91.
[86] Riesen SC, Kovacevic A, Lombard CW, Amberger C. Echocardiographic screening of purebred cats: an overview from 2002 to 2005. Schweiz Arch Tierheilkd 2007;149:73–6.
[87] Liu SK, Tilley LP. Dysplasia of the tricuspid valve in the dog and cat. J Am Vet Med Assoc 1976;169:623–30.
[88] Robinson NA, Armíen AG. Tubular hypoplasia of the aorta and right atrioventricular valve dysplasia in a Bulldog. J Vet Diagn Invest 2010;22:667–70.
[89] Diana A, Guglielmini C, Acocella F, et al. Chylothorax associated with tricuspid dysplasia and atrial septal defect in a Bullmastiff. J Am Anim Hosp Assoc 2009;45:78–83.
[90] Famula TR, Siemens LM, Davidson AP, Packard M. Evaluation of the genetic basis of tricuspid valve dysplasia in Labrador Retrievers. Am J Vet Res 2002;63:816–20.
[91] Andelfinger G, Wright KN, Lee HS, et al. Canine tricuspid valve malformation, a model of human Ebstein anomaly, maps to dog chromosome 9. J Med Genet 2003;40:320–4.
[92] Choi R, Lee SK, Moon HS, et al. Ebstein's anomaly with an atrial septal defect in a Jindo dog. Can Vet J 2009;50:405–10.
[93] Takemura N, Machida N, Nakagawa K, et al. Ebstein's anomaly in a Beagle dog. J Vet Med Sci 2003;65:531–3.
[94] Brambilla PG, Di Marcello M, Tradati F. Complex congenital heart disease: prevalence and clinical findings. Vet Res Commun 2003;27(Suppl. 1):735–8.
[95] Chetboul V, Tran D, Carlos C, et al. Congenital malformations of the tricuspid valve in domestic carnivores: a retrospective study of 50 cases. Schweiz Arch Tierheilkd 2004;146:265–75.
[96] Hoffmann G, Amberger CN, Seiler G, Lombard CW. Tricuspid valve dysplasia in fifteen dogs. Schweiz Arch Tierheilkd 2000;142:268–77.
[97] Patterson DF, Pyle RL, Van Mierop L, et al. Hereditary defects of the conotruncal septum in Keeshond dogs: pathologic and genetic studies. Am J Cardiol 1974;34:187–205.
[98] Heaney AM, Bulmer BJ. Cor triatriatum sinister and persistent left cranial vena cava in a kitten. J Vet Intern Med 2004;18:895–8.
[99] Gordon B, Trautvetter E, Patterson DF. Pulmonary congestion associated with cor triatriatum in a cat. J Am Vet Med Assoc 1982;180:75–7.
[100] Koie H, Sato T, Nakagawa H, Sakai T. Cor triatriatum sinister in a cat. J Small Anim Pract 2000;41:128–31.
[101] Nakao S, Tanaka R, Hamabe L, et al. Cor triatriatum sinister with incomplete atrioventricular septal defect in a cat. J Feline Med Surg 2011;13:463–6.
[102] Wander KW, Monnet E, Orton EC. Surgical correction of cor triatriatum sinister in a kitten. J Am Anim Hosp Assoc 1998;35:383–6.
[103] Stern A, McClure RC, Holmberg D, et al. Cor triatriatum dexter in a dog. Compen Contin Educ Pract Vet 1986;8:401–2.
[104] Tobias AH, Thomas WP, Kittleson MD, Kometebedde J. Cor triatriatum dexter in two dogs. J Am Vet Med Assoc 1993;202:285–90.
[105] Johnson MS, Martin M, De Giovanni JV, et al. Management of cor triatriatum dexter by balloon dilatation in three dogs. J Small Anim Pract 2004;45:16–20.
[106] Duncan RB, Freeman LE, Jones J, Moon M. Cor triatriatum dexter in an English Bulldog puppy: case report and literature review. J Vet Diagn Invest 1999;11:361–5.
[107] Brayley KA, Ettiger SJ, Lunney J. Cor triatriatum dexter in a dog. J Am Anim Hosp Assoc 1994;30:153–6.
[108] Mitten RW, Edwards GA, Rishniw M. Diagnosis and management of cor triatriatum dexter in a Pyrenean Mountain Dog and an Akita Inu. Aust Vet J 2001;79:177–80.

[109] Linde-Sipman JS, Stokhof AA. Triple atria in a pup. J Am Vet Med Assoc 1974;165:539–41.

[110] Chanoit G, Bublot I, Viguier E. Transient tricuspid valve regurgitation following surgical treatment of cor triatriatum dexter in a dog. J Small Anim Pract 2009;50:241–5.

[111] Szatmári V, Sótonyi P, Fenyves B, et al. Doppler-ultrasonographic detection of retrograde pulsatile flow in the caudal vena cava of a puppy with cor triatriatum dexter. Vet Rec 2000;147:68–72.

[112] Nieuwland J, Beijerink N, Szatmári V. Resolution of ascites after successful balloon dilatation of cor triatriatum dexter in a dog. Tijdschr Diergeneeskd 2010;135:330–3.

[113] From AH, Mazzitello WF, Judd AS, Edwards JE. Ebstein's malformation of the tricuspid valve associated with valvular stenosis and cor triatriatum. Chest 1973;64:248–51.

[114] Hansing CE, Young WP, Rowe GG. Cor triatriatum dexter: persistent right sinus venosus valve. Am J Cardiol 1972;30:559–63.

[115] Atwell RB, Sutton RH. Suspect three chambered right atrium in a pup. Vet Rec 1983;113:86–7.

[116] Poanta L, Albu A, Fodor D. Chiari network: case report and brief literature review. Med Ultrason 2010;12:71–2.

[117] Slight RD, Nzewi OC, Buell R, Mankad PS. Cor triatriatum sinister presenting in the adult as mitral stenosis: an analysis of factors which may be relevant in late presentation. Heart Lung Circ 2005;14:8–12.

[118] Lee HM, Sung HS, Kim SY. Anesthetic management of non-cardiac surgery with adult onset type of cor triatriatum sinister: a case report. Korean J Anesthesiol 2011;60:444–8.

[119] Sevimli S, Gundogdu F, Arslan S, Senocak H. Cor triatriatum sinister in a 19-year-old patient. Turk Kardiyol Dern Ars 2008;36:259–62.

[120] Fossum TW, Miller MW. Cor triatriatum and canal anomalies. Semin Vet Med Surg (Small Anim) 1994;9:177–84.

[121] Hoffmann DE, Tobiass HA. What is your diagnosis? Cor triatriatum dexter. J Am Vet Med Assoc 2003;223:951–2.

[122] Tanaka R, Hoshi K, Shimizu M, et al. Surgical correction of cor triatriatum dexter in a dog under extracorporeal circulation. J Small Anim Pract 2003;44:370–3.

[123] Adin DB, Thomas WP. Balloon dilation of cor triatriatum dexter in a dog. J Vet Intern Med 1999;13:617–9.

[124] Johnson MS, Martin M, De Giovanni JV, et al. Management of cor triatriatum dexter by balloon dilatation in three dogs. J Small Anim Pract 2004;45:16–20.

[125] Nakayama T, Wakao Y, Uechi M, et al. A case report of surgical treatment of a dog with atrioventricular septal defect (incomplete form of endocardial cushion defect). J Vet Med Sci 1994;56:981–4.

[126] Santamarina G, Espino L, Vila M, Suarez ML. Partial atrioventricular canal defect in a dog. J Small Anim Pract 2002;43:17–21.

[127] Monnet E, Orton EC, Gaynor J, et al. Diagnosis and surgical repair of partial atrioventricular septal defects in two dogs. J Am Vet Med Assoc 1997;211:569–72.

[128] Akiyama M, Tanaka R, Maruo K, Yamane Y. Surgical correction of a partial atrioventricular septal defect with a ventricular septal defect in a dog. J Am Anim Hosp Assoc 2005;41:137–43.

[129] Benson DW, Sund KL. Looking down the atrioventricular canal. Cardiovasc Res 2010;88:205–6.

[130] Person AD, Klewer SE, Runyan RB. Cell biology of cardiac cushion development. Int Rev Cytol 2005;243:287–335.

[131] Jiao K, Langworthy M, Batts L, et al. Tgfbeta signaling is required for atrioventricular cushion mesenchyme remodeling during in vivo cardiac development. Development 2006;133:4585–93.

[132] Barnett JV, Desgrosellier JS. Early events in valvulogenesis: a signaling perspective birth defect res. Part. C. Embryo Today 2003;69:58–72.

[133] Sakabe M, Matsui H, Sakata H, et al. Understanding heart development and congenital heart defects through developmental biology: a segmental approach. Congenit Anom (Kyoto) 2005;45:107–18.

[134] Saponaro V, Staffieri F, Franchini D, Crovace A. Complete atrioventricular canal in a dog. J Vet Cardiol 2010;12:135–40.

[135] Ohad DG, Baruch S, Perl S. Incomplete atrioventricular canal complicated by cardiac tamponade and bidirectional shunting in an adult dog. J Am Anim Hosp Assoc 2007;43:221–6.

[136] Amberger CN, Boujon CE, Amberger C, Boujon C. Atrioventricular canal defect (incomplete form of endocardial cushion defect) and ostium secundum type interatrial septal defect in a dog. J Vet Cardiol 2002;4:37–41.

[137] Konstantinov IE, Rosapepe F, Dearani JA, et al. A tribute to Giancarlo Rastelli. Ann Thorac Surg 2005;79:1819–23.

[138] Blieden LC, Randall PA, Castaneda AR, et al. The "goose neck" of the endocardial cushion defect: anatomic basis. Chest 1974;65:13–7.

[139] Gotsman MS, Beck W, Schrire V. Left ventricular cineangiocardiography in endocardial cushion defects. Br Heart J 1968;30:182–6.

[140] Yamano S, Uechi M, Tanaka K, et al. Surgical repair of a complete endocardial cushion defect in a dog. Vet Surg 2011;40:408–12.

20

Echocardiographic Evaluation of Congenital Cardiopathies Before and After Intervention

CLAUDIO BUSSADORI IN COLLABORATION WITH DANITZA PRADELLI

Pulmonic Valve Stenosis, 324
Patent Ductus Arteriosus, 331
Ventricular Septal Defect, 336
Atrial Septal Defect, 339

Pulmonic Valve Stenosis

Pulmonic stenosis (PS) is one of the three most common congenital heart defects in dogs [1,2]. Initially described in 1982, pulmonic balloon valvuloplasty (PBV) is now the treatment of choice for congenital valvular PS in humans and in dogs [3-9]. Factors determining successful PBV include appropriate patient selection and choice of the method. The balloon-to-annulus ratio is an important factor that influences PBV results [10]. Traditionally, the pulmonic annulus diameter (PAd) is measured by angiography and/or transthoracic echocardiography (TTE). The morphologic characterization of PS is performed by TTE [7,11].

Evaluation Prior to Valvuloplasty

Preinterventional evaluation of dogs with PS referred for PBV is traditionally performed by TTE. In some cases, the use of transesophageal echocardiography (TEE) and/or angiography is also advocated. The pulmonic valve morphology, PAd measurement, degree of right ventricular (RV) hypertrophy and/or dilatation, extent of the hypertrophy (global or of the right ventricular outflow tract), and tricuspid valve leakproofness are assessed using bidimensional (2D) TTE in most cases. The pressure gradient and the obstruction characteristics (fixed or dynamic) are evaluated in Doppler mode.

Stenosis Type Identification

Using TTE, valvular PS can be classified as either type A or type B as described in Chapter 19. Some stenoses are considered to be intermediate, with pulmonic valve cusp fusion and mild narrowing of the pulmonic valve annulus. A variant of valvular PS, described as hourglass PS, has also been described. It is characterized by mildly fused or nonfused pulmonic valve cusps, deep bottle-shaped sinuses, and a narrower proximal diameter of the main pulmonary artery than that of the right ventricular outflow tract (RVOT) [11,12]. The diagnosis of PS associated with a type R2A coronary anomaly can be suggested by TTE but often must be confirmed by angiocardiography. In our experience, an anomalous coronary artery must be suspected when the pulmonic valve is impossible to identify using TTE. This anomalous coronary artery can at times be seen by TTE right above the valve (subvalvular stenosis) (see Chapter 19). TEE has been found to be very useful in these cases (Figure 20-1).

Types A and B and intermediate PS can be treated by PBV but the results will differ depending on the type of

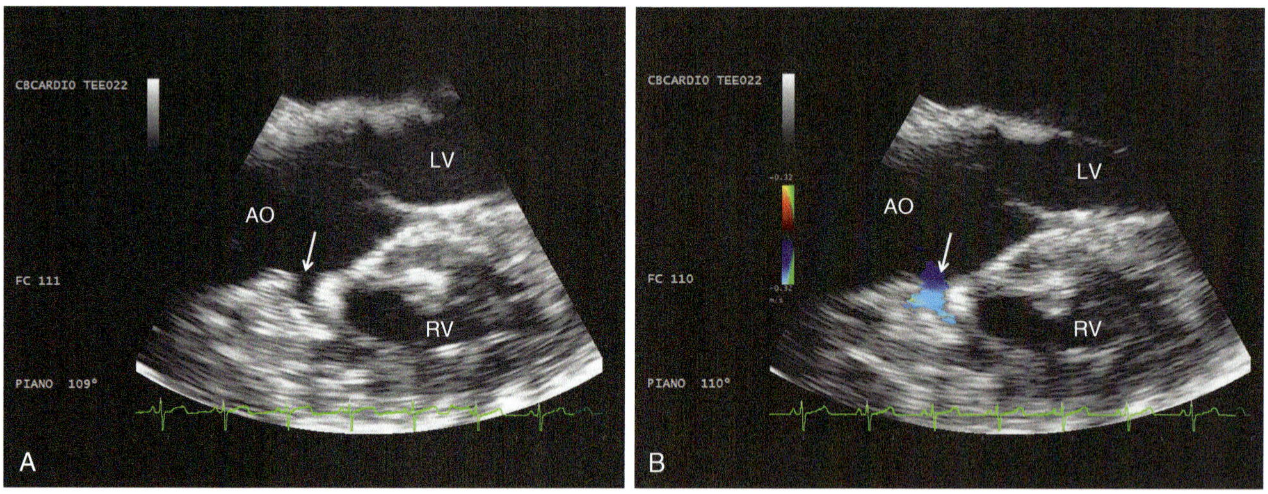

• Fig. 20-1 Transesophageal echocardiogram (longitudinal median view centered on the aorta) in a dog with an anomalous origin of the coronary arteries. A, This image of the aorta shows a large right coronary artery with a bifurcation *(arrow)*. B, The bifurcation, which is the origin of the right and left anomalous coronary arteries, is better visualized in color Doppler mode. *Ao,* Aorta; *LV,* left ventricle; *RV,* right ventricle. (Photo credit: Claudio Bussadori.)

PS. The presence or absence of annulus hypoplasia and the degree of pulmonic cusp fusion are important factors to consider during evaluation, since severe hypoplasia and absence of fusion of the commissures are associated with poor results [7,13]. PBV is unanimously considered contraindicated in cases of hourglass morphology, due to the risk of tear or dissection of the arterial wall during balloon inflation (see Chapter 6) [14]. PBV is also contraindicated for PS resulting from coronary artery anomaly. Some authors have suggested the possibility of using less aggressive PBV, using a lower balloon-to–pulmonic annulus diameter (B/PAd) ratio [15,16]. In our experience and that of other teams, we do not recommend this, partly because of the risk of coronary artery compression inducing myocardial ischemia during balloon dilation and partly because this stenosis is the result of annulus strangulation by the anomalous coronary artery and not the result of pulmonic cusp fusion [7,17,18].

PV Annulus Diameter Measurement

Pulmonic valve (PV) annulus diameter measurement must be performed at the level of insertion of the pulmonic valve cusps on the annulus, in systole, using the right parasternal short axis transaortic and left cranial views. The average of the values is then calculated (Figure 20-2).

Evaluation of the Tricuspid Valve

The tricuspid valve must be evaluated carefully. In fact, the tricuspid valve annulus deforms when right ventricular dilation becomes significant or when RV hypertrophy causes malalignment of the papillary muscles. In the latter situation, distinction between these changes and those resulting from tricuspid dysplasia becomes difficult. The presence of tricuspid regurgitation is associated with a poorer prognosis [19].

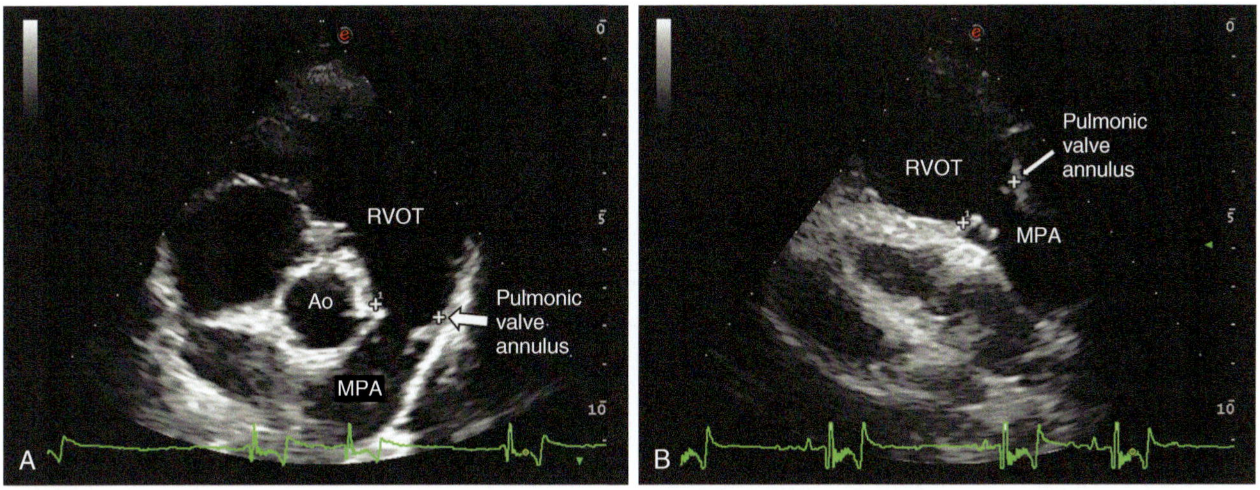

• **Fig. 20-2** Bidimensional (2D) transthoracic echocardiogram showing how to measure the dimensions of the pulmonic valve annulus. A, Right parasternal short axis transaortic view. B, Left cranial view. Measurements must be taken in systole at the level of the pulmonic valve insertion point on the annulus, as shown in these images. *Ao,* Aorta; *MPA,* main pulmonary artery; *RVOT,* right ventricular outflow tract. (Photo credit: Claudio Bussadori.)

Evaluation of Right Ventricular Hypertrophy

An accurate evaluation of the type of RV hypertrophy (severity and localization) must be done prior to PBV. Significant RV hypertrophy (Figure 20-3) could interfere with the passage of catheters. In addition, severe RVOT hypertrophy (Figure 20-4) can predispose to a specific complication such as "suicide right ventricle," characterized by a severe and potentially fatal subvalvular obstruction occurring immediately following valvular dilation. This complication is the result of ventricular hypercontractility associated with severe RVOT hypertrophy. It is significantly correlated to the transvalvular pressure gradient, the degree of RV hypertrophy, and RVOT hyperactivity [20-23]. Treatment with an intravenous beta blocker such as esmolol can effectively reduce the contractility of the right ventricle and its RVOT, thus reducing the dynamic component of the obstruction at the outflow tract level. This leads to an immediate improvement in arterial oxygenation. When such a predisposition is suspected, we recommend prophylactic administration of beta blockers prior to PBV.

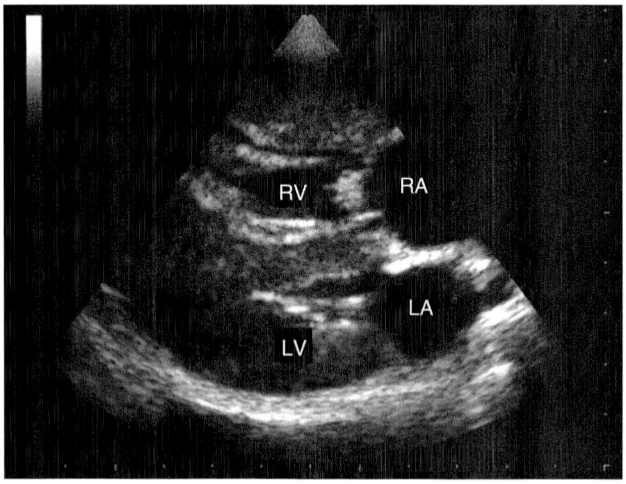

• **Fig. 20-3** Transthoracic echocardiogram (right parasternal long axis 4 chambers view) in a dog with pulmonic stenosis (PS). The right ventricle (RV) is rarely hypertrophied. *LA,* Left atrium; *LV,* left ventricle; *RA,* right atrium. (Photo credit: Claudio Bussadori.)

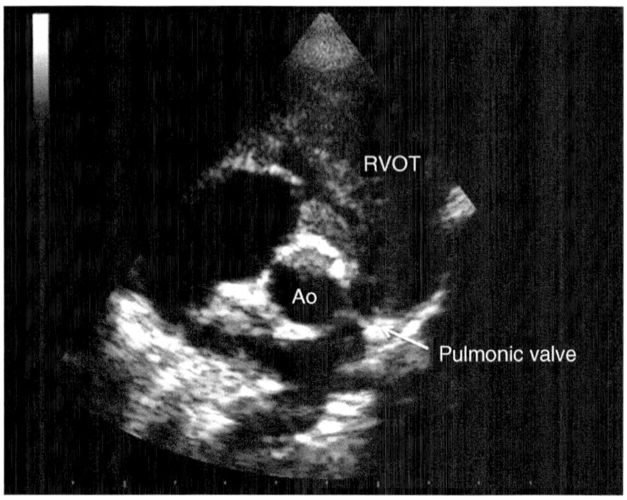

• **Fig. 20-4** Bidimensional (2D) transthoracic echocardiogram (right parasternal short axis view at the heart base level) in a dog with pulmonic stenosis (PS). The right ventricular outflow tract (RVOT) appears to be severely hypertrophied. *Ao,* Aorta. (Photo credit: Claudio Bussadori.)

Evaluation of the Degree of Right Ventricular Dilation

Right ventricular dilation must be taken seriously since it can indicate systolic dysfunction. Although several quantitative methods for evaluating right ventricular function have been described (see Chapter 10), examination of the right ventricle structure and function remains largely qualitative in current practice. The complexity of the right ventricle morphology, with its bellow shape and trabeculations, makes the calculation and ejection fraction difficult. New parameters based on strain measurement (see Chapter 10) seem to hold more promise for the evaluation of right ventricular function, an important determinant for postintervention prognosis [24-26]. Inclusion and exclusion criteria of right ventricle function status could be established, thus avoiding performing PBV in dogs with irreversible right ventricular dysfunction.

Evaluation of Other Associated Congenital Lesions

Finally, the goal of preintervention evaluation is to identify any associated congenital lesions. We have reported that one third of the dogs with PS also suffered from another congenital cardiopathy [27]. The most frequent of these was ventricular septal defect. Persistent left cranial vena cava (PLCVC) is a hemodynamically benign anomaly but it potentially complicates the vascular approach for PBV (the right jugular vein is the best venous access in such a case). PLCVC is suspected when a circular hypoechoic structure is identified between the left atrium and the pericardium on the right parasternal long axis 4 chambers view. If the transducer is rotated counterclockwise, an elongated structure appears entering the atrioventricular groove, between the left atrium and left ventricle (Figure 20-5). This structure represents a dilated coronary sinus due to the left cranial vena cava draining into it.

Transesophageal Echocardiography

As discussed earlier, TEE can be useful in the diagnosis of specific morphologic anomalies, such as abnormal coronary arteries and hourglass stenoses. This technique is also useful to obtain a good view of the pulmonic valve and its annulus in dogs with limited echographic window, such as Bulldogs (see Chapter 5).

Tridimensional Echocardiography

Tridimensional (3D) echocardiography is a new technology, providing high-quality images of the pulmonic valve [28]. The morphology of the stenotic valve can be assessed accurately and the area of the stenotic orifice can be calculated prior to PVB (see Chapter 6).

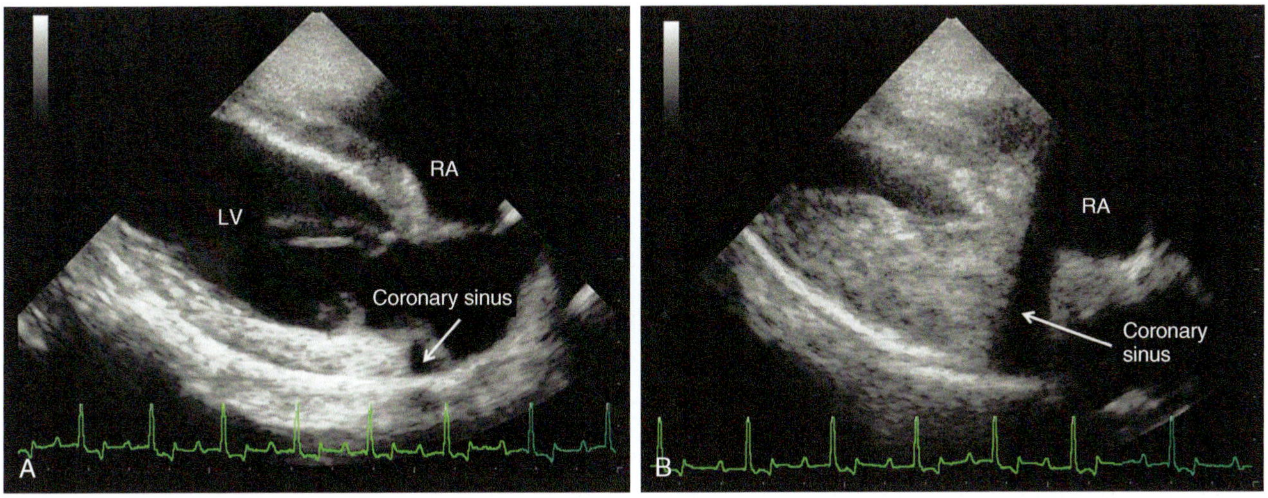

• **Fig. 20-5** Transthoracic bidimensional (2D) echocardiogram (right parasternal long axis 4 chambers view) showing the coronary sinus. A, The coronary sinus is visible between the left atrium posterior wall and the pericardium. B, By rotating the transducer counterclockwise, the coronary sinus appears as an elongated, anechoic structure between the left atrium and the left ventricle, along their posterior surfaces. *LV,* Left ventricle; *RA,* right atrium. (Photo credit: Claudio Bussadori.)

Postvalvuloplasty Assessment

In our practice, postvalvuloplasty evaluation is performed using TTE immediately or 24 hours following the procedure and then 1, 3, 6, and 12 months later. We have evaluated pulmonic valve mobility using 2D mode (which should be much improved if the dilation was good), along with thickness ("posttraumatic" pulmonic valve thickening can occur following PBV; Figure 20-6) and changes in the right and left ventricles. The post-PBV transventricular pressure gradient (Figure 20-7) and the characteristics of residual stenosis (stationary versus dynamic) can

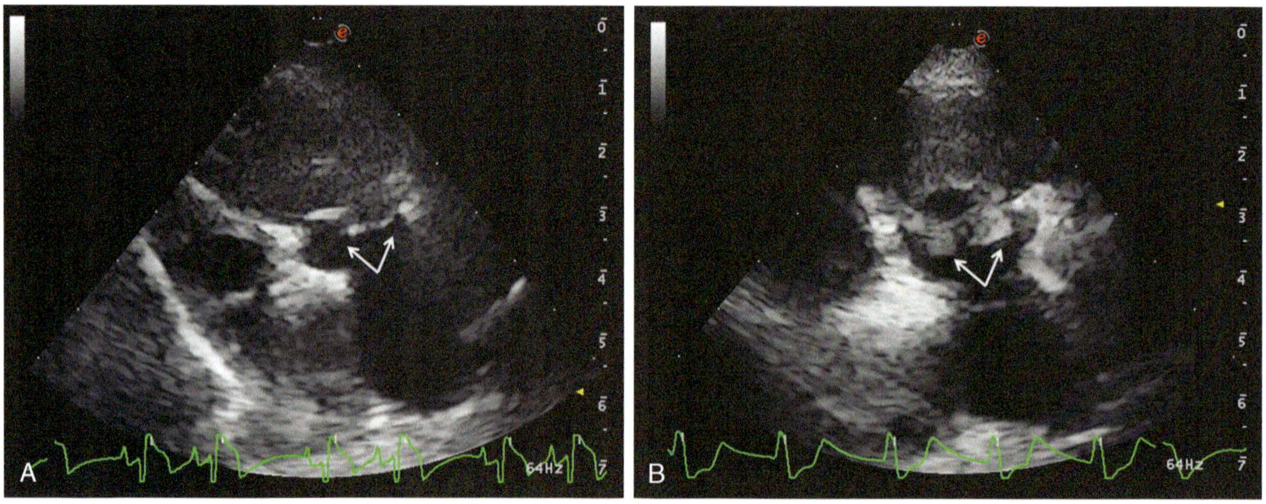

• **Fig. 20-6** Bidimensional (2D) transthoracic echocardiogram (left parasternal cranial view centered on the pulmonic valve) in a dog with pulmonic stenosis (PS) before (A) and after (B) valvuloplasty. The pulmonic valve cusps *(arrows)* appear fused prior to and very thickened following intervention (postdilation trauma). (Photo credit: Claudio Bussadori.)

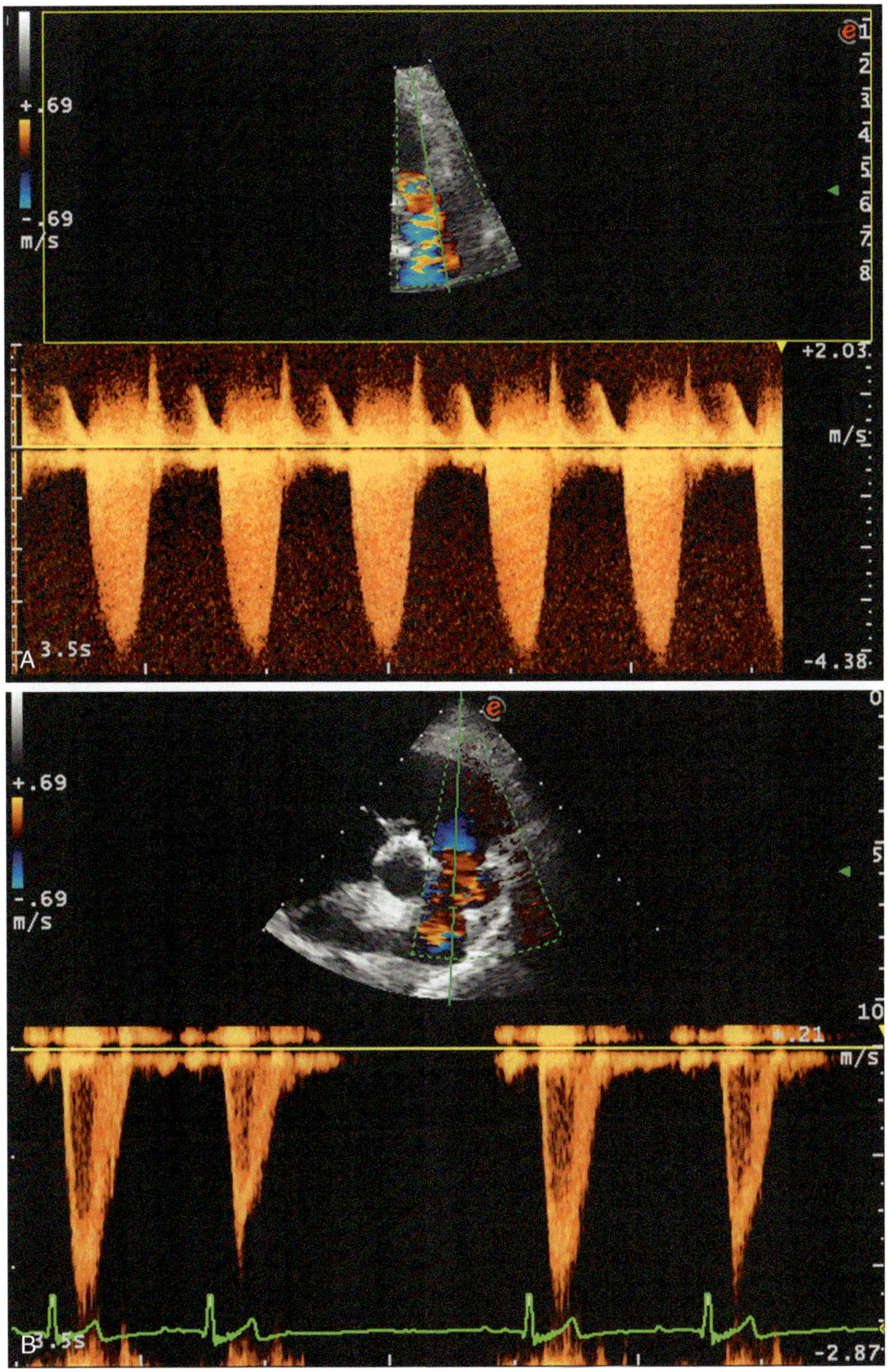

• **Fig. 20-7** Pulsed spectral Doppler in a dog with pulmonic stenosis (PS) before (A) and following (B) valvuloplasty. The flow before valvuloplasty has a high velocity and is turbulent. Continuous wave Doppler is required to record the maximum velocities. Following the valvuloplasty, the flow becomes laminar and the marked reduction of its maximum velocity allows it to be recorded in pulsed Doppler mode. (Photo credit: Claudio Bussadori.)

be appreciated using Doppler mode (Figure 20-8). The importance of post-PBV pulmonic regurgitation and the degree of tricuspid regurgitation are also studied.

In veterinary medicine, the definition of immediate and long-term success of a PBV varies according to different authors. Proposed criteria include a reduction of the preintervention pressure gradient ≥50%, a postsurgical gradient <50 to 80 mm Hg, or a pressure gradient <50 mm Hg immediately following PBV and 75 mm Hg 1 year later [7,9,13,29,30]. Even in human medicine, the definition of immediate and long-term success varies according to the literature. In all cases, the threshold value of the gradient was arbitrarily selected based on a gradient above which medical or interventional follow-up would be reasonably advised. These values can range from 25 to 50 mm Hg [4,5,31].

The success of PBV can be underestimated when only immediate results are taken into consideration. In fact, a dynamic RVOT obstruction as well as pulmonic valve edema can increase the pressure gradient. Delayed gradient reduction is possible with regression of the RVOT hypertrophy and disappearance of postoperative pulmonic valve thickening. This phenomenon has been well documented in human medicine [5,20,21]. A study has shown that the long-term outcome of patients after a PBV depends on the site of the residual gradient pressure: RVOT gradients decreased significantly over time whereas valvular gradients increased slightly [32].

In our study, the pre-PBV pulmonic gradient was identified as being an independent criterion for predicting immediate and long-term success of the intervention. Animals in which gradient reduction was disappointing (immediately and long term) had a significantly higher pre-PBV gradient than that of the dogs in which PBV was considered satisfactory. Another predictive criterion, which is independent of long-term success, was the 24-hour residual gradient following PBV [13].

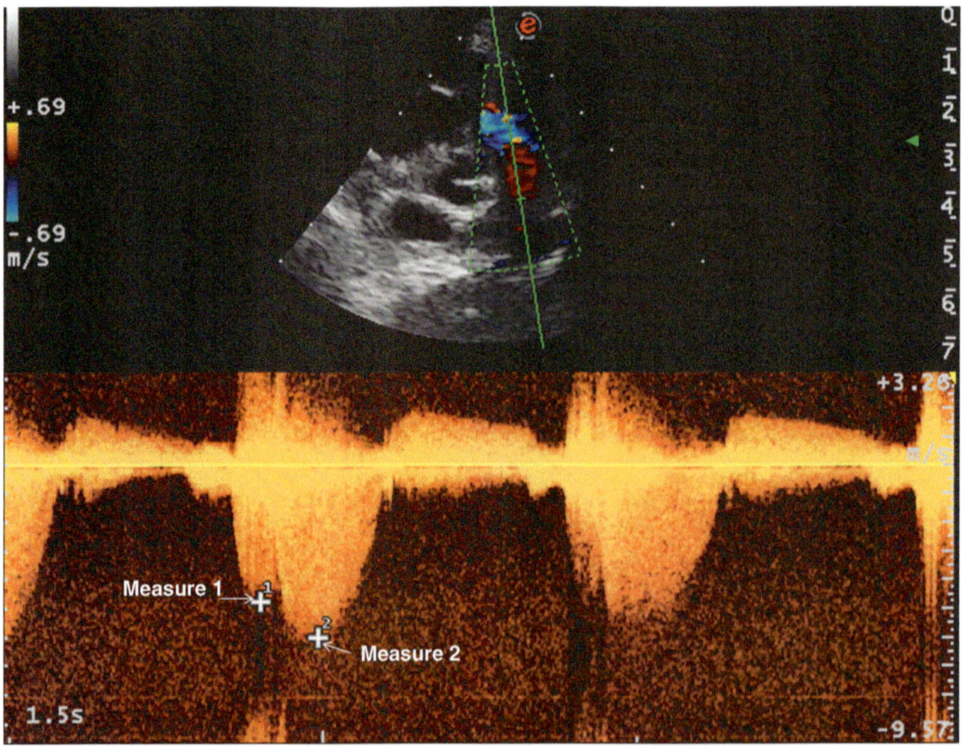

• **Fig. 20-8** Pulsed spectral Doppler in a dog with pulmonic stenosis (PS) following valvuloplasty. The dynamic stenosis bladelike signal (Measure 2) is superimposed on the fixed stenosis signal (Measure 1). The dynamic stenosis seems to be more severe than the fixed stenosis. (Photo credit: Claudio Bussadori.)

Pulmonic regurgitation either appears or is increased following PBV, suggesting effective valve dilation (commissurotomy). In our experience, this regurgitation is rarely significant. Tricuspid regurgitation generally decreases following intervention, except when tricuspid dysplasia is present.

In our experience, TEE allows visualization during the intervention of the immediate increase in pulmonic cusp mobility after dilation.

3D echocardiography allows evaluation of the changes in the pulmonic cusps and calculation of the area of the post-PBV valvular orifice. This can be compared to the pre-PBV area and gives a good idea of the enlargement of the orifice. The 3D echocardiography can also help to reveal post-PBV complications such as arterial wall dissection (see Chapter 6).

Patent Ductus Arteriosus

Patent ductus arteriosus (PDA) surgical ligature or occlusion with an endovascular device at a young age is associated with an excellent prognosis [33-35]. However, occlusion of a reverse PDA is not recommended because it leads to a sudden increase in the right heart afterload, usually resulting in acute right heart failure followed by the death of the animal [36,37]. Reverse PDA must be distinguished from PDA with pulmonary arterial hypertension but still associated with a left-to-right shunt. Recent studies have demonstrated that the occlusion of the latter type of PDA can lead to favorable results [38]. PDA occlusion offers important clinical benefits but the best occlusion method still remains to be identified. Occlusion by surgical ligature of PDA in a dog was reported as early as 1952 [39]. This remains a common approach for treating PDA in dogs. Endovascular device occlusion (placement by catheter) is increasingly being used in veterinary medicine. Several devices, such as coils, plugs (Amplatzer®), or specific PDA Amplatzer occlusion devices for dogs (Amplatz® canine duct occluder, or ACDO), have been used. The ACDO is the most recently developed endovascular device for dogs and has become the current treatment of choice. The procedure (surgical or interventional) and device choices are based on a combination of factors, including the PDA morphology, the minimal ductal diameter (MDD), and the size of the patient. ACDO has been found to be effective in the occlusion of PDA of different shapes and sizes [40-43]. The cylindrical shape of type III PDA (see below) has proven to be problematic because the ACDO is difficult to anchor in this case. This type of PDA is fortunately very infrequent. Larger diameter PDAs in very small dogs can also present a challenge due to their small femoral artery diameters. In these cases, surgical ligature should be considered.

Evaluation Prior to Occlusion

TTE is useful to confirm the presence of PDA, evaluate volume overload and state of myocardial function, and determine the presence or absence of any concomitant cardiopathies.

Degree of Volume Overload and Systolic Function of the Left Ventricle

To evaluate the degree of volume overload and the systolic function, echocardiographic measures must include at least end-systolic and end-diastolic diameters, indexed end-systolic and end-diastolic volumes (ESVI and EDVI, respectively), ejection fraction, and left ventricular sphericity index.

Evaluation of the systolic function prior to the procedure is important in order to determine whether systolic dysfunction is present and whether functional and clinical postintervention recovery is possible. Several groups of PDA patients can be distinguished: those in which left ventricular function will return to normal following a PDA occlusion; those in which ventricular dysfunction will persist irreversibly following the intervention; and those in which acute left heart failure will develop postoperatively, requiring intensive treatment for several days. To date, we do not have specific threshold values to distinguish PDA cases with preserved systolic function from those with irreversible systolic dysfunction. However, in our experience, an EDVI <300 mL/m^2 and an ESVI <200 mL/m^2 indicate a preserved systolic function.

New echocardiographic methods, such as left ventricular myocardial tissue Doppler and strain measurements using speckle tracking, could potentially help to obtain more accurate parameters [44,45].

Minimal Ductal Diameter

TTE may not provide reliable MDD measurements and PDA morphologic classification. Angiography and/or TEE should be used as ancillary testing. According to a study, MDD measurements using TTE can significantly differ from those obtained using angiography [45]. However, in another study, TTE measurements of the MDD (not including the ampulla) done using a left cranial parasternal view correlated well with those obtained using angiocardiography [46].

Overall, the average difference between the two methods is small but the divergence between the TTE MDD measurements and those obtained by angiography can often be large for a given individual [47].

In our experience, 3D echocardiography seems to be the most reliable method to accurately measure the MDD. In a single view, the two orthogonal MDDs can be measured (see Chapter 6). This is important because, in some cases, the ostium is elliptical and not circular. Therefore there is a risk of underestimating the size of the occlusion device to use if only one diameter measurement is taken into account.

PDA Morphology

Angiography is the gold-standard method to determine PDA morphology and dimensions. PDAs can be grouped into three main types:

- Type I: The PDA diameter progressively decreases from the aorta to its junction with the main pulmonary artery.
- Type IIA: This type of PDA has essentially parallel walls, until a sudden reduction in its diameter (MDD <50% of the ductal diameter) at the level of insertion in the main pulmonary artery.
- Type IIB: This type of PDA is characterized by a diameter markedly decreasing from the aorta toward the main pulmonary artery, the narrowest point being at the level of insertion into the main pulmonary artery.
- Type III: This type of PDA presents a constant diameter throughout its length, giving it a tubular aspect [48].

Angiographic images are classically recorded on a single plane, which does not always render the best spatial representation of PDA anatomy. This is improved by viewing the PDA over several planes. Our experience suggests that TEE is just as good a technique as angiography to determine PDA morphology and to measure the MDD as well as the diameter of the ductal ampulla. The MDD and ampulla diameter measurements are obtained using a longitudinal cranial view (Figure 20-9). A multiplane TEE can also help to determine whether the PDA ostium is elliptic rather than circular (short axis view), which can affect the selection of the occlusion device. Finally, TEE is useful for monitoring the occlusion procedure [49]. This technique allows real-time observation of the occlusion device deployment within the PDA (Figure 20-10) as well as evaluation of the flow through the PDA before and after placement of the occlusion device (Figure 20-11). This can help with decision making during the procedure. In addition, the amount of contrast product injection needed to verify the position of the device and proper occlusion of the PDA is reduced with the use of TEE during the occlusion procedure.

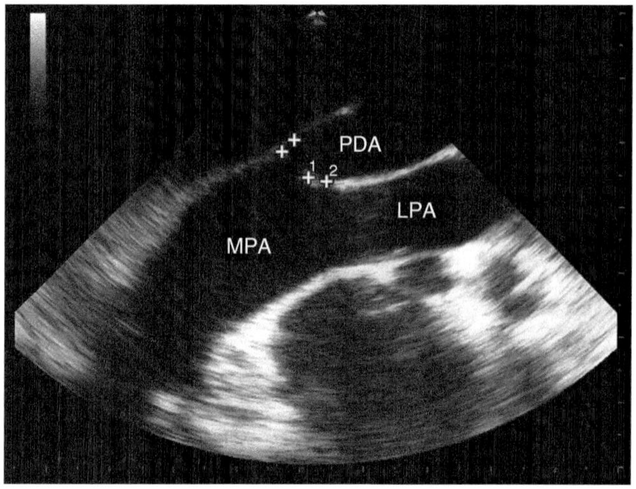

• **Fig. 20-9** Transesophageal echocardiogram in a dog with patent ductus arteriosus (PDA) (longitudinal cranial view centered on the duct). This is an enlarged view of the ductus (PDA), allowing accurate measurement of the minimum diameter (measurement 1) and the ampulla width (measurement 2). *LPA,* Left pulmonary artery; *MPA,* main pulmonary artery. (Photo credit: Claudio Bussadori.)

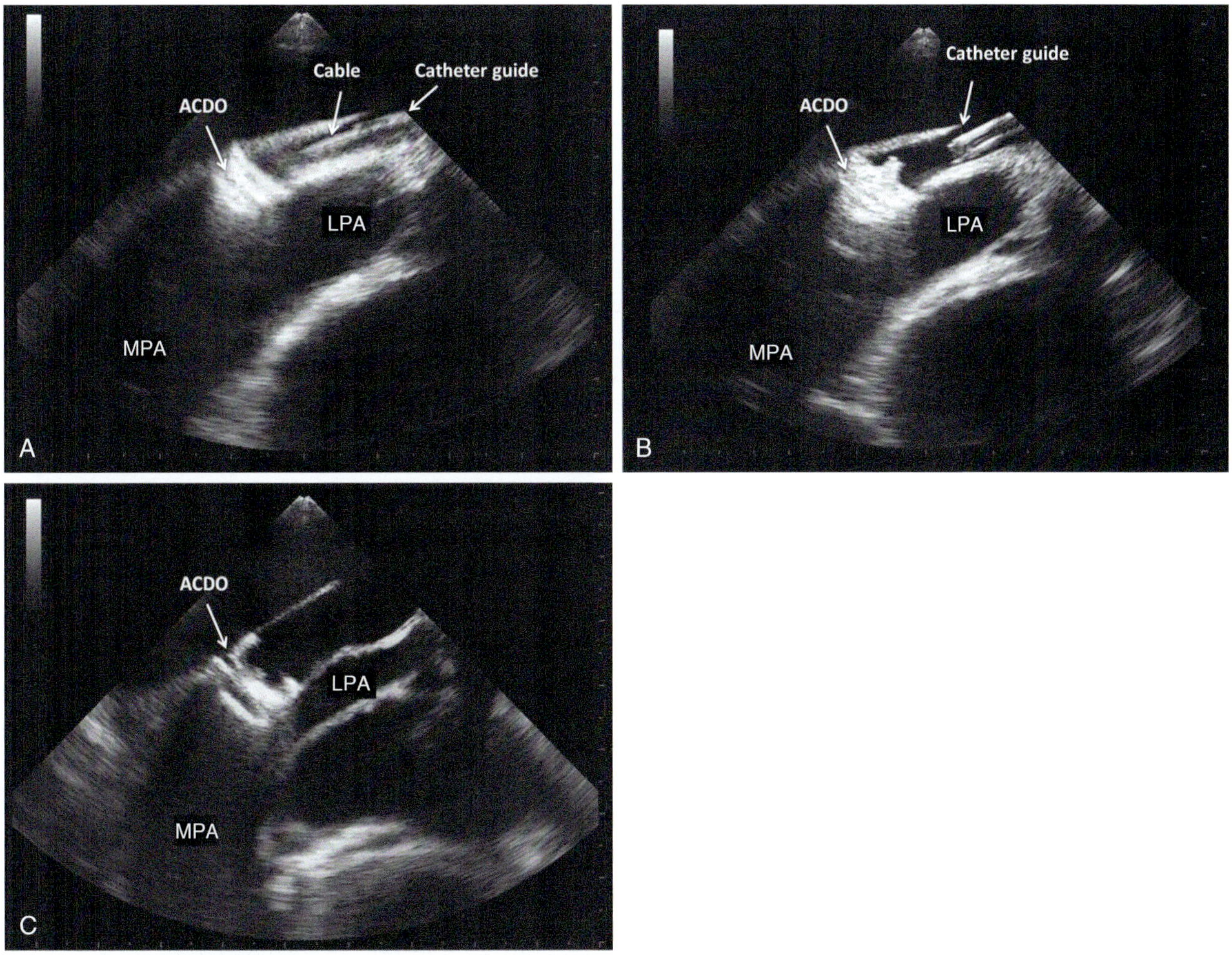

• **Fig. 20-10** Transesophageal echocardiogram in a dog with patent ductus arteriosus (PDA) (longitudinal cranial view centered on the duct). These three views were taken during the occlusion procedure using an Amplatz® canine duct occluder (ACDO). A, ACDO deployment at the level of the minimal ductal diameter. The ACDO is still attached to its cable. B and C, ACDO release. *LPA,* Left pulmonary artery; *MPA,* main pulmonary artery. (Photo credit: Claudio Bussadori.)

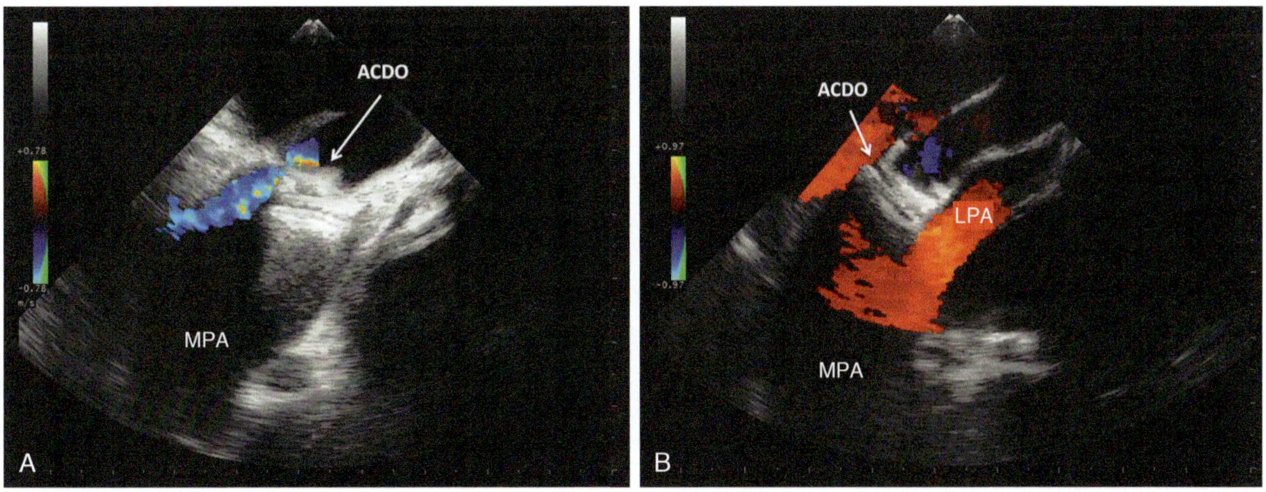

• **Fig. 20-11** Transesophageal echocardiogram in a dog with patent ductus arteriosus (PDA) (longitudinal cranial view centered on the duct). A, The Amplatz® canine duct occluder (ACDO) is not yet released. Color Doppler shows the presence of an overly significant residual flow, suggesting that the ACDO diameter was too small. B, A larger diameter ACDO is inserted. No residual flow is observed. *LPA,* Left pulmonary artery; *MPA,* main pulmonary artery. (Photo credit: Claudio Bussadori.)

Evaluation of Pulmonary Arterial Pressure

Eccentric or concentric RV hypertrophy, flattening or paradoxic motion of the interventricular septum, and dilation of the main pulmonary artery are echocardiographic signs compatible with pulmonary artery hypertension (PAH) (see Chapter 18) [50,51].

Doppler parameters that must be evaluated prior to PDA occlusion include the aortopulmonary gradient, pulmonic-to-systemic stroke volume ratio (Qp/Qs), and pulmonic and/or tricuspid regurgitation velocity measurements. The first parameter allows the detection of possible PAH (reduction of the gradient indicating elevated pulmonary artery pressure). This gradient is estimated by measuring the maximum velocity of the flow through the PDA. Proper alignment with the flow is necessary to obtain a correct measurement.

The measurement of the pulmonic and tricuspid regurgitation flow velocities allows the estimation of the systolic and diastolic pulmonary artery pressures, respectively [50-52]. The normal right atrial physiologic pressure is <6 mm Hg. It ranges from 10 to 15 mm Hg when right-sided congestive heart failure is present. Systolic and diastolic pulmonary artery pressures are obtained by adding the estimated right atrial pressure to the systolic tricuspid regurgitation and diastolic pulmonic regurgitation pressure gradients, respectively. The maximal pulmonic regurgitation pressure gradient is well correlated with the mean pulmonary artery pressure [53].

Evaluation of the Significance of the Shunt

The shunt through the PDA is considered to be minimal if Qp/Qs is <1.5 (assuming a normal pulmonary arterial pressure, with a high pressure gradient between the aorta and the main pulmonary artery), moderate with left diastolic overload if Qp/Qs is between 1.5 and 2, and large with diastolic overload and possible PAH when Qp/Qs is >2.

Associated Congenital Cardiopathies

One of the important goals of preocclusion evaluation is to ascertain that the cardiopathy is indeed a PDA and not associated with concomitant congenital cardiopathies.

Persistence of the Left Cranial Vena Cava

Persistence of the left cranial vena cava does not have any hemodynamic impact but it is important to be aware of it prior to surgical ligature.

Aortopulmonary Window

The main differential diagnosis of PDA is aortopulmonary window (APW). In this rare malformation, the aorta and main pulmonary artery are directly connected [54]. An APW is the result of defective fusion of the conotruncal crests. This congenital anomaly is to be distinguished from the truncus arteriosus. Unlike the latter, APW is generally associated with normal pulmonic and aortic valves. The window begins most often just above the sinuses of Valsalva sinuses and extends over a variable distance to the aortic arch. The left atrium and left ventricle are dilated due to the significant left-to-right shunt.

Concomitant Subaortic Stenosis

The aortic flow velocity can be elevated due to left volume overload. The transaortic pressure gradient is even greater when concomitant subaortic stenosis is present. The true gradient related to the stenosis will be appreciated only after PDA occlusion.

Postintervention Assessment

In our practice, PDA postocclusion evaluation is performed by TTE immediately or 24 hours following the procedure and then 1, 3, 6, and 12 months later. TTE reevaluation following occlusion allows the assessment of volume and contractility changes, identification of potential ischemic lesions, verification of the position of the occlusion device, and quantification of any residual flow.

In most cases, PDA occlusion results in an immediate reduction of the left volume overload, followed in most cases by disappearance of left ventricle eccentric hypertrophy in the long term [55]. End-systolic and end-diastolic left ventricular volumes as well as aortic flow maximum velocity will decrease progressively. Immediately following the occlusion, the shortening and ejection fractions appear decreased. However, the stroke volume and cardiac output remain adequate due to the large diastolic left ventricular volume (Figure 20-12).

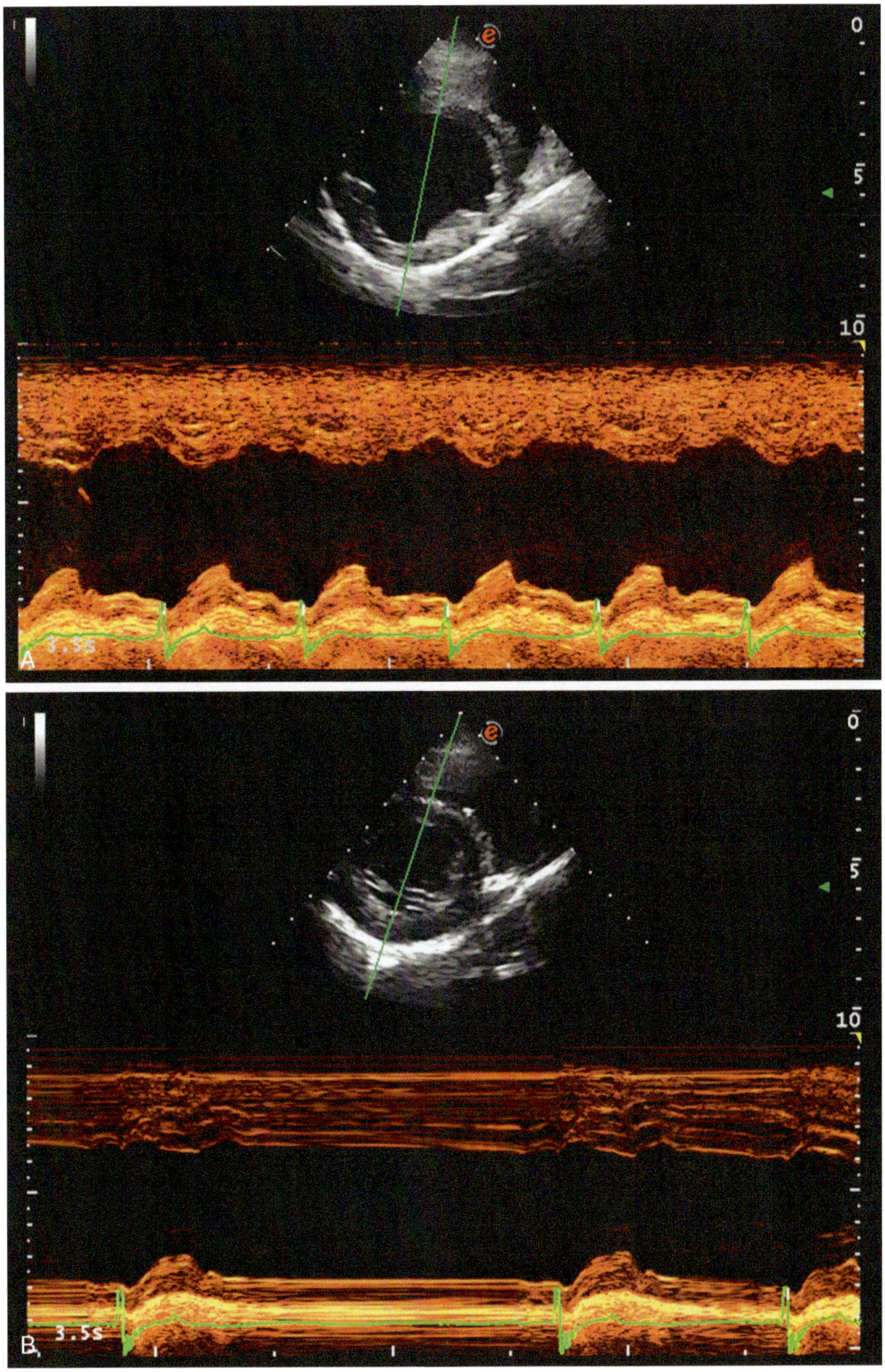

• **Fig. 20-12** Time-motion (TM) echocardiogram (transventricular view) in a dog before (A) and after (B) patent ductus arteriosus (PDA) occlusion using an Amplatz® canine duct occluder (ACDO). Prior to occlusion, the end-diastolic volume index was 218 mL/m^2, the end-systolic volume index was 65 mL/m^2, the shortening fraction was 40%, and the ejection fraction was 70%. Following occlusion, the end-diastolic volume index fell to 156 mL/m^2, the end-systolic volume index to 63 mL/m^2, the shortening fraction to 31%, and the ejection fraction to 60%. (Photo credit: Claudio Bussadori.)

In cases of chronic volume overload, as in the case of tardively diagnosed PDA, ventricular dysfunction is present and often becomes irreversible even following PDA occlusion.

Finally, TTE allows one to check the ACDO device position (2D mode) and to detect any residual shunt (color Doppler mode) (Figures 20-13 and 20-14).

Ventricular Septal Defect

Small ventricular septal defects (VSDs) do not require any intervention. However, VSD occlusion becomes necessary if left ventricular volume overload is present (moderate or large VSD). Treatment options include palliative banding of the main pulmonary artery,

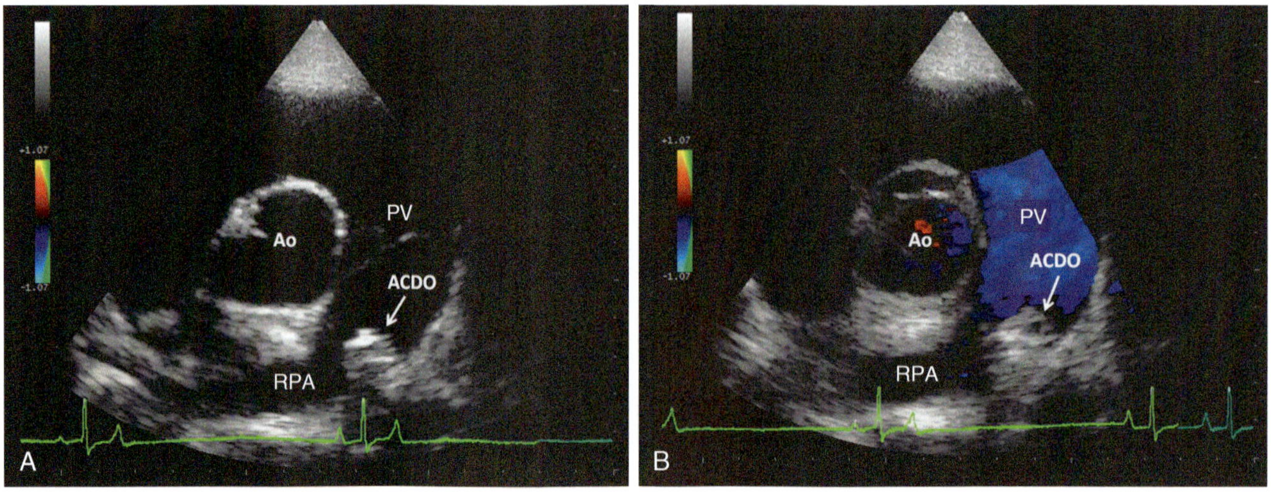

• **Fig. 20-13** Transthoracic echocardiogram (right parasternal short axis view at the level of the heart base) after Amplatz® canine duct occluder (ACDO) occlusion of a patent ductus arteriosus (PDA) in a dog. A, The occlusion device is positioned correctly. B, No residual flow is detectable. *Ao,* Aorta; *PV,* pulmonic valve; *RPA,* right pulmonary artery. (Photo credit: Claudio Bussadori.)

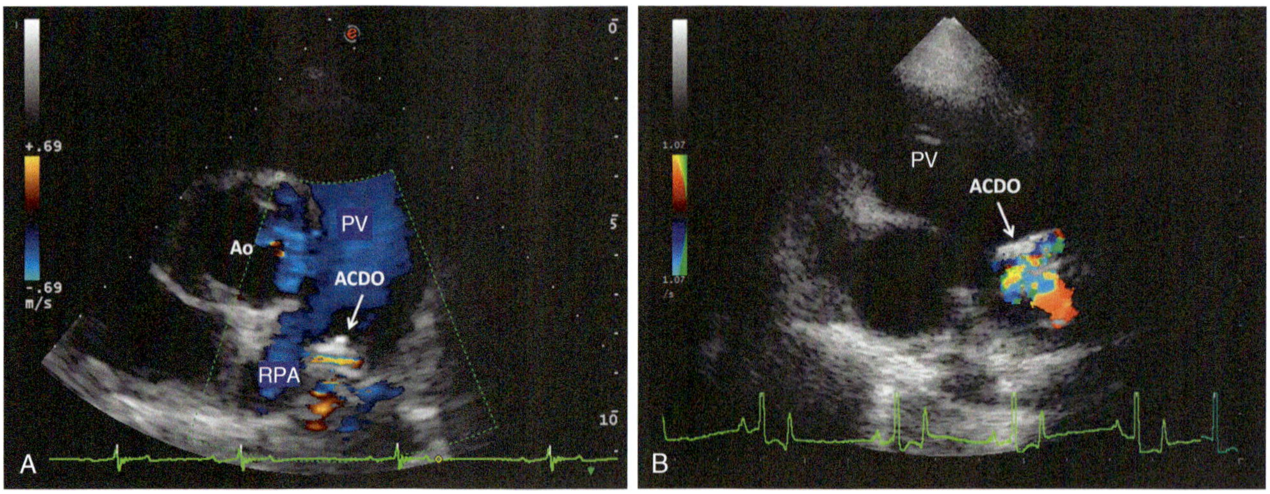

• **Fig. 20-14** Transthoracic echocardiograms [parasternal short axis view at the level of the heart base (A) and left cranial view (B)] 1 month after Amplatz® canine duct occluder (ACDO) occlusion of a patent ductus arteriosus (PDA) in a dog. A small residual flow through the occlusion device is present. *Ao,* Aorta; *PV,* pulmonic valve; *RPA,* right pulmonary artery. (Photo credit: Claudio Bussadori.)

surgical repair, and endovascular occlusion using different types of devices (coils or perimembranous or muscular VSD Amplatzer® occlusion devices) [56-60]. Two types of Amplatzer® devices are available: one designed for muscular VSD and another for supracristal VSD located at least 1 to 2 mm from the aortic valve. The first has a symmetric form whereas the second is elliptically shaped, allowing deployment without creating any interference with the aortic valve. Amplatzer® muscular VSD occlusion devices have been used to occlude perimembranous VSD located at least 5 mm from the aortic valve (Figure 20-15).

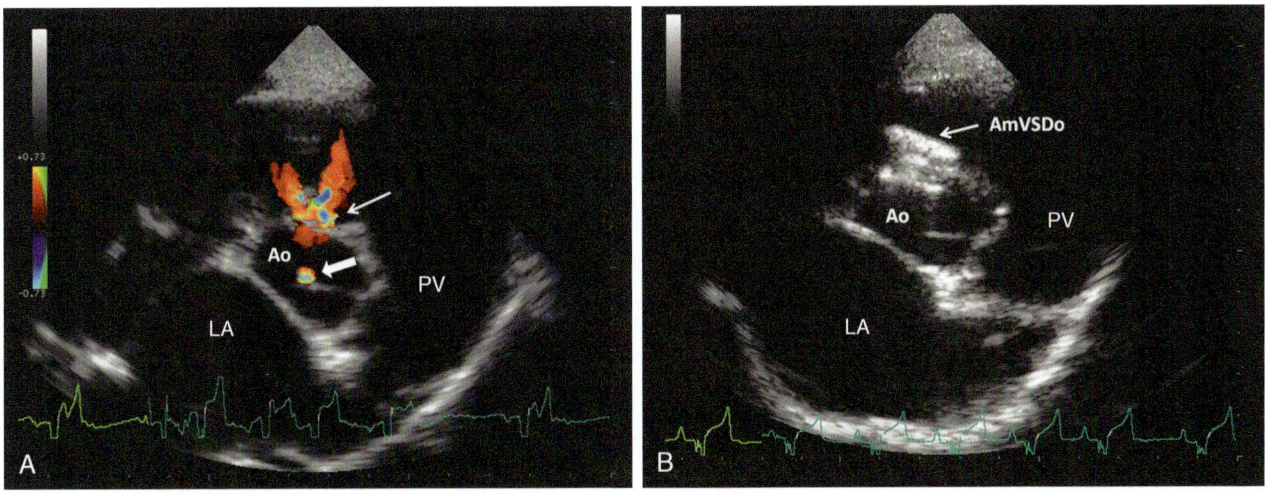

• **Fig. 20-15** Transthoracic echocardiogram (right parasternal short axis view at the level of the heart base) in a dog with a perimembranous VSD *(thin arrow)*. A, Color Doppler shows the flow through the ventricular septal defect (VSD) as well as mild aortic regurgitation *(thick arrow)*. B, View following VSD occlusion using an Amplatzer® (AmVSDo) muscular VSD occlusion device. *Ao,* Aorta; *LA,* left atrium; *PV,* pulmonic valve. (Photo credit: Claudio Bussadori.)

When evaluating a VSD with occlusion in mind, it is important to examine the neighboring structures thoroughly, especially the ones next to the aortic, mitral, and tricuspid valves and the atrioventricular node [61].

Muscular VSDs are relatively remote from any structure. Juxtaarterial VSDs or those associated with anomalies such as double outlet right ventricle (doubly committed VSD) are closely linked to the valvular tissue (aortic or pulmonary). In these cases, occlusion with an Amplatzer® device is impossible.

The posteroinferior edge of all perimembranous VSDs contains the atrioventricular node, which should not be injured. In addition, perimembranous inlet VSDs are very close to the mitral and/or tricuspid valves. Finally, supracristal (outlet) VSDs are difficult to occlude satisfactorily if there is only a small separation between the rim of the defect and the aortic valve (Figure 20-16). Septal malalignment or aortic valve prolapse through the VSD is a formal contraindication for device VSD closure (Figure 20-17).

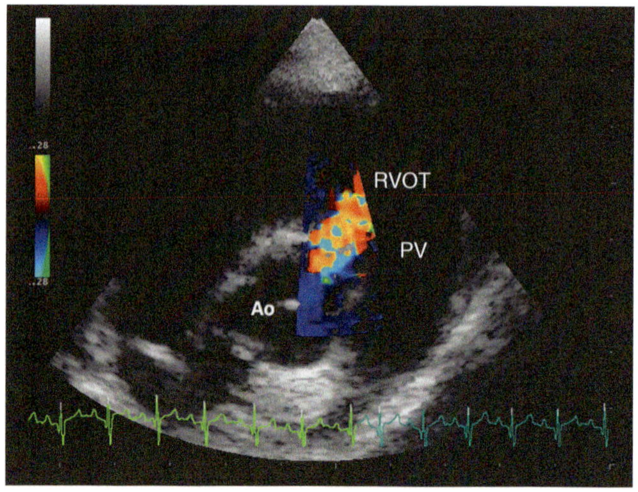

• **Fig. 20-16** Transthoracic echocardiogram (right parasternal short axis view at the level of the heart base) in color Doppler mode in a dog with a supracristal ventricular septal defect (VSD). *Ao,* Aorta; *PV,* pulmonic valve; *RVOT,* right ventricular outflow tract. (Photo credit: Claudio Bussadori.)

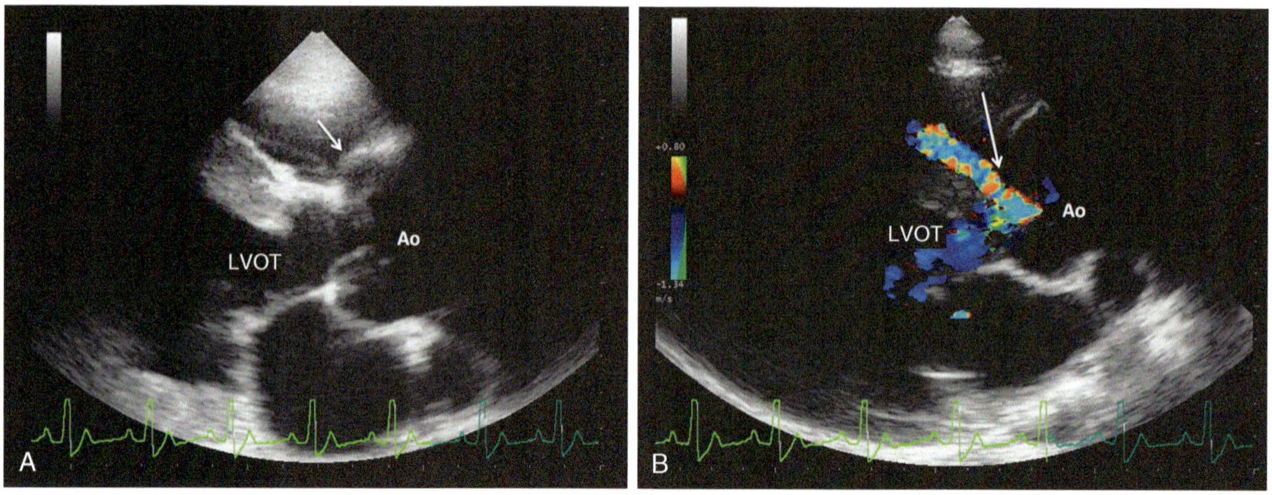

• **Fig. 20-17** Transthoracic echocardiogram (right parasternal long axis 5 chambers view) in a dog with a ventricular septal defect (VSD), septal misalignment, and aortic regurgitation. A, The arrow shows the prolapse of one of the aortic cusps through the VSD. B, Color Doppler reveals the aortic regurgitation associated with the VSD *(arrow)*. *Ao,* Aorta; *LVOT,* left ventricular outflow tract. (Photo credit: Claudio Bussadori.)

The selection of the occlusion device is based on the angiographic and/or TTE measurement of the VSD size. The largest diameter is selected. TTE allows monitoring of the occlusion procedure.

As discussed in Chapter 18, the Qp/Qs ratio can be calculated. The VSD is considered to be small if Qp/Qs is ≤1.5, moderate if it is between 1.5 and 2.5, and large if it is >2.5. The degree of PAH associated with large VSD can be calculated by subtracting the pressure gradient of the shunt flow through the VSD to the systemic systolic arterial pressure. Values ranging between 50 and 80 mm Hg indicate moderate PAH. Values <50 mm Hg suggest severe PAH.

Atrial Septal Defect

Atrial septal defects (ASDs) with significant left-to-right shunt can be occluded using an endovascular approach with an occluding device (Amplatzer® septal occluder, or ASO) or repaired by open heart surgery using a patch. A hybrid approach has been described recently [62-64]. The catheter approach is not appropriate for all types of ASD. It can be considered in cases of persistent ostium secundum and foramen ovale ASD but not in ostium primum, sinus venosus, or coronary sinus ASD (Figures 20-18 and 20-19). When evaluating an ASD with occlusion with an ASO in mind, evaluation of the neighboring structures (especially the atrioventricular valves, right pulmonary veins, and coronary sinus) is important. One will have to ensure that the size of the ASO needed for the ASD occlusion will not interfere with these structures. Furthermore, there also must be enough septal tissue to support the device (≥4 mm), as well as an adequate rim (surrounding at least 75% of the ASD circumference), to ensure proper support for the device once released. Evaluation of these criteria requires the use of TTE, TEE, and fluoroscopy to measure the ASD diameter using balloon catheters at the time of the procedure [65-71]. More recently, the usefulness of real-time 3D TTE or TEE echocardiography was reported in humans. It allows better characterization of the morphology of these defects [72,73]. As with VSD, the Qp/Qs ratio can be calculated for ASD. An ASD is considered to be small if this ratio is ≤1.5, moderate if it is between 1.5 and 2.5, and large if it is >2.5.

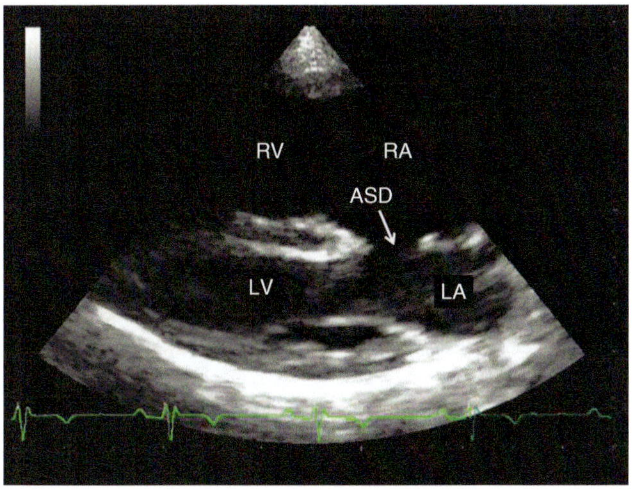

• **Fig. 20-18** Transthoracic echocardiogram (right parasternal long axis 4 chambers view) in a dog with a large ostium primum atrial septal defect (ASD). Note that the atrioventricular valves insert on the lower rim of the ASD and that the right cavities are dilated due to the right volume overload associated with the shunt. *LA*, Left atrium; *LV*, left ventricle; *RA*, right atrium; *RV*, right ventricle. (Photo credit: Claudio Bussadori.)

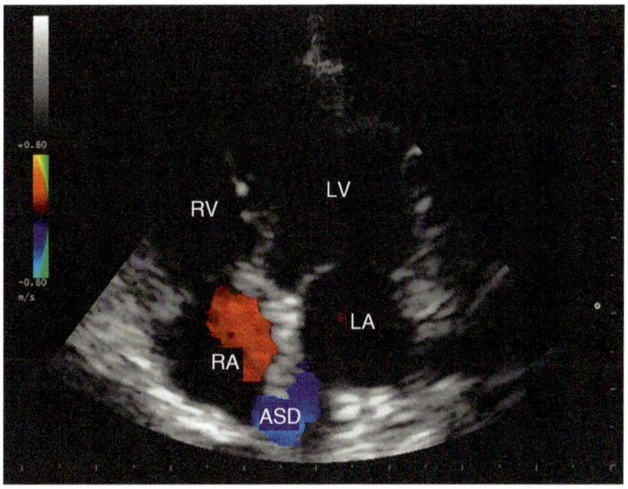

• **Fig. 20-19** Transthoracic echocardiogram in color Doppler mode (apical 4 chambers view) in a dog with a large sinus venosus atrial septal defect (ASD). The flow through the ASD appears in blue, indicating a left-to-right shunt. Notice the dilation of the right cavities due to the right volume overload. *LA*, Left atrium; *LV*, left ventricle; *RA*, right atrium; *RV*, right ventricle. (Photo credit: Claudio Bussadori.)

REFERENCES

[1] Oliveira P, Domenech O, Silva J, et al. Retrospective review of congenital heart disease in 976 dogs. J Vet Intern Med 2011;25:477–83.

[2] Buchanan JW. Causes and prevalence of cardiovascular disease. In: Kirk RW, Bonagura JD, editors. Kirk's current veterinary therapy XI. Philadelphia: WB Saunders; 1992, p. 647–55.

[3] Kan JS, White RI, Mitchell SE, Gardner TJ. Percutaneous balloon valvuloplasty: a new method for treating congenital pulmonary valve stenosis. N Engl J Med 1982;307:540–2.

[4] Rao PS. Percutaneous balloon pulmonary valvuloplasty: state of the art. Catheter Cardiovasc Interv 2007;69:747–63.

[5] McCrindle BW. Independent predictors of long-term results after balloon pulmonary valvuloplasty. Circulation 1994;89:1751–9.

[6] Gudausky TM, Beekman RH. Current options, and long term results for interventional treatment of pulmonary valvar stenosis. Cardiol Young 2006;16: 418–27.

[7] Bussadori C, DeMadron E, Santilli RA, Borgarelli M. Balloon valvuloplasty in 30 dogs with pulmonic stenosis: effect of valve morphology and annular size on initial and 1-year outcome. J Vet Intern Med 2001; 15:553–8.

[8] Johnson MS, Martin M, Edwards D, et al. Pulmonic stenosis in dogs: balloon dilation improves clinical outcome. J Vet Intern Med 2004;18:656–62.

[9] Johnson MS, Martin M. Results of balloon valvuloplasty in 40 dogs with pulmonic stenosis. J Small Anim Pract 2004;45:148–53.

[10] Estrada A, Moise NS, Erb HN, et al. Prospective evaluation of the balloon-to-annulus ratio for valvuloplasty in the treatment of pulmonic stenosis in the dog. J Vet Intern Med 2006;20:862–72.

[11] Bussadori C, Amberger C, Le Bobinnec G, et al. Guidelines for the echocardiographic studies of suspected subaortic and pulmonic stenosis. J Vet Cardiol 2000;2:15–22.

[12] Milo S, Fiegel A, Shem-Tov A, et al. Hour-glass deformity of the pulmonary valve: a third type of pulmonary valve stenosis. Br Heart J 1988;60:128–33.

[13] Locatelli C, Domenech O, Silva J, et al. Independent predictors of immediate and long-term results after pulmonary balloon valvuloplasty in dogs. J Vet Cardiol 2011;13:21–30.

[14] Ho SY, Rigby ML, Anderson RH. Echocardiography in congenital heart disease made simple. In: Cardiopulmonary medicine from Imperial College Press. The ventricular outflow tract 2001, p. 104–19.

[15] Fonfara S, Martinez Pereira Y, Swift S, et al. Balloon valvuloplasty for treatment of pulmonic stenosis in English Bulldogs with an aberrant coronary artery. J Vet Intern Med 2010;24:354–9.

[16] Fonfara S, Martinez Pereira Y, Dukes McEwan J. Balloon valvuloplasty for treatment of pulmonic stenosis in English Bulldogs with an aberrant coronary artery—2 years later. J Vet Intern Med 2011;25:771.

[17] Kittleson M, Thomas W, Loyer C, Kienle R. Letter to the editor. J Vet Intern Med 1992;6:250–1.

[18] Buchanan JW. Pathogenesis of single right coronary artery and pulmonic stenosis in English Bulldogs. J Vet Intern Med 2001;15:101–4.

[19] Francis AJ, Johnson MJ, Culshaw GC, et al. Outcome in 55 dogs with pulmonic stenosis that did not undergo balloon valvuloplasty or surgery. J Small Anim Pract 2011;52:282–8.

[20] Fontes VF, Esteves CA, Sousa JE, et al. Regression of infundibular hypertrophy after pulmonary valvuloplasty for pulmonic stenosis. Am J Cardiol 1988;62:977–9.

[21] Thapar MK, Rao PS. Significance of infundibular obstruction following balloon valvuloplasty for valvar pulmonic stenosis. Am Heart J 1989;118:99–103.

[22] Thapar MK, Rao PS. Use of propanolol for severe dynamic infundibular obstruction prior to balloon pulmonary valvuloplasty. Cathet Cardiovasc Diagn 1990;19:240–1.

[23] Khambatta HJ, Velado M, Gaffney JW, et al. Management of right ventricular outflow tract reactivity following pulmonary valve dilatation under general anesthesia: experience of a medical mission. Paediatr Anaesth 2006;16:1087–9.

[24] Bussadori C, Oliveira P, Arcidiacono C, et al. Right and left ventricular strain and strain rate in young adults before and after percutaneous atrial septal defect closure. Echocardiography 2011;28:730–7.

[25] Jurcut R, Giusca S, Ticulescu R, et al. Different patterns of adaptation of the right ventricle to pressure overload: a comparison between pulmonary hypertension and pulmonary stenosis. J Am Soc Echocardiogr 2011;24:1109–17.

[26] Jurcut R, Giusca S, La Gerche A, et al. The echocardiographic assessment of the right ventricle: what to do in 2010? Eur J Echocardiogr 2010;11:81–96.

[27] Toschi Corneliani R, Locatelli C, Domenech O. Retrospective study of pulmonic stenosis in 259 dogs. In: ECVIM Congress Proceeding 2008.

[28] Anwar AM, Soliman O, van den Bosch AE, et al. Assessment of pulmonary valve and right ventricular outflow tract with real-time three-dimensional echocardiography. Int J Cardiovasc Imaging 2007;23: 167–75.

[29] Thomas WP, De Lellis LA, Sisson D. Balloon dilation of congenital outflow obstruction in dogs: mid-term results 1990. In: Proceedings of the 8th ACVIM forum. Washington DC, p. 907–9.
[30] Gordon SG, Miller MW, Baig S. A retrospective review of balloon valvuloplasty for the treatment of pulmonic stenosis in 50 dogs 2002. In: Proceedings of the First International Symposium for Veterinary Cardiology. Prague; June 14–15.
[31] Mendelsohn AM, Banerjee A. Ra Meyer, Schwartz DC. Balloon pulmonary valvuloplasty: a differing view. Catheter Cardiovasc Interv 1997;40:429–30.
[32] Gupta D, Saxena A, Kothari SS, Juneja R. Factors influencing late course of residual valvular and infundibular gradients following pulmonary valve balloon dilatation. Int J Cardiol 2001;79:143–9.
[33] Eyster GE, Eyster JT, Cords GB, Johnston J. Patent ductus arteriosus in the dog: characteristics of occurrence and results of surgery in one hundred consecutive cases. J Am Vet Med Assoc 1976;168:435–8.
[34] Bureau S, Monnet E, Orton EC. Evaluation of survival rate and prognostic indicators for surgical treatment of left-to-right patent ductus arteriosus in dogs: 52 cases (1995–2003). J Am Vet Med Assoc 2005;227:1794–9.
[35] Campbell FE, Thomas WP, Miller SJ, et al. Immediate and late outcomes of transarterial coil occlusion of patent ductus arteriosus in dogs. J Vet Intern Med 2006;20:83–96.
[36] Pyle RL, Park RD, Alexander AF, Hill BL. Patent ductus arteriosus with pulmonary hypertension in the dog. J Am Vet Med Assoc 1981;178:565–71.
[37] Oswald GP, Orton EC. Patent ductus arteriosus and pulmonary hypertension in related Pembroke Welsh Corgis. J Am Vet Med Assoc 1993;202:761–4.
[38] Seibert RL, Maisenbacher HW, Prosek R, et al. Successful closure of left-to-right patent ductus arteriosus in three dogs with concurrent pulmonary hypertension. J Vet Cardiol 2010;12:67–73.
[39] Walters B, Bramer CN. Patent ductus arteriosus. North Am Vet 1952;33:252–5.
[40] Gordon SG, Saunders AB, Achen SE, et al. Transarterial ductal occlusion using the Amplatz Canine Duct Occluder in 40 dogs. J Vet Cardiol 2010;12:85–92.
[41] Nguyenba TP, Tobias AH. Minimally invasive per-catheter patent ductus arteriosus occlusion in dogs using a prototype duct occluder. J Vet Intern Med 2008;22:129–34.
[42] Nguyenba TP, Tobias AH. The Amplatz canine duct occluder: a novel device for patent ductus arteriosus occlusion. J Vet Cardiol 2007;9:109–17.
[43] Tobias AH, Stauthammer CD. Minimally invasive per-catheter occlusion and dilation procedures for congenital cardiovascular abnormalities in dogs. Vet Clin North Am Small Anim Pract 2010;40: 581–603.
[44] Chetboul V, Serres F, Gouni V, et al. Noninvasive assessment of systolic left ventricular torsion by 2-dimensional speckle tracking imaging in the awake dog: repeatability, reproducibility, and comparison with tissue Doppler imaging variables. J Vet Intern Med 2008;22:342–50.
[45] Saunders AB, Miller MW, Gordon SG, Bahr A. Echocardiographic and angiographic comparison of ductal dimensions in dogs with patent ductus arteriosus. J Vet Intern Med 2007;21:68–75.
[46] Schneider M, Hildebrandt N, Schweigl T, Wehner M. Transthoracic echocardiographic measurement of patent ductus arteriosus in dogs. J Vet Intern Med 2007;21:251–7.
[47] Nguyenba TP, Tobias AH. Minimally invasive per-catheter patent ductus arteriosus occlusion in dogs using a prototype duct occluder. J Vet Intern Med 2008;22:129–34.
[48] Miller MW, Gordon SG, Saunders AB, et al. Angiographic classification of patent ductus arteriosus morphology in the dog. J Vet Cardiol 2006;8: 109–14.
[49] Saunders AB, Achen SE, Gordon SG, Miller MW. Utility of trans-esophageal echocardiography for transcatheter occlusion of patent ductus arteriosus in dogs: influence on the decision-making process. J Vet Intern Med 2010;24:1407–13.
[50] Johnson LR, Boon JA, Orton EC. Clinical characteristics of 53 dogs with Doppler-derived evidence of pulmonary hypertension: 1992–1996. J Vet Intern Med 1999;13:440–7.
[51] Pyle RL, Abbott LA, MacLean HN. Severe pulmonary hypertension and cardiovascular sequelae in dogs. Vet Med 2004;99:530–41.
[52] Schober KE, Baade H. Doppler echocardiographic prediction of pulmonary hypertension in West Highland White Terriers with chronic pulmonary disease. J Vet Intern Med 2006;20:912–20.
[53] Masuyama T, Kodama K, Kitabatake A, et al. Continuous wave Doppler echocardiographic detection of pulmonary regurgitation and its application to noninvasive estimation of pulmonary artery pressure. Circulation 1986;74:484–92.
[54] Margiocco ML, Domenech O, Bussadori CM. Aorticopulmonary window in a dog. Veterinaria 2003;17:27–32.

[55] Stauthammer CD, Nguyenba TP, Tobias AH. Short and long term cardiac changes following complete occlusion of uncomplicated patent ductus arteriosus in dogs [abstract]. J Vet Intern Med 2007;21:609.
[56] Shimizu M, Tanaka R, Hoshi K, et al. Surgical correction of ventricular septal defect with aortic regurgitation in a dog. Aust Vet J 2006;84:117–21.
[57] Shimizu M, Tanaka R, Hirao H, et al. Percutaneous transcatheter coil embolization of a ventricular septal defect in a dog. J Am Vet Med Assoc 2005;226(69–72):52–3.
[58] Fujii Y, Fukuda T, Machida N, et al. Transcatheter closure of congenital ventricular septal defects in 3 dogs with a detachable coil. J Vet Intern Med 2004;18:911–4.
[59] Margiocco ML, Bulmer BJ, Sisson DD. Percutaneous occlusion of a muscular ventricular septal defect with an Amplatzer muscular VSD occluder. J Vet Cardiol 2008;10:61–6.
[60] Bussadori C, Carminati M, Domenech O. Transcatheter closure of a perimembranous ventricular septal defect in a dog. J Vet Intern Med 2007;21:1396–400.
[61] Ho SY, McCarthy KP, Rigby ML. Morphology of perimembranous ventricular septal defects: implications for transcatheter device closure. J Interv Cardiol 2004;17:99–108.
[62] Gordon SG, Miller MW, Roland RM, et al. Transcatheter atrial septal defect closure with the Amplatzer atrial septal occluder in 13 dogs: short- and mid-term outcome. J Vet Intern Med 2009;23:995–1002.
[63] Gordon SG, Nelson DA, Achen SE, et al. Open heart closure of an atrial septal defect by use of an atrial septal occluder in a dog. J Am Vet Med Assoc 2010;236:434–9.
[64] Sanders RA, Hogan DE, Green HW, et al. Transcatheter closure of an atrial septal defect in a dog. J Am Vet Med Assoc 2005;227:430–4.
[65] Bennhagen RG, McLaughlin P, Benson LN. Contemporary management of children with atrial septal defects. Am J Cardiovasc Drugs 2001;1:445–53.
[66] Lammers A, Hager A, Eicken A, et al. Need for closure of secundum atrial septal defect in infancy. J Thorac Cardiovasc Surg 2005;129:1353–7.
[67] Saxena A, Divekar A, Soni NR. Natural history of secundum atrial defect revisited in the era of transcatheter closure. Indian Heart J 2005;57:35–8.
[68] Moake L, Ramaciotti C. Atrial septal defect treatment options. AACN Clin Issues 2005;16:252–66.
[69] Masura J, Gavora P, Podnar T. Long-term outcome of transcatheter secundum-type atrial septal defect closure using Amplatzer septal occluders. J Am Coll Cardiol 2005;45:505–7, 453.
[70] Yew G, Wilson NJ. Transcatheter atrial septal defect closure with the Amplatzer septal occluder: five year follow-up. Catheter Cardiovasc Interv 2005;64:193–6.
[71] De Ridder S, Suttorp MJ, Ernst S, et al. Percutaneous transcatheter closure of atrial septal defects: initial single-center experience and follow-up results. Initial experience with three-dimensional echocardiography. Acta Cardiol 2005;60:171–8.
[72] Roberson DA, Cui W, Patel D, et al. Three-dimensional trans-esophageal echocardiography of atrial septal defect: a qualitative and quantitative anatomic study. J Am Soc Echocardiogr 2011;24:600–10.
[73] Chen FL, Hsiung MC, Hsieh KS, et al. Real time three-dimensional transthoracic echocardiography for guiding Amplatzer septal occluder device deployment in patients with atrial septal defect. Echocardiography 2006;23:763–70.

Index

A

ACDO (Amplatz® canine ductal occluder), 105f, 331, 333f, 335f–336f
AFI (automated function imaging), 77f–78f, 79, 198f
Age (influence on diastolic function), 129
Aliasing, 4–5
Anemia
  and high cardiac output heart failure, 254–255
  hyperdynamic state, 255
  left ventricular dilation, 255f
Angle between interventricular septum and aorta
  in hypertrophic obstructive cardiomyopathies, 209
  in subaortic stenosis, 286
Annulus
  mitral
    dilation of, 298
    movement of the. *see* Motion, of the annulus, mitral
    pulmonic (measurements), 100–101
    S′ wave velocity of the, 118–119, 215
    tissue Doppler of the, 118–119, 132, 144f, 146f, 215, 215f
  tricuspid, 152
    tissue Doppler of, 152
Aortic dissection, 248
Aorto-pulmonary fistula, 291f
Aortopulmonary window, 334
Area
  aortic, 298
  of the distal regurgitant jet (quantification), 172
  of the left atrium, 30
  length (method), 117f
  of the regurgitant orifice (regurgitant orifice area: ROA), 172
Arterial hypertension
  pulmonary, 229–240
    conventional echocardiography in, 231–233, 231f
    etiology and pathogenesis of, 230–231, 230f
    indirect Doppler signs, 231f–234f, 234
    new imagery techniques in, 237–240
    prevalence of, 166, 166t, 175
    in reverse PDA, 331
  systemic
    canine, 249–252
    feline, 246–249
Artery
  aberrant coronary, 293–294
  aorto-pulmonary collateral, 90
ASO *(Amplatz® Septal Occluder)*, 339
Asynchony (intra - and inter-ventricular), 192, 192f, 198f
Atrial septal defect, 167f, 305–307, 306f–307f, 339, 339f
  echocardiographic characteristics of, 306–307
  types of, 306
Atrial systole, 118, 128
Atrioventricular canal
  complete, 316, 317f
  echocardiographic aspects, 317–318
  partial, 317, 317f

B

Bacterial endocarditis
  aortic regurgitation secondary to, 176, 176f
  of the aortic valve, 101, 102f, 177f
  of the mitral valve, 101, 175, 175f
Base
  apex
    gradient, 61, 190
    length, 184
  of the heart, 294f
    heart base tumors, 275–278, 276t
Bernoulli (modified equation of), 32
Breed. *see* Effect of breed
Bull's eye, 78f, 198f

C

Cardiac metastases, 280
Cardiac tamponade (echocardiographic signs), 261–265, 263f–266f
Cardiac valve (3D evaluation of the), 100–102
Cardiomyopathy
  arrhythmogenic right ventricular cardiomyopathy in the Boxer, 201, 201f
  atypical, 224–225
  dilated cardiomyopathy in the cat, 222, 223f–224f
  hypertrophic
    in the cat, 133f, 149f, 208–218, 208f–212f, 214f–217f
    in the dog, 202, 203f
    evaluation of the diastolic function in, 213–215
    obstructive, 212
  primary dilated cardiomyopathy in the dog, 182
    in the Doberman, 187
    echocardiographic diagnosis of
      asymptomatic or occult forms, 187
      major criteria, 187
      minor criteria, 187
    in the Irish Wolfhound, 187
  restrictive, 218–222, 220f–222f, 226f, 267f
    speckle tracking in, 217–218
  right ventricular cardiomyopathy in the cat, 224–225
  undetermined in the cat, 224
  uremic cardiomyopathy, 202, 202f
Chemodectoma, 276f–277f, 276t
Chiari (network), 314
Chordae tendinae (rupture of), 160–162
Circumference
  aortic, 30
  atrial, 30
Coefficients of variation, 40, 41f
Compliance, 128–129
Congestive heart failure, 149f, 183f, 247f
  high cardiac output, 252
Contraction
  isovolumic, 128, 217
  post-systolic, 252
    radial, 194

Note: Page numbers followed by "b", "f" and "t" indicate boxes, figures, and tables respectively.

Convergence area, 172. *see also* PISA
Cor triatriatum, 313–316
  dexter, 314, 315f–316f
  sinister, 314, 314f–315f
Coronary sinus, 306–307, 315–316, 327f
Cysts
  intrapericardial, 268
  pericardial, 275

D

DCM. *see* Cardiomyopathy, dilated, in the cat; Cardiomyopathy, primary dilated, in the dog
Deceleration
  deceleration time of the E wave, 131
  slope, 309–310
Degenerative mitral valve disease (DMVD), 162f–164f, 167f, 171f–172f, 188
  in large dogs, 160, 175
Descent
  x, 140
  y, 140
Detorsion, 112
Diameter
  of the aortic root, 30
  aorto-lateral of the left atrium, 30
  diastolic of the right ventricular base, 26t, 31, 32t
  left ventricular internal
    end-diastolic, 24
    end-systolic, 24
  minimal ductal, 331–332
  of the pulmonic valve annulus, 325, 325f
  septo-lateral of the left atrium, 30
  TM of the left atrium, 28
Diastasis, 128, 140
Diastole, 130f
  determinants of, 128–129, 131t–132t
  phases of, 128f
    atrial systole, 128
    isovolumic relaxation, 132
    rapid filling, 128
    slow filling, 128
  pseudo-normal, 130
  pseudo normalization, 134
Diastolic anomalies
  in dilated cardiomyopathies in dogs, 182
  in hypertrophic cardiomyopathies in cats, 208–218
  in restrictive cardiomyopathies in cats, 218–222, 220f–222f, 226f, 267f
Diastolic pulmonic regurgitation, 188, 334
Dilation
  aortic, 248, 248f, 251, 251f
  of the left atrium, 162, 247f
  of the left ventricle, 162
  of the main pulmonary artery, 334
  of the mitral annulus, 160
  of the pulmonary veins, 162
  of the right chambers, 166
  of the right ventricle, 166f, 326
Dirofilaria, 242, 242f
Doming
  diastolic of pulmonic cusps, 231
  at the end of diastolic mitral anterior leaflet movement, 186
  systolic doming in pulmonic stenosis, 295
Doppler
  color, 6f, 18f, 98f, 168f, 177f, 293f
    amplitude analysis, 5
    turbulent flows, 5
    variance, 5
Doppler *(Continued)*
  spectral, 142f, 226f–227f
    continuous, 5, 148f, 168f, 174f
    normal values, 32–35
    pulsed, 4–5, 132
      aliasing, 4–5
      ambiguous velocity. *see* Aliasing
      high recurrence frequency (high PRF), 4–5
      Nyquist limit, 4–5
      recurrence frequency, 4–5
      sample volume, 4–5
      of the transaortic flow, 17
      of the transmitral flow, 17, 131
      of the transpulmonic flow, 17, 34f
      of the tricuspid flow, 17
  Tissue Doppler (TDI)
    of the annulus
      mitral, 118–119, 132
      tricuspid, 152
    in dilated cardiomyopathies, 62
    in hypertrophic cardiomyopathies, 215–217
    in mitral regurgitation, 169–171
    myocardial, 50–62, 248–249
      bidimensional color TDI mode, 53–54, 53f–54f
      color TM mode, 52–53, 52f
      influence of heart rate on, 61
      inter-day variability, 61
      intra-day variability, 61
      pulsed TDI mode, 169–171
    in systemic arterial hypertension, 249
Duchenne (myopathy of), 196
Dysfunction
  diastolic, 135t–136t, 137f, 213t
    delayed relaxation, 129
    pseudo-normal diastole, 130, 135f
    pseudo-normalization of diastole, 134
    restrictive, 130, 136f
  left longitudinal, 190
  myocardial, 248–249
  radial, 190
  structural analysis
    restrictive, 134
  systolic
    in dilated cardiomyopathies, 183
    in hypertrophic cardiomyopathies, 217
    in mitral regurgitation, 117
    in patent ductus arteriosus, 299
    in systemic hypertension, 248–249
    in aortic stenosis, 289f
Dysplasia
  of the mitral valve, 308f–310f
    anatomopathology of, 308–310
    echocardiographic aspects of, 308–310
  of the tricuspid valve, 310–312, 310f–312f
Dystrophin, 62

E

Early diastolic stretching, 223f
Ebstein (anomaly of), 310
Echocardiography
  three-dimensional (3D)
    in evaluation of the cardiac valves, 100–102
    modes, 96–98
    in patent ductus arteriosus, 103–104
    in pulmonic valvuloplasty, 327
    technology of, 96
    transesophageal, 102–105, 103f
    in ventricular volume measurements, 99–100

Echocardiography *(Continued)*
transesophageal (TEE), 287
3D TEE, 102–105, 105f–106f
complications of, 87
protocol of, 87–89
EDVI. *see* End-diastolic volume index
Effect
of breed
on the shortening fraction, 114
on tissue Doppler of the left ventricle wall, 58t–59t
of phenotype on normal values, 22
Effusion
pericardial, 166, 167f, 209, 260–268, 261f–263f
etiology, 260t, 266–268
secondary to a cardiac tumor, 268
pleural, 209
Elastic recoil, 128
End-diastolic volume index, 116t–117t, 164–166
End-systolic volume index, 116t–117t, 164
End-systolic wall stress, 114–115
circumferential, 114
Endocardial cushion. *see* Endocardial cushion defect
Endocardial cushion defect, 316–318
ES separation (increase of), 186
ESVI. *see* End-systolic volume index
Excessive moderator bands, 224, 224f–225f

F

Fallot (tetralogy of). *see* Tetralogy of Fallot
Feline hypertrophic muscular dystrophy, 209
Filling phases
rapid, 128
slow, 128
Filters
high-pass, 50, 50f
low-pass, 50
Flow
alignment with, 32
laminar, 5, 32–33
pulmonary venous, 18, 35, 35f, 35t
transaortic, 17, 189f
transmitral, 17, 34f, 141f, 144f, 146f, 169f
transpulmonic, 17
tricuspid, 17, 33, 34t–35t
turbulent, 32–33
Fraction
ejection, 117–118
regurgitant, 174–175
shortening, 112–115
endocardial, 112–114, 113f, 114t
Midwall shortening fraction, 114
of the right ventricle, 152
systolic, 35
Function, 260
atrial, 225–226
diastolic. *see* Diastole; Diastolic anomalies
systolic. *see also* Systolic dysfunction
global of the left ventricle, 109–126
of the left atrium, 129
longitudinal (evaluation of), 152–154
radial, 152, 191f
of the right ventricular wall, 152

G

Gradient
base-apex, 59–60
intramyocardial
longitudinal, 59–60
radial, 59
mean, 290
peak systolic, 290
pressure gradients, 290, 305
GRMD (Golden Retriever muscular dystrophy), 196, 196f–200f

H

HCM. *see* Cardiomyopathy, hypertrophic
Heart rate, 27
Heart rate (influence on)
diastolic filling, 129
shortening fraction, 112
TDI parameters, 61
Helix
subendocardial, 48, 57t
subepicardial, 48, 57t
Hemangiosarcoma, 273–275, 273f–274f
Hepatic venous congestion, 166, 185, 201
Hydration (influence of the state of), 28
Hyperthyroid cardiopathy, 254, 254f–255f
Hypertrophy
of the left ventricle, 208–210, 247f, 250f
in athlete physiology, 62
in hypertrophic cardiomyopathies, 202, 208–210
"inappropriate" eccentric hypertrophy in MR, 163
pathologic, 62
in systemic arterial hypertension, 246, 246f
in uremic cardiomyopathy, 202
of the right ventricle, 326
in PAH, 231–232
in pulmonic stenosis, 295, 326f
in the tetralogy of Fallot, 313

I

Index
of sphericity. *see* Sphericity index
of volume
end-diastolic volume index, 164–166
end-systolic volume index, 164
of myocardial performance, 121, 121f, 155t
(echocardiographic) of left atrial pressure, 141–147
Tei, 120–121, 153–154, 171, 235f
Interatrial septum (rupture of), 166–167
Intra- and interventricular synchrony, 55f–56f
Intrahepatic portosystemic shunt, 86–87, 93f
Isovolumic relaxation time, 132, 145–147, 147f, 215
IVRT. *see* Isovolumic relaxation time

L

Leading edge, 22
Left atrium
degree of dilation, 174
diameter
aortolateral, 30
septolateral, 28
TM, 28
systolic function of, 129
wall rupture of, 266, 267f
Lymphomas, 278

M

Main pulmonary artery, dilation of, 231, 231f
Malalignment of the papillary muscles, 325

Mesothelioma, 280, 280f
Midwall layer, 48
Mitral valve prolapse, 160, 160b, 161f
Mode
  bidimensional, 4, 31t, 185f
  3D
    in real-time, 96, 97f
    volume, 97, 98f
    zoom, 96, 97f
  spectral Doppler
    Doppler effect, 4
    frequency shift, 4
    laminar flow, 4
  time-motion
    anatomic ("free angle"), 4, 22
    color TM of the diastolic mitral flow, 133
  tissue Doppler
    bidimensional, 50–51, 53–54, 53f–56f, 60f
    color TM, 52–53, 52f
    myocardial, 50–62
    pulsed wave, 51–52, 51f
    single-gated pulsed wave, 51, 51f
Motion
  of the annulus
    mitral, 118, 119f, 119t
      amplitude of the, 118
      relative contribution of, 118
    tricuspid, 152
  longitudinal, 48, 49f, 73t
    of the left ventricular wall, 57t, 59–60
  paradoxical septal motion, 166
  radial, 48, 49f, 57t, 72t
  systolic anterior motion of the mitral valve, 233
Multiplane reconstruction, 97–98, 99f, 102f
Myocardial fibers, 48, 48f
  longitudinal, 112
  radial, 112
Myocardial infiltration, 274
Myocardial motion
  left longitudinal, 62
  left radial, 62
  segmental, velocity of, 62, 63f
"Myocardial stunning," 65f
Myocardium, active relaxation of, 128
Myxomas, 279
Myxosarcomas, 279

N

Nyquist limit, 4–5

O

Obstruction
  dynamic, 210–211
    of the right ventricular outflow tract in cats, 211
    of the RV outflow tract in pulmonic stenosis, 293
  of the left ventricular outflow tract in cats, 286

P

PAH. *see* Pulmonary arterial hypertension (PAH)
Papillary muscle atrophy, 184, 184f
Papillary muscles, malalignment of, 325
Patent ductus arteriosus, 103–104, 104f–105f, 298–303, 299f–302f, 331–336
  echocardiographic aspects of, 298–303
  minimum diameter measurement, 332f
  morphology, 332
Patent ductus arteriosus *(Continued)*
  Qp/Qs in, 334
  reverse, 301–303, 302f–303f
PDCM. *see* Primary dilated cardiomyopathy in the dog, 182
Pericarditis
  constrictive, 268–269
  hemorrhagic, 268, 268f
Pericardium
  anatomy and function of, 260
  congenital anomalies of, 269
  cysts, 269
  diseases of, 259–270
  effusions. *see also* Effusion, pericardial
    etiology of, 260t, 266–268
  pericardoperitoneal diaphragmatic hernia, 269
  pressure in the, 260
  total or partial absence of, 269
  ventricular interdependence, 260
Pericardoperitoneal diaphragmatic hernia, 269
Phenotype, influence of, 22
  allometric approach, 22
  ratios
    aortic, 22
    weight, 22
Physiologic heterogeneity of wall motion, 61
PISA (proximal isovelocity surface area)
  factors affecting, 173
  zones, 172
PISA method. *see* PISA (proximal isovelocity surface area)
Pressure
  atrial
    echocardiographic indices of, 141–147
    left, 129f, 140, 140f, 140t, 143f, 143t
    right, 236
  filling pressure
    elevated and abnormal relaxation, 213
    of the left ventricle, estimation of, 139, 147t
    normal and delayed relaxation, 213
  intrapericardial, 260
  pulmonary arterial, 236f, 334
    diastolic, estimation of, 237, 237f–238f
    systolic, estimation of, 236, 236f
  pulmonary capillary wedge, 140, 140f
  systolic right ventricular, 295–296
Proximal isovelocity surface area (PISA). *see* PISA
Pulmonary arterial hypertension (PAH), 166t, 169f–170f, 188f, 229–240, 235f, 238f–239f, 267f
Pulmonary interstitial fibrosis in the West Highland White terrier, 234
Pulmonary veins, dilation of, 162
Pulmonic valve cusps, post valvuloplasty thickening of, 328, 328f

R

Radial segmental asynchrony, 194, 194f, 195f
Ratio
  Adur/ARdur, 142
  AT/ET, 33, 234
  E/A, 33
    of the transmitral flow, 131
  E/IVRT, 145–147, 147f
  LVd/RVd, 32t
  of maximal velocities
    of the E wave and propagation velocity (E/Vp), 145, 145f
    of the transmitral E and mitral annulus E' wave, 142–144
  PEP/ET
    of the left ventricle, 120t
    of the right ventricle, 155t

Ratio *(Continued)*
RJarea/LAarea, 172
Sm/Dm, 35, 132
RCM. *see* Restrictive cardiomyopathy
Regurgitant flow rate (RFR), 172
Regurgitant orifice area (ROA), 172
Regurgitation
aortic, 176–177, 176f, 248f, 251f
secondary to bacterial endocarditis, 176
mitral, 103f, 123f, 142–144, 143f, 145f, 147, 148f, 160–175, 173f, 211–212, 266, 267f
by dilation of annulus, 160
quantification of the severity of, 165t
pulmonic, 177–178, 178f
tricuspid, 175–176
Relaxation
abnormal, with elevated filling pressure, 213
active myocardial relaxation, 128
delayed, 129, 129f, 133f–134f, 214f–215f
with normal filling pressure, 213
isovolumic, 56–59, 128
time, 132, 145–147
Remodeling
left ventricular, 174, 246–247
mitral valve, 160, 160f
myocardial, 209
Repeatability, 40, 61
Reproducibility, 40, 61
Restrictive cardiomyopathy, 218–222, 220f–222f, 226f, 267f
Rhabdomyosarcoma, 279, 279f
Rotation
axial, 48
left ventricular systolic, 79, 80t
Rupture
of the atrial wall, 266, 267f
of the chordae tendineae, 160–162, 161f
of the interatrial septum, 166–167

S

Simpson method, 116, 116f
monoplane, 184f
Sonomicrometry, 65f
Speckle tracking imaging, 74–82, 74f–76f, 79f–81f
in cardiomyopathies
dilated, 194f–195f
hypertrophic, 217–218, 218f–220f
restrictive, 222, 223f
in DMVD, 171, 171f
of the left ventricle, 218f, 223f
Speckles, 74
Sphericity index, 28, 28f
changes of the, 163
Spontaneous echocardiographic contrast, 210, 225t
Stationary reverberation artifacts, 70
zones of, 61
Stenosis
pulmonic, 105f, 291–298, 296f–297f
echocardiographic aspects of, 294–298
severity of, 296
subaortic, 286–291, 286f–291f
afterload mismatch in, 289–290
echocardiographic aspects of, 287–291
severity of, 290
types of, 287–288
subvalvular pulmonic, 292f, 293
in double-chambered right ventricle, 293
suicide right ventricle, 326

Stenosis *(Continued)*
supravalvular pulmonic, 292
valvular pulmonic, 292, 295f
Strain
imaging, 64–72, 67f, 71f, 155t, 193f, 253f
myocardial, velocity profile of, 63f
peak systolic, 66–69, 76f
rate, imaging, 64–72, 69f–71f
relative, 66f
velocity, 79
Systolic dysfunction, 123t, 144
Systolic notching of the pulmonic flow, 234
Systolic torsion, left ventricular, 79

T

Tau time constant, 128
TDI (tissue Doppler imaging), 50–62, 190f–191f, 249f–250f, 252f–253f
TEE. *see* Transesophageal echocardiography (TEE)
TEE views
caudal
longitudinal, 89, 90f–91f
transverse, 89, 90f
cranial
longitudinal, 91f–92f
for aorta and PDA, 88–89, 88f
for pulmonary artery, 89, 89f
transverse, 88, 88f
median
longitudinal, 89, 89f
transverse, 89, 89f, 91f
Tei index
left ventricular, 171
of the right ventricle, 154, 154f, 155t
Teichholz method, 115t, 116–117, 163–164
Tetralogy of Fallot, 312–313, 313f
echocardiographic aspects of, 313
overriding aorta in, 313
Thickness
of the interventricular septum, 41, 42f
of the left ventricular free wall, 24
of the right ventricular free wall, 31
Thrombosis
neoplastic, 274
risk assessment of, 225–226
Thrombus, 186f, 278f
intraventricular, 209
organized, 274, 275f, 278f
Time
E wave deceleration time, 131, 141, 141f
of isovolumic relaxation time (IVRT), 132, 145–147
of the left heart base descent, 119, 120f, 120t
of pre-ejection, 120
systolic time intervals, 120, 120f, 120t
of the right ventricle, 153–154
of ventricular ejection (ET), 120
Tissue tracking imaging, 62–64, 64f–65f
Transducer, 5
Transesophageal echocardiography (TEE), 85–94, 86f, 324f
Translation, 48
Tumors
atrial, 279, 279f
cardiac, 271–282, 272f
ectopic thyroid, 277–278, 278f
heart base, 275–278, 276f–277f, 276t
intracardiac, 278–280
metastatic, 280
myocardial, 279

U

UCM. *see* Cardiomyopathy, undetermined

V

Valve
  mitral
    bacterial endocarditis of the, 175, 175f
    remodeling of the, 160, 160f
  tricuspid, 314, 315f
Valvuloplasty
  postvalvuloplasty assessment, 328–331, 328f–330f
  pulmonic, 104–105
Variability
  interday, 40, 61
  interoperator, 40, 42f
  intraday, 40, 61
Variation, coefficients of, 40
Vegetation, 175
Velocities
  intraatrial, 226
  longitudinal, of the left ventricular free wall, 56–59, 67f–68f, 153t
  maximal, 33b
    of A wave, 33
    of E wave, 33, 141
    of transaortic flow, 33f
    of transpulmonic flow, 34f
  radial velocities of the left ventricular free wall, 56–59, 60f
  regional myocardial velocities, 74
  of the right ventricular free wall, 153
  of the S′ wave of the mitral annulus, 118–119
  of segmental myocardial motion, 62
  strain velocities, 79
  of transmitral flow propagation, 145
Velocity profiles
  longitudinal, 56–59
  of myocardial strain, 63f
  radial, 56–59
Velocity-time integral (VTI), 33
Ventricle
  left, 112f–113f
    global systolic function of, 109–126
    kinetics of, 174
    noncompaction of, 225
    normal values of, 22–28
    remodeling of, 174
  right
    cardiomyopathy of the, 224–225
    diastolic diameter of the base of the, 31
    evaluation of radial systolic function of, 152
    free wall velocities of the, 153
    indices derived from speckle tracking of, 121
    shortening fraction of, 152
    suicide of the, 326
    systolic thickness of the wall of, 31
    systolic time intervals of, 153–154
Ventricular hyperkinesis, 164f
Ventricular septal defects, 86–87, 303–305, 304f–305f, 336–339, 337f–338f
  echocardiographic aspects of, 304–305
  pulmonary arterial pressure in, 305
Ventricular septal defects *(Continued)*
  Qp/Qs in, 305
  types of, 303
Ventricular suction, 128
Views
  left parasternal
    apical, 10–11
      2 chambers view, 11, 13f
      4 and 5 chambers views, 11, 11f–12f
    caudal, 10–11
    cranial, 14, 14f–15f, 294f, 300f
  normal TM, 16–17
    transaortic, 17
    transmitral, 17
      A point, 17
      E point, 17
      F point, 17
      CD segment, 7f
    transventricular, 16–17
  right parasternal
    long axis, 6–8, 23f, 99f–100f
      4 chambers, optimized for atria, 6, 7f, 18f, 175f
      5 chambers, optimized for aorta, 8, 8f, 29f, 318f
    short axis, 9–10, 293f
      aorta-main pulmonary artery level (transaortic), 10, 10f, 30f–31f
      apex level (transapical), 9, 9f
      chordae tendineae level (transventricular), 9, 9f, 23f, 184f
      mitral valve level (transmitral), 9f, 10
      papillary muscle level (transpapillary), 9, 9f
  subcostal (or subxiphoid), 16, 16f, 290f
Volume
  end-diastolic volume index, 116, 164–166, 183–184
  end-systolic volume index, 116–117, 163–164, 183–184
  regurgitant (RV), 172
  ventricular
    left ventricular volume, measurement of, 99–100, 101f
    methods of estimation of, 115–117
      area-length, 116, 117f
      geometric, 115–116
      planimetric, 116–117
      Simpson method, 116, 116f
      Teichholz, 115, 115t
      Wyatt area-length method, 115

W

Wave
  A
    duration of, 33
    maximum velocity of, 33
  AR, 132
    maximum velocity of, 35
  Dm, 35, 132
  E, 134f
    deceleration time of, 131, 141, 141f
    duration of, 33
    maximal velocity of, 141
  pre-A, 140
  S′, velocity of the mitral annulus, 118–119
  Sm, 35, 132
  V, 140
Wyatt area-length method, 115